Healthcare Ethics in a Diverse Society

Healthcare Ethics in a Diverse Society

MICHAEL C. BRANNIGAN
Center for the Study of Ethics,
La Roche College

JUDITH A. BOSS
Brown University School of Medicine

Mayfield Publishing Company
Mountain View, California
London • Toronto

Library of Congress Cataloging-in-Publication Data

Brannigan, Michael C.
   Healthcare ethics in a diverse society/Michael C. Brannigan, Judith A. Boss
      p. cm.
         Includes bibliographical references and index.
         ISBN 1-55934-976-X
         1. Medical ethics.   2. Social ethics.   I. Boss, Judith A.
            II. Title.
      R724.B72   2000
         174′.2—dc21   00-042716

Manufactured in the United States of America

10   9   8   7   6   5   4   3   2   1

Mayfield Publishing Company
1280 Villa Street
Mountain View, CA 94041

Sponsoring Editor, Ken King; production editor, Melissa Williams; manuscript editor, Mary Roybal; design manager, Glenda King; text designer, Linda Robertson; permissions editor, Marty Granahan; manufacturing manager, Randy Hurst. The text was set in 9.5/12 New Baskerville by UG/GGS Information Services and printed on acid-free 45# Highland Plus by R. R. Donnelley & Sons Company.

To the Boys of Rhode Island: Ted, Jim, and Ron, My Lifelong Buddies
  —Michael Brannigan

To My Daughter Alyssa and Son-In-Law Bill, in Celebration of Their Wedding
  —Judith Boss

Preface

The Ryoanji Zen temple in Kyoto is known for its famous rock garden. Displaying clusters of rocks separated by wide expanses of raked sand, the garden harbors a curious feature in that the spectator sees a disparate number of rocks, depending on the angle and perspective. From a sitting position close to the temple door one counts twelve rocks, but from a spot near the center thirteen rocks appear. Moving to the end farthest from the temple door, the viewer counts eleven. No matter where one sits, the viewer cannot take in all the rocks.

In the same way, our viewpoints on most matters will always be limited, and they shift according to our point of reference. Location often justifies disposition, particularly with perspectives in healthcare. Thus, the mainstream views of healthcare ethics in the United States are a product of its tradition, just as South Asian countries sustain traditional Buddhist perspectives.

This text performs two tasks. First, it provides a sound, comprehensive overview of conventional U.S. healthcare ethics. This overview is the backbone of the book and is reflected in the chapter summaries below. Second, it introduces readers to cross-cultural perspectives on several issues. In combining the conventional and the cross-cultural, the text is a solid house with many windows, offering alternative ways of perceiving and resolving healthcare ethical issues along with the more mainstream approaches in the United States. Moreover, it enables readers to further appreciate the complexities of ethical issues by situating them within the backdrop of the interplay of culture and medicine.

We do not attempt to take a stand on the relative merits of any of the cross-cultural perspectives we present. A comparative analysis would take us far beyond the scope of this book. We simply offer windows on other perspectives so that readers can become more aware of worlds outside their own. These windows include scenes from the religious traditions of Islam, Hinduism, Buddhism, Roman Catholicism, and Judaism, along with some European, African, Asian, and Native-American viewpoints, in a way that complements the analysis in the commentary.

The underlying premise of the text is that our vision is healthier if it has more breadth. This is a simple truth. The more we learn about our setting, the more we can appreciate where we live. The more we learn about what lies outside our dwelling, the more we can value what lies inside. The more aware we are of other cultures, the more we can appreciate our own—for a defining quality of America is precisely its rich diversity.

Diversity . . . no other term more aptly describes the backgrounds, milieus, and perspectives of our students. This diversity shows itself in the world students inhabit, which is quite different from the world of two decades ago. For instance, there is a growing interest not only in other cultures, but also in alternative ways of healing. Here in the United States, we are becoming more aware of our own unique, internal diversity. Visit any major metropolitan hospital in the United States and you will encounter hospital staff and patients who represent a wide variety of cultures and beliefs. For example, not only is Islam the fastest-growing major religion today, but Islamic patients constitute a powerfully growing segment of our healthcare professional and patient population.

Indeed, this diversity lends itself to rich classroom dialogue. However, there is a clear gap between students' needs in light of such diversity and what conventional biomedical ethics texts presently offer. Understandably, most texts, including our own, discuss issues within the context of Western philosophical theories and principles, such as the high premium we place on patient autonomy. Yet, even though the discipline of healthcare ethics is becoming more significant and widespread in many other cultures, there is a dearth of discussion in classroom texts as to how these cultures address some of the same issues. Most other texts do not address this diversity and therefore do not sufficiently address the world that today's students inhabit. Our book intends to squarely address this need for cross-cultural perspectives in healthcare ethics.

Caveats

This treatment of ethical issues requires some measure of caution. The reader must be careful not to think that any window encapsulates the essence of a culture's or religious tradition's viewpoint. For example, we provide cultural windows on Hindu beliefs, yet Hinduism is not homogeneous. The "untouchables," the outcasts of the Indian caste system, for example, adhere generally to Hindu beliefs, but quite a few of their beliefs and practices are outside Hindu orthodoxy.

Along these lines, we need to be careful to avoid associating a country and its peoples with one single medical tradition. Often, a plurality of therapeutic systems exists in various cultures. Not all Japanese, for example, are committed to one exclusive healthcare approach. As in China, patients in Japan will shop around for the approach that is more suitable and convenient for them, whether it be modern "cosmopolitan" medicine or traditional Chinese medicine, known as *kanpo*.

We also need to refrain from thinking of "other" traditions as completely alien from the more "orthodox" Western positions. For example, not only does the Islamic worldview share the monotheistic perspective of Judaism and Christianity, but the Islamic system eventually incorporated teachings from the ancient Greek philosophical texts of Plato and Aristotle as well as the medical texts of Hippocrates and Galen. Nevertheless, there remain distinct differences. Muslim teachings do not conceive of a strict mind/body distinction, therefore Muslim medical teachings posit a firm link between bodily and spiritual healing, between a healthy life and a moral life.

Our cultural windows make it clear that we have no grounds for assuming that the predominant principles, values, and moral assumptions concerning healthcare in the United States are universally accepted. On the other hand, in no way are we proposing that the healthcare values and principles in the United States are wrongheaded and that we should adopt wholesale the perspectives and values of other cultures. We simply believe that there is no better way to examine an issue than to broaden our perspectives on that issue.

The Book's Organization

Chapter 1   Moral Theory   This opening chapter provides a solid introduction to a wide spectrum of moral theories, including a discussion of the role of moral theory in healthcare ethics and an in-depth analysis and critique of cultural relativism. In addition to examining standard moral theories ranging from natural law theory to utilitarianism and deontology, it explores viewpoints such as care perspectives, virtue ethics, communitarian ethics, the relation between morality and religion, and the principlism/casuistry debate. Unlike many other texts, it contains selections from the classic works of Aristotle, Immanuel Kant, and John Stuart Mill.

Chapter 2   Critical Thinking: The Basis for Ethical Reasoning   This chapter offers a concise introduction to critical reasoning. It covers fundamental topics such as *is* and *ought* statements, levels of thinking, the anatomy of arguments, logical reasoning, and fallacies. It then applies the rules of critical thinking to reasoning in the area of healthcare ethics. The chapter concludes with highlights from the classic article by Judith Jarvis Thomson, "A Defense of Abortion." Using her arguments, the chapter illustrates rules of argumentation and an analysis of fallacies.

Chapter 3   The Relationship Between Healthcare Professionals and Patients   The physician/patient relationship lies at the heart of healthcare ethics. The nature of this relationship is examined against the backdrop of managed care and other facets of the healthcare system. Special attention is given to the role of nurses along with that of physicians. The dynamics of the healthcare professionals' roles are studied in view of the crucial importance assigned to matters of disclosure, confidentiality, and informed consent.

Chapter 4   Abortion and Maternal-Fetal Conflicts   Abortion continues to be one of the most contentious moral controversies. After reviewing various procedures, the chapter examines various perspectives from law and religion. It then looks more closely at secular arguments regarding both the moral status of the fetus and the rights of women. After examining selective abortion, maternal-fetal conflicts, and partial-birth abortion, the chapter closes with a discussion of the obligations of healthcare professionals regarding abortion.

Chapter 5   Genetic Engineering, Reproductive Technologies, and Cloning   The issues examined in this chapter represent the new frontier in medical and scientific technologies. They also raise critical questions regarding human purpose and identity. After reviewing the history of eugenics research, the chapter offers a detailed study of the Human Genome Project, perhaps the most far-reaching and adventurous scientific project in human history. This study is followed by a critical examination of questions surrounding genetic screening and genetic engineering. Various types of reproductive technologies are examined, with special attention given to issues surrounding human cloning.

Chapter 6 Human and Animal Experimentation   After offering a history of medical experimentation, this chapter presents a thorough analysis of the most pressing questions related to various aspects of experimentation, including the involvement of the state and conflicts of interest. Special attention is given to human subjects with respect to informed consent, the criteria for selection, and the effects on vulnerable and marginalized groups such as children and fetuses. A section deals with experimentation on nonhuman animals and addresses questions regarding their moral and legal status.

Chapter 7 Organ Transplantation   Issues surrounding organ transplants highlight a broad spectrum of moral concerns: defining death, fair distribution of organs to potential recipients, personal responsibility for health, and the socioeconomic context of the free market. This chapter examines the key issues involved in both procuring and allocating organs, including the practice of multiple listing. It closes with a discussion of xenografts, or cross-species tissue transplantation.

Chapter 8 Euthanasia: End-of-Life Decisions   Euthanasia remains one of the most difficult and painful issues in healthcare. This chapter explores prominent themes and questions and takes a closer look at the definition of death and its relation to notions of the person. After giving a typology of euthanasia, the chapter addresses the question of whether there is a moral difference between active and passive euthanasia. It then discusses issues concerning decision making for incompetent patients, including sections on advance directives and medical futility. It pays special attention to the controversial subject of physician-assisted suicide.

Chapter 9 HIV and AIDS: Prejudice and Policies   This chapter opens with a discussion of AIDS exceptionalism, illustrating how prejudices can affect policy-making. It then addresses the sensitive issue of HIV screening, highlighting the arguments for and against. Even after testing, a number of ethical concerns remain, such as contact tracing. These concerns are examined along with other strategies. The chapter ends with an analysis of whether mandatory disclosure of the HIV status of both patients and healthcare professionals is justified.

Chapter 10 Challenges in Healthcare Policy and Reform   The text concludes with an examination of the most pressing issues regarding healthcare policy and reform. It addresses the most prominent challenges in both macroallocation and microallocation, particularly within the context of managed care and HMOs. After exploring theories relevant to a just healthcare system, the chapter pays special attention to the problem surrounding the notion of "healthcare needs," including a discussion of cosmetic surgery and Viagra. It concludes by presenting the pros and cons of three options for healthcare reform: the existing free-market approach, national health insurance, and a multitiered system.

Readings   Readings have been judiciously selected from the writings of many of the most prominent scholars in the field. Many reflect both supporting and opposing arguments concerning specific issues such as truth-telling to patients, abortion, reproductive technologies, alcoholics and liver transplantation, physician-assisted suicide, and national health insurance. The readings also represent a broad base of perspectives, from the classic works of Aristotle, Kant, and Mill to legal rulings on confidentiality, views on genetic engineering within a marketing context, Christian views regarding fetal transplants, and feminist perspectives on the physician/patient relationship. The readings have been edited to facilitate comprehension by students. They are followed by "Comprehension and Reflection" questions to help students focus on central ideas in the reading, to act as a tool for review, and to help generate classroom discussion.

Additional Resources   A resource section at the end of the text contains valuable supplemental material, including a Glossary/Index that offers a succinct review of the most important terms in the text and serves as a useful tool for study and review. Also included are samples of living wills and other critical documents. Endnotes covering all the chapters are listed.

Additional Features   1. This text intends to deliver a clear and readable introduction to healthcare ethics for the beginning student. It does not presuppose a background in philosophy but gives a clear and concise treatment of the most essential topics in healthcare ethics. Students are exposed to the basic issues without being sidetracked by cutting-edge topics peripheral to an introductory text.

2. One feature of students' diversity is their work experience. The healthcare professionals who take courses in medical ethics include nurses, nurse practitioners, nurse anesthetists, nurse managers, radiologists, radiographers, medical students, pre-med students, physician assistants, social workers, physical therapists, pharmacists, and hospital administrators. Their interests will remain diverse as they continue to specialize in these fields.

Despite this broad diversity in health-related fields, most texts approach healthcare ethics primarily from the perspective of the dynamics between physician and patient. Many students—whether nurses, social workers, radiologists, anesthetists, or hospital administrators—face moral conflicts that stem essentially from their occupational roles within the hospital bureaucracy, with all its institutional constraints. We therefore address ethical issues within this broader context of the healthcare professional, not just the physician.

3. Another aspect of students' diversity is their educational preparation. Students often comprise an assortment of healthcare professionals along with an array of traditional undergraduates who represent a vast spectrum of majors. Since quite a few students come to our classes equipped with little philosophical training, it is all the more imperative that they be exposed to and critically examine the fundamental issues of medical ethics in terms that are palatable.

Herein lies the special feature of Chapter 2, "Critical Thinking." A principal goal in teaching healthcare ethics is to enable students to become sensitive to the key ethical issues in bioethics and to appreciate various positions, particularly ones they themselves may not share. This can occur only if students have the requisite skills for evaluating evidence given for the various positions. Studying ethics, therefore, is inseparable from knowing the components of sound reasoning. Ethical analysis presupposes a sound measure of critical-thinking skills.

4. The text covers important and timely issues, such as:

- A broad range of ethical theories incorporating virtue ethics, feminist viewpoints, and communitarian theories
- Methodological issues pertaining to casuistic (case-oriented) and principles approaches

- Ethical implications of genome research
- A timely discussion of the ethical issues surrounding human cloning
- Ethical issues pertaining to healthcare organizations and how these issues affect the relationship between healthcare professionals and patients
- The impact of managed care on the healthcare profession
- Landmark legal cases throughout the chapters, such as the key ruling in the *Tarasoff* case
- Various issues arising from cost-containment pressures
- Medical futility, one of the most common issues faced by hospital ethics committees
- Issues of individual responsibility for well-being and health, a running theme throughout the book; for example, discussion of the controversy surrounding liver transplants for alcoholics

5. At the end of each issues chapter are eight Cases for Analysis. These are followed by Discussion Questions to facilitate class discussion.

This text addresses healthcare ethics by utilizing the prevailing philosophical-ethical traditions prominent in the United States and throughout much of Western culture, yet it does so while acknowledging other currents that compel us to look beyond our borders. We consider this to be the first order of business in this new century. In a world that is growing smaller, we cannot afford to limit our vision.

Acknowledgments

We would like to thank our colleagues who served as reviewers for their valuable suggestions: Kathleen Cook, Ohio State University; Hal Walberg, Mankato State University; Anne Donchin, Indiana University—Indianapolis; Eric Kraemer, University of Wisconsin, LaCrosse; Dr. Thomas R. McCormick, University of Washington School of Medicine, Seattle; Richard Noble, University of Michigan, Ann Arbor; Betty J. Odello, Pierce College; William Sewell, Michigan Technological University; and Barbara C. Thornton, University of Nevada, Reno.

Our heartfelt thanks go to our editor Ken King for his ongoing encouragement and support and for making the vision behind the book become a reality, to Melissa Williams Kreischer, production editor, for her cheerfulness and efficiency managing the production of the book, and to Marty Granahan, permissions editor, for her able assistance in obtaining permissions for the readings. We also wish to express appreciation to the librarians at Brown University and La Roche College, especially Michael Jackson and Cole Puvogel, for their assistance in our research. We express our sincere gratitude to our colleagues, especially Rev. Patrick O'Brien, Gen Ohi, Kazumasa Hoshino, Akira Akabayashi, Carol Moltz, Barbara Coyne, and Susan Klimcheck, for their invaluable feedback. We would like to thank our assistants, James Nuzum, Cindy Speers, and Leslie Kirby for their unflagging enthusiasm and invaluable assistance in the preparation of this manuscript. Also profound thanks to our families, especially Michael's wife, Brooke and Judy's daughter, Alyssa.

Contents

CHAPTER 2   **Critical Thinking: The Basis for Ethical
Reasoning 54**

CHAPTER 3   The Relationship Between Healthcare Professionals and Patients   108

CHAPTER 4   Abortion and Maternal-Fetal Conflicts   174

CHAPTER 5   Genetic Engineering, Reproductive Technologies, and Cloning   249

Chapter 6   Human and Animal Experimentation   327

CHAPTER 7   Organ Transplantation   409

CHAPTER 8   Euthanasia: End-of-Life Decisions   473

CHAPTER 9 **HIV and AIDS: Prejudice and Policies   549**

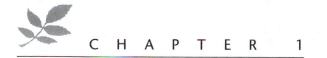

Moral Theory

The systematic attempt of the Nazis during World War II to exterminate European Jews is one of the most abhorrent events in the history of humankind. Even more disconcerting is the realization that the Holocaust was not the act of a few deranged sadists but apparently had the support of many German people.[1] The medical profession, in particular, played a crucial and willing role throughout the Holocaust, both in fostering Nazi ideology and in carrying out the Final Solution. By 1933, the year Hitler came to power, there were already 2,800 members in the Nazi Physicians' League. Indeed, physicians were three times more likely than the general public to be members of the Nazi Party, and fifteen times more likely than judges. These physicians and other medical professionals were apparently convinced that they were acting ethically in sterilizing and destroying people who posed a threat to the racial health of the German nation.

The mass killings began in 1939 with the euthanasia, or "mercy killing," of what was deemed useless life. The people first slated for Hitler's "humane euthanasia" program were the mentally ill and "incurably sick persons [who] should be granted a mercy death."[2] The gassing of the mentally ill was stopped because of protests from the public and from a few church dignitaries. When the target of the program was switched to the Jews, however, no similar outcry occurred.

Thousands of Jews were used as subjects in medical experiments of a most atrocious nature. What was perhaps most disconcerting about these physicians and scientists was, with a few exceptions, their normalcy. Like American slaveholders and the cavalrymen who hunted down and massacred thousands of American Indians, these Nazis were, for the most part, "good" family men and upstanding members of the community. According to a U.S. medical consultant who investigated Nazi medical war crimes following the war, the medical profession readily adopted the Nazi ideology in exchange for "security and social recognition."[3] Dr. Josef Mengele, chief medical officer of the Auschwitz-Birkenau concentration camp, was one of the most notorious of these medical war criminals. His medical experiments on the inmates of Auschwitz are believed to have caused 400,000 deaths.

In the early 1960s, Yale psychologist Stanley Milgram conducted an experiment on obedience to determine whether Americans would follow orders as readily as had the Germans in Nazi Germany. Milgram's subjects, many of whom were professionals, were led to believe that they were delivering a series of increasingly painful electric shocks as

MEDICINE IN NAZI GERMANY:
Dr. Mengele's Experiments on Twins

Nine-year-old Eva Mozes Kor was one of the few children who survived Dr. Mengele's infamous twin experiments. Her story follows.

I often say that we, the Mengele Twins, are the children without a childhood because when we look back on our wonder years, we remember the huge chimneys, the smell of burned flesh, the shots, the blood taking, the endless tests in Mengele's labs, the rats, lice, and dead bodies that were everywhere. . . . the emotional scars are so deep that only now, more than 40 years later, are we attempting to face our past and come to terms with it. . . .

In the spring of 1944, when I arrived at Auschwitz-Birkenau with my family, my twin sister and I were torn away from my mother's arms and we became part of some 1500 sets of twins used by Mengele in his many deadly experiments. . . .

Three times a week we were taken to the blood lab. There they tied both my arms to restrict the blood flow. In one arm, they gave me shots; from the other they took blood, a lot of blood. . . . On a few occasions, I saw twins faint from loss of blood. They wanted to learn how much blood we could lose and still survive.

Once a week we were taken to the shower room, given a bar of soap, and our clothes were disinfected in a fruitless effort to rid us of lice; we were covered from head to toe. Three times a week we were taken (always accompanied by an SS guard) to the Auschwitz I labs for experiments. These would last from 8–10 hours. They would strip us naked and put a group of us, all children, in a big room. Every part of our body was measured, photographed, marked, and compared to charts. Every movement we made was noted. I felt like a piece of meat. . . . These experiments were emotionally very difficult to deal with, but the deadly ones were done in the blood lab.

In early July, 1944, I was injected with some kind of germ. By evening I became very ill. I had a very high fever and I was trembling. I could hardly move or think. . . . I was desperately trying to hide the fact that I was ill because there was a rumor that no one came back from the hospital alive. My fever was very high and I was sent to the hospital. Mengele came to see me twice a day with four other doctors. They checked my fever chart but never examined me. I was given no food, no water, no medication. I remember one of the doctors said sarcastically, "Too bad she has only two weeks to live," but I was determined to get well and be reunited with my twin sister, Miriam. I made a silent pledge to fight with all my being to survive. Today I know that if I would have died, Mengele would have killed my twin sister with a phenol shot to the heart, and then performed autopsies on our bodies, comparing my diseased organs with Miriam's. I remember waking up on the barracks floor, fading in and out of consciousness, and saying to myself, "I must survive!" I was crawling to the other end, to reach a faucet with water. After two weeks my fever broke and I was reunited with Miriam. Six months later, on January 27, 1945, we were liberated in Auschwitz by the Russian army.[4]

part of an experiment on the effect of punishment on learning. In fact, the person playing the role of the learner was an accomplice of the experimenter and was not actually receiving the shocks.

When subjects balked on hearing the screams of pain from the learner, they were urged to continue by an experimenter wearing a white lab coat. Despite the feigned protests of the learner, about two-thirds of the subjects obeyed the experimenter and continued delivering what they believed were potentially fatal electric shocks. The findings of this experiment suggest that people can be persuaded to torture, and perhaps even kill, another person at the urging of an authority figure. Milgram wrote of his findings:

> Ordinary people, simply doing their jobs, and without any particular hostility on their part, can become agents in a terribly destructive process. Moreover, even when the destructive effects of their work become patently clear, and they are asked to carry out actions incompatible with fundamental standards of morality, relatively few people have the resources needed to resist.[5]

The Nazi experiment and the human propensity to uncritical conformity illustrate the need for a carefully thought-out healthcare ethics. We will examine the moral reasoning of Dr. Mengele later in this chapter. Fortunately, the moral reasoning adopted by the Nazi physicians is the exception rather than the rule. For the most part, medical professionals have adhered to moral codes.

THE DISCIPLINE OF HEALTHCARE ETHICS

Healthcare ethics in Europe and North America has been influenced primarily by the Hippocratic Oath. Modern codes of ethics in Western medicine modeled on the Hippocratic Oath include the American Medical Association (AMA) Codes of Ethics, the Declaration of Geneva (1948), and the International Code of Medical Ethics (1949). The Hippocratic tradition, which began as a movement among ancient Greek physicians, emphasizes individual relationships and paternalism. Under **paternalism,** the physician, because of his or her greater medical knowledge and authority, decides what is best for the patient. The oath is divided into two parts: (1) the duties of the medical student to his teacher and his teacher's family and to transmit medical knowledge, and (2) the rules to be observed by physicians in the treatment of patients.

Challenges to the individualism and paternalism inherent in the Hippocratic tradition have come from both Western and non-Western traditions. Healthcare ethics in most cultures is closely tied to the major religious and philosophical traditions. For example, the practice of medicine for both the Hindu and the Buddhist is a virtuous lifestyle intimately connected with the search for enlightenment and release from the cycle of birth and rebirth.

Socialist countries place more emphasis than does the United States on community and social concerns. For example, the Soviet Medical Oath begins by requiring physicians to solemnly swear "to dedicate all my knowledge and strength to the preservation and improvement of the health of mankind and to the treatment and prevention of disease, and to work in good conscience wherever it is required by society."[6] The communal aspect of healthcare is also emphasized in countries with socialized medicine, such as Canada and Australia. The nursing profession likewise has always re-

THE HIPPOCRATIC OATH[7]

I swear by Apollo Physician, by Asclepius, by Health, by Panacea and by all the gods and goddesses, making them my witnesses, that I will carry out, according to my ability and judgment, this oath and this indenture. To hold my teacher in this art equal to my own parents; to make him my partner in livelihood. . . . I will use treatment to help the sick according to my ability and judgment, but never with a view to injury and wrong-doing. Neither will I administer a poison to anybody when asked to do so, nor will I suggest such a course. Similarly I will not give to a woman a pessary to cause abortion. But I will keep pure and holy both my life and my art. I will not use the knife, not even, verily, on sufferers from stone, but I will give place to such as are craftsmen therein. Into whatsoever house I enter, I will enter to help the sick, and I will abstain from all intentional wrong-doing and harm, especially from abusing the bodies of man or woman, bond or free. And whatsoever I shall see or hear in the course of my profession . . . if it be what should not be published abroad, I will never divulge, holding such things to be holy secrets. . . .

garded social ethics as central to its profession. The Code for Nurses, which was endorsed by the International Council of Nurses in 1973 and reaffirmed in 1989, includes a section "Nurses and Society," which states that "the nurse shares with other citizens the responsibility for initiating and supporting actions to meet the health and social needs of the public."

Modern healthcare ethics in the United States was born in the civil rights era of the 1960s. It developed in response to publicity on abuses in medical research, such as the Tuskegee syphilis study (discussed later in this chapter) and to moral dilemmas raised by the development of new technologies that could prolong life—or the dying process. While the paternalism inherent in the Hippocratic tradition has been called into question, the concern for individual rights and **autonomy,** the ability to make free and rational choices, continues to dominate healthcare ethics in the United States. Few non-Western traditions, in contrast, regard the isolated individual as the focus of medicine. Instead, the self is viewed in the social context. Consequential arguments, that is, those that judge the morality of a particular course of action based on the consequences of that action, are also prominent in modern Western healthcare ethics. This is especially evident in the justification of medical experimentation on nonconsenting human subjects in the early and mid-twentieth century and on nonhuman animals today.

The task of healthcare ethics is to identify and resolve moral issues that arise, or may arise, within medical practice and biomedical research. Is a physician morally obligated to tell a patient that he is dying of cancer? Does our right to life entail the right to choose when to end our life? Should laws prohibit physician-assisted suicide? Is selective abortion morally justified? Is using nonhuman animals in experiments designed to benefit humans morally justified? On the other hand, is it morally obligatory to use nonhuman animals in experiments if doing so brings significant benefits to humans?

INDIA:
The Upanishad Tradition in Healthcare Ethics

The physicians' oath contained in the Hindu Upanishads predates the Hippocratic Oath by two centuries. The Hindu oath emphasizes right conduct, respect for the sanctity of life, knowledge and discipline, and reverence. It also reflects the importance of the concepts of dharma (right action) and karma (habit-energy) in Indian life. **Karma** is grounded in the theory of rebirth and the belief that "the direction of one's action—including the direction of one's efforts at acquiring knowledge and understanding—determines one's status in this lifetime and even in lifetimes to come."[8]

Following are excerpts from the *Atreya Anushasana* (seventh century B.C.):

1. The physician should first investigate the patient and his disease thoroughly and on correct diagnosis, should think of treatment. Treatment however efficient is bound to fail if the diagnosis is wrong. . . .

7. Physician who by his conduct allows the disease to progress or adopts hasty measure even before the right time is to be considered a "sinner" and stands liable for punishment. . . .

10. Aim of treatment is not merely to relieve the suffering but to restore health; strive to maintain and promote health but do not undermine the natural strength of the patient.

11. The scope of medical science is merely to lend a helping hand to those who are sinking in the quagmire of disease; it is just an aid. Physician should not assume too much either to himself or to his science in case of cure.

12. Physician is not the controller of life, (neither its saviour nor its remover) proper diagnosis and suitable therapy are the only two on which he has control. . . .

17. No charity is greater than saving a life. Treatment never goes to waste, in some it brings wealth, with some others fame, friendship with some others but with every one it brings experience to the physician.

18. Medical science should not be used for selfish gains nor for money, but should be for the service of all creatures. . . .

23. Practicing the profession on the principles of philosophy of life, looking after the health of the deserving and the needy, showing kindness and compassion to all beings is the Dharma for the medical man; accepting from the rich just enough money to meet the minimum needs, his life and his dependents is the Artha; respecting the elders, scholars, professional brethren and nobles and receiving honors from them, winning love and affection of all by sympathetic service is the Karma; by practicing thus the physician is sure to attain salvation Maksha.[9]

What system is most just for allocating medical resources? Is human cloning morally acceptable? If so, under what circumstances?

Healthcare ethics today, at least in the United States, is for the most part academic in its orientation. Since 1970, healthcare ethics has become one of the most, if not the most, prestigious and lucrative fields in philosophy. Many colleges and universities have centers devoted to the study of healthcare ethics. Most large hospitals and medical schools also have professional medical ethicists on their staff to act as professional advice givers when moral problems arise.

On one hand, this shift from ethicists as theoreticians to ethicists as participants in practical decision making should be applauded. On the other hand, because medical ethicists are hired and paid by hospitals, they are under pressure to work within the paradigm of the status quo. Thus, it is all the more important that we learn about and remain open to views outside our tradition rather than simply accepting uncritically the way things are.

THE ROLE OF MORAL THEORY IN HEALTHCARE ETHICS

Despite the differences in healthcare traditions around the world, these traditions have many shared moral concerns as well as common theoretical underpinnings. Moral philosophy is generally divided into theoretical ethics and applied ethics. **Theoretical ethics** appraises the logical foundations and internal consistencies of ethical systems.[10] **Applied ethics** uses these theories to give practical guidelines or behavioral norms.[11] Healthcare ethics generally emphasizes applied ethics by applying general moral theories and principles to problems arising in the context of medical practice and biomedical research.

Most students, if given a choice, would prefer to skip moral theory and move on to discussions of real-life moral issues in healthcare ethics, often contrasting theory and action. This is a false dichotomy, since it is theory that informs our actions. Knowing how to ground discussions of controversial moral issues—such as abortion, euthanasia, and cloning—in moral theory and good moral reasoning makes us less vulnerable to the type of persuasive but misleading thinking that the subjects in the Milgram study engaged in.

A good theory offers guidance for thinking about and resolving moral issues. Although we might happen to come upon a good solution without it, a moral theory, like a road map, makes us more likely to reach our destination with the least amount of wrong turns and aggravation. By providing guidelines, moral theories help us identify conflicts and contradictions in our thinking and make more satisfactory moral decisions. For example, a film made of the Milgram experiment revealed that those who were most likely to give in to the urgings of the authority figure knew that what they were doing was wrong but were unable to articulate *why* it was wrong. Those who were able to resist the authority figure, on the other hand, were able to provide justifications for their refusal in the form of moral principles and moral theory; they were able to say why continuing to deliver the shocks was wrong.

In other words, theories provide a framework for discussing real-life moral issues and making real-life decisions. However, like maps, not all theories are equally good. Some may be good as far as they go but leave out too much. In this case, we may want to combine them with other theories. Some theories may lead us down dead ends.

Knowing the strengths and weaknesses of different moral theories can save us from going down these dead ends.

Moral theories fall into two main categories: (1) ethical relativism and (2) universalism or objectivism. **Ethical relativism** argues that morality is different for different people. Universalist theories, in contrast, state that there are fundamental, objective moral principles and values that are universally true for all people, independent of their personal beliefs or cultures.

ETHICAL RELATIVISM

Some people think that abortion is a personal decision; others think it is wrong despite what the individual may think about it. Some people think that experimentation on nonhuman animals is not morally problematic; others, including Buddhists and Hindus, think it is morally reprehensible no matter what benefits it brings to humans. Who is right, and who is wrong? Cultural and individual disagreement creates serious doubts in many people's minds about whether moral issues can ever be resolved or whether meaningful dialogue between those holding opposing positions is even possible.

Ethical relativists maintain that moral differences cannot be resolved. According to ethical relativists, there are no independent or universal moral standards. Instead, morality is created by people; it is a human invention. Humans, either individually or collectively, are seen as the ultimate measures and arbitrators of what is right and wrong. Ethical relativism can be subdivided into ethical subjectivism and cultural relativism.

Ethical Subjectivism

Ethical subjectivists claim that individuals create their own morality. There are no objective moral truths—only individual opinions. Unlike reason, **opinion** is based on feelings rather than on analysis or facts. What is wrong for you may be right for me, depending on our respective feelings. You may feel that abortion is murder; I may feel that it is morally acceptable. You may feel that it is morally acceptable, and perhaps even obligatory, to conduct medical experiments on nonhuman animals; I may feel that it is terribly wrong. You may feel that racism is wrong; I may feel that white supremacy is morally right and that women of color should be sterilized. You may believe that euthanasia should be mandatory once a person reaches an age at which he or she is no longer socially productive; I may be opposed to involuntary euthanasia because I feel that human life has intrinsic value. You may feel that taking sexual advantage of pediatric patients while they are unconscious is immoral; I may feel that it is morally acceptable. The rightness or wrongness of our actions depends solely on how each of us *feels* about it. In other words, my action in sterilizing women of color or in euthanizing elderly patients without their knowledge or consent is morally commendable, and perhaps even morally obligatory, as long as I personally *feel* that what I am doing is right. Ethical subjectivism is not merely a "live and let live" moral code whereby we resolve moral differences by admitting and respecting their legitimacy. Under ethical subjectivism, no overarching principles require us to respect others or their points of view.

Dr. Hannibal "the Cannibal" Lecter, in Thomas Harris's novel *The Silence of the Lambs*, is a true ethical subjectivist. Dr. Lecter is a psychiatrist who is highly respected in professional circles, particularly for his accurate professional evaluations of the criminal mind. When more and more of his patients join the missing persons list, a police investigation reveals that this brilliant man who seems to have such keen insight into human nature also has a taste for human flesh. Why did he cannibalize those who trusted him most? For fun. Lecter, it turns out, has no remorse; indeed, as the author points out, he is a man with a free mind and a clear conscience unfettered by either guilt or kindness. Of course, not all ethical subjectivists are serial killers or abusers. However, ethical subjectivism recognizes no moral difference between Dr. Lecter and Dr. Schweitzer or Mother Teresa.

Do not confuse ethical subjectivism with the obviously true and trivial statement that "whatever a person believes is right for him or her is what that person believes is right for him or her." Ethical subjectivism goes beyond this by claiming that sincerely believing or feeling that something is right *makes* it right for the individual. Because morality is merely a matter of personal opinion, we can never be mistaken about what is right and what is wrong. In other words, my action in sterilizing women of color without their knowledge or consent or in taking sexual advantage of my pediatric patients is morally acceptable as long as I personally feel that what I am doing is right. How *they* might feel about the matter is morally irrelevant.

Like his counterpart Dr. Lecter, convicted serial killer Craig Price, when asked if he thought what he did was wrong, calmly replied, "Morality is a private choice." If morality is simply a matter of personal opinion, there is no point in trying to use rational arguments to convince the racist gynecologist or the pediatric pedophile that what they are doing is wrong, any more than it would make sense to try to convince me that I really don't like cashew nuts.

Similarly, there would be no point in proceeding any further in a moral issues course if morality is simply a matter of personal feeling rather than of reason or shared values. When viewpoints come into conflict, those people who are strongest or have the most power will be able to impose their agenda on others. Ethical subjectivism is not the same as tolerance for another's beliefs; under ethical subjectivism, we do not have to tolerate other people's views or even their lives unless we feel that tolerance is right for us.

Ethical subjectivism is one of the weakest moral theories. If taken seriously, it would permit people to exploit and hurt others without having to justify their actions. As a theory, it does not provide a correct explanation for why certain actions are wrong. In real life, we generally make moral judgments independently of anyone's feelings toward the action. Indeed, the fact that serial killers such as Dr. Lecter enjoy torturing and killing their hapless victims or that the pediatrician gets great pleasure out of taking sexual advantage of his unconscious patients only makes their actions more horrific. If ethical subjectivism were true, our moral heroes would be psychopaths, such as Dr. Hannibal "the Cannibal" Lecter, who act solely on their feelings without concern for any universal moral principles.

Cultural Relativism

The majority of American adults equate morality with cultural norms. Like ethical subjectivists, cultural relativists maintain that standards of right and wrong are created by people. However, according to **cultural relativism,** morality is based on cultural norms and laws rather than on the opinions of isolated individuals. Public opinion, not private

SUB-SAHARAN AFRICA:
Infant Circumcision

Seventeen-year-old Fauziy Kasinga fled her native home in Togo, Africa, and sought asylum in the United States to avoid an arranged marriage and female circumcision, which are customs in her culture. Currently, asylum is granted in the United States to people who can show that they have a well-grounded fear of persecution based on race, religion, nationality, political belief, or membership in a social group. Female circumcision, also known as clitorectomy or female genital mutilation, involves removing the clitoris and sometimes other genital tissue to curtail the woman's sexual pleasure. No anesthetic is used, and the procedure, especially if it is not carried out under sterile conditions, sometimes causes serious health problems and even death.

Female circumcision is common in most sub-Saharan African nations, where the rates range from 10 percent to 98 percent.[12] Like male circumcision in the United States, which is supported by most men, female circumci-sion is supported by most women in countries where the practice is prevalent, even women who have undergone the procedure.[13]

Female circumcision has been banned in most states of the United States. However, routine (as opposed to therapeutic or religiously based) male circumcision, which was intro-duced in the late nineteenth century to discourage masturbation, is still widely practiced. Although routine male circumcision is on the decline since many of its purported medical benefits have been discredited, about half of all newborn boys in the United States are still circumcised. In many in-stances, the surgical procedure is carried out without anesthesia. Routine circumcision of males has been discon-tinued in all other Western nations and is even illegal as a form of child abuse in some countries, such as France. Neither male nor female cir-cumcision is practiced in Asia or by Asian Americans.

opinion, determines what is right and what is wrong. There are no objective, universal moral standards that hold for all people in all cultures, only different cultural customs. For example, in the United States, most boys are circumcised after birth; that is, the foreskin around the genitals is surgically removed. In almost all other Western nations routine **circumcision** of males is considered immoral, and in countries such as France it is considered child abuse. Female circumcision, on the other hand, is considered highly immoral in the United States but morally acceptable in many African cultures. Who is right, and who is wrong?

Do not confuse cultural relativism with sociological relativism. **Sociological rela-tivism** is simply the observation that disagreement exists among cultures regarding moral values. Unlike cultural relativism, sociological relativism leaves open the possibil-ity that a culture, such as Nazi Germany, may be mistaken about a moral value. Cultural relativists argue that this is impossible, since culture alone is the source of moral values.

Cultural relativists, in other words, argue not merely that some moral values are relative to culture but that *all* moral values are nothing more than cultural customs. Because there are no universal moral standards, the moral values of one culture cannot be judged to be better or worse than those of any other culture. Head-hunting, for example, is right or wrong only within a particular cultural context. In some New Guinea cultures, it is morally commendable for a young man to give his sweetheart a shrunken head as a trophy. In Western cultures, however, such an action would be regarded as highly immoral and as evidence of a serious psychiatric disorder. According to the cultural relativist, head-hunting is morally right for the New Guinea man but morally wrong for an American.

Similarly, a cultural relativist would argue that women in a culture that believes women should be kept in subjection have a moral obligation to be submissive to their fathers or husbands. In such cultures, it is the men who control the reproductive functions of the women. Should a woman refuse to bear a child for her husband, her husband would have a moral right, and perhaps even a moral duty, to force his wife to comply with cultural standards. According to a cultural relativist, in our culture it is wrong for a man to use brute force on his wife only because it goes against our cultural norms. There are no other standards by which to gauge the morality of people's actions. In highly patriarchal cultures, women who refuse to be submissive or to turn control of their reproductive functions over to their husbands are immoral.

Morality may also change within a culture over time, much as laws and fashions change. Slavery is now considered highly immoral in the United States. Two hundred years ago, however, not only was slavery believed to be morally acceptable by the majority; according to cultural relativists it was morally acceptable. Likewise, during and prior to World War II, that Jews were morally inferior and a threat to the well-being of Aryans was generally accepted in Germany, and in much of Europe for that matter. If morality is synonymous with conformity to cultural norms, the abolitionists and the freedom fighters, not the slaveholders and Nazis like Dr. Mengele, were immoral.

Cultural relativism, like ethical subjectivism, is wrought with problems and contradictions. For example, morality can change over time, but because cultural relativism identifies morality with the status quo there is no such thing as moral progress even though most people believe that abolishing slavery, stopping the Nazi experiments on Jews, and granting women fuller reproductive freedom represent moral progress, not simply changing fads. Most of us believe that the Nuremberg Tribunal was appealing to a moral law that superseded human laws when it declared Nazi war criminals guilty of "crimes against humanity." We believe, as did some Germans, including the Jews who survived, that what the Nazis did was wrong, regardless of their cultural norms and laws. Cultural relativism, however, precludes critiquing one's own cultural norms. It cannot account for the fact that most people believe there are ways in which their own society can be improved.

Cultural relativism also legitimates the exclusion of certain groups of people—such as Jews, women, and people of color—from the full respect and protection of the community. In the United States, for example, women and people of color do not receive the same quality of healthcare as do white men. If morality is a cultural creation, humans, as well as nonhuman animals, have moral value only if their society grants them moral status. The cultural definition of the moral community is, to a large extent, politically and economically motivated. Cultural relativism, in other words, supports a definition of the moral community that serves primarily to maintain the status quo. By doing so, it protects the interests of those in power while morally sanctioning the marginalization and exploitation of other groups.

In his book *Hitler's Willing Executioners*, Harvard scholar Daniel Goldhagen argues that the persecution of the Jews in Germany before and during World War II was not the act of a few Nazis. Anti-Semitism and the exclusion of the Jews from the moral community was the prevailing norm in German culture. The removal of the Jews from the moral community was a gradual process built on decades of anti-Semitism among the Germans. Not only was the exclusion of the Jews from the moral community supported by popular opinion, but the German Supreme Court itself ruled in 1936 that "the Jew is only a rough copy of a human being, with humanlike facial traits but nonetheless . . . lower than any animal . . . otherwise nothing. For all that bear a human face are not equal." Because it was culturally acceptable to be anti-Semitic, the majority of Germans, according to Goldhagen, willingly participated in the Holocaust. If cultural relativism is a correct description of morality, then Dr. Josef Mengele behaved morally since in Nazi Germany Jews legally were nonpersons. Jews had no rights that Dr. Mengele and other physicians who used them in medical experiments were bound to respect.

Between 1930 and 1953, the U.S. Department of Health Services conducted a study on syphilis known as the Tuskegee Study. It used as subjects, without their informed consent, poor black men living in six different Southern states. Despite the discovery in the late 1940s that penicillin could cure syphilis, treatment was withheld from the nearly three hundred men participating in the study. As a result, many of the men whose lives could have been saved by penicillin died simply for the sake of increasing scientific knowledge about the progression of the disease. According to a cultural relativist, the Tuskegee Study was not immoral at the time, although it would be immoral now. Like passing fashions, U.S. cultural norms have changed with the passing of civil rights legislation and the establishment of review boards for medical research.[14] What was moral fifty years ago is now immoral. Perhaps times will change and it will once again be moral to experiment on certain groups of humans—for example, clones bred for this purpose.

Modern cultural relativism came of age in the late nineteenth and early twentieth centuries with the study of so-called "simple" cultures by anthropologists, who were impressed with the vast differences in customs among different cultures. Cultural relativism was also proposed as a corrective to the prevailing view of social evolutionists, who ranked groups of people and cultures as more or less developed, both culturally and morally. Ruth Benedict, one of the foremost proponents of cultural relativism, wrote, "We recognize that morality differs in every society, and is a convenient term for socially approved habits."[15]

The early cultural relativists failed to take into account that generally the so-called dominant cultural values are simply the values held by a small group of people who happen to hold the power in the culture. People who are oppressed by cultural values that disadvantage them rarely agree that this is the way things ought to be. Instead, they often hold values that conflict with those of the majority culture. The views of the majority may also conflict with the law as well as with the views of healthcare professionals, who generally hold a privileged place in society.

In other words, ideas about what is moral can differ *within* a culture, a phenomenon that cultural relativism has difficulty explaining. For example, ideas about the morality of selective abortion vary widely within cultures such as India, China, and the United States. When differences of opinion about what is right and wrong exist within a culture or when the majority of people disagree with the law of the land, what standards are we to use to determine what is moral and what is immoral?

In our rapidly changing modern world, it is becoming more and more difficult to draw sharp distinctions between cultures, or even to define our own cultural norms. Just as "no man is an island," so, too, "no culture is an island." A practice in one culture has repercussions in other cultures. For example, the rejection in 1938 by the American Medical Association of a request by 5,000 black physicians to join the organization was widely reported in German medical journals as affirmation of the importance of programs of racial hygiene. On a more positive note, the recent emphasis in American medicine on patient autonomy in making informed decisions about personal healthcare is having a ripple effect in both Japan and Muslim countries, which traditionally tend to be paternalistic. Exposure to the perspective of another culture can help healthcare professionals break through cultural paradigms that neglect certain moral aspects of healthcare.

Furthermore, cultural relativism leaves us with no guidance for deciding what is moral or immoral when disagreement arises over the morality of a particular practice within a culture. The belief that there are no shared universal moral values can also lead to suspicion and mistrust of people from other cultures or subcultures, rather than to tolerance and a sense of community. We may feel that "they" do not share our respect for life or for personal autonomy and even that people from other cultures have dangerous values. Because cultural relativism rules out the possibility of rational discussion when cross-cultural values come into conflict and persuasion fails, groups may resort either to apathy or isolationism, when the values of other cultures are not a threat, or to violence, when another culture's values or actions create a threat to their way of life. We need to critically examine any moral feelings we might have that are based more on cultural tradition than on sound reasoning.

Most theories, even though they may not stand up under the scrutiny of critical analysis, contain at least a grain of truth. In disavowing cultural relativism, too many ethicists have divorced morality from the actual historical and cultural settings in which we make our moral decisions. Cultural relativism reminds us that context is important in moral decision making. Our traditions, our religious values, and our political and social institutions all shape the way in which we apply moral principles. However, while the application and interpretation of universal moral principles and ideals may be relative to society, the moral principles themselves are not solely the invention of society.

If morality is a cultural creation, we have no justifiable grounds for labeling the Nazi culture immoral, since our norms apply only to those living within our culture. All we can say is that it was no better and no worse than our culture, just different. Cultural relativism, as a moral theory, fell out of favor among ethicists and social scientists following World War II. The horrors of the Holocaust made it hard for them to maintain the belief that there are no basic standards of right and wrong outside of cultural norms.

Reasons for Moral Disagreement

If ethical relativism is incorrect, how can we explain disagreement among individuals and cultures over moral values? The fact that people disagree does not necessarily mean that there are no objective moral principles. People can disagree for a number of

THE KABLOONA:
Euthanasia in the Arctic

The Kabloona are an Eskimo culture in the Canadian Arctic. In Kabloona society, children had a moral obligation to honor their elderly and ailing parents' requests to die. The following description was published in 1941 by Gontran de Poncins:

One observer was told of an Eskimo who was getting ready to move camp and was concerned about what to do with his blind and aged father, who was a burden to the family. One day the old man expressed a desire to go seal hunting again, something he had not done for many years. His son readily assented to this suggestion, and the old man was dressed warmly and given his weapons. He was then led out to the seal grounds and was walked to a hole in the ice into which he disappeared.[16]

Is cultural relativism the only way to explain the difference between the Kabloona and modern Americans?

Americans can hire caregivers or put their ailing parents or grandparents in nursing homes. The Kabloona, on the other hand, were a nomadic people; there were no nursing homes or hospitals or spare bedrooms for grandparents. As nomadic people, their lives depended on following the seal herds. To take a blind and ailing parent on one of the treks could have resulted in the starvation not just of the elderly parent, but of the whole family. The son respected his father's autonomy, waiting until the father requested the "hunting" trip.

What is different here is not the fundamental moral value of respect for life, family loyalty, and personal autonomy, but conditions that place limitations on how these values can best be applied. Saving the lives of many took precedence over prolonging the father's life.

reasons. They may be mistaken about the facts. For example, it was once believed that excessive masturbation caused blindness and insanity. Also, American physicians used to routinely lie to dying cancer patients, believing that the truth would be so upsetting that it might produce more harm than good and maybe even kill the patients. Recent studies have shown both of these beliefs to be mistaken.

Disagreement can also occur because natural conditions or religious beliefs influence the expression of a particular moral value. In some societies, such as the Kabloona Eskimos, children had a moral obligation to euthanize their elderly and ailing parents if their parents requested it. In American society, it is considered immoral for children to euthanize their parents. The question of when, if ever, it is morally permissible to assist an elderly or terminally ill person in taking his or her life is not limited to the Kabloona culture. The introduction of medical technology that can prolong the lives of the elderly and the dying has brought the issue of death with dignity and assisted suicide to the forefront in most industrialized cultures.

Morality is similar to language. At first glance, all languages appear to be different. When we first hear a foreign language, it seems to make no sense. However, the many different languages in the world all share a common syntax; that is, the fundamental grammatical structure of all human languages is the same, even though the specific words may differ from language to language. Understanding the morality of other cultures requires that we become familiar with the context in which the moral principles are applied and moral decisions made. Only when we take the time to discover our underlying commonalities can true cross-cultural communication among healthcare professionals begin.

The Moral Community and Personhood

Variations in cultural norms can also occur because of differences in how cultures define their moral communities. According to anthropologist Clyde Kluckholn, some universal moral values are recognized by all cultures. No culture, for example, approves of indiscriminate lying, cheating, or stealing. Random violence is also universally prohibited. Every culture also makes arrangements for the care of its children. These moral values, however, apply only to members of a particular culture's **moral community,** that is, to those who are seen as having moral value. Beings who have moral worth are known in ethics as **persons.** Persons are worthy of respect in themselves, rather than because of their usefulness or value to someone else. Nazi physicians, such as Dr. Josef Mengele, did not use healthy Aryans of Nazi persuasion in their atrocious medical experiments. Headhunters always select their victims from outside their immediate community.

Traditional Western ethics does not give clear guidance with regard to the important question of just who, or what, is a person, although it is generally agreed that rational adult humans are persons. Definitions of persons as autonomous and rational moral agents seem too restrictive or vague. Sentience is similarly vague and difficult to measure.

The identification of the term *person* with *human being* in most Western societies and the exclusion of humans from the category *animal* (although humans are clearly a species of animal) betray our **anthropocentric** bias in defining the moral community. Likewise, the use of the term *man* for all humans reflects a patriarchal bias. In cultural relativism, moral status is granted by one's community; there are no rights independent of those created by culture. Those who are considered closer to the center of the moral community—such as white males in American culture—receive more privileges and protection. Those who are **marginalized**—such as women, homosexuals, blacks, and Hispanics—have less access to economic and social benefits. This situation is reflected in the wide discrepancies in access to healthcare and in the quality of healthcare received by members of different groups in the United States. Beings who are outside of the moral community can be treated as a "means only" and be killed, exploited for their organs, or used as subjects in medical experiments solely for the benefit of those within the moral community.

Some cultures have a much more inclusive definition of the moral community. In Buddhist and Hindu healthcare ethics, the moral community is defined very broadly to include all living beings. Other definitions of the moral community include ancestral spirits. How a culture defines moral community, as well as the individual's relationship to the moral community, has a profound effect on medical practices. In the United States, the moral community is seen primarily as a collection of autonomous persons, a view reflected in the nature of the physician/patient relationship and our emphasis on patient autonomy and privacy.

In some cultures, personhood is defined primarily in relational terms: To be a member of a moral community means to be part of a larger entity that itself commands more respect. In the Afro-Caribbean healing tradition of Haiti, the individual patient is defined by a web of relationships that includes not only the extended family but also ancestors and spirits. Healing is aimed at healing and readjusting relationships rather than at simply curing the physical disorder.[17] Similarly, among the Akan of Ghana, healing is aimed at restoring the harmony of relationships as well as at restoring the body.[18] Medical performances such as chants are aimed at healing the universe as well as curing the body.

The cultural definition of the moral community is, to a large extent, politically and economically motivated and serves to maintain the status quo, especially in cultures that tend to define the moral community rather narrowly. For a being or a group of beings to be excluded from the moral community, it first must be "depersonalized." Before embarking on the Final Solution, the German Supreme Court first ruled that the Jew was a nonperson. By protecting the interests of those in power and morally sanctioning the marginalization and exploitation of other groups, cultural relativism promotes ethnocentrism and legitimates hatred and discrimination. Problems such as sexism and racism, which are based on long traditions of discrimination against women and people of color, exist in our culture in part because the majority of American adults, according to developmental psychologist Lawrence Kohlberg, define morality primarily in terms of cultural mores and values.[19]

While Dr. Mengele eluded capture, his compatriot Adolf Eichmann was found guilty of crimes against humanity under the Nuremberg Charter. When asked if he had moral doubts about the extermination program, Eichmann replied, "Who am I to judge?" The quintessential cultural relativist, Eichmann illustrates the dangers of cultural relativism. According to him, his conscience was at peace because he had always been a good, law-abiding citizen whose chief standard was the "good society" as defined by his culture.[20]

BEYOND ETHICAL RELATIVISM: MORAL DEVELOPMENT AND HEALTHCARE PROFESSIONALS

The Stage Theory of Moral Development

According to Lawrence Kohlberg and other developmental psychologists, there are innate cognitive structures that are fundamental to all humans. These structures include causality, time and space, and moral excellence. Although the specific content of moral codes can vary depending on a person's culture, the difference is only on the surface. The conceptual structures from which these specific codes are formulated are universal.

In his research, Kohlberg found that humans, with the exception of psychopaths and other severely impaired people, have an inherent potential for growth from the lower (earlier) to the higher stages of moral development. Kohlberg identified three main stages of **moral development:** the preconventional, the conventional, and the postconventional. At the preconventional stage, people are motivated by egotistical concern. At the conventional stage, people's moral reasoning is influenced mainly by their peers or their cultures; in other words, they are cultural relativists. Ninety percent of American adults are at this stage of moral development; their primary concern is to please others and, like the people in Milgram's study, to respect authority and social rules. The third, or postconventional, stage is that of autonomous, principled moral reasoning based on universal principles such as justice and respect.

These states are universal or transcultural and represent "transformations in the organization of thought, rather than increasing knowledge of cultural values."[21] Studies from more than forty Western and non-Western countries support Kohlberg's theory that the stages of moral development are universal. These studies also lend support to the theory that some cultures are better than others at promoting virtue and moral development. For example, people in the United States tend to score lower on tests of moral development than people from Canada and Iceland, but higher than people living in Taiwan.

Each stage represents a different pattern or system of logic for determining the just and right way to solve a moral conflict. Higher stages are more complex than earlier stages. People at higher stages of moral development tend to be more satisfied with their moral decisions, and people in general prefer a solution to a moral problem that uses the highest stage of moral reasoning conceptually available to them. A person will stay at a stage until it is replaced by a new stage. Transition to a new stage is generally prompted by social and cognitive disequilibrium, in which a person encounters a crisis that his or her current mode of thinking is unable to satisfactorily resolve.

Women and the Care Perspective

Because Kohlberg's early research was done exclusively on men, his gender-biased research was understandably unacceptable to many researchers and feminist philosophers. Carol Gilligan, who had studied with Kohlberg, decided it was time to correct this bias. In her interviews with women, Gilligan concluded that women's moral development tends to follow a path different from that of men. Men tend to be duty- and principle-oriented; women are more context-oriented and tend to view the world in a more emotional and personal way. Women's moral judgment, Gilligan found, is characterized by a concern for themselves and others; women accept and maintain responsibility within relationships, attachment, and self-sacrifice. Gilligan calls this the "care perspective," in contrast to Kohlberg's "justice perspective." In her research with women, Gilligan postulated three stages of moral development moving from self-centered moral reasoning to self-sacrifice at the conventional level to mature care ethics, in which a person is able to balance her own needs and the needs of others. Gilligan's position is alluded to in Hilde Lindemann Nelson's article on a feminist standpoint on the healthcare relationship at the end of Chapter 3.

Although Gilligan's and Kohlberg's theories emphasize different aspects of moral development and Kohlberg subdivides each stage into two levels, their stages are roughly parallel. For example, the preconventional stage in both theories includes egoists and ethical subjectivists. Similarly, people at the conventional stage are cultural relativists who look to their culture for moral guidance. The different descriptions of the conventional stage are not surprising, given the different ways in which men and women are socialized in our culture. Men, for the most part, are socialized to be the upholders of law and order and to believe that maleness carries certain privileges. Women, on the other hand, are taught that being a good woman involves self-sacrifice and placing the welfare of others before her own. In her article "A Feminist Critique of

🍂 THE STAGES OF MORAL REASONING

Stage	Kohlberg's Description	Gilligan's Description
Preconventional	*Avoid punishment:* Fear of punishment is primary motive. *Egoist:* Satisfy one's needs; consider the needs of others only if it benefits you. "You scratch my back, I'll scratch yours."	*Self-centered:* Viewing one's own needs as all that matters.
Conventional	*Good boy/nice girl:* Please and help others; earn others' approval; conform to group and peer norms. *Society-maintaining:* Respect authority and social rules; maintain the existing social order.	*Self-sacrificing:* Viewing others' needs as more important.
Postconventional	*Social contract or legalistic:* Obey useful, albeit arbitrary, social rules; appeal to social consensus and majority rule as long as minimal basic rights are safeguarded. *Conscience and universal principles:* Autonomously recognize universal principles, such as justice and equality, that are rational and logically consistent and reflect a respect for equal human rights and dignity.	*Mature care ethics:* Able to balance one's own needs and the needs of others.

Physician-Assisted Suicide" (see Chapter 8), Susan Wolf argues that the belief in self-sacrifice as a womanly virtue places women under greater pressure to choose euthanasia when they become a burden to their family.

In both Kohlberg's and Gilligan's theories, the postconventional stage is represented by autonomous moral reasoning in which the person looks to transcultural values, whether in the form of principles of justice and respect or of sentiments such as compassion and empathy. More recent studies suggest that both men and women draw from both the justice perspective and the care perspective and that moral maturity involves the ability to use both in making moral decisions.

Medical students tend to be at a higher level of conventional reasoning or a lower level of postconventional reasoning as measured by the Defining Issues Test (DIT), which is based for the most part on Kohlberg's stages of moral development.[22] However, while physicians are better at moral reasoning than the average adult, they consistently score lower in moral reasoning than clinical medical ethicists.[23]

Later researchers have questioned Gilligan's claim that men and women have different moral orientations. Indeed, several research studies have found that women in medical school score higher than male medical students on justice-oriented tests such as the DIT, which measures primarily moral reasoning.[24] On the other hand, in a study of graduating medical students, 66.7 percent of the men showed a preference for the justice perspective while 72.2 percent of the women showed a preference for the care perspective.[25] Female physicians are also more likely to integrate the justice and the care orientations than to show a strong preference for only one orientation.[26] Of course, the research results don't mean that women in general score high on scales of justice orientation, but simply that women who choose to become physicians do. It is possible that women (and men) who prefer a care orientation may choose to go into different fields in healthcare. Also, not everyone accepts a developmental theory of moral behavior. Clearly, more research needs to be done on the dimensions of the orientation of care among healthcare professionals.

The Four Components of Moral Behavior

While one's level of moral development is positively correlated to moral behavior, moral reasoning is not the only determinant or component of moral behavior. Moral behavior is a complex phenomenon that cannot be represented as a single variable. Psychologist James Rest identified four components of moral behavior: (1) moral judgment or reasoning, (2) moral sensitivity, (3) moral motivation, and (4) moral character.[27] A deficiency in any of these components, Rest notes, can result in a failure to act morally.

In the 1991 movie *The Doctor*, a successful surgeon who is lacking in moral sensitivity and compassion for his patients learns the difference between treating patients as machines to be fixed and caring for his patients when he becomes seriously ill. Moral sensitivity is the awareness of how our actions affect others. It involves the ability to empathize and to imagine ourselves in another person's shoes. There are striking differences in people's sensitivity to the needs and welfare of others. People like Mother Teresa and Albert Schweitzer, for example, are highly sensitive to the suffering of others. Florence Nightingale "was so ready with her sympathy for all who suffered or were in trouble" that, even as a teenager, people referred to her as an "angel in the homes of the poor."[28] In contrast, people who are deficient in the moral sensitivity component of moral behavior, like Dr. Josef Mengele, are often unable to recognize a moral situation. They may fail to act or may make offensive comments not out of malice, but simply because they are unaware of the effect of their behavior on others.

Many healthcare professionals know what is right and are sensitive to people's needs and the moral issues involved but lack the moral motivation to put this knowledge into action. Instead, they put nonmoral values—such as money, popularity, and conformity to cultural or peer norms—above what they know to be right. They may fail to follow up on their dream to serve the very needy as Nightingale and Schweitzer did, choosing instead a high-paying, less fulfilling job. Or they may fail to report a peer who is operating on patients while intoxicated. People who fail to act on what they know is right are known as weak-willed. Many of the subjects in Milgram's experiment on obedience were weak-willed; they were sensitive to the supposed suffering of the person they were shocking and knew it was wrong, but they put obedience to authority above what they knew was right. In contrast, healthcare professionals who are highly motivated morally are more likely to act on their beliefs about what is right. They put moral values above nonmoral values. For example, dentists who score high on a measure of moral motivation are far more likely to treat a patient who has tested positive for HIV and to agree that healthcare professionals have a responsibility to treat patients known to be infected with other blood-borne diseases.[29]

Moral character is related to integrity and virtue. This aspect of moral behavior is emphasized in Confucian and Buddhist healthcare ethics, which hold the development of moral character to be one of the primary duties of a healthcare professional. A person of high moral character is able to integrate the other three components of moral behavior into his or her personality. Moral character predisposes us to act morally. People of high moral character are more likely to persevere in accomplishing their goals, even in the face of strong pressure to do otherwise.

Ethics Education and Moral Maturity

Both Gilligan and Kohlberg agree in their later work that the most adequate moral orientation is one that takes both the justice and care perspectives into consideration; the two perspectives, rather than being mutually exclusive, complement and enrich each other.[30] While the majority of graduating medical students in one study used both justice and care in resolving moral conflicts, only 15 percent showed a balanced approach, in which neither justice nor care was predominant.[31]

Effective moral decision making is a holistic rather than a fragmented, either/or process. People who are strong in one component of moral behavior tend to be strong in the others. For example, there is a strong correlation between higher scores on tests of moral reasoning and greater sensitivity to family opposition regarding aggressive treatment of a critically ill family member.[32] Physicians who score lower in moral reasoning, in contrast, are more likely to treat dying patients aggressively despite a patient's or family's wishes to the contrary.

Professional training, on its own, does not facilitate—and may even inhibit—moral development. In the mid-1970s, primarily in response to moral issues arising because of new technology, both medical and nursing schools began introducing formal courses in healthcare ethics. Within a decade, the majority of these schools offered ethics courses. The addition of formal courses in healthcare ethics to the curriculum has been found to promote growth in moral reasoning among medical students.[33] Furthermore, longitudinal studies show that positive changes in moral reasoning skills are retained.[34] This may account for the finding that the level of moral development of graduating medical students in the 1980s was slightly higher than that of practicing physicians and staff nurses.[35]

In a study of moral sensitivity among dentists, researchers found that sensitivity could be enhanced through professional training.[36] An ethics curriculum that includes role playing to promote moral sensitivity has also been found to enhance moral reasoning. Studies also show that healthcare professionals, such as nurses, who have high levels of empathy and are able to take the perspective of others are more likely to exhibit moral sensitivity in actual clinical situations.[37] Ethics education also counteracts tendencies toward the goals of "exclusiveness" and "privilege" that too often characterize professionals in high-status fields such as healthcare.[38]

The study of ethics and the promotion of moral development, in other words, have real-life consequences. In a study of the relationship between moral reasoning and clinical performance as measured by the number of malpractice claims, it was found that physicians with few or no claims per year had higher levels of moral development than those with multiple claims. Physicians at higher levels of moral reasoning were also open to peer reviews and professional relationships. The researchers concluded that higher-level postconventional moral reasoning provides a "protective element" against malpractice resulting from poor medical decisions.[39]

Not surprisingly, there is a positive correlation between a faculty's overall rating of residents' performance and their stage of moral development.[40] Medical students and physicians who score high on tests of moral reasoning are also more likely to live up to their commitments and to be able to manage morally problematic cases.[41] The positive relationship between level of moral reasoning and professional performance has led at least one medical school in Israel to consider assessed level of moral reasoning as a criterion for admission to medical school.[42]

HEALTHCARE ETHICS AND RELIGION

Many people look to their clergy not only as religious authorities, but also as moral authorities. Some of the earliest bioethicists in the United States came out of the Protestant tradition, with its faith in scientific knowledge and its emphasis on human freedom. In particular, Paul Ramsey's book *The Patient as Person: Explorations in Medical Ethics* (1970) led to what has been called the "renaissance of healthcare ethics."[43] Today many, if not most, hospital ethics boards have at least one clergy member. Clergy are also asked to testify before Congress on ethics issues such as cloning and healthcare.

Judaism regards medicine as a covenant between God and the physician. Because the physician is God's messenger for healing people in need, Jewish doctors cannot refuse to help someone in need of medical care. "The Torah gave permission to the physician to heal; moreover, this is a religious precept. . . . if the physician withholds his services it is considered as shedding blood."[44] Healing is also important in the Christian tradition. Indeed, much of the mission of Jesus involved healing and caring for those in need.

The concept of God in the major world religions—Judaism, Christianity, Hinduism, and Islam—is so intimately connected to the concept of moral goodness that the moral code is incorporated directly into the doctrine of these religions. However, this does not imply that religion or scripture is the only source of moral guidance or that morality is relative to religion. Judaism, Hinduism, and most Christian denominations teach that the basic moral principles in the scriptures are universal and discoverable through other means, such as reason or intuition. Others, including some Muslims and fundamentalist Christians, maintain that ethics is inseparable from religion and is built entirely on it.

In Islamic countries religion plays a central role in healthcare, while in the United States religion is often regarded as irrelevant to medical practice. In societies committed to medical care based on a mechanistic model, religious groups such as Christian Scientists and Jehovah's Witnesses, who turn to prayer for healing, have come into conflict with the medical establishment and the courts.

CULTURAL WINDOWS

THE ISLAMIC TRADITION IN HEALTHCARE ETHICS

Islamic culture grounds healthcare ethics in religious doctrine, as revealed by Allah in the Quran. Medical knowledge, like all knowledge, is regarded as part of the knowledge of God. According to the Islamic tradition, "The study of Medicine entails the revealing of God's signs in His creation. . . . The practice of Medicine brings God's mercy unto His subjects. Medical practice is therefore an act of worship and charity on top of being a career to make a living."[45] Islamic physicians in non-Islamic cultures, such as the United States and Canada, are also bound to the Islamic code of ethics.

Following are excerpts from the Islamic Organization of Medical Sciences 1981 *Islamic Code of Medical Ethics Kuwait Document*:

The Oath of the Doctor
I swear by God . . . The Great
To regard God in carrying out my profession

To protect human life in all stages and under all circumstances, doing my utmost to rescue it from death, malady, pain and anxiety . . .
To keep people's dignity, cover their privacies and lock up their secrets . . .

To be, all the way, an instrument of God's mercy, extending my medical care to near and far, virtuous and sinner and friend and enemy . . .
To strive in the pursuit of knowledge and harness it for the benefit but not the harm of Mankind . . .
To revere my teacher, teach my junior, and be brother to members of the Medical Profession joined in piety and charity . . .
To live my Faith in private and in public, avoiding whatever blemishes me in the eyes of God, His apostle and my fellow Faithful
And may God be witness to this Oath.

Divine Command Theory

On March 22, 1997, thirty-nine members of Heaven's Gate, a California cult, left their earthly bodies to ascend to a "Higher Level." According to cult members, the physical body is merely an earthbound vessel for the soul. Do, the "sainted one" and leader of the cult, had received the command that it was time to move to a "Higher Level" from his companion Ti, a nurse who died in 1985 and communicated the divine will to him from the higher, spiritual level. The command came to leave this earth and join a spaceship in the tail of the Hale–Bopp comet, which was passing Earth. The mass suicide of the cult members took place in stages, with those who chose to go last helping the others administer poison. Was the mass suicide morally justified? Does the fact that an action was divinely commanded, as those who participated in it believed, morally justify it?

In Plato's *Euthyphro,* Socrates asks, "Do the gods love holiness because it is holy, or is it holy because the gods love it?" The **divine command theory** claims the latter: Something is holy, or moral, simply because God loves it. The divine command theory,

CHRISTIAN SCIENTISTS:
Refusing Medical Treatment

Christian Scientists believe that reality consists solely in the mind. Illnesses are mental in origin, and prayer is the proper antidote to suffering. For Christian Scientists, seeking medical care runs contrary to their faith. To place their faith in both prayer and medicine is hypocrisy and as such, it is believed, greatly diminishes the power of prayer.

In 1990, the health of Colin Newmark, the three-year-old son of Christian Scientists, began to deteriorate rapidly. His parents reluctantly took him to a nearby hospital. Diagnostic tests indicated that Colin suffered from an intestinal blockage. His parents agreed to surgery to remove the blockage because they considered the procedure to be purely mechanical rather than medical.

A pathological report on tissue taken during the surgery revealed that Colin was suffering from non-Hodgkin's lymphoma. The doctors in charge of the case recommended chemotherapy and radiation therapy. Without medical intervention, Colin would probably die within eight months. On the other hand, the therapy, which gave Colin a 40 percent chance of survival, would be painful and debilitating to Colin and could result in kidney failure, immunological and neurological problems, and sterility.

The Newmarks refused treatment and attempted to have Colin removed from the hospital into the care of a Christian Scientist practitioner. The hospital in turn sued for custody of Colin so the physicians could treat him. The Delaware Supreme Court ruled in favor of the parents.[46]

Not all court rulings have supported the religious freedom of minors. In 1999, seventeen-year-old Alexis Demos refused to undergo a blood transfusion following a snowboarding accident. Jehovah's Witnesses, Demos and her family refused the procedure because it was against their religious beliefs. The case ended up in a Massachusetts court, where the judge ruled in favor of the physicians. The Academy of Pediatrics, which opposes religious exemptions to child-protection laws, supports such rulings, pointing to the emotional toll on healthcare providers if a patient dies after refusing treatment. Doctors and nurses grieve the loss of their young patients long after the media attention has faded.[47]

in other words, is a type of ethical relativism, since morality is dependent on or relative to the will of God. There are no independent, universal moral standards by which to judge God's commands. No justification other than God's commanding it is necessary for an action to be right.

If our response to Do and his followers is that God would not have commanded this mass suicide, we are implying that independent moral standards exist by which we can appraise the morality of God's commands. However, the divine command theory leaves us without any criteria for judging actions. A believer in this theory can simply reply to our protests that no support is needed—that it's just a matter of faith. The divine command theory is not the same as ethical subjectivism, in which each person follows his or her own feelings. While the mass suicide of the members of Heaven's Gate involved only those who consented, the divine command theory would also justify the mass killing of nonconsenting people—such as a healthcare professional's systematically euthanizing residents of a nursing home or hospital ward—as long as the person carrying out the killing had received a "divine command" to do so.

Natural Law Ethicists

Natural law ethicists disagree with the divine command theory. They maintain that God commands an action because it is moral beforehand, independent of God's commanding it. Natural law ethics is one of the oldest and most persistent moral theories. Aristotle, Thomas Aquinas, Thomas Jefferson, Martin Luther King, Jr., Elizabeth Cady Stanton, and Mahatma Gandhi all incorporated aspects of natural law ethics into their philosophies. Variations of natural law ethics are espoused by moral philosophers throughout the world. African philosopher Kwame Gyekye is a member of the Akan tribe in Ghana. Akan moral philosophy is a blend of natural law and utilitarian ethics. Gyekye writes, "The response of the Akan moral thinker would be that God approves of the good because it is good. . . . the event of a breach of the moral law clearly suggests the Akan conviction that God approves of the good because it is good and eschews the evil because it is evil."[48]

UNIVERSAL MORAL THEORIES

Like natural law ethicists, most moral philosophers and healthcare ethicists subscribe to the existence of universal and objective moral principles. There are several different universalist theories, including natural law theory, utilitarianism, deontology, rights ethics, and virtue ethics. All these theories agree that universal moral principles exist that are binding on all people regardless of their personal opinion, culture, or religion and that these moral principles are discovered rather than created by people. Although individual interests or cultural customs, as noted in the Kabloona case, can influence how a particular moral principle or theory is applied, fundamental moral principles are universal and transcultural.

Unlike ethical subjectivism and cultural relativism, which are mutually exclusive theories, universalist theories are all based on the presumption that universal and objective moral principles exist. Conflicts obviously arise between the different universal theories. However, the distinctions are not nearly as black-and-white as many academic philosophers have made them out to be. Rather than being exclusive or embracing the whole picture, for the most part the different theories fit together, with each reinforcing or building on the others. Moral judgment is a whole into which we must fit principles, character and intentions, cultural values, circumstances, and consequences.

Natural Law Theory

According to **natural law theory,** morality is grounded in rational human nature. While physical nature is fixed and determined, human nature is free and autonomous.

Accepting natural law theory does not entail knowing the origin of natural law. Just as not all physicists agree on the origin of the laws of physics, not all natural law ethicists agree on the origin of natural law. Aquinas believed that God created natural or moral law as part of His divine plan for the universe. Aristotle, on the other hand, maintained that the moral law has always existed as part of the natural order. Whatever the origin of moral law, all natural law ethicists agree that moral law exists outside of cultural norms and personal preferences. It is embedded in our rational nature and is the same for all humans. God and humans, religious people and atheists alike, are all bound by the same moral principles and sentiments.

These natural laws exist in the form of very general or formal moral laws or principles such as "respect for other persons" and the Golden Rule, which are contained in the moral codes of all major religions. These very general principles form the basis of normative moral rules that contain specific content and guidelines for action, for example, "Euthanasia is immoral" and "Honor your mother and your father."

Unlike cultural relativism, which equates morality with conformity and obedience to human laws and customs, natural law theory, like all nonrelativistic theories, may call for civil disobedience if a human law conflicts with natural or moral law. Members of animal liberation groups break into laboratories to set the animals free; antiabortionists block women from entering Planned Parenthood clinics; before the legalization of abortion, women formed cooperatives to assist other women in getting abortions; Dr. Jack Kevorkian—after five arrests, a murder conviction, and what he says are more than 130 assisted suicides, one of which was broadcast on national television—continues to advocate for physician-assisted suicide.[49] Are these people justified, on the grounds of a higher moral law, in breaking the law of the land? Natural law theorists respond with a qualified yes. A person is justified in breaking a human law if it is unjust and if breaking it does not create more harm than obeying it would.

Natural law is also **teleological,** meaning that it is grounded in a vision of the purpose or goal of the natural order. As we move toward that goal, interpretations of the application of natural law may change. For example, some Roman Catholic natural law ethicists argue that, while the prohibition on contraception may have been appropriate at one time because of the command for humans to go forth and multiply, it is no longer morally required because of overpopulation.

Some weaknesses of natural law are its generality and its assumption that all rational beings will agree on the content of natural law. In addition, the specific normative rules, because they are interpretations of the more general natural law, are subject to human error and cultural biases. Despite these perhaps unavoidable shortcomings, natural law theory is one of the most popular moral theories.

In light of the widespread acceptance of natural law ethics, it is not surprising that it is used by the United Nations. According to the U.N. Nuremberg Charter, rulers and citizens—regardless of their particular religious affiliation or lack thereof—are responsible "under God and [natural] law." Natural laws, the charter continues, include prohibitions against "crimes against humanity," "torture," and "waging or preparing for an unjust war." Each person, according to the charter, has an individual responsibility to not take refuge in the laws and customs of his or her culture. Because of all people's ultimate responsibility to a universal moral code, people can be tried under international law when they obey cultural customs that are contrary to natural law. Nazis such as Dr. Mengele, while models of morality under the standard of cultural relativism, were found sadly wanting according to natural law ethics as interpreted by the United Nations.

Religious teachings may help clarify one's moral position or motivate one to behave morally; however, most philosophers, as well as most theologians, agree that morality exists independent of religion. When people who are religious use the terms *right* and *wrong*, they generally mean the same thing as someone who is not religious. Religious differences tend to fall away in most serious discussions of moral issues, such as cloning, euthanasia, or abortion, not because religion isn't important to the participants but because moral disputes can be discussed, and resolved, without bringing religion into the discussion.

Even though most healthcare ethicists may agree that morality does not depend on religion, we are still left with the question of to what extent faith strengthens one's moral resolve and to what extent faith can actually enhance the healing process. If healings based on prayer or other acts of faith were rare, there would be less reason to give a second thought to court cases in which believers and medical professionals come into conflict. However, medical science has been unable to explain several significant cases of faith healing.[50]

On the other hand, several children have died because their parents refused medical treatment on religious grounds when a simple operation could have saved their life. How are the religious beliefs of patients and their families and the moral obligation of medical professionals to act in the best interests of their patients to be weighed in cases like these? We'll return to this question in the discussion of autonomy and paternalism.

Utilitarianism

During the 1960s, there were not enough kidney dialysis (hemodialysis) machines in the United States for everyone who needed one. According to one estimate, about 800 people were on hemodialysis in 1967, and between 60,000 and 90,000 people with chronic kidney failure needed the treatment.[51] This raised the question of who should be selected to receive hemodialysis. After examining various options, the Seattle Artificial Kidney Center at the University of Washington turned the decision over to a specially appointed, anonymous committee. This committee, later dubbed the "God Committee" because it had the power of life and death, evaluated each candidate according to his or her social worth. In addition to being otherwise healthy, each candidate selected for dialysis had to be under forty years of age, self-supporting, and a resident of Washington. Other factors being equal, priority was given to candidates who had dependents, who were stable in their behavior and emotionally mature, and who had a record of public service.

Basing moral decisions on a cost/benefit calculation of social worth is an example of the application of **utilitarianism.** According to utilitarians, the morality of an action is determined solely by its consequences. The desire for happiness, they argue, is universal, and we intuitively recognize it as the greatest good. Happiness is synonymous with pleasure, unhappiness with pain. Actions are right, therefore, to the extent that they tend to promote overall happiness and wrong to the extent that they tend to promote overall unhappiness. Utilitarian theory is not the same as ethical egoism. What counts in utilitarianism is not just individual or even human happiness, but the sum of the happiness of the whole community of **sentient beings**—that is, beings capable of experiencing pleasure and pain.

In determining which action or policy produces the greatest happiness, we cannot rely on a majority vote, since people's choices are not always well informed. Nor can we rely on feelings, such as sympathy, alone, because feelings can also mislead us. Instead we need a rational principle to guide our actions and choices. This principle, known as the principle of utility or the greatest happiness principle, states that "actions are right in proportion as they tend to promote happiness, wrong as they tend to produce the reverse of happiness."[52]

The principle of utility is sometimes broken down into two separate principles: the no-harm principle and the duty to promote good. The no-harm principle is also known as **nonmaleficence** or, in Eastern ethics, **ahimsa.** The duty to promote good is also known as the principle of **beneficence** or, in Eastern ethics, *jen.*

Bentham and Mill   English philosopher Jeremy Bentham (1748–1832) promoted utilitarianism primarily as a practical tool of social reform. To this end, he developed the utilitarian calculus (also known as the calculus of pleasures or the hedonic calculus) as a means of scientifically determining which action or policy is morally preferable. He listed seven factors that he believed should be considered when measuring the total amount of pleasure:

1. *Intensity*, the strength of pleasure or pain
2. *Duration*, the amount of time the pleasure or pain lasts
3. *Certainty*, the probability that the pleasure or pain will occur
4. *Propinquity*, the nearness in time of the pleasure or pain
5. *Fecundity*, how productive the pleasure will be in producing further pleasure
6. *Purity*, the likelihood that the pleasure does not also produce pain
7. *Extent*, the number of people affected by the action

These factors were used at the Seattle Artificial Kidney Center. For example, duration meant preferential treatment for younger applicants and the elimination from the program of older people who did not have long to live; certainty meant including only people who were most likely to survive dialysis; fecundity was a factor in selecting people whose continued lives would, in turn, bring the most good to society; extent entailed giving preference to applicants with families.

The application of utilitarian theory to the allocation of scarce healthcare resources is also found in the cost/benefit analysis used in 1993 by the state of Oregon in deciding how to best distribute federal health funds. Should healthcare resources go to those who can afford to pay for them, as in the American system? Or should they be distributed in a more equitable manner that spreads the benefits over more people, as in Canada and, to some extent, the Oregon Health Plan, even if this means that some people will be denied expensive healthcare treatments?

John Stuart Mill challenged Bentham's formulation of utilitarian theory. Despite his great admiration for Bentham, Mill disagreed with him on several points. While Bentham was a fervent believer in equality, Mill maintained that not all pleasures are equal. According to Bentham, the happiness of any one sentient being is no more important than that of any other. Mill, in contrast, argued that some pleasures are more desirable than others; the intellectual pleasures of a human, for example, are qualitatively better than the physical pleasures of nonhuman animals.

The debate over the quality of pleasures is played out in healthcare ethics in the context of both animal experimentation and euthanasia. Some researchers justify animal experimentation, even while acknowledging that it causes animals pain, because of the benefits to humans. The continued enjoyment of the "higher" human pleasures, they argue, outweighs the pain experienced by the animals. Others, such as Australian utilitarian Peter Singer, maintain that for medical researchers to not grant equal consideration to nonhuman animal subjects with sentience and cognitive ability equal to those of certain groups of humans whom we would not use as subjects in medical research is to engage in speciesism.

The quality of pleasures is also an issue in nonvoluntary euthanasia and selective abortion. It has been argued that the quality of life, that is, the capacity to experience any higher pleasures, of some humans—such as infants who are severely mentally retarded or handicapped, the senile, and the comatose—is so low that they do not have a life worth living. Singer, for example, argues in favor of optional euthanasia of babies born with Down syndrome or spina bifida because of their compromised "quality of life."[53]

Rule-Utilitarianism Versus Act-Utilitarianism   Some modern utilitarians divide utilitarianism into two major types, act and rule, although it is doubtful whether either Bentham or Mill drew this distinction. Rule-utilitarians are concerned with the morality of particular classes of actions, such as human cloning, active euthanasia, and mandatory AIDS testing. According to them, we should, in any particular situation, follow the rule that *in general* brings about the greatest happiness for the greatest number. A rule-utilitarian, for example, might agree that a particular case of active euthanasia is morally justified; however, the rule-utilitarian would still argue that this class of actions should be forbidden since the overall harm of policies or laws that permit active euthanasia would outweigh any benefits to the few.

Act-utilitarians, in contrast, are more concerned with the morality of particular actions. In their view, no action—be it infanticide, cloning, or animal experimentation—is inherently immoral. Establishing absolute moral rules against these actions fails to take into account that there may be situations, albeit rare, when active euthanasia, for example, might be the best way to maximize happiness. Most objections against utilitarian theory are directed against act-utilitarianism.

Because rule-utilitarians regard obedience to rules as more important than utility, rule-utilitarians are not considered true utilitarians by some philosophers. It does not follow that, because a particular rule may in general bring about greater utility, we ought to follow this rule always, even in those rare cases where it does not. Most utilitarians accept a position somewhere between rule- and act-utilitarianism. Bentham himself pointed out that, while the utilitarian calculus should always be kept in mind, it need not be carried out before every moral judgment or act.

Criticisms of Utilitarianism   One of the primary criticisms of utilitarian theory is that it does not take into account the dignity and rights of each individual person. Instead it permits the sacrifice of the few to benefit the many if doing so would increase the overall happiness. Nazi physicians and scientists justified their experiments on the inmates of concentration camps on the grounds that it was morally justifiable to sacrifice the interests of the few to benefit the many.[54] Do the long-term benefits of these experiments outweigh the pain and suffering of hundreds of people used in the study? Under utilitarian theory, these experiments might be not only morally acceptable, but morally required—provided they were carried out on "useless" people. Just as people who contribute less to the social good should have lower priority when it comes to allocating scarce medical resources, so too should the interests of people with limited social utility count less when it comes to using them as research subjects. What matters is not the pain or pleasure of the individual person, but that of society as a whole.

On the other hand, many ethicists believe that, even if we can justify using the findings of such experiments based on the principle of utility, we still ought not to. Instead, we should make a commitment never to use data from experiments that violated human rights and dignity. To use a purely utilitarian calculus, they argue, is to stoop to the level of Dr. Mengele. Eva Mozes Kor, a survivor of Dr. Mengele's experiments, appeals to all scientists and doctors to make a pledge to promote a universal ideal that states, "Treat the subjects of your experiments in the manner that you would want to be treated if you were in their place."[55]

Despite the shortcomings of utilitarianism, rather than rejecting it, most health-care ethicists combine the principle of utility with other universal principles and ideals, such as justice and respect for autonomy. The problem of suffering, along with the related concepts of compassion and beneficence, is central to the ethics of many cultures. For example, Chinese philosopher Mo-tzu (c. 470–391 B.C.), like his British counterpart Jeremy Bentham, taught that the standard of utility, or what he called universal love, should be applied equally to all people. Only by striving to maximize happiness and minimize suffering, by loving everyone as our own family, can we achieve a world of peace and harmony. Mo-tzu developed his utilitarian philosophy primarily as a challenge to what he saw as the passivity of Confucianism. However, Confucianism, with its emphasis on deontology and virtue, won out in the end.

Deontology

On August 15, 1996, Judith Curren, a forty-two-year-old mother of two young daughters, committed suicide with the assistance of Dr. Jack Kevorkian. Unlike most of Kevorkian's clients, Curren was not terminally ill. However, she was suffering from depression, chronic fatigue syndrome, and fibromyalgia—a benign inflammation of fibromuscular tissue. Was Curren's suicide morally justified? Did Kevorkian have a duty to assist her, or did he have a duty to refuse his assistance? Many deontologists would say that Curren's suicide was not morally justified. Her pain and suffering were not relevant; what counted was both Curren's and Kevorkian's duty to respect her intrinsic worth as a rational, autonomous person. This intrinsic worth entails a moral duty to not destroy rational life.

Deontology regards duty—doing what is right for its own sake—as the foundation of morality. Strong strands of deontology are evident in Confucianism and Hindu ethics, as well as in many Western philosophies. The high standards of excellence put forth by deontologists have inspired psychologists such as Lawrence Kohlberg to study moral development and to map the transition from preconventional moral reasoning to postconventional, principled moral reasoning. Kohlberg was especially influenced by the work of German philosopher Immanuel Kant (1724–1804).

The Categorical Imperative   Kant believed that we should do our duty purely out of the good will, not because of rewards or punishments or other consequences. If there is a universal moral law and if it is morally binding, it must be based on reason. While actions based on sympathy or other sentiments may be praiseworthy, they have no moral value.

According to Kant, the most fundamental moral principle is the **categorical imperative.** He stated two formulations of the categorical imperative. The first formulation is:

> Act only on that maxim by which you can at the same time will that it should become a universal law.

The categorical imperative is a general formal principle that provides a framework for deriving moral maxims or specific duties, such as "Do not lie" or "Help others in distress." Both the Golden Rule in Judeo-Christian ethics and the Law of Reciprocity in Confucian ethics are similar to the categorical imperative. The Golden Rule states, "Do unto others as you would have them do unto you." Similarly, when Confucius (551–479 B.C.) was asked if there was a single principle that could be used as a guide to conduct in our lives, he replied, "Do not impose on others what you yourself do not desire." In other words, according to deontologists, while cultural differences may influence how medical professionals carry out a moral principle, the underlying moral principle is universal. Moral maxims or duties, by their very nature, apply to everyone and under all circumstances.

Studies of physicians' lying to patients with terminal cancer (early studies in the United States and a more recent study in the United Arab Emirates) found that many physicians considered it morally acceptable to lie to patients.[56] However, what is striking in these studies is that almost all of these physicians also stated that it would be wrong if they were dying of cancer and their own physician did not tell them. According to deontologists, healthcare professionals have a moral duty to ask themselves in their dealings with patients, "Would I want to be treated this way?" It is inconsistent for a physician to argue that it is wrong for others to lie but okay for him or her. If we can make an exception of ourselves whenever it is to our advantage, the moral rule "Do not lie" is meaningless.

Kant believed that all rational beings would recognize the categorical imperative as universally binding. The idea that reason provides the foundation of morality makes humans and other rational beings very special in Kant's mind. Whereas rational beings have free will, everything else in nature operates according to physical laws. Because autonomy is essential for dignity, only rational beings have intrinsic worth. Rational beings, therefore, can never be treated as expendable but must be treated with dignity. This ideal is summed up in Kant's second formulation of the categorical imperative, also known as the practical imperative.

> So act as to treat humanity, whether in thine own person or in that of any other, in every case as an end in itself, never as a means only.

Unlike the categorical imperative itself, specific moral maxims or rules are subject to debate. For example, we may want to modify the rule "Do not lie" to "Do not lie except to save a life." Many healthcare ethicists also question Kant's rule against committing suicide. According to Kant, suicide is an abomination because it involves the misuse of our freedom of action to destroy ourselves and our freedom or autonomy. My life may seem worthless or I may be a burden to others, but this is not a sufficient reason for me to seek to end my life. Kant, of course, was writing in the days before medical technology could artificially extend the dying process. Some people believe that refusing to help someone die who is suffering terribly and is unable to carry out his or her own suicide is disrespectful and hence violates the second formulation of the categorical imperative. What specific moral maxims, then, do we come up with for formulating a just policy on euthanasia and physician-assisted suicide? Would we want to universalize a maxim that states, "Physicians have a duty to carry out the request of their patient"? This may seem appropriate in some situations, but in others it might not be. Consider a student who is temporarily depressed because of a poor grade on an exam and requests medical assistance in committing suicide. Does depression, suffering, or severe pain sometimes compromise our autonomy to such an extent that others, out of respect, should override our request? Throughout the process of formulating specific moral maxims, we should be continually asking ourselves if the proposed maxim is consistent with the requirements of the categorical imperative. Does it respect persons? Are we willing to universalize it?

Kant argued that universalizing moral maxims requires that they be absolutely binding in all circumstances. For example, if it is wrong to commit suicide, then it is *always* wrong to commit suicide or to assist someone in committing suicide, no matter what the circumstances. While other deontologists, for the most part, accept the categorical imperative as universally binding and agree with Kant that we have an **absolute duty,** independent of circumstances, to respect the intrinsic worth of autonomous moral agents, they disagree that the maxims or duties derived from the categorical imperative are also absolute. Instead they argue that moral duties are **prima facie duties,** that is, duties that may on occasion be overridden by stronger moral claims.

Ross's Seven Prima Facie Duties   Scottish philosopher W. D. Ross (1877–1971) listed seven prima facie duties that he claimed we intuitively recognize. Unlike Kant, Ross included in his list the future-oriented duties of nonmaleficence and beneficence, which arise because of the consequences of our actions. Three duties stem from past obligations: fidelity, gratitude, and reparation. There are also two ongoing duties: self-improvement and justice.

The duty of **fidelity,** or loyalty, arises from past promises and commitments. The duty of fidelity or filial piety is particularly strong in Confucian ethics. Healthcare professionals sometimes have divided loyalties. Physicians who work for a health maintenance organization (HMO) may have competing loyalties of providing the best care possible to their patients and holding down costs for their employers. In some countries, loyalty to the state and loyalty to the patient may come into conflict. In the former Soviet Union, psychiatrists were often used by the state as instruments of social coercion. An even more extreme example of divided loyalties is that of doctors working in the Nazi death camps, who often acted completely contrary to their professional commitments in carrying out the orders of the state.

The duty of **gratitude** is evoked when we receive gifts or unearned favors and services from others. In cultures in which medical expertise is regarded as a divine gift, healthcare professionals have a duty of gratitude toward God to treat those in need without expectation of remuneration.

Reparation, the third duty based on past actions, requires that we make up for past harm we have caused others. Healthcare professionals who cause harm to their patients, either through direct action or through neglect, have a duty to try to repair the damage or to compensate the patient. The purpose of medical malpractice insurance is to ensure that this duty is carried out.

Finally, we have two ongoing duties: self-improvement and justice. **Self-improvement,** as a moral duty, entails striving to improve our moral knowledge and our virtue. It requires that we work to overcome our ignorance by becoming well informed about moral issues. Being virtuous also requires using our moral knowledge to make this world a better place. Kant, for example, regarded duties to ourselves as our most important moral duties, since respect for others is grounded in proper self-esteem or self-respect, which in turn is based on strength of character. Judith Curren's request for suicide, Kant would probably argue, reflected a lack of proper self-respect on her part. While contemporary Western healthcare ethics tends to separate healthcare professionals' personal and professional lives, most Eastern healthcare ethics regard self-improvement as one of the primary duties of the healthcare professional.

Justice, the seventh prima facie duty, is an ongoing duty that requires giving each person equal consideration. Especially relevant in the allocation of healthcare resources is **distributive justice,** which requires the fair distribution of benefits and burdens in a society. Because there are not enough healthcare resources for everyone, the distribution of this good is an issue of justice. For example, minorities and women in the United States are more likely to lack medical insurance or access to adequate medical care than are white males. Only half of all low-income, full-time workers are insured. In 1999, while 16.3 percent of all Americans lacked health insurance coverage, 35 percent of Hispanics, 22 percent of blacks, and 21 percent of Asians were uninsured.[57] Also, a disproportionate percentage of medical resources are spent during patients' last few years of life. According to some healthcare ethicists, it is unjust that those who are dying long, lingering deaths receive such a disproportionate share of medical and other resources when other people lack access to even basic healthcare.

Distributive justice requires impartiality. The Baby Doe Law, for example, requires that medical treatment be offered to newborns with disabilities if it would be offered if the child were not disabled. Peter Singer also argues that impartiality requires that we not carry out medical experiments on nonhuman animals if we would not be willing to carry out the same experiment on a human of similar cognitive ability.

Rawls's Theory of Justice   According to American philosopher John Rawls, justice requires not only impartiality, but also treating people fairly and in proportion to their needs as well as their merits. Rawls bases his theory of justice on an unbiased and impartial social contract. To devise principles of justice that are fair, Rawls proposed that we use a conceptual device he calls the "veil of ignorance." Under the veil of ignorance, everyone is ignorant of the advantages or disadvantages he or she will receive in this life. Rawls argues that, under these conditions, all rational people would agree on the following two principles of justice:

1. Each person is to have an equal right to the most extensive basic liberty compatible with a similar liberty for others.

2. Social and economic inequalities are to be arranged so that both are (a) reasonably expected to be to everyone's advantage and (b) attached to positions and offices open to all.

Inequalities of birth and natural endowment (what Rawls calls the "natural lottery") and historic circumstances such as slavery create undeserved disadvantages for certain people. Simply redistributing opportunities or wealth does not solve the root problem as long as the underlying conditions that disadvantage certain people remain. What is needed, according to Rawls, is a change in the social system to prevent these injustices from occurring in the first place. Opponents of legalized euthanasia in the United States, for example, have argued that we must alleviate the extraordinary inequalities in the way medical care is distributed before we can think of moving toward legalizing voluntary euthanasia. Otherwise, people without adequate medical insurance or support will be disproportionately pressured into requesting euthanasia.

Weaknesses of Deontology   A primary weakness of deontology is that it sacrifices community in the name of individual autonomy. This tendency is particularly evident in American healthcare ethics, which is strongly influenced by Kantian ethics. The deontologist's overriding concern with duty and justice fails to take into account the role of sentiment and care within specific relationships. Feminist care ethicists, in particular, argue that practical morality is constructed through interaction with others, not merely by an autonomous examination of the dictates of reason. We will look more closely at the contribution of care ethics to healthcare ethics later in this chapter.

Finally, Kantian deontology ignores consequences, although this weakness has been rectified by Ross's addition of nonmaleficence and beneficence to the list of duties. Indeed, John Stuart Mill points out that the categorical imperative, by its very nature, requires that we take consequences into account when we adopt moral rules. According to Mill, rational people would not universalize a moral rule that would harm rather than benefit the moral community.

Few philosophers accept deontology in its entirety, but despite its shortcomings the strengths and richness of deontology far outshine its weaknesses. It would be a mistake to consider any philosophical, or even scientific, theory to be a finished or complete statement about a particular phenomenon. One characteristic of a good theory is that it is amenable to revision and generates further thought. Deontology, with its emphasis on autonomy and the dignity of the individual, has had a major influence on the development of rights ethics in both Western and non-Western philosophies.

Rights Ethics

Moral rights are not the same as legal rights, although in a perfectly just society the two would overlap. For example, it was several years after the outbreak of the AIDS epidemic in the United States before the moral rights of people infected with HIV not to be tested without their consent and not to be discriminated against by healthcare providers were finally acknowledged by legislators.

Moral rights are generally seen as either natural and existing independently or derived from duties. Most philosophers agree that moral rights do not stand on their own but are derived from duties; for example, utilitarians, deontologists, natural law ethicists, and Buddhist ethicists all see rights as entailing duties. John Stuart Mill argues that rights are derived from the principle of utility; we have a right not to be harmed. According to deontologists, rights are important because they protect our dignity as persons. Because we are entitled to certain rights, others have a duty to honor these rights.

Unlike deontologists, who regard duty as the foundation of rights, rights ethicists, such as John Locke (1632–1704), believe that moral rights stand on their own. According to **rights ethics,** moral rights stem from our human nature and are self-evident and God-given. Furthermore, humans alone have moral rights, because of our creation in the image of God. The influence of natural rights ethics on healthcare ethics in the United States is particularly evident in the way rights are depicted as existing independent of any duties or concerns regarding the harm to others caused by the exercise of an individual's rights or freedom.

Welfare (Positive) Rights Versus Liberty (Negative) Rights   Moral rights are generally divided into liberty rights and welfare rights. **Welfare (positive) rights** entail the right to receive basic social goods such as education, medical care, and police protection, as well as a duty on the part of others such as the government to provide these social goods. Welfare rights are important because we cannot pursue our legitimate interests without a minimal standard of living or of health. **Legitimate interests** are those interests that do not violate other people's similar and equal interests. For example, a racist may have an interest in preventing black physicians from joining the American Medical Association (AMA). However, doing so violates black physicians' right to equal opportunity.

Liberty (negative) rights, in contrast, entail the right to be left alone to pursue our legitimate interests without interference from the government or from other people. Liberty or negative rights include autonomy, privacy, freedom of speech, and freedom from harassment, confinement, unwanted medical treatment, or participation in experiments without our informed consent. Healthcare ethics in the United States places more emphasis on liberty rights than on welfare rights.

People who emphasize liberty rights are known as libertarians. **Libertarians** believe that personal autonomy—the freedom to make our own decisions—is the highest moral value. For example, Dr. Jack Kevorkian, a libertarian, considers the decision to commit suicide to be one of our most fundamental rights. Deontologists, in contrast, maintain that our liberty rights are limited by our duty to respect ourselves; thus, we do not have a right to harm ourselves or neglect our own welfare. The emphasis on liberty rights at the expense of welfare rights tends to seriously handicap those who are unable to assert their liberty rights either because of natural disadvantages or because of traditional roles that limit their options. In most countries, healthcare is considered a welfare right, and the government has a moral obligation to provide at least minimal healthcare to its citizens. The World Health Organization (WHO) also holds that "health is one of the fundamental rights of every human being without distinction of race, religion, political belief, economic or social conditions."

In the United States, in contrast, where healthcare is considered a liberty right except in the case of the elderly and the poor, for whom it is a welfare right, the government's only obligation is to refrain from interfering with a citizen's choice of healthcare provider. One question addressed by the Clinton administration was whether the current healthcare system in the United States is just or whether all citizens have a welfare right to healthcare.

The separation of rights from duties by many libertarians fails to take into account the limitations placed on marginalized groups by social traditions and prejudices. While the United States boasts some of the most advanced medical technology in the world, the average life span of Americans (73.6 years for men and 79.2 years for women)[58] and the infant mortality rate compare unfavorably to those in countries such as England, Japan, Australia, Canada, and most European countries where healthcare is seen as a welfare right rather than distributed according to the free market. A woman living in Japan or Canada, for example, lives an average of four years longer than a woman living in the United States.[59] Black Americans and those who cannot afford to purchase private health insurance or healthcare are especially disadvantaged. The average life span of a black American in 1997 was four years less than that of a white American, and the mortality rate of black infants was more than double that of white infants.[60]

Healthcare Issues and Rights   A widely debated right in healthcare ethics is the "right to life." Euthanasia also raises the question of whether we have a "right to die." Another controversial topic is the "right to procreation," or reproduction. Do people have a right to have children? If so, is procreation a liberty right? That is, should the state refrain from interfering even though the prospective parent may be unfit to be a parent or there is a serious problem with overpopulation? Or is procreation a welfare right as well? In the United States, with its emphasis on autonomy, people have a liberty right to have children—although this was not always the case. In China, on the other hand, the right to have children is weighed against the social good, and the state may restrict a person's childbearing options after the birth of the first child. Reproduction as a welfare right comes into play most poignantly in the case of infertility. Do health insurance carriers, including those funded by tax money, have a moral obligation to provide coverage for infertility treatment?

What are the rights of children? As nonrational beings, do young children have any rights other than those their parents and society claim on their behalf? Do parents have the right to volunteer their children as subjects in medical experiments? What about the right of parents to make medical decisions for their children, especially decisions that may result in pain and disfigurement, as in the case of circumcision, or even death, as in the case of Christian Scientists who refuse medical treatment? Do unborn children have a right to live in a drug-free environment, or does the woman's right to control her body override any rights or interests an unborn child might have?

Another healthcare issue is the rights, if any, of nonhuman animals. Tom Regan argues that rights are grounded in interests; since nonhuman animals have interests, they also have rights. Buddhist ethicists go even further and extend the concept of rights to all of nature. Carl Cohen disagrees; he maintains that only humans can be the bearers of rights. Nonhuman animals cannot have rights since they lack the capacity to claim rights.

Like utilitarianism and deontology, rights ethics is problematic if it is used as a complete explanation of morality. However, while ethicists may disagree on the origin of rights and on who or what is a bearer of rights, few would deny the importance of rights in healthcare ethics. Likewise, almost all ethicists acknowledge the importance of virtue and character development in healthcare.

Virtue Ethics

Virtue ethics emphasizes right being over right action. More important than the rules or principles we follow is the sort of person we are. Moral principles are not like a computer program that can be fed a moral issue or dilemma and calculate an answer. The language of principles, rights, and duties does not exist in isolation but rather stems

from the character and motives of good persons. When we speak of a morally good action or a principled person, we are speaking of the motives or intentions of a virtuous
person.

Confucianism, Buddhism, feminist care ethics, and the moral philosophies of
David Hume, Aristotle, and Jesus are often classified as virtue ethics. Nursing ethics also
places a high value on virtue. Since the founding of nursing by Florence Nightingale in
the mid-1800s, nurses have been taught that strong moral values and strength of character are essential ingredients of the nursing profession. The importance of virtue
ethics in nursing is reflected in the Florence Nightingale Pledge and in early versions
of the American Nurses Association Code.

Virtue and Morality   A **virtue** is an admirable character trait or a disposition to habitually act in a manner that benefits ourselves and others. The actions of virtuous people
stem from a respect and concern for the well-being of themselves and others. Compassion, courage, generosity, loyalty, and honesty are all examples of virtues. Although
virtues are often spoken of as distinct, individual traits, virtue is more correctly defined
as an overarching quality of goodness that gives unity and integrity to a person's character. According to Aristotle, virtuous people are those who "desire and act in accordance
with a rational principle."[61]

Virtue ethics is a component of almost all moral theories. Rather than being an alternative to ethical theories that stress right conduct, virtue ethics complements theories of right action. Kant, for example, devoted a considerable portion of his *Metaphysics of Morals* to virtue ethics. Rather than ignoring the role of emotions, he simply
makes it clear that mere feeling is not sufficient. Utilitarians also acknowledge that virtuous and caring people are more likely to perform good actions and abstain from
harming others. For this reason, John Stuart Mill argued, we should cultivate a virtuous
and benevolent disposition. The blend of virtue ethics with theories of right action is
probably strongest in Eastern healthcare ethics.

CHINESE HEALTHCARE ETHICS:
A Blend of Many Traditions

Chinese healthcare ethics is currently in a state of flux due to several competing influences. Traditional Chinese healthcare ethics is a virtue ethics supported by deontology. Character-building is one of the primary moral duties of healthcare professionals, and the purpose of medical treatment is to restore harmony in the patient. This requires first establishing a harmonious relationship between the patient and the healthcare professional. In Chinese culture, wisdom and the cultivation of a virtuous character, rather than rules and laws, are the preferred method of achieving this goal.

This tradition arose out of the Three Teachings—Confucianism, Buddhism, and Taoism—which provide a framework for the explanation and treatment of disease. Of the three, Confucianism has had the most profound influence.[62] Bian Que (fifth century), a contemporary of Hippocrates, sought to eliminate reliance on witchcraft and sorcery by establishing a medical ethics that emphasized the moral character of the physician. Confucian physicians were required to put justice before personal gain and to treat honesty as a duty.

According to legend, Confucian physician Dong Feng (third century A.D.) "treated people without charge. Five apricot trees were to be planted when one was cured of a serious illness and one apricot tree was to be planted when one was cured of a minor disease. Several years later, a forest of 100,000 apricot trees appeared."[63] The apricots were exchanged for grain, which was distributed to the poor. The expression "warm spring in the apricot wood" is still used to praise the noble moral character of a physician.

During the Ming dynasty (1368–1644), principles of medical ethics were established. The Five Commandments and Ten Tenets for physicians put forward by Gong Jiongxian are similar to present-day ethical codes for physicians. These principles include having respect for human life, doing one's best to rescue the dying and heal the wounded, showing concern for those who suffer from disease, employing honesty in the practice of medicine, studying medical skills painstakingly, avoiding carelessness in one's work, acting in a dignified manner, respecting local customs and being polite, and treating all patients, whether noble or humble, equally.[64]

The introduction of Marxism into China, with its emphasis on the community good and the future rather than on the individual and the present, has had an influence on Chinese healthcare. Article 1 of the People's Republic of China's 1988 "Regulations on Criteria for Medical Ethics and Their Implementation" states that "the purpose of the criteria is to strengthen the development of a society based on socialist values, to improve the quality of professional ethics of healthcare workers and to promote health services."[65] More recently, Western influences have led to an increasing concern for autonomy and individual well-being.

Kant emphasized the importance of developing a virtuous character—what he called a "good will"—not because virtue tells us what to do but because it ensures that we will be more likely to do our duty. Virtue ethicists, however, want to go further than this. It is not only particular types of moral action that are morally relevant, but also the character and intentions of the moral agent. It is having certain feelings, as well as acting in certain ways, that makes an action morally right. Only caring people can act in truly caring ways. In a healthcare situation, the person being cared for should feel that he or she really matters. Hospice is based on an ethics of care. While some healthcare givers will be attentive to a patient as long as they are able to offer medical assistance, truly caring persons continue to care even after it is clear that they can do nothing more medically. They care because they empathize with the patient's suffering, not simply because they can offer technical medical assistance. Because virtuous people are motivated to act in ways that benefit others, the cultivation of a virtuous character is important for healthcare professionals in many cultures.

Aristotelian and Confucian Ethics   "If the will be set on virtue," Confucius taught, "there will be no practice of wickedness." We acquire virtue, according to Aristotle, through repetition of good acts, or what he called **habituation:** "By doing what is just a man becomes just, and temperate by doing what is temperate, while without doing thus he has no chance of ever becoming good."[66] Virtue, in other words, develops through practical interaction with the world. Aristotle's theory on the importance of practical experience to morality is supported by empirical studies. A study conducted in Spain on informed consent, for example, revealed that the more experience a healthcare professional has in providing palliative care to the terminally ill, the more likely he or she is to believe that the terminally ill have a right to be informed of their condition.[67]

Both Aristotle and Confucius taught that virtue in most instances entails finding the mean between excess and deficit. For example, courage is the mean between cowardice (a deficit) and foolhardiness (an excess); truthfulness lies between irony and boastfulness. The **doctrine of the mean** should not be misinterpreted as advising us to be wishy-washy or to compromise our moral standards. Rather, it tells us to seek what is reasonable.

Buddhist Ethics   The doctrine of the mean is also found in Buddhist ethics, which, like Confucianism, teaches that the mean, or Middle Path, is that which is consistent with harmony and equilibrium, or the Way. Suffering plays a central role in Buddhist philosophy. Only through the Eightfold Path—which consists of right understanding, right thought, right speech, right action, right livelihood, right effort, right mindfulness, and right concentration—can one overcome suffering. Buddha, known also as the "Great Physician," believed that the health of the body and the health of the spirit cannot be separated. Buddhist monks have long been active in the field of healthcare. In fact, many early Chinese and Japanese hospitals were attached to Buddhist monasteries.

Buddhism rejects individualism as illusory; we exist only as members of the community of all living beings. We cannot resolve the problems that plague modern society by encouraging an individualism that allows people to pursue their concept of the good at the expense of other human and nonhuman beings. Because we are all part of the same being, being virtuous and true to ourselves involves extending respect and compassion to everything that lies in our path of experience. Buddhists, therefore, are opposed to medical experimentation and organ transplants that use nonhuman animals, although they advocate the development of artificial organs for transplant.

Healthcare, however, is more than just the application of medical technology and knowledge. Healthcare ethics in countries strongly influenced by the Confucian and Buddhist traditions are more often rooted in the quality of relationships than in the advancement of medical technology and knowledge. Because the primary cause of human suffering in these traditions is the corruption of the human mind, harmony and an end to suffering depend primarily on the moral development of the members of society. Without moral progress and moral wisdom, modern Buddhists warn, our rapid technological advances could lead us down the path to disaster. Healthcare professionals are expected to constantly strive to improve their character. Dr. Wang Chin-ta of the Tianjin First Central Hospital in China writes, "No matter how good doctors and nurses are technically, if they do not have noble [virtuous] thinking, they cannot serve the patient, the people, and the country."[68]

Like Confucian and Buddhist ethics, contemporary Western care ethics emphasizes the virtues of care and empathy over reason, of context over abstract moral principles, and of communal relationships and friendships over individual rights. According to Scottish philosopher David Hume, while reason may help us discover universal moral principles, it is sympathy, rather than reason, that motivates us to behave morally.

Feminist Care Ethics   Feminist care ethics developed primarily out of Gilligan's study of women's moral reasoning. Gilligan found that, in making abortion decisions, women are more likely to think in terms of relationships and their responsibility to care for and avoid hurting others than in terms of applying abstract moral principles. Care ethics is intended for public policy as well as personal relationships. In many African communities, women are very active in healthcare as doctors and healthcare providers. It is believed that women, because they carry human life in their bodies, are more connected to the spiritual dimension of health and more sensitive to the needs of patients. Indeed, caring has been called the primary "moral art" for nursing practice.[69]

Feminist care ethicists claim that we are at our moral best when we are caring and being cared for. Care, not rational calculations or an abstract sense of duty, creates moral obligation. Since being attentive is a key element of care, to take care of a patient is to be attentive to his or her needs. Indeed, the term *respect* literally means "to look again." Respectful attention means finding out what is causing a person's suffering and responding in a caring manner. Thus, an ethics of care requires that we improve our communication skills and moral sensitivity and pay more attention to how healthcare decisions affect everyone—patients as well as family and friends of the patient. This is no easy task, especially when so many healthcare professionals, like the doctor from the movie *The Doctor*, are pressed for time and burdened by other concerns.

One criticism of feminist care ethics is that it reinforces cultural patterns of male dominance and female subordination by legitimating the belief that nurturing and self-sacrifice are feminine virtues. This pattern is often played out in the traditional physician/nurse relationship. Because feminist care ethics was modeled on the mother/child relationship, it can also easily be co-opted by a healthcare system that places physicians and patients in a parent/child relationship. Attention to oneself and to values such as fairness is needed to place limits on caring.

Feminist care ethicists are aware that an inclination to care is not always enough and that caring can be exploited to maintain the patriarchal power structure. Furthermore, when our inclination to care is lacking, our commitment to an ideal or to principles of caring can motivate us to do what is right. Therefore, most care ethicists acknowledge the need to harmonize the care perspective with the justice perspective. On this point, care ethicists and deontologists find common ground. Indeed, contemporary ethics education for nurses focuses on integrating skill in making principled moral judgments with fostering the legacy of care in the profession.

Justice also has to be tempered by care. The assumption that justice requires impartiality conflicts with the almost universal belief that we have a greater moral obligation to care for and support our family and friends. In particular, the implication of utilitarian theory that utility requires forgoing family fun times and instead devoting our time to helping needier children seems counterintuitive. Justice and care, rather than being incompatible, need to be balanced and even integrated depending on the context. Partiality may be morally appropriate when it comes to specific relationships such as parents and children, or doctors and patients. Indeed, while at first glance paying more attention to one's children or one's patients may not seem just, in the greater scheme of things impartiality in particular relationships may end up causing harm and injustice. Parents who refuse to give their own children more attention or more food than other children in the world or a doctor who refuses to give his or her patients better care than people in the poorest parts of the world receive and instead tries to be everything to everyone generally ends up being too exhausted to be of any help to anyone. On the other hand, a doctor who hoards medical supplies for his or her own patients, thus preventing other patients from getting much-needed medical supplies, has behaved unjustly and has carried care ethics too far.[70]

THE FOUR MORAL PRINCIPLES APPROACH TO HEALTHCARE ETHICS

In the early 1970s, the U.S. Congress established the National Commission for the Protection of Human Subjects of Biomedical and Behavioral Research. Their 1979 report (known as the Belmont Report) stated that four basic principles should be observed in research using human subjects: beneficence, nonmaleficence, justice, and respect for autonomy.[71] These four principles have since become the backbone of contemporary Western healthcare ethics.

Tom Beauchamp and James Childress, in *Principles of Biomedical Ethics* (1979), argue that useful rules for healthcare ethics can be formulated using these four principles, along with other moral considerations such as rights and virtues. This approach, also known as **principlism,** makes the claim that these principles are compatible with many, if not most, moral theories and thus provide a common language for healthcare ethicists from diverse cultures and philosophical backgrounds.

One drawback of this approach is lack of agreement about the meaning of the four principles. Some ethicists argue that the first two principles, beneficence and nonmaleficence, are really one principle. In traditions in which doing good is regarded as a moral obligation, bringing about benefits for the patient and avoiding any harm that may prevent this goal are part of the same duty. Utilitarians also subsume justice under this unitary principle. Other traditions hold to a prima facie moral duty only to avoid harm; while beneficence is an ideal, the physician does not have a moral duty to benefit a patient (other than providing appropriate medical care), especially when the patient does not want a particular beneficial treatment. Physicians, however, do have a duty to refrain from treatment that will harm the patient, even if the patient may desire it.

While beneficence and nonmaleficence dominate the Hippocratic tradition, in contemporary Western healthcare ethics respect for patient autonomy and liberty rights are usually more important than beneficence. This is especially true in the United States, which subscribes to what Beauchamp and Childress refer to as an "autonomy model" that gives autonomy moral priority over beneficence. A central problem under this model is authority, or physician paternalism versus patient autonomy. The Hippocratic tradition places the authority to make medical decisions primarily in the hands of the physician; the autonomy model, in contrast, focuses on the patient as the decision-maker. Under the autonomy model, physicians who fail to inform their patients of a pessimistic prognosis or of all treatment options or who fail to get informed consent for medical treatment and research can come under heavy criticism.

Paternalists maintain that if patients are likely to cause serious harm to themselves or fail to secure important benefits for themselves, then physicians are justified in restricting patients' autonomy. Unlike the Hippocratic tradition, the autonomy model allows paternalism only when a patient is not fully rational or may harm another person. A rational or competent person is one who is deemed capable of choosing the best means to achieve a chosen end. A patient who chooses self-destructive goals or refuses treatment may be considered irrational. Autonomy may also be impaired if a person is not fully informed, whether because of the absence of information, because of laziness, or because of resistance and denial. Some ethicists also question just how much the suffering and pain associated with illness compromise a person's autonomy. In the case of children or other incompetent patients, parents or legal surrogates can make medical choices on their behalf. This raises the question of the limits of parental power. Does parental autonomy, for example, give parents the right to authorize nontherapeutic surgery, such as routine circumcision, for their children?

Many healthcare ethicists reject the autonomy model. In Islamic healthcare ethics, paternalism takes precedence when a conflict arises between autonomy and paternalism. The focus on the isolated physician/patient relationship in the autonomy model also ignores the communal nature of healthcare decision making found in many, if not most, cultures. In Japanese society, autonomy is viewed not in individualist terms, but in what Japanese ethicist Rihito Kimura refers to as "related-autonomy," whereby decisions are made in the context of extended relationships rather than by the individual patient. A woman, for example, may represent ailing family members, even though they may be grown and married, often describing her children's or husband's symptoms to the physician and asking for treatment.[72]

In traditional Buddhist ethics, autonomy plays only a minor role except to the extent that self-improvement requires autonomous responsibility for one's karma. Beneficence as compassion, on the other hand, is a fundamental principle in Buddhist healthcare ethics. Beneficence and respect for the sanctity of life are also more important than autonomy in Jewish law. In China, while autonomy is recognized, individual wishes are subordinated to the common good. Medical decisions are made not by physicians in consultation with their individual patients, but by all those in authority.

Giving moral priority to patient autonomy also raises the question of the autonomy of healthcare professionals. In the United States, physicians are increasingly seen as being "on tap," highly educated technicians whose services are at the disposal of their clients.[73] More and more, physicians are expected to serve the desires of their patients.

Indeed, many Arab immigrants in the United States view American doctors' offering them choices, rather than telling them the best course of treatment, as a sign of weakness and lack of competence.

To what extent does respect for patient autonomy require healthcare professionals to compromise their own beliefs and integrity? Does respect for patient autonomy, for example, impose a duty on a physician or counselor opposed to abortion for sex selection to provide prenatal diagnosis for a couple who wish to know the gender of their unborn child so they can seek an abortion if the fetus is female? Does a physician have a moral obligation to provide a dying patient with medical treatment that the physician believes will be futile or, at the other extreme, to accede to a patient's request for euthanasia or assisted suicide? The question of the autonomy of healthcare workers also arises in the context of providing healthcare to patients with contagious diseases such as AIDS. In 1987, the AMA, which supports patient autonomy, stated that physicians are obliged to treat patients "without regard to risks" and that refusing to treat patients with HIV was "invidious discrimination."[74]

Promoting patient autonomy by informing patients of all their options does not always increase their freedom. The wide choice of reproductive technologies now available, for example, may put pressure on people to use them, thus infringing on their autonomy. Furthermore, not all information is welcomed by a patient. Navahos, for example, believe that negative words have the power to bring about events; advance directives, rather than increasing patient self-determination and autonomy, are regarded as dangerous, much like self-fulfilling prophecies.

The current focus on patient autonomy also ignores issues of justice associated with global health issues such as famine, war, epidemics, and environmental degradation. The expectation that physicians will honor patient confidentiality may even put pressure on a physician to lie or withhold important information, even though doing so may harm others. The individualism underlying the autonomy model is based on an inaccurate description of human behavior. Behavior such as smoking, promiscuity, or using drugs while pregnant affects more than just the person engaging in the behavior. Respect for autonomy can be costly for those who are directly harmed by the behavior as well as for those who are expected to foot the bill because of others' destructive lifestyles.

In the United States, autonomy is so important that social values and justice are sometimes overlooked. For people unable to pay for healthcare, autonomy is meaningless. Allowing people free access to the marketplace of healthcare is not the same as allowing people to take advantage of this access. Increasing autonomy for some may decrease it for others, a formula often overlooked in discussion of the reduction of autonomy in individual physician/patient relationships.

All this does not mean that respect for patient autonomy is an unimportant value in healthcare ethics but rather that it needs to be harmonized with concern for justice and the well-being of society. Healthcare takes place within a social context. Failure to consider the political and economic context in which discussions of justice take place can severely disadvantage certain groups of people.

Proponents of the four principles approach recognize its weaknesses. However, they also maintain that it provides a useful, though incomplete, framework for healthcare ethics. Rather than offering a comprehensive moral theory or guideline for moral decision making, principlism establishes the moral perimeters within which particular moral decisions should be made. Within these parameters, however, decisions may vary.

For example, kidney dialysis at the Seattle Artificial Kidney Center at the University of Washington could be allocated based on utilitarian considerations, on a first-come first-served model, on need, or on a combination of all three. Each solution falls within the parameters set by the four principles. Even within these parameters, however, some solutions will be better than others, so dialogue is important in resolving a moral conflict. On the other hand, the allocation of dialysis only to those who secretly pay off members of the committee or promise them some sort of favor, such as sex, falls outside the parameters of moral acceptability.

THE PRINCIPLISM/CASUISTRY DEBATE

The emphasis on universal principles as the deciding factor in the resolution of moral conflicts has become an issue among healthcare ethicists. For principlists, the four principles of beneficence, nonmaleficence, autonomy, and justice provide the primary guidance in moving toward moral resolution. The dominant challenge to the overarching status of principles comes from **casuistry,** an approach that is grounded in a type of practical reasoning. Aristotle used the term *phronesis* to refer to this type of practical, contextual judgment. Casuists urge us to consider the specific facts in each particular situation. In this respect, casuistry operates inductively, starting with specific cases rather than general principles, whereas principlism works deductively, starting with general principles and then applying these principles to specific cases. Casuists caution us against thinking that the mere application of general moral principles and norms is sufficient for the resolution of a moral conflict.

Consider, for example, the principle of utility. Supporters of casuistry contend that, as neat as this principle may seem as a universal norm, because each situation is unique and involves several types of variables the principle cannot be applied as an absolute standard. Otherwise, we would have what philosopher Stephen Toulmin calls the "tyranny of principles." Each case, according to the casuist, needs to be judged on its own merits. The principle of utility may work in some cases but, as we noted earlier in this chapter, not in all cases. Moral resolution instead comes from making specific judgments concerning the specific aspects of each case.

Supporters of principlism argue that even casuists, despite their objection to the role of principles, imply the validity of certain principles. Specific judgments within each case still suggest some underlying rules and principles, even though they may not be articulated as such. To rely on only one approach poses a false dichotomy. Framing a debate in healthcare ethics solely in terms of either principlism or casuistry results in an incomplete analysis of the issue at hand. Good moral reasoning entails a dialectical relationship rather than one in which viewpoints are seen as mutually exclusive. Just as casuists assume certain basic moral principles, so too must principlists acknowledge that each context is unique and that context influences the way principles are applied. The degree to which we apply rules and assign priorities to principles that are in conflict depends on the particular situation. Thus, the most productive approach to resolving moral conflicts is one in which the two approaches, casuistry and principlism, work dialectically, with each informing, supporting, and correcting the other.

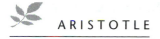
ARISTOTLE

Nicomachean Ethics

The Greek philosopher Aristotle (384–322 B.C.) is one of the most important thinkers of all times. In *Nicomachean Ethics,* Aristotle argues that living the good life— the life of virtue—is our most important human activity. Because the function of humans is to exercise reason, virtue involves living according to reason. Only by living in accord with reason can we achieve happiness, inner harmony, and a well-ordered society.

Book I

CHAPTER 1

Every art and every inquiry, and similarly every action and pursuit, is thought to aim at some good; and for this reason the good has rightly been declared to be that at which all things aim. But a certain difference is found among ends; some are activities, others are products apart from the activities that produce them. Where there are ends apart from the actions, it is the nature of the products to be better than the activities. Now, as there are many actions, arts, and sciences, their ends also are many; the end of the medical art is health, that of shipbuilding a vessel, that of strategy victory, that of economics wealth. But where such arts fall under a single capacity—as bridle-making and the other arts concerned with the equipment of horses fall under the art of riding, and this and every military action under strategy, in the same way other arts fall under yet others—in all of these the ends of the master arts are to be preferred to all the subordinate ends; for it is for the sake of the former that the latter are pursued. It makes no difference whether the activities themselves are the ends of the actions, or something else apart from the activities, as in the case of the sciences just mentioned. . . .

CHAPTER 7

Let us again return to the good we are seeking, and ask what it can be. It seems different in different actions and arts; it is different in medicine, in strategy, and in the other arts likewise. What then is the good of each? Surely that for whose sake everything else is done. In medicine this is health, in strategy victory, in architecture a house, in any other sphere something else, and in every action and pursuit the end; for it is for the sake of this that all men do whatever else they do. Therefore, if there is an end for all that we do, this will be the good achievable by action, and if there are more than one, these will be the goods achievable by action.

So the argument has by a different course reached the same point; but we must try to state this even more clearly. Since there are evidently more than one end, and we choose some of these (e.g. wealth, flutes, and in general instruments) for the sake of something else, clearly not all ends are final ends; but the chief good is evidently something final. Therefore, if there is only one final end, this will be what we are seeking, and if there are more than one, the most final of these will be what we are seeking. Now we call that which is in itself worthy of pursuit more final than that which is worthy of pursuit for the sake of something else, and that which is never desirable for the sake of something else more final than the things that are desirable both in themselves and for the sake of that other thing, and therefore we call final without qualification that which is always desirable in itself and never for the sake of something else.

Now such a thing happiness, above all else, is held to be; for this we choose always for itself and never for the sake of something else, but honour, pleasure, reason, and every virtue we choose indeed for themselves (for if nothing resulted from them we should still choose each of them), but we choose them also for the sake of happiness, judging that by means of them we shall be happy. Happiness, on the other hand, no one chooses for the sake of these, nor, in general, for anything other than itself. . . .

Presumably, however, to say that happiness is the chief good seems a platitude, and a clearer account of what it is is still desired. This might perhaps be given, if we could first ascertain the function of man. For just as for a flute-player, a sculptor, or any artist, and, in general, for all things that have a function or activity, the good and the 'well' is thought to reside in the function, so would it seem to be for man, if he has a function. Have the carpenter, then, and the tanner certain functions or activities, and has man none? Is he born without a function? Or as eye, hand, foot, and in general each of the parts evidently has a function, may one lay it down that man similarly has a function apart from all these? What then can this be? Life seems to be common even to plants, but we are seeking what is peculiar to man. Let us exclude, therefore, the life of nutrition and growth. Next there would be a life of perception, but it also seems to be common even to the horse, the ox, and every animal. There remains, then, an active life of the element that has a rational principle; of this, one part has such a principle in the sense of being obedient to one, the other in the sense of possessing one and exercising thought. And, as 'life of the rational element' also has two meanings, we must state that life in the sense of activity is what we mean; for this seems to be the more proper sense of the term. Now if the function of man is an activity of soul which follows or implies a rational principle, and if we say 'a so-and-so' and 'a good so-and-so' have a function which is the same in kind, e.g. a lyre-player and a good lyre-player, and so without qualification in all cases, eminence in respect of goodness being added to the name of the function (for the function of a lyre-player is to play the lyre, and that of a good lyre-player is to do so well): if this is the case, [and we state the function of man to be a certain kind of life, and this to be an activity or actions of the soul implying a rational principle, and the function of a good man to be the good and noble performance of these, and if any action is well performed when it is performed in accordance with the appropriate excellence: if this is the case,] human good turns out to be activity of soul in accordance with virtue, and if there are more than one virtue, in accordance with the best and most complete.

But we must add 'in a complete life'. For one swallow does not make a summer, nor does one day; and so too one day, or a short time, does not make a man blessed and happy. . . .

Book II

CHAPTER 1

Virtue, then, being of two kinds, intellectual and moral, intellectual virtue in the main owes both its birth and its growth to teaching (for which reason it requires experience and time), while moral virtue comes about as a result of habit, whence also its name *ethike* is one that is formed by a slight variation from the word *ethos* (habit). From this it is also plain that none of the moral virtues arises in us by nature; for nothing that exists by nature can form a habit contrary to its nature. For instance the stone which by nature moves downwards cannot be habituated to move upwards, not even if one tries to train it by throwing it up ten thousand times. . . . Neither by nature, then, nor contrary to nature do the virtues arise in us; rather we are adapted by nature to receive them, and are made perfect by habit.

. . . The virtues we get by first exercising them, as also happens in the case of the arts as well. For the things we have to learn before we can do them, we learn by doing them, e.g. men become builders by building and lyre-players by playing the lyre; so too we become just by doing just acts, temperate by doing temperate acts, brave by doing brave acts.

This is confirmed by what happens in states; for legislators make the citizens good by forming habits in them, and this is the wish of every legislator, and those who do not effect it miss their mark, and it is in this that a good constitution differs from a bad one.

Again, it is from the same causes and by the same means that every virtue is both produced and destroyed, and similarly every art; for it is from playing the lyre that both good and bad lyre-players are produced. And the corresponding statement is true of builders and of all the rest; men will be good or bad builders as a result of building well or badly. For if this were not so, there would have been no need of a teacher, but all men would have been born good or bad at their craft. This, then, is the case with the virtues also; by doing the acts that we do in our transactions with other men we become just or unjust, and by doing the acts that we do in the presence of danger, and being habituated to feel fear or confidence, we become brave or cowardly. The same is true of appetites and feelings of anger; some men become temperate and good-tempered, others self-indulgent and irascible, by behaving in one way or the other in the appropriate circumstances. Thus, in one word, states of character arise out of like activities. This is why the activities we exhibit must be of a certain kind; it is because the states of character correspond to the differences between these. It makes no small difference, then, whether we form habits of one kind or of another from our very youth; it makes a very great difference, or rather *all* the difference.

CHAPTER 2

Since, then, the present inquiry does not aim at theoretical knowledge like the others (for we are inquiring not in order to know what virtue is, but in order to become good, since otherwise our inquiry would have been of no use), we must examine the nature of actions, namely how we ought to do them; for these determine also the nature of the states of character that are produced, as we have said. . . .

But though our present account is of this nature we must give what help we can. First, then, let us consider this, that it is the nature of such things to be destroyed by defect and excess, as we see in the case of strength and of health (for to gain light on things imperceptible we must use the evidence of sensible things); both excessive and defective exercise destroys the strength, and similarly drink or food which is above or below a certain amount destroys the health, while that which is proportionate both produces and increases and preserves it. So too is it, then, in the case of temperance and courage and the other virtues. For the man who flies from and fears everything and does not stand his ground against anything becomes a coward, and the man who fears nothing at all but goes to meet every danger becomes rash; and similarly the man who indulges in every pleasure and abstains from none becomes self-indulgent, while the man who shuns every pleasure, as boors do, becomes in a way insensible; temperance and courage, then, are destroyed by excess and defect, and preserved by the mean.

But not only are the sources and causes of their origination and growth the same as those of their destruction, but also the sphere of their actualization will be the same; for this is also true of the things which are more evident to sense, e.g. of strength; it is produced by taking much food and undergoing much exertion, and it is the strong man that will be most able to do these things. So too is it with the virtues; by abstaining from pleasures we become temperate, and it is when we have become so that we are most able to abstain from them; and similarly too in the case of courage; for by being habituated to despise things that are terrible and to stand our ground against them we become brave, and it is when we have become so that we shall be most able to stand our ground against them. . . .

CHAPTER 5

Next we must consider what virtue is. Since things that are found in the soul are of three kinds—passions, faculties, states of character, virtue must be one of these. By passions I mean appetite, anger, fear, confidence, envy, joy, friendly feeling, hatred, longing, emulation, pity, and in general the feelings that are accompanied by pleasure or pain; by faculties the things in virtue of which we are said to be capable of feeling these, e.g. of becoming angry or being pained or feeling pity; by states of character the things in virtue of which we stand well or badly with reference to the passions, e.g. with reference to anger we stand badly if we feel it violently or too weakly, and well if we feel it moderately; and similarly with reference to the other passions.

Now neither the virtues nor the vices are *passions,* because we are not called good or bad on the ground of our passions, but are so called on the ground of our virtues and our vices, and because we are neither praised nor blamed for our passions (for the man who feels fear or anger is not praised, nor is the man who simply feels anger blamed, but the man who feels it in a certain way), but for our virtues and our vices we *are* praised or blamed.

Again, we feel anger and fear without choice, but the virtues are modes of choice or involve choice. Further, in respect of the passions we are said to be moved, but in respect of the virtues and the vices we are said not to be moved but to be disposed in a particular way.

For these reasons also they are not *faculties;* for we are neither called good nor bad, nor praised nor blamed, for the simple capacity of feeling the passions; again, we have the faculties by nature, but we are not made good or bad by nature; we have spoken of this before.

If, then, the virtues are neither passions nor faculties, all that remains is that they should be *states of character.*

Thus we have stated what virtue is in respect of its genus.

CHAPTER 6

We must, however, not only describe virtue as a state of character, but also say what sort of state it is. We may remark, then, that every virtue or excellence both brings into good condition the thing of which it is the excellence and makes the work of that thing be done well; e.g. the excellence of the eye makes both the eye and its work good; for it is by the excellence of the eye that we see well. Similarly the excellence of the horse makes a horse both good in itself and good at running and at carrying its rider and at awaiting the attack of the enemy. Therefore, if this is true in every case, the virtue of man also will be the state of character which makes a man good and which makes him do his own work well. . . .

Virtue, then, is a state of character concerned with choice, lying in a mean, i.e. the mean relative to us, this being determined by a rational principle, and by that principle by which the man of practical wisdom would determine it. Now it is a mean between two vices, that which depends on excess and that which depends on defect; and again it is a mean because the vices respectively fall short of or exceed what is right in both passions and actions, while virtue both finds and chooses that which is intermediate. Hence in respect of its substance and the definition which states its essence virtue is a mean, with regard to what is best and right an extreme.

But not every action nor every passion admits of a mean; for some have names that already imply badness, e.g. spite, shamelessness, envy, and in the case of actions adultery, theft, murder; for all of these and suchlike things imply by their names that they are themselves bad, and not the excesses or deficiencies of them. It is not possible, then, ever to be right with regard to them; one must always be wrong. Nor does goodness or badness with regard to such things depend on committing adultery with the right woman, at the right time, and in the right way, but simply to do any of them is to go wrong. It would be equally absurd, then, to expect that in unjust, cowardly, and voluptuous action there should be a mean, an excess, and a deficiency; for at that rate there would be a mean of excess and of deficiency, an excess of excess, and a deficiency of deficiency. But as there is no excess and deficiency of temperance and courage because what is intermediate is in a sense an extreme, so too of the actions we have mentioned there is no mean nor any excess and deficiency, but however they are done they are wrong; for in general there is neither a mean of excess and deficiency, nor excess and deficiency of a mean. . . .

QUESTIONS FOR COMPREHENSION AND REFLECTION

1. What is the goal, according to Aristotle, toward which every act and inquiry aims? Does "the good," as defined by Aristotle, justify regulation of the medical field in areas such as the patient/physician relationship, euthanasia, human experimentation, and genetic engineering? Support your answers.

2. According to Aristotle, what is the relationship between morality and happiness? What are the implications of this relationship for healthcare practice? Do healthcare professionals have a moral duty to make their patients happy even if it means doing something they regard as immoral or medically unsound? Can a patient ever be mistaken about what will make him or her happy? If so, does the healthcare professional then have a paternalistic duty to override the patient's request? Support your answers. Discuss how Aristotle, were he alive today, might answer these questions.

3. What is a virtue, and how do people become more virtuous? Do healthcare professionals have a duty to cultivate virtue in themselves? Support your answers. Discuss how a physician might apply the doctrine of the mean in his or her practice.

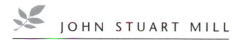

JOHN STUART MILL

On Liberty

John Stuart Mill (1806–1873) carried on the utilitarian tradition of Jeremy Bentham. Like Bentham, Mill was interested in applying utilitarian principles to political matters and social reform. Mill believed that the protection of individual rights from social coercion by the majority or by government was essential for moral progress and individual happiness. Applying the principle of utility, Mill concluded that there are only two legitimate grounds for social coercion: (1) to prevent someone from harming others (the no-harm principle) and (2) to prevent people from interfering with other people's legitimate interests.

CHAPTER 1

. . . The object of this essay is to assert one very simple principle, as entitled to govern absolutely the dealings of society with the individual in the way of compulsion and control, whether the means used be physical force in the form of legal penalties or the moral coercion of public opinion. That principle is that the sole end for which mankind are warranted, individually or collectively, in interfering with the liberty of action of any of their number is self-protection. That the only purpose for which power can be rightfully exercised over any member of a civilized community, against his will, is to prevent harm to others. His own good, either physical or moral, is not a sufficient warrant. He cannot rightfully be compelled to do or forbear because it will be better for him to do so, because it will make him happier, because, in the opinions of others, to do so would be wise or even right. These are good reasons for remonstrating with him, or reasoning with him, or persuading him, or entreating him, but not for compelling him or visiting him with any evil in case he do otherwise. To justify that, the conduct from which it is desired to deter him must be calculated to produce evil to someone else. The only part of the conduct of anyone for which he is amenable to society is that which concerns others. In the part which merely concerns himself, his independence is, of right, absolute. Over himself, over his own body and mind, the individual is sovereign. . . .

. . . I regard utility as the ultimate appeal on all ethical questions; but it must be utility in the largest sense, grounded on the permanent interests of man as a progressive being. Those interests, I contend, authorize the subjection of individual spontaneity to external control only in respect to those actions of each which concern the interest of other people. If anyone does an act hurtful to others, there is a *prima facie* case for punishing him by law or, where legal penalties are not safely applicable, by general disapprobation. There are also many positive acts for the benefit of others which he may rightfully be compelled to perform, such as to give evidence in a court of justice, to bear his fair share in the common defense or in any other joint work necessary to the interest of the society of which he enjoys the protection, and to perform certain acts of individual beneficence, such as saving a fellow creature's life or interposing to protect the defenseless against ill usage—things which whenever it is obviously a man's duty to do he may rightfully be made responsible to society for not doing. A person may cause evil to others not only by his actions but by his inaction, and in either case he is justly accountable to them for the injury. . . .

But there is a sphere of action in which society, as distinguished from the individual, has, if any, only an indirect interest: comprehending all that portion of a person's life and conduct which affects only himself or, if it also affects others, only with their free, voluntary, and undeceived consent and participation. When I say only himself, I mean directly and in the first instance; for whatever affects himself may affect others through himself: and the objection which may be grounded on this contingency will receive consideration in the sequel. This, then, is the appropriate region of human liberty. It comprises, first, the inward domain of consciousness, demanding liberty of conscience in the most comprehensive sense, liberty of thought and feeling, absolute freedom of opinion and sentiment on all subjects, practical or speculative, scientific, moral, or theological. . . . Secondly, the principle requires liberty of tastes and pursuits, of framing the plan of our life to suit our own character, of doing as we like, subject to such consequences as may follow, without impediment from our fellow creatures, so long as what we do does not harm them, even though they should think our conduct foolish, perverse, or wrong. Thirdly, from this liberty of each individual follows the liberty, within the same limits, of combination among individuals; freedom to unite for any purpose not involving harm to others: the persons combining being supposed to be of full age and not forced or deceived.

No society in which these liberties are not, on the whole, respected is free, whatever may be its form of government; and none is completely free in which they do not exist absolute and unqualified. The only freedom which deserves the name is that of pursuing our own good in our own way, so long as we do not attempt to deprive others of theirs or impede their efforts to obtain it. Each is the proper guardian of his own health, whether bodily *or* mental and spiritual. Mankind are greater gainers by suffering each other to live as seems good to themselves than by compelling each to live as seems good to the rest. . . .

1. How would Mill most likely respond to the Nazi concentration camp experiments? Are these experiments justified under the principle of utility if it can be shown that many people have benefited as a result of these experiments?
2. Discuss whether the principle of utility, as interpreted by Mill, justifies physician-assisted suicide. Would Mill support Dr. Kevorkian? Support your answer.
3. Utilitarian theory is frequently used to formulate social policies regarding issues such as AIDS testing and the distribution of social benefits such as medical care. Discuss what positions Mill would most likely take on mandatory AIDS testing and on socialized medicine.

IMMANUEL KANT

Fundamental Principles of the Metaphysic of Ethics

Unlike the utilitarians, Immanuel Kant (1724–1804) was more concerned with establishing a metaphysical foundation for morality than in coming up with an ethical system that could be used for formulating social policy. Like Aristotle, Kant believed that only reason could provide this foundation. If a moral law is to be morally compelling, it must be logically consistent as well as absolutely binding. The most fundamental moral principle—the categorical imperative—requires us to do something regardless of the consequences.

Nothing can possibly be conceived in the world, or even out of it, which can be called good without qualification, except a Good Will. Intelligence, wit, judgment, and the other *talents* of the mind, however they may be named, or courage, resolution, perseverance, as qualities of temperament, are undoubtedly good and desirable in many respects; but these gifts of nature may also become extremely bad and mischievous if the will which is to make use of them, and which, therefore, constitutes what is called *character*, is not good. It is the same with the *gifts of fortune*. Power, riches, honour, even health, and the general well-being and contentment with one's condition which is called *happiness*, inspire pride, and often presumption, if there is not a good will to correct the influence of these on the mind, and with this also to rectify the whole principle of acting, and adapt it to its end. . . .

A good will is good not because of what it performs or effects, not by its aptness for the attainment of some proposed end, but simply by virtue of the volition, that is, it is good in itself, and considered by itself is to be esteemed much higher than all that can be brought about by it in favour of any inclination, nay, even of the sum total of all inclinations. Even if it should happen that, owing to special disfavour of fortune, or the niggardly provision of a step-motherly nature, this will should wholly lack power to accomplish its purpose, if with its greatest efforts it should yet achieve nothing, and there should remain only the good will (not, to be sure, a mere wish, but the summoning of all means in our power), then, like a jewel, it would still shine by its own light, as a thing which has its whole value in itself. Its usefulness or fruitlessness can neither add to nor take away anything from this value. . . .

To be beneficent when we can is a duty; and besides this, there are many minds so sympathetically constituted that, without any other motive of vanity or self-interest, they find a pleasure in spreading joy around them, and can take delight in the satisfaction of others so far as it is their own work. But I maintain that in such a case an action of this kind, however proper, however amiable it may be, has nevertheless no true moral worth, but is on a level with other inclinations, *e.g.* the inclination to honour, which, if it is happily directed to that which is in fact of public utility and accordant with duty, and consequently honourable, deserves praise and encouragement, but not esteem. For the maxim lacks the moral import, namely, that such actions be done *from duty*, not from inclination. Put the case that the mind of that philanthropist were clouded by sorrow of his own: extinguishing all sympathy with the lot of others, and that while he still has the power to benefit others in distress, he is not touched by their trouble because he is absorbed with his own; and now suppose that he tears himself out of this dead insensibility, and performs the action without any inclination to it, but simply from duty, then first has his action its genuine moral worth. . . .

The moral worth of an action does not lie in the effect expected from it, nor in any principle of action which requires to borrow its motive from this expected effect. For all these effects—agreeableness of one's condition, and even the promotion of the happiness of others—could have been also brought about by other causes, so that for this there would have been no need of the will of a rational being; whereas it is in this alone that the supreme and unconditional good can be found.

The pre-eminent good which we call moral can therefore consist in nothing else than *the conception of law* in itself, *which certainly is only possible in a rational being*, in so far as this conception, and not the expected effect, determines the will. . . .

But what sort of law can that be, the conception of which must determine the will, even without paying any regard to the effect expected from it, in order that this will may be called good absolutely and without qualification? As I have deprived the will of every impulse which could arise to it from obedience to any law, there remains nothing but the universal conformity of its actions to law in general, which alone is to serve the will as a principle, *i.e.* I am never to act otherwise than so *that I could also will that my maxim should become a universal law.* Here now, it is the simple conformity to law in general, without assuming any particular law applicable to certain actions, that serves the will as its principle, and must so serve it, if duty is not to be a vain delusion and a chimerical notion. The common reason of men in its practical judgments perfectly coincides with this, and always has in view the principle here suggested. Let the question be, for example: May I when in distress make a promise with the intention not to keep it? I readily distinguish here between the two significations which the question may have: Whether it is prudent, or whether it is right, to make a false promise. The former may undoubtedly often be the case. . . . The shortest way, however, and an unerring one, to discover the answer to this question whether a lying promise is consistent with duty, is to ask myself, Should I be content that my maxim (to extricate myself from difficulty by a false promise) should hold good as a universal law, for myself as well as for others? and should I be able to say to myself, "Every one may make a deceitful promise when he finds himself in a difficulty from which he cannot otherwise extricate himself"? Then I presently become aware that while I can will the lie, I can by no means will that lying should be a universal law. For with such a law there would be no promises at all, since it would be in vain to allege my intention in regard to my future actions to those who would not believe this allegation, or if they over-hastily did so would pay me back in my own coin. Hence my maxim, as soon as it should be made a universal law, would necessarily destroy itself.

. . . I do not indeed as yet *discern* on what this respect [for the natural law] is based (this the philosopher may inquire), but at least I understand this, that it is an estimation of the worth which far outweighs all worth of what is recommended by inclination, and that the necessity of acting from *pure* respect for the practical law is what constitutes duty, to which every other motive must give place, because it is the condition of a will being good *in itself,* and the worth of such a will is above everything. . . .

Everything in nature works according to laws. Rational beings alone have the faculty of acting according *to the conception* of laws, that is according to principles, *i.e.* have a *will.* Since the deduction of actions from principles requires *reason,* the will is nothing but practical reason. . . .

The conception of an objective principle, in so far as it is obligatory for a will, is called a command (of reason), and the formula of the command is called an Imperative.

All imperatives are expressed by the word *ought* [or *shall*], and thereby indicate the relation of an objective law of reason to a will, which from its subjective constitution is not necessarily determined by it (an obligation). They say that something would be good to do or to forbear, but they say it to a will which does not always do a thing because it is conceived to be good to do it. . . .

Now all *imperatives* command either *hypothetically* or *categorically.* The former represent the practical necessity of a possible action as means to something else that is willed (or at least which one might possibly will). The categorical imperative would be that which represented an action as necessary of itself without reference to another end, *i.e.* as objectively necessary.

Since every practical law represents a possible action as good, and on this account, for a subject who is practically determinable by reason, necessary, all imperatives are formulae determining an action which is necessary according to the principle of a will good in some respects. If now the action is good only as a means *to something else,* then the imperative is *hypothetical;* if it is conceived as good *in itself* and consequently as being necessarily

the principle of a will which of itself conforms to reason, then it is *categorical.* . . .

. . . an imperative which commands a certain conduct immediately, without having as its condition any other purpose to be attained by it . . . is Categorical. It concerns not the matter of the action, or its intended result, but its form and the principle of which it is itself a result: and what is essentially good in it consists in the mental disposition, let the consequence be what it may. This imperative may be called that of Morality. . . .

When I conceive a hypothetical imperative in general I do not know beforehand what it will contain until I am given the condition. But when I conceive a categorical imperative I know at once what it contains. For as the imperative contains besides the law only the necessity that the maxims* shall conform to this law, while the law contains no conditions restricting it, there remains nothing but the general statement that the maxim of the action should conform to a universal law, and it is this conformity alone that the imperative properly represents as necessary.

There is therefore but one categorical imperative, namely this: *Act only on that maxim whereby thou canst at the same time will that it should become a universal law.*

Now if all imperatives of duty can be deduced from this one imperative as from their principle, then, although it should remain undecided whether what is called duty is not merely a vain notion, yet at least we shall be able to show what we understand by it and what this notion means. . . .

A man reduced to despair by a series of misfortunes feels wearied of life, but is still so far in possession of his reason that he can ask himself whether it would not be contrary to his duty to himself to take his own life. Now he inquires whether the maxim of his action could become a

_____

*A maxim is a subjective principle of action, and must be distinguished from the *objective principle,* namely, practical law. The former contains the practical rule set by reason according to the conditions of the subject (often its ignorance or its inclinations), so that it is the principle on which the subject *acts;* but the law is the objective principle valid for every rational being, and is the principle on which it *ought to act,* that is, an imperative.

universal law of nature. His maxim is: From self-love I adopt it as a principle to shorten my life when its longer duration is likely to bring more evil than satisfaction. It is asked then simply whether this principle founded on self-love can become a universal law of nature. Now we see at once that a system of nature of which it should be a law to destroy life by means of the very feeling whose special nature it is to impel to the improvement of life would contradict itself, and therefore could not exist as a system of nature; hence that maxim cannot possibly exist as a universal law of nature, and consequently would be wholly inconsistent with the supreme principle of all duty. . . .

If then there is a supreme practical principle or, in respect of the human will, a categorical imperative, it must be one which, being drawn from the conception of that which is necessarily an end for every one because it is *an end in itself*, constitutes an *objective* principle of will, and can therefore serve as a universal practical law. The foundation of this principle is: *rational nature exists as an end in itself*. Man necessarily conceives his own existence as being so: so far then this is a *subjective* principle of human actions. But every other rational being regards its existence similarly, just on the same rational principle that holds for me: so that it is at the same time an objective principle, from which as a supreme practical law all laws of the will must be capable of being deduced. Accordingly the practical imperative will be as follows: *So act as to treat humanity, whether in thine own person or in that of any other, in every case as an end withal, never as means only*. We will now inquire whether this can be practically carried out.

To abide by the previous examples:

Firstly, under the head of necessary duty to one-self: He who contemplates suicide should ask himself whether his action can be consistent with the idea of humanity *as an end in itself*. If he destroys himself in order to escape from painful circumstances, he uses a person merely as a *mean* to maintain a tolerable condition up to the end of life. But a man is not a thing, that is to say, something which can be used merely as means, but must in all his actions be always considered as an end in himself. I cannot, therefore, dispose in any way of a man in my own person so as to mutilate him, to damage or kill him. (It belongs to ethics proper to define this principle more precisely so as to avoid all misunderstanding, *e.g.* as to the amputation of the limbs in order to preserve myself; as to exposing my life to danger with a view to preserve it, &c. This question is therefore omitted here.)

Secondly, as regards necessary duties, or those of strict obligation, towards others; he who is thinking of making a lying promise to others will see at once that he would be using another man *merely as a mean*, without the latter containing at the same time the end in himself. For he whom I propose by such a promise to use for my own purposes cannot possibly assent to my mode of acting towards him, and therefore cannot himself contain the end of this action. This violation of the principle of humanity in other men is more obvious if we take in examples of attacks on the freedom and property of others. For then it is clear that he who transgresses the rights of men, intends to use the person of others merely as means, without considering that as rational beings they ought always to be esteemed also as ends, that is, as beings who must be capable of containing in themselves the end of the very same action. . . .

QUESTIONS FOR COMPREHENSION AND REFLECTION

1. What is "the good will"? What is the relevance of the good will in making medical decisions? Discuss the characteristics of a physician with a good will.
2. Kant formulated his views on suicide long before the development of medical technology that could be used to extend the dying process. Is euthanasia always incompatible with the categorical imperative? What would Kant's position most likely be on physician-assisted suicide? What would Kant's position most likely be on the eu-

thanasia of terminally ill people who request euthanasia or of people in comas or with severe brain damage who are unable to give their consent? Support your answers.

3. The categorical imperative requires that we treat persons as ends in themselves and never as a means only. Using the categorical imperative, develop policies on human cloning and on the use of humans as subjects in medical experiments.

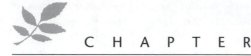

C H A P T E R   2

Critical Thinking
The Basis for Ethical Reasoning

Until recently, most physicians routinely lied to patients who were dying of terminal diseases such as cancer. In a 1961 study, over two-thirds of the American physicians surveyed reported that they infrequently or never disclosed a cancer diagnosis to a patient.[1] More recently, a 1989 study at a major hospital in Rhode Island revealed that the majority of doctors were willing to use deception in certain circumstances. Three-quarters of them said they would not report a case of gonorrhea to the health department, even though they were required to do so by law, if an infected husband was worried that his wife would leave him upon learning that he had been unfaithful. In addition, about two-thirds stated that, if questioned by the wife, they would back up the husband's story that he was taking antibiotics for another problem. Even more disturbing was the finding that 40 percent of doctors would engage in deception if they accidentally killed a patient by giving an overdose of medicine.[2]

THE IMPORTANCE OF CRITICAL THINKING SKILLS

We have probably all heard the expression "The road to hell is paved with good intentions." Without correct reasoning, a person with good intentions may end up actually causing more harm than good. Although people may be strongly motivated to do what is right, they cannot always figure out the best way to achieve this goal.

While the intentions of the healthcare professionals in the above studies who lied may have been good, their moral analysis of when it is appropriate to lie to patients was probably not. Until the 1970s, when healthcare ethics came into its own as a field of study, it was generally accepted that physicians should withhold the truth when it might cause harm to the patient. It was also assumed that most patients did not want to know the truth about serious illnesses and that physicians had a duty to shield them from despair through the use of benevolent falsehoods.

While beneficence in some cases may justify paternalism, the practice of paternalism must be consistent with the underlying principle of respect for persons. Many physicians who lied to patients out of paternalistic concern adopted a double standard that placed them above their patients, thus violating both the principle of autonomy and the principle of equal respect for the dignity of others. Physicians expected their patients to respond truthfully to their questions; however, they did not feel bound to respond truthfully to patients' queries about their prognosis.

Critical thinking involves the ability to identify moral problems as well as to resolve them. Because most physicians were so steeped in paternalism, they saw nothing wrong with lying to patients with terminal cancer. Not until the practice was identified as morally problematic did researchers begin looking into the effects of lying on patients dying of cancer. Physicians who condoned lying to patients on paternalistic grounds failed to take into account the long-term effects the practice would have on the erosion of trust between patients and physicians.

Given the recent rapid advances in medical technology, honing our critical thinking skills is even more important. Circumstances can get out of control because of failure to foresee potential moral issues. For example, bioethicists are trying to predict possible problems and create effective policies regarding the uses of human cloning. By applying critical thinking skills to hypothetical scenarios, they hope to curtail potential disasters—or at least to be able to effectively deal with any problems that should arise. An examination of how healthcare professionals in other cultures handle moral problems can widen our scope of thinking and alert us to solutions or potential problems we might not have considered.

The development of critical thinking skills also gives us the tools to analyze our own worldviews. Some people are so emotionally invested in certain moral issues that they may unwittingly manipulate their arguments in order to "prove" a conclusion that does not follow logically from their argument. When confronted with objections to their positions, such people often resort to resistance and fallacies to shield their "argument" from critical analysis. An understanding of logic and moral reasoning can help us break through these patterns of resistance. By sharpening our analytical skills, we can become more independent in our thinking and less susceptible to opinions that foster narrow-mindedness and bigotry.

THE ROLE OF *IS* AND *OUGHT* STATEMENTS IN HEALTHCARE ETHICS

Morality is more than a list of moral rules. Healthcare ethics, in particular, requires the rational use of both descriptive statements and prescriptive statements. **Descriptive statements** tell us what *is*, while **prescriptive statements** tell us what *ought* to be. Unlike science, which is descriptive, ethics is primarily prescriptive, with descriptive statements playing a supporting role.

Descriptive Statements

Healthcare decisions are made within a real-world, as opposed to a merely hypothetical, context. Therefore, descriptive statements in the form of medical judgments, scientific findings, information about the particular context in which the decision will be made, and sociological or political observations play a key role. Following are some examples of descriptive statements:

> "Each year an estimated 2,000 poor but healthy Indians, looking for enough money to provide a dowry or build a house, sell one of their kidneys to a rich person in need."[3]

"By the tenth week [the fetus] already has acquired a face, arms and legs, fingers and toes . . ."[4]

"Karen Quinlan is in a persistent vegetative state."

"About 40 percent of college students engage in binge drinking."[5]

"Some laboratory experiments cause pain to nonhuman animals."

Descriptive statements can be true or false. Statistics or other findings cited in an argument should be backed up by reliable sources. Incorrect or missing information can lead to the misapplication or misordering of moral principles. For example, the assumptions that (1) people with terminal cancer did not want to know they had cancer and (2) people who were told they had terminal cancer suffered more as a result of knowing than those who were not told led to the playing down of the principle of autonomy and to overemphasis on the principles of paternalism and nonmaleficence. Both assumptions are descriptive, or factual, statements that were later proved to be false.

Sometimes we need to make moral decisions without having all the necessary factual information. For example, in deciding whether to withdraw life support from a person in a coma or persistent vegetative state, as in the case of Karen Quinlan, we may not know his or her wishes regarding the withdrawal of life support. Nor do we know what it is like for people in a persistent vegetative state. Are they conscious at all? Are they in pain? In such cases, we need to do our best to garner whatever information we can from friends and family about the wishes of the comatose patient, as well as any information available about the chances of recovery. Similarly, in cases in which a technology is still being developed, such as cloning, the best we can do is conjecture about the future impact of the technology.

Prescriptive Statements

Prescriptive statements deal with values. They tell us what *ought* to be and what we *ought* to do. Moral principles and norms, such as those we studied in Chapter 1, are prescriptive statements. Following are some examples of prescriptive statements:

"Every person has a right to life."

"Try your best to treat others as you would wish to be treated yourself."

"Do not lie."

"Do no harm."

"Maximize pleasure and minimize pain."

When making moral judgments, healthcare ethicists use descriptive statements about the world and human nature along with prescriptive statements about moral values. Moral values are only one of many types of values. There are also aesthetic values; economic values; social values such as power, fame, and popularity; and political values such as national integrity and solidarity. The increasing pressure on health insurance companies and HMOs to cut costs, for example, has created conflicts between economic values and the moral value of providing quality medical care. Only moral values, however, carry the force of the *ought*. Although it would be nice to be beautiful, wealthy, popular, and intelligent, moral values, by their very nature, demand that we give them precedence over nonmoral values.

FIGURE 2.1   The Three Levels of Thinking

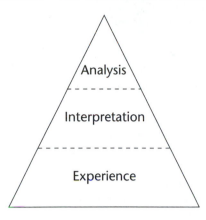

In making moral decisions, we use descriptive statements about the world and about human nature along with prescriptive statements about moral values. When we apply critical thinking skills to healthcare ethics, it is important that we first get our facts straight, but ethics goes beyond science and observation. We cannot go directly from a descriptive statement about how things are to a statement about how things ought to be. A description of a particular practice, such as the technique used to clone mammals, cannot in itself tell us whether human cloning is moral or immoral. We need to bring in prescriptive statements for moral guidance in order to make such a judgment.

THE THREE LEVELS OF THINKING

The thinking process used in ethical reasoning can be broken down into three levels: experience, interpretation, and analysis (Figure 2.1). Keep in mind that this division is artificial; for example, we never have *pure* experience or engage in *pure* analysis. All three levels overlap and interact with one another. All experiences are filtered through our interpretations of the world. All analysis occurs within a real-life context.

Experience

Experience, the first level of thinking, forms the foundation of moral reasoning. For this reason, critical thinking requires that we first have our facts straight. Experience goes beyond the five senses; it also includes indirect experience. We may have seen a news show about someone whose life was saved because he received a kidney from a person living in India; we may have read an article on the Karen Quinlan case; we may have a friend who is a binge drinker; we may have a family member who is dying of cancer; we may experience moral repugnance when we see pictures of animals being used in lab experiments; we may have to forgo a certain medical treatment because we lack health insurance; we or someone close to us may have struggled over whether to have an abortion. All these experiences inform our moral decision making.

At this level of moral reasoning, we simply describe our experiences in the form of descriptive statements. We do not, at least in theory, pass judgment on these experiences or draw any conclusions from them.

Interpretation

Interpretation involves trying to make sense out of our experiences. Figure 2.2 lists some possible interpretations of the experience that "some lab experiments cause pain to nonhuman animals."

Our interpretations of our experience, taken together, form what is known as our **worldview.** A worldview that is held by a particular profession or discipline is known as a **paradigm.** A paradigm delineates what is "normal" and, in the medical profession, sets boundaries for what is acceptable medical practice and research. Anything that falls outside of or is at odds with the accepted or dominant paradigm is regarded as suspect, frivolous, or even dangerous.

Physicist and philosopher Thomas Kuhn notes that paradigm shifts that involve openness to new ways of thinking are more likely to occur in times of crisis when the prevailing paradigm is unable to solve a particular pressing problem. The rapid development of new technologies that create new life in ways previously unimaginable and that, at the other end of the spectrum, can prolong life almost indefinitely may precipitate just such a crisis. The focus in Western medicine on the human body as mechanical may be inadequate for answering questions that arise as a result of these new technologies.

Most people like to think that they acquired their worldview on their own. In reality, our worldviews, or interpretations of different moral issues, are strongly influenced by our upbringing, our peers, our profession, and our culture. Not only do our experiences contribute to our worldview, but our worldview, or interpretation of events, also shapes the way we experience the world. Our interpretations are, in turn, grounded in certain metaphysical assumptions about the nature of reality. What does it mean to be a human? What is the relationship between humans and the rest of nature? Are humans different, in a morally relevant sense, from all other animals? What is the relationship between mind and body? Are we purely physical beings, or do we have nonmaterial souls as well? Do we have free will, or is all of our behavior subject to causal laws?

FIGURE 2.2 Interpretation

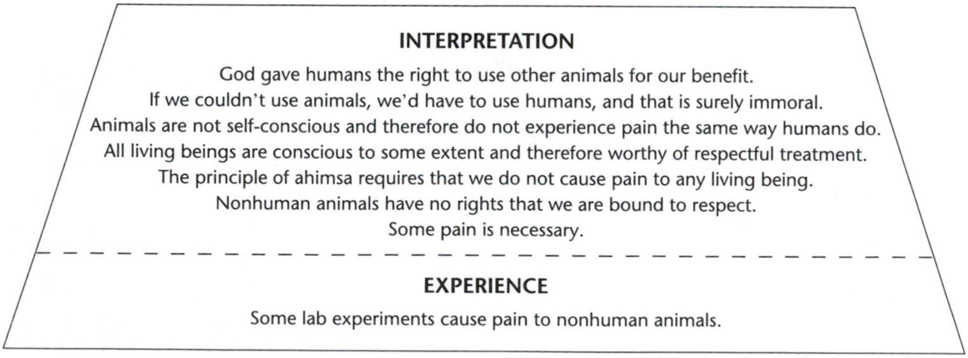

INTERPRETATION

God gave humans the right to use other animals for our benefit.
If we couldn't use animals, we'd have to use humans, and that is surely immoral.
Animals are not self-conscious and therefore do not experience pain the same way humans do.
All living beings are conscious to some extent and therefore worthy of respectful treatment.
The principle of ahimsa requires that we do not cause pain to any living being.
Nonhuman animals have no rights that we are bound to respect.
Some pain is necessary.

EXPERIENCE

Some lab experiments cause pain to nonhuman animals.

Dualism Versus Materialism   How we define illness and well-being, how we experience illness, and how we respond to illness are bound up with our concept of personhood. In most Western cultures, reality is divided into two distinct substances: the material, or physical, body and the nonmaterial mind, also referred to as the soul or spirit. This view is known as **metaphysical dualism.** The body, being material, is subject to causal laws of mechanics. The mind, in contrast, possesses free will because it is nonmaterial and rational.

Some scientists and physicians deny the existence of a soul or mind and recognize only matter in the universe. **Scientific materialism** reduces the human to purely body. In 1672, British philosopher and scientist Robert Boyle (1627–1691) expressed the following view of the human body: "I think the physician is to look upon the patient's body as an engine that is out of order, but yet so constituted that, by his concurrence with . . . the parts of the automaton itself, it may be brought to a better state." Because all phenomena in the universe, according to metaphysical materialism, are matter, including the human mind, they are subject to the same physical laws and can be understood by the same type of scientific analysis. One criticism of the Human Genome Project, discussed in Chapter 5, is that it risks reducing people to a genetic code. Reductionism removes the human body from its social and personal context and reduces it to an object to be studied and manipulated. The idea that the entire human body, including the mind, can be reduced to an elaborate organic machine continues to dominate Western medicine and medical research. The reduction of mental illness, alcoholism, learning problems, and even character flaws such as nastiness to chemical imbalances or physical dysfunction and the current faith in the ability of genetic engineering to produce a "perfect" child are both examples of the power of this particular worldview.

Practically speaking, both the dualistic and the materialist worldviews have similar effects on healthcare practices. Healing is a mechanical process in both, because it is the body (including the brain) that gets sick, separate from the mind or spirit—if such an entity exists. The compartmentalization of humans into body and soul ensured harmony between medicine and mainstream Christian religion by relegating the care of the body to the physician and the care of the soul to the clergy. Indeed, Protestantism shared science's confidence in the ability to gain power over nature as the means to securing human well-being.

The Technological Imperative   The view of the body as a machine and confidence in the ability of science to solve human problems gave rise to the **technological imperative**, which impels us "to use the capacities [technology] provides us without adequate reflection on whether they will lead to the humane goals of medical care."[6] Thus, technology becomes an end in itself rather than a means to humane, ethically informed ends. The relationship between technology and its ends is circular rather than linear. New technologies arise in response to problems identified by the current paradigm (e.g., the need for "better" prenatal diagnostic techniques, cosmetic surgery, infertility treatments, organ transplant technologies, and other life-sustaining technologies). New technologies, in turn, may suggest or even impose new ends, such as genetic enhancement or preconception gender selection. Because technologies permit the manipulation of the genetic code prior to birth as well as extension of the dying process, they can also give rise to new ethical issues. One of these issues is the extent to which medical technology impinges on the human experience.

TIBET:

Death and Dying Within a Buddhist Context

Tibetan Buddhist Sogyal Rinpoche suggests that Westerners can learn from the Buddhist view of death and dying. In Buddhist philosophy, nothing has permanence or inherent existence of its own; death is viewed as a transition into a new life or state of consciousness. All things, when viewed in their true relation, are not independent but instead are interdependent with all other things.

In *The Tibetan Book of Living and Dying*, which is based on the ancient teachings connected with the *Tibetan Book of the Dead*, Sogyal Rinpoche maintains that people who believe that this life is the only one and deny death and the afterlife will develop no long-term vision. "What the masters must suspect is that there is a danger that people who have no strong belief in a life after this one will create a society fixated on short-term results, without much thought for the consequences of their actions." He blames the fear of dying evident in Western medicine for the current obsession with youth, the stigma attached to those dying of AIDS and cancer, and the discarding of old people "into old people's homes, where they die lonely and abandoned."[7]

According to Rinpoche, if we are to take life seriously, we all need to ask ourselves, "What if I were to die tonight?" and imagine our own deaths. In sharp contrast to the typical Western experience of impending death, the moment of death for the Tibetan Buddhist is one of freedom rather than emotional trauma. People are prepared for this moment through meditation and instruction under a master. Near-death experiences, so often maligned in Western medicine as simply hallucinations, are viewed in both ancient and modern Tibetan teachings as moments of great inspiration and potential enlightenment.

The proper atmosphere for dying is one of trust and spiritual inspiration in the loving presence of one's master or spiritual friends, not the impersonal at-

Death and Dying Death and genetic disorders that cannot be fixed are the bane of the medical profession. Dying and death signal failure. In the traditional Western paradigm, the mechanistic view of humans is in conflict with the Christian belief in an afterlife. This may explain why the Hospice movement, which ministers to dying patients, has occurred outside the mainstream hospital and physician relationship, at least in the United States. In Western medicine, death is an embarrassment, an evil to be avoided. In 1986, a group of social scientists writing on the technological imperative predicted that "death prevention may become the purpose of health care."[8] Their prediction may soon come true. Considerable attention is given to developing technology to deter death, often at considerable expense, in terms of both monetary cost and prolonged suffering of those who are dying.

According to a recent study, dying, not old age, is to blame for the high costs of healthcare. About 25 percent of the healthcare dollar is spent on medical treatment of people in their last few years of life. In the Netherlands, despite the acceptance of eu-

mosphere of a hospital ward. The *Tibetan Book of the Dead* is read repeatedly, and the practices in it are carried out in order to achieve peace of mind. Ritual purifications are also performed, and mantras are chanted following the death. Sogyal Rinpoche writes:

What is essential, you see, is to realize now, in life, when we still have a body, that its apparent, so convincing solidity is a mere illusion. . . . The deepening perception of the body's illusory nature is one of the most profound and inspiring realizations we can have to help us to let go.

Inspired by and armed with this knowledge, when we are faced at death with the *fact* that our body is an illusion, we will be able to recognize its illusory nature without fear, to calmly free ourselves from all attachment to it, and to leave it behind willingly, even gratefully and joyfully, knowing it now for what it is. In fact, you could say, we will be able, really and completely, to die when we die, and so achieve ultimate freedom.[9]

In Tibet, death is celebrated as an opportunity for attaining liberation. Tibetan Buddhist tradition celebrates the day of the death of masters, rather than their birthdays as in the West. In the ancient teachings of the *Dzogchen Tantras,* the symbol of death as a moment of rebirth is the mythical bird garuda, which is born fully grown, bursting out of its shell and soaring into the sky.

So if, at the moment of death, we have already a stable realization of the nature of mind, in one instant we can purify all our karma. And if we continue that stable recognition, we will actually be able to end our karma altogether, by entering the expanse of the primordial purity of the nature of man, and attaining liberation.[10]

The concept of death embraced by many Buddhists is radically different from that held by most Western healthcare practitioners. It is interesting to note that, following a near-death experience, people tend to lose their fear of death as well as move toward Buddhism and away from more dualistic religions and philosophies. Because near-death experiences do not fit within the Western medical paradigm, it is not surprising that the majority of people who have these life-changing experiences in American hospitals do not tell their physicians.[11]

thanasia, between 30 and 40 percent of the healthcare dollar is spent on those who are dying. Much of this money goes toward "strenuous medical efforts" in controlling terminal illnesses and keeping patients alive—regardless of their age.[12]

Even though most North Americans and Europeans profess a belief in a better life after death, they still have trouble accepting death and everything associated with it. In most Latin American and South American cultures, in contrast, death represents a new beginning. In Mexico, most people die at home surrounded by family and friends rather than in a hospital isolated from the community. Death is regarded as a natural part of existence and is both celebrated and mourned. On the Day of the Dead, one of Mexico's most important annual holidays, Mexico City is decked out for a gala night of celebration to receive the spirits of the dead that return to eat with their living relatives. In Hindu and Buddhist cultures, death is the end of the body but not the end of life itself; instead, death represents a transition into the next life.

CULTURAL WINDOWS

THE HEALING POWER OF PRAYER

In many cultures, such as the Arab world, religion, prayer, and the practice of medicine are inseparable. The shaman, who acts as an intermediary between the spirit world and the physical world, also plays an important role as a healer in many Southeast Asian, African, and Latin and South American cultures.

In Western medicine, ancient Jewish sources include prayers to inspire the physician's healing. The best known of these is the Daily Prayer of a Physician. Once ascribed to the Jewish philosopher and physician Moses Maimonides (1135–1204), this prayer is now believed to have been written in the eighteenth century by Jewish-German physician Marcus Herz.[13]

There are also many examples of Christian prayers used by physicians. Indeed, much of the Gospel of Luke, who was a physician, focuses on the role of faith and prayer in healing. In some denominations, such as Christian Science and Jehovah's Witnesses, prayer is regarded as the most powerful tool of healing. Many Catholics also turn to prayer when traditional medicine fails. Indeed, many documented cases seem to be miracle healings.

It wasn't long ago that, despite the professed belief of the majority in God, an almost schizophrenic divide existed in Western medicine between the spiritual and the physical worlds. However, in the past few years, interest in the role of spirituality has grown dramatically, along with a growth in alternative and complementary medicine.[14] In a recent survey of 296 family physicians in the United States, 75 percent stated that they believed "prayers of others could promote a patient's recovery."[15] This figure is more than double that of earlier surveys.

In 1988, cardiologist Randolph Byrd of the University of California at San Francisco carried out a study of the effect of prayer on healing that caught the attention of the medical community. Byrd randomly divided 393 heart patients into two groups. One group received only the standard medical care. The second group, in addition to receiving the standard medical care, was prayed for daily, by first name, by a group of volunteers who described themselves as born-again Christians. Dr. Byrd, the patients, and the hospital staff were not aware of which patients were in which group. At the conclusion of the study, the medical records of the patients were assessed. Byrd found that those who were part of the prayed-for group "received fewer antibiotics, suffered less congestive heart failure, and were less likely to develop pneumonia." He concluded, "These data suggest that intercessory prayer to a Judeo-Christian God has a beneficial effect in patients admitted to a coronary care unit."[16]

However, because the results of other studies have been weak or inconsistent, medical associations are hesitant to prescribe prayer as a medical procedure. "It is premature," states an article in the prestigious British medical journal *Lancet*, "to promote faith and religion as adjunctive medical treatments."[17] But more Western medical professionals are now open to the possibility that spirit and body may not be as separate as they once thought.

Prayer and Healing Because Westerners see the body as a separate entity from the soul, religion and spirituality have no part in the Western medical paradigm. In the Muslim medical paradigm, in contrast, prayer and faith in Allah play a central role in the healing process. According to Islam, Muhammad said, "Seek treatment, for God has created a cure for every illness; some already known and others yet to be known."[18] Only very recently has the role of prayer in healing been investigated by Western scientists. However, such research is peripheral, since prayer cannot be explained in the context of the mechanistic medical paradigm.

Cultural Paradigms and the Patient/Physician Relationship For the most part, the dominant medical paradigm reflects the paradigm of the wider culture. Sometimes, however, there is a clash within a culture between medical paradigms and the world-views of patients, as happens with Jehovah's Witnesses who refuse medical treatment for their children. Medical professionals' views on euthanasia, selective abortion, organ transplants, and animal experimentation also differ from those of the general population, with medical professionals tending to be more in favor of these practices.

Buddhists believe that mind and body are not separate substances but rather manifest one substance, referred to in Buddhist philosophy as the One. Because all reality is interconnected, most Buddhists oppose the taking of life, including the destruction of nonhuman animals in medical experiments. Healing in Buddhist cultures, rather than being a mechanical process, is tied in with the quest for enlightenment and spiritual growth.

Many Native Americans also emphasize our interconnectedness with the earth as well as with one another. They do not divide the world into animate and inanimate objects but rather see everything, including the earth itself, as having a self-conscious life. While the traditional Western paradigm tends to be individualistic and focused on the physician/patient relationship, respect for the environment is an important health issue in Native American medicine. Because humans are part of nature rather than separate from nature, practices that harm the earth also harm humans.

Autonomy Versus Community Assumptions about human nature also vary from culture to culture. Most Westerners view people as autonomous, independent beings. The primary moral obligation of healthcare providers is to respect and promote the moral autonomy of the patient. This worldview, in turn, affects how healthcare decisions are made. Family and community members are generally excluded from medical decisions, including life and death decisions, made by competent adults. Both the United States and Canada have seen a shift in the past thirty years toward truth telling and information disclosure in cases involving cancer. However, the information is disclosed only to the patient. The family is for the most part excluded from the decision-making process, unless the patient requests that they be included. This shift reflects an increasing emphasis on patient autonomy and the individual as the focal point of decision making.

In many other cultures, however, personhood is a holistic concept defined in terms of relationships with the living and the dead, human and nonhuman, that continue after death. The Chinese and Japanese, as noted in the discussion in Chapter 8 on euthanasia, see people primarily as members of a wider community rather than as isolated individuals. Healing involves the nurturing or restoring of harmony and relationships as well as the physical cure. Hence, the family and the community play a much greater

CULTURAL WINDOWS

UNITED STATES:
"Healthy Babies Only, Please"

American medical professionals have a strong bias for healthy children and tend to be overly pessimistic in their prognoses of untreatable genetic disorders. They are also likely to approve of selective abortion for genetic disorders and to say that they would have an abortion should their child have a minor disorder such as a deformed hand or the chance of mild mental retardation. Thus, while paying lip service to "nondirective genetic counseling," they put considerable pressure on pregnant women to have prenatal diagnosis for genetic disorders.[19]

One of the greatest frustrations reported by parents following the birth of a child with a severe genetic disorder is not an ignorant public but the insensitivity of physicians and other medical personnel and their inability to see the child's life as worthwhile.[20] Physicians tend to judge social worth based on their own achievement-oriented value system. A life defined by a physician or geneticist as a "wrongful life," or one not worth living, might be defined very differently by parents. One woman writes: "Many doctors believe it would be better if all children with neural tube defects were never born and they are likely to communicate this attitude to parents. . . . Physicians and parents often have quite different views of the value of life for spina bifida children."[21]

role in medical decisions. This difference needs to be considered in any analysis of the morality of different medical practices, such as truth telling.

Polynesians carry the concept of community even further. They believe that human beings, natural and man-made objects, and nature itself make up a related, sentient totality. The sky and the mountains are persons, not things. Healing, therefore, involves the readjustment of relationships not just between humans, but also between humans and the rest of the world.

Cultural Hierarchies   The Western medical paradigm, like Western culture in general, is hierarchical. Despite the focus on patient autonomy and empowerment, most of the power in medicine still rests with professionals—mainly male physicians. The patriarchal hierarchy is embedded in the Western medical paradigm. Women traditionally have been underrepresented in medical research and receive poorer medical treatment than men. Practices such as lying to wives and girlfriends to protect men, illustrated in the Rhode Island study mentioned at the beginning of this chapter, have only added fuel to feminists' claim that they are discriminated against by healthcare providers.

A cultural paradigm that places white males at the top of the human hierarchy also shortchanges so-called minorities. Race is a cultural construction, rather than one based on scientific fact. Beliefs about fundamental biological differences based on racial lines developed in Europe, primarily in England and Germany, in the eighteenth and nineteenth centuries. These beliefs, in turn, justified colonization, slavery, and

NATIVE AMERICANS:
"We Are All Related"

Eagle Man, an Oglala Sioux writer and lawyer, argues for a return to or the adoption of what he considers traditional Native American values. While not rejecting modern medicine, he points out that good health includes more than just attention to the proper functioning of the body. We need to take a less dualistic approach to health and well-being.

According to Native Americans, bioethics involves paying attention to the wholeness, or totality, of the ethical life lived in thoughtful harmony with the seasons and the biosphere. Health involves more than simply looking after our individual bodies. Practices that disrespect this harmony by disrupting cosmic principles and the natural balance can lead to disease and sickness. "The plight of the non-Indian world," Eagle Man writes, "is that we have lost respect for Mother Earth from whom and where we all come."[22] Practices that threaten and pollute the earth and poison the atmosphere are a great danger to our health. Indeed, he argues, our very survival as a species depends on giving up dualism, recognizing our interconnectedness, and cultivating a respect toward the earth and toward each other.

Healing in traditional Native American culture focuses on the goodness of generation and restoration of the whole. In addition to possessing the wisdom needed to restore harmony and the power of the earth, medicine is connected to knowledge of the healing power of the biosphere and the natural world, especially the plant world. According to the Winnebago of Wisconsin:

. . . ask those who possess plants to take pity on you. If they take pity on you, they will give you one of the good plants that give life and thus you can use them to encourage you in life. However, one plant will not be enough for you to possess. All [the plants] that are to be found on your grandmother's hair, all those that give life, you should try to find out about, until you have a medicine chest [full]. Then you will indeed have great reason for being encouraged.[23]

Among the Navaho, witchcraft as well as disrespect for the natural world can disrupt harmony. To reestablish health in the ailing person, cosmological ceremonies called "chantways" are conducted by ritual specialists.

Recently, indigenous people such as Eagle Man have united in their protest against pollution and destruction of the natural world. Western medicine is also paying more attention to environmental factors in disease.

---

anti-Semitism. The ancient Egyptian, Mesopotamian, Greek, and Roman civilizations did not subscribe to similar beliefs about racial differences. While they were aware that people differed in appearance, they did not see this as evidence of the moral superiority of one group over another or of immutable differences among humans.

Ideas of race still play a central role in medicine and research. Among the first things a patient is asked are his or her race, gender, and age. A person's racial classification,

JAPAN:
Truth Telling and Cancer Patients

In Japan, the patient is treated not as an isolated, autonomous individual but as part of a family and a community, an attitude shaped by the Confucian emphasis on family and community. *Kyokan* (the feeling of togetherness) and *ningen* (the human person in relationship to others) are more important in Japan than the isolated individual.[24]

Because of the emphasis on relationship and sharing, key family members, rather than the individual cancer patient, are the focal point of decision making. Rihito Kimura refers to this as "related-autonomy."[25] Family members are expected to play an integral role in the care and protection of the patient; therefore, negative information related to a diagnosis may be given only to the immediate family and not to the patient.[26] The medical team communicates with family members by speaking to them directly, as well as through written communication, regarding the problem, possible treatments and decisions, and their feelings about the situation.

Adult children remain an integral part of their family of origin. A woman will sometimes visit a physician on behalf of her adult child or husband to explain the problem and make decisions about treatment.

Only since the 1980s have ideals of autonomy and individual rights become part of healthcare ethics in Japan.[27] Although the younger generation in Japan is beginning to question some of the tradition, especially regarding withholding the truth of diagnosis from the patient, young people still respect traditional family values and prefer shared decision making. Thus, the notion of autonomy and withholding information from a patient in Japan has a very different meaning than in more individualistic countries such as the United States, where the power of disclosure is placed in the hands of the physician.

furthermore, is based on the heritage of their "least desirable" parent according to the prevailing culture. A person of primarily European descent with some "black" blood is classified as African American—the tacit belief being that the nonwhite heritage has left him or her tainted.

Certain diseases, such as sickle cell disease, are considered race-specific. In fact, only people from West Africa, rather than Africans in general, are more likely to have sickle cell disease, and it is also found in people who are not of African descent. Thus, it is not a racial disease but a disease found in people from certain localities. Similarly, Tay-Sachs disease is labeled a Jewish disease by the medical profession, despite the fact that Jews are not a racial but a religious group. In fact, Tay-Sachs is a genetic disorder found in people from a particular locale in Eastern Europe, including Arabs, and is very rare among Jews who are not from this part of Eastern Europe. It is also commonly assumed by the medical profession that being of African descent predisposes a person to diabetes, high blood pressure, and kidney failure. Yet there are very few cases of diabetes in West Africa, the place of origin of most African Americans.

Why do healthcare professionals continue to classify diseases as "race-specific" or certain groups of people as "high risk" for certain diseases? The medical profession exists within a cultural context of racism and reflects this worldview. Atwood Gaines writes, "Affliction is attributed to the fact that the individuals are 'minority,' by which is meant biologically different and therefore 'defective.' " Racism, combined with a mechanistic, individualistic view of the body, leads healthcare professionals to ignore the role of oppression and discrimination in disease.

In addition, nonwhites are also more likely than whites to be used in medical research without their informed consent. The Tuskegee Study, discussed in Chapter 6, is one of the most blatant examples of racism in medical research. There is also a tacit assumption that nonwhites and women are less rational and more "animal-like" than white males. Thus, they are more likely to be diagnosed as having a mental disorder and to be treated with powerful psychotropic drugs.[28]

The heavy reliance on nonhuman animals in medical research is another expression of a hierarchical worldview that places men over women, Europeans over non-Europeans, and humans over nonhuman animals. The belief that humans are the central or most significant reality of the universe is known as anthropocentrism. Unlike the Christian, Jewish, and Muslim worldview, which privileges humans, Hindus, Buddhists, and Jains do not draw a sharp distinction between humans and other animals. Karma and reincarnation link all living beings into a united One. Both Peter Singer and Judith and Alyssa Boss, in their articles on the use of nonhuman animals in research, challenge the traditional Western paradigm, arguing that the current division between human and nonhuman animals cannot be morally justified.[29]

Analysis

Analysis lies at the heart of moral reasoning. We may not be able to know with certainty what is right, but we can know with certainty when something is wrong. We know it is wrong to sexually exploit or torture children purely for enjoyment. Analysis helps us sort out the limits of what is morally acceptable. By eliminating certain alternatives, we can move closer to a satisfactory moral decision.

As members of a culture or a particular profession, we tend to be enmeshed in a particular worldview and set of metaphysical assumptions about the world. Because interpretations can be one-sided or distorted, we must remain open-minded when we listen to different interpretations of and assumptions about the nature of reality and human nature. Of course, some interpretations may turn out to be better than others, but we should base measurements of their worth on analysis rather than on tradition or prejudice.

Many people rely on opinion or on a blend of fact and opinion in formulating their views on moral issues. It is important to learn how to distinguish between opinion and analysis. An opinion is a statement that is based on feeling rather than on fact. We may feel that a certain practice or position is morally justified yet be unable to support or give reasons for our opinion. People who engage in **rhetoric,** instead of using logical arguments, use only statements that support their opinion and disregard any statements that do not support it. However, unless we can back up our interpretations with good reasons, they are merely opinions—whether they are those of the majority or simply personal opinions.

Analysis of moral issues requires beginning with correct facts and examining the possible interpretations of our experiences in light of fundamental moral principles and sentiments. In critical thinking, we need to examine our basic assumptions rather than simply uncritically accept them. Analysis requires that we provide good reasons for why we support or reject a particular interpretation or worldview. It also requires a willingness to engage in self-critical analysis and to challenge our own views as well as those of others. Experiences and interpretations that can stand up under critical analysis can become part of our argument. Those that cannot should be discarded, no matter how dear to our heart they may be. By not critically analyzing our worldview, we can become caught up in a sort of self-fulfilling prophecy whereby we interpret our experience through the filter of a particular worldview, and our "experience," in turn, further confirms our distorted worldview. For example, at the beginning of the AIDS crisis, the disease was associated with homosexuals and drug addicts, reflecting our culture's homophobia. This prejudice not only fueled homophobia but caused medical professions to overlook the spread of AIDS among the heterosexual population and children.

According to Kuhn, challenges to traditional paradigms generally come from outside the profession or from people new to the profession. Those who question the prevailing paradigm, such as feminists or non-Westerners, are often considered to be irrational or on the fringes. Research findings that cannot be explained within the traditional paradigm are often dismissed, no matter how remarkable their results. For example, when Dr. Dan Blazer, dean of medical education at Duke University, was asked regarding the findings of the studies on the healing power of prayer, "What would even the most dramatic results really mean?" he replied, "Frankly, it's hard to see how studies like this can tell us anything."[30] The problem, he explained, was that prayer can't be scientifically measured. In other words, under the Western scientific paradigm, a legitimate scientific study would have to "measure the 'dose' of prayer each subject receives—impossible without some kind of prayer meter."[31] The separation of the material and the spiritual characteristic of Western medicine is summarized in the following statement by Dr. Blazer, who describes himself as a devout Christian: "I pray for my patients every day. But that's not a matter of medical science for me. It's a matter of faith."[32]

Nontraditional healthcare professionals and the experience of healthcare systems outside our cultural paradigm can greatly enrich our moral analysis and provide us with new perspectives on ways to resolve problems in healthcare. Paradigms from other cultures involve viewing the world in radically different ways. They require that we interpret our experiences in new ways and reevaluate our traditional modes of moral analysis. Most large hospitals around the world serve patients with widely diverse backgrounds who may not share the assumptions of many of the medical professionals. The study of other cultural worldviews plays an important role in breaking down our resistance to different ideas and promoting serious analysis of moral issues.

Analysis requires open-mindedness and a willingness to look beyond the box of the traditional paradigm. The prevailing paradigm establishes limits on the range of acceptable answers to healthcare problems. If we remain stuck in a particular paradigm, certain problems can seem unsolvable; if we can break out of the box, a solution might be obvious.

ANCIENT MEDICINE

Primitive and ancient medicine conjures up images of magical, mystical rituals in which medicine men in exotic costumes called forth supernatural powers to exorcise spirits and demons thought to cause illness. However, much ancient medicine was quite sophisticated and employed empirical treatment. Indeed, some sources conjecture that ancient cultures in Greece, Egypt, Asia, and the Americas may have derived their ideas about medicine from a common source.

In most ancient cultures, health and disease were considered religious as well as physical phenomena. Medicine and surgery were used in conjunction with religious ritual in both ancient Egypt and Mesopotamia. Egyptian papyri from 2000–1500 B.C. describe the course of various illnesses and relate them to parts of the body. The great Greek physician Galen (A.D. 129–199) developed a model of disease based on anatomy and physiology as well as temperament and time of the year.

The Aztecs in Mexico were familiar with the healing properties of certain minerals and many local plants. During a 1576 epidemic, a Catholic missionary, Father Sahagun, used a stone called eztetl (bloodstone) to stop bleeding through the nose. According to him, this remedy saved many lives.[33] In 1570, Philip II of Spain sent his physician, Dr. Hernandez, to Mexico to learn from the Aztecs. Dr. Hernandez compiled a considerable body of knowledge, including about twelve hundred plants used for medicinal purposes. However, he died before he could publish his work.

For a long time, modern scientists ignored the medicine and medical practices of the ancients. While many medical practices of ancient cultures have not stood up to scientific scrutiny, others have much to offer. Modern research, for example, has revealed that many of the plants used by ancient healers have curative powers. Western physicians are also beginning to look at ancient Asian medical practices such as acupuncture.

RESISTANCE

Most of us hate to be proved wrong. To avoid having our views or interpretations challenged, we may resort to a type of immature defense mechanism known as **resistance.** Everyone uses resistance at times to keep from feeling overwhelmed. A problem arises, however, when resistance becomes a habitual way of responding to challenges to our views. When this happens, resistance acts as a barrier to any critical analysis of our worldview (Figure 2.3).

Resistance can interfere with our ability to make good moral decisions. A study of moral reasoning among physicians found that those at higher levels of moral reasoning, as measured by the Defining Issues Test,[34] were more open to peer review and less

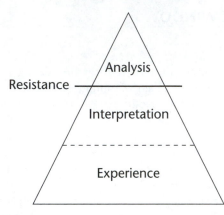

FIGURE 2.3   Resistance

likely to use resistance and had fewer malpractice claims brought against them.[35] In order to move past interpretation to analysis of issues in healthcare ethics, we need to break down the barrier of resistance. We may rely primarily on one type of resistance, or we may employ a wide repertoire of types depending on the situation. Resistance can take several forms. We will look at just a few of the types of resistance that people may use when their moral views are challenged.

Ignorance

In some situations, we are ignorant because information is not available. For example, we do not know if people in comas are suffering, nor do we know what the long-term effects of cloning may be. The best we can do in these cases is gather what information is available and then make an educated guess. Sometimes, however, we avoid learning about particular issues because we just do not want to know, rationalizing that not knowing excuses us from having to think about the issue or to take a stand. Jews were used as unwilling research subjects during the Holocaust because most Germans chose to remain ignorant about the extent of the atrocities taking place in their own back-yards. Similarly, we may prefer to remain comfortably ignorant about the suffering of animals used in medical research or the effects of a free-market healthcare system on those who cannot afford healthcare. However, ignorance does not let us off the hook. An act of omission—failure to act or take a stand—is as much a moral decision as taking action.

Avoidance

Rather than welcoming feedback from people with different points of view, we may avoid people who disagree with us. Some people who hold strong opinions about certain moral issues, such as abortion, yet are insecure in the face of challenges to their position read only literature that supports their opinion and associate only with people who agree with them. Many healthcare professionals read only literature that fits with the traditional Western medical paradigm and summarily dismiss nontraditional healthcare practices or those of other cultures. The tendency to avoid controversial or unfamiliar viewpoints can lead to a serious lack of communication and even to hostility between people who hold widely opposing views.

We can also avoid having to make a decision by engaging in denial. People who are dying or have just lost a loved one may engage in denial. This type of resistance has been interpreted by doctors as a genuine lack of interest on the part of terminal cancer patients in knowing the truth about their condition. Bioethicists may deny the possibility of cloning or other new medical technologies being misused, thus avoiding the need to think about the issue.

Anger

We cannot always avoid people who disagree with us, especially if we are taking a class in ethics! Confronted with a challenge to our views, we may respond by getting angry. Anger may be expressed overtly in physical violence or threats or by storming out of the room, or it may be expressed more subtly in glares, snubs, sarcastic remarks, or angry replies such as "Don't force your views on me." Anger, as a form of resistance, is most effective in thwarting disagreement when the angry person has greater social or physical power that leaves the more vulnerable person feeling threatened and intimidated.

Clichés

"It's all relative." "To each his own." "Things always work out for the best." "There are two sides to every story." "I have a right to my own opinion." Used sparingly, clichés can be useful in illustrating a point; however, the habitual use of clichés in response to challenges to our views trivializes issues and hence acts as a barrier that keeps us from thinking about them.

Technical/Professional Jargon

This type of resistance also involves the use of language to shield our views from critical analysis. However, instead of engaging in trite clichés, the person uses language that is esoteric and difficult for laypeople to understand. Professionals such as physicians and academics are particularly prone to this type of resistance. Healthcare professionals frequently use Latin or lengthy scientific terms for simple medical conditions. Many logicians also use Latin rather than vernacular names for the various fallacies. In healthcare ethics, generally accepted moral principles such as "Do no harm" are given more difficult names, such as nonmaleficence. The use of language that is understandable only to a select group of professionals creates the illusion that the user has a special knowledge or expertise by confusing mastery of the terminology with mastery of the concepts. This, in turn, discourages people from outside the field from questioning the professionals' "expertise."

Conformity/Superficial Tolerance

Many people are afraid that they will not be accepted by their peers. Even though they may actually disagree, they go along with the group or class rather than risk rejection. Bioethicists who are employees of a hospital or members of an ethics committee may refrain from straying too far from conventional moral thinking out of fear of losing their jobs. Susan Sherwin argues that conformity to traditional medical and philosophical views is a prerequisite of being hired as a bioethicist or being appointed to a health-care ethics committee. This conformity, in turn, perpetuates the traditional power hierarchy that currently characterizes the Western medical establishment and prevents the development of new ideas and creative solutions to problems. Increasingly, physicians are demanding "clinical ethicists" with MDs, rather than ethicists from outside the medical profession such as medical ethicists and theologians.

Other people who engage in superficial tolerance do not have a point of view of their own or confuse fairness with not taking sides. The statement "I can see both sides of the issue" sometimes masks a reluctance to analyze the often contradictory sides of a moral issue.

"I'm Struggling"

During the Nazi occupation of France, the thirty-five hundred people of the village of Le Chambon provided refuge to Jews who were fleeing the Nazis. Many years later, villagers were asked by a television reporter from the United States why they did this when other people in France were still struggling with the issue. One elderly gentleman replied, "Those who struggle don't act; those who act don't struggle." It is appropriate to wrestle with a moral issue such as abortion or physician-assisted suicide before reaching at least a tentative stand, but for some people the struggle is a means of avoiding taking a stand while creating an appearance of concern.

Overcoming Resistance

People who habitually engage in resistance may unwittingly become caught up in "doublethink," a term coined by George Orwell in his novel *1984*. **Doublethink** involves holding two contradictory views at the same time and believing both to be true. College students often hold certain contradictory views regarding morality. For example, in a study of how college students judge social issues, 35 percent of students stated that abortion is immoral because life starts at conception.[36] While they stated that abortion was morally wrong because the fetus was a person, many of the students in the pro-life group also argued that abortion should be legal because it is a personal choice. This is doublethink, since by definition a person is valued as an end in him- or herself and deserves the protection of the community. Similarly, many medical professionals who claim to be scientific materialists and also value patient autonomy subscribe to two contradictory views of human nature: that human nature is mechanical and determined, and that human nature is autonomous and free.

Putting aside our resistance may bring up uncomfortable feelings and ideas. Consequently, breaking through resistance can create disequilibrium and confusion. While we may believe that avoiding conflict will make our life more tranquil and enjoyable, in fact habitual resistance takes a lot of energy. When we shut out ideas and experiences that conflict with our cherished worldview, we also miss opportunities. Resistance can numb us to the needs of others and leave us unprepared to make effective moral decisions.

RECOGNIZING AND BREAKING DOWN ARGUMENTS

Before we can engage in critical analysis, we first need to know how to recognize arguments and how to distinguish between good and bad arguments.

The Components of an Argument

An **argument** is made up of two or more propositions, one (the conclusion) of which is supported by the others (the premises). A **proposition** in logic is a statement that expresses a complete thought and can be true or false. The same proposition can be stated in different ways. For example, "Torturing children is wrong," "It is wrong to torture children," and "Kinder zu quälen ist unmoralisch" are all the same proposition, even though they are different statements, because they all express the same thought.

The **conclusion** is the proposition that is affirmed or denied on the basis of the other propositions. The conclusion of an argument can appear anywhere in the argument. The **premises** are those propositions that provide reasons or support for the conclusion. An argument may or may not contain premise indicators and conclusion indicators, terms that can help us identify the premises and conclusion. Words such as *because, for, since*, and *as shown by* can serve as premise indicators. Words such as *therefore, thus, hence,* and *consequently* can serve as conclusion indicators. The words that serve as indicators can also appear in other contexts; for example, *because* and *therefore* are also used in explanations.

The process by which we move from the premise(s) to the conclusion in an argument is known as **inference.**

$$\text{Premise(s)} \xrightarrow{\text{Inference}} \text{Conclusion}$$

The premises form the foundation of the argument. In a good argument, the premises must be strong enough to support the conclusion. Premises can take several forms, including descriptive statements, prescriptive statements, definitions of key terms, and analogies. A well-constructed argument, like a well-built house, must be able to withstand challenges to its integrity. If the premises are weak, the whole argument may collapse like the proverbial house built on sand.

Breaking down an argument into its component parts makes it easier for you to analyze the argument. In breaking down an argument, look for any premise and conclusion indicators. If there are no indicators, begin by identifying the conclusion. The conclusion can appear anywhere in an argument. In identifying the conclusion, ask yourself, "What is this person trying to prove? What position is this person defending?" Next identify the premises. Ask yourself, "What support is this person offering for his or her conclusion?"

The following argument has been broken down into its component parts.

Causing unnecessary pain is immoral. Therefore, it is wrong to use rabbits in cosmetic experiments, since animals such as rabbits are capable of feeling pain.
Conclusion indicator: Therefore
Conclusion: it is wrong to use rabbits in cosmetic experiments
Premise 1: Causing unnecessary pain is immoral
Premise indicator: since
Premise 2: animals such as rabbits are capable of feeling pain

Premise 1 in the above argument is a prescriptive statement; premise 2 is a descriptive statement. Of course, we may not agree with the conclusion of the argument because we may disagree with one of the premises.

An argument may be expressed in a single sentence or may take up several pages. The conclusion may appear anywhere in the written or spoken argument. In the above example, the conclusion comes in the middle of the argument. Although the conclusion in an argument follows from the premises, some people prefer to state the conclusion early on in the argument for the sake of clarity.

Avoiding Rhetoric

Many people mistake rhetoric for logical argumentation. Rhetoric is a means of defending a particular worldview or opinion rather than a means of analyzing it.[37] In logical arguments, the inference process begins with a set of premises and ends with the conclusion. Rhetoric, in contrast, begins with a pseudo-conclusion or opinion. Rhetoricians use only statements that support their particular opinion and disregard any statements or facts that do not. The purpose of rhetoric is to win over your opponents through the power of persuasive speech; the purpose of a logical argument is to discover the truth. Debates of moral issues in which each side begins with a particular position are often based on rhetoric, with each side presenting only "arguments" that support its particular position.

Defining Key Terms

Clearly defined key terms that are used in a consistent manner throughout the argument are essential to a well-constructed argument. Sometimes it is fairly easy to define key terms. For example, *binge drinking* is defined as consuming more than five drinks in a short period of time. *Elective abortion* is defined as the termination of a pregnancy at the request of the pregnant woman for nontherapeutic reasons.

However, at other times defining key terms is not as easy as it may first appear, and some ethicists need to devote considerable time to defining their key terms and explaining the rationale behind the definitions. For example, the term *unnecessary pain* in the previous argument is notoriously vague. What one person may consider unnecessary pain—using rabbits in experiments to verify the results of a previous experiment—another person may find necessary. In the euthanasia debate, the terms *death* and *extraordinary treatment* are both notoriously ambiguous. Some people consider the use of feeding tubes for a comatose patient ordinary treatment; others consider it extraordinary treatment. The definition of *personhood* affects decisions about euthanasia, as well as those concerning abortion, organ transplantation, reproductive technologies, and the use of human and nonhuman animals in research. Without clear, nonarbitrary criteria, definitions of *personhood* can be molded to benefit those in power, as when the U.S. Supreme Court declared that the slave was not a person and when the German Supreme Court declared that the Jew was not a person. Because Jews were not persons, it was morally justified to use them as nonconsenting subjects in medical experiments. Even seemingly simple terms such as *harm* have many shades of ethical meaning. Some people think of harm in the sense of physical injury; others include emotional, social, and even spiritual or karmic setbacks in their definition of *harm*.

Thus, while two people may agree with the premises of an argument, their different understanding of the key terms may lead them to disagree with the conclusion. This can result in confusion over the nature of the disagreement. When disagreement stems from an ambiguous key term, we have what is known as a verbal dispute, rather than a genuine disagreement. In order to avoid verbal disputes, key terms should be clearly defined from the outset.

Emotive Language

The words we choose in formulating an argument send a message as much as does the argument itself. While there is nothing wrong with using expressive language, emotionally charged words can distract from the argument. For example, terms such as *vegetable, playing God, test-tube babies, genetic roulette,* and *anti-choice* tend to alienate participants rather than encourage a search for common ground. On the other hand, the use of highly technical or medical terms, such as *neonate* rather than *baby* or *newborn,* in discussions of newborns and euthanasia tends to commodify the baby and distract from the fact that we are talking about a human life. Sometimes, however, it is difficult to settle on a neutral term. In the abortion debate, for example, pro-life activists prefer the term *unborn or preborn child,* while pro-choice activists prefer the term *fetus.*

At other times, emotive, or emotionally charged, language might be an appropriate means of making a point. Debates on the real-life effects of the new reproductive technologies on the lives of real women and men, including humiliation and dashed hopes, or on the horrors of certain medical experiments might be better expressed through the use of appropriate emotive language. In any case, the point is to choose our words carefully in order to clarify our argument rather than distract and hinder progress toward a resolution of the debate.

The Slippery Slope

Beware of the slippery slope (also known as the wedge), the hypothetical path (or foot in the door) that leads from the morally acceptable to the unacceptable. Taking that fateful first step onto the path, we are warned, is dangerous, and one step may inevitably lead to more steps that send us sliding helter-skelter to the bottom. Kant, for example, warned that, once we begin lying, each subsequent lie becomes easier and easier. If we condone lying to patients with terminal cancer, will physicians then be more likely to lie in other cases?

Keep in mind that the slippery slope is simply a metaphor. In determining whether we are in any real danger of tumbling out of control to the bottom of the slippery slope, we need to seek empirical evidence by asking ourselves: "Are there safety nets that can be put in place, usually in the form of public policy or legislation, to catch us should we start down the precipitous descent?" For example, in giving the go-ahead to new gene technologies, we first need to ascertain whether these technologies might be misused and whether the probabilities of misuse are reasonable. If so, we then have to determine whether we can place a safety net between morally acceptable uses of gene therapy and morally unacceptable uses of gene therapy and gene enhancement. If we can make a distinction, can we be fairly sure that the safety net will hold, or will permitting genetic engineering lead us down the slippery slope to Frankenstein?

On the other hand, we need to resist the temptation to go to the opposite extreme. Not all concerns about heading down the slippery slope are warranted. Alarmists as well as traditionalists often use the slippery slope argument to deflect debate on an issue. For example, the current struggle for equal consideration of the interests of women in medical treatment is based on a long history of institutional oppression of women. When Mary Wollstonecraft published *Vindication of the Rights of Woman* in 1792, her views were received by most people with ridicule. One critic, Thomas Taylor, wrote in response to her book that, if equality should apply to women, then why should it not be applied also to dogs, cats, horses, and other "brutes"? Since this, he suggested, was patently absurd, it would be ludicrous to extend equal rights to women. Taylor's response may seem absurd to us today, but at the time it seemed to make good sense to most people.

The **slippery slope argument** has also been used against the legalization of euthanasia. It is too easy, the argument goes, for legalized voluntary euthanasia to slide down the slope toward a nonvoluntary euthanasia in which the timing of our demise falls under the control of medical bureaucrats or conniving relatives. Similarly, visions of an army of cloned Hitlers taking over the world may make sense to and alarm some people who are unfamiliar with the technology of cloning, despite the fact that such a scenario is very unlikely.

DEDUCTIVE AND INDUCTIVE REASONING

Arguments have traditionally been divided into two types: deductive and inductive. Only deductive arguments can provide decisive proof for their conclusions. Inductive arguments, in contrast, can provide only some support for their conclusions.

Deductive Arguments

Deductive Arguments in healthcare ethics, as elsewhere, generally begin with a moral theory or a set of general ethical principles, along with relevant general observations about the world. These general premises are then applied to a particular decision or medical practice.

General premises ⟶ Specific conclusion

For example, we would decide whether or not lying to patients with terminal cancer is morally acceptable by first seeking a moral theory or general principle on lying. According to Kantian ethics, which we studied in Chapter 1, lying is always wrong. By applying this general principle, we could come up with a conclusion regarding the specific practice in question.

Lying is morally wrong.

Physicians who intentionally give incorrect prognoses to patients with terminal cancer are lying.

Therefore, physicians who intentionally give incorrect prognoses to patients with terminal cancer are morally wrong.

If we agree with the premises in this argument and if the argument is valid (that is, the logical form of the argument is correct), as it is in the above example, then we must accept the conclusion as true.[38]

Our next task in analyzing a deductive argument is to examine the premises. Do we accept the Kantian claim that all lying is wrong? If we believe that the duty not to lie is only a prima facie, rather than an absolute, moral duty, then we have to reject the first premise. If either premise is deemed false, then the conclusion, even though it may still be true, does not logically follow from these two premises. On the other hand, if we accept both premises as true, then we have to accept the conclusion.

Inductive Arguments

Inductive arguments proceed in the opposite direction. They begin with particular cases and from there move to general principles. In other words, they develop a set of principles based on judgments in particular situations rather than on abstract philosophical theories.

Specific premises ⟶ General conclusion

The following is an example of an inductive argument regarding the moral permissibility of lying to patients with terminal cancer:

According to Dr. Collins, most people with terminal cancer would prefer not to know that they are dying.

There have been cases in which patients went into a deep depression after learning they had terminal cancer.

Physicians should do what is in the best interests of their patients.

Therefore, it is (probably) morally acceptable to lie if the benefits of lying outweigh the harm of lying.

In inductive logic, the conclusion is not decisively true or false. Instead it is just *probably* true or false, depending on the strength of the premises. Generally, the more true, relevant premises we can garner in support of our conclusion, the stronger the argument. The three main types of inductive reasoning are analogy, causal connection, and generalization.

Analogy   An **analogy** draws a comparison between two similar things or events. Analogies are used to argue that because things are similar in some important respects, they are also similar in other respects. Analogies clarify important points in an argument and help in explanation. For example, people have made analogies between the structure of an atom and that of the solar system, between a moral theory and a road map, between the fetus and an acorn or an unconscious violinist, and between the brain and a computer.

One of the more popular analogies used in modern healthcare ethics is the analogy between Nazi medicine and contemporary medical practices. Some pro-life advocates compare the Holocaust (the killing of millions of innocent Jews) to abortion (the killing of millions of innocent babies). Analogies have also been drawn between the killing of handicapped people by Nazi physicians and the nonvoluntary euthanasia of people such as Nancy Cruzan, a young woman who was in a persistent vegetative state in a Missouri nursing home, as well as between the current Human Genome Project and the Nazi eugenics program.

To determine the strength of an analogy, we need to examine the number of ways in which the two things being compared are similar or dissimilar and the relevance of the analogy to the case under debate. Are Jews and fetuses sufficiently similar? Are the motives of the physicians, and the social policies supporting the practices, similar enough to draw conclusions based on an analogy between the killing of handicapped people in Germany and the withdrawal of the feeding tube from Nancy Cruzan? If the dissimilarities between two things being compared outweigh the similarities, the analogy is probably not a good one. In addition, the conclusion should not go beyond what one can logically infer from the analogy. For example, in Judith Jarvis Thomson's article at the end of this chapter, the situation of the unconscious violinist who needs temporary use of our kidneys in order to survive has been criticized as being too dissimilar to the normal circumstances of pregnancy for the analogy to be used to morally justify abortion.

Causal Connection   Inductive reasoning using causal connections plays an important role in the formulation of arguments in healthcare ethics. This type of reasoning infers a predictable effect from what is assumed to be its cause. Causal laws are discovered through the use of observation and properly controlled empirical studies. For example, double-blind studies[39] with a treatment group and an untreated control group have shown the placebo effect to be responsible for recovery in some cases where medications and medical procedures were previously assumed to be causal factors in a patient's recovery.

The dominant paradigm generally dictates which presumed cause/effect relationships are worthy of scientific investigation. Assumptions that have become part of established medical practice, such as the routine circumcision of infant boys in the United States and of girls in some African nations, often go unchallenged. On the other hand, practices that fall outside traditional medicine, such as the use of herbal remedies or prayer, are often deemed too trivial to be subjected to scientific investigation. While we may attribute too much causal power to medicine and surgical procedures, we should also be aware of the opposite danger of dismissing without proper investigation possible cause/effect relationships in nontraditional forms of medicine or in the medical practices of other cultures.

Generalization   Generalization, the third type of inductive reasoning, arrives at a general rule or conclusion based on particular experiences. Again, we can engage in faulty generalization because we fail to question the dominant paradigm. Many medical practices in the West are based on research that used only male subjects, the assumption being that males are the quintessential humans and females are deviations from this norm. Similarly, the current Human Genome Project, which is touted as an international collaboration, uses only European families as models in its formulation of a "representative" human genome.

In order to avoid bias, logically sound use of generalization should be based on genuinely representative samples. Representative samples are usually generated by randomly selecting members from the particular group under study. Thus, a study of the effects of a particular medicine on humans would include a roughly even number of male and female subjects, and a typical human genome would be based on the genomes of people from all over the world.

Combining Deductive and Inductive Reasoning

Western moral analysis has traditionally focused on abstract, deductive reasoning. Those who favor an inductive approach to healthcare ethics argue that the particulars of a case—the persons, the circumstances, and the relationships between people—and not abstract philosophical principles form the foundation of ethical analysis; rather than being absolutely binding, the moral principles need to be weighed against the concrete particulars. Those who favor a deductive approach, in contrast, argue that moral principles are more important and that individual cases should be judged in light of these principles.

Inductive and deductive logic, however, are not mutually exclusive methods of critical thinking. Moral analysis makes use of multiple methods of analysis, including both deductive and inductive reasoning. The relationship between deductive and inductive reasoning in healthcare ethics is dialectical rather than exclusive. *Dialectic* is a term derived from the Greek word meaning "to converse" and was used by Socrates in his pursuit of the Truth. We touched on the relationship between deductive and inductive logic in our discussion in Chapter 1 on the principlism/casuistry debate.

Resolving Moral Conflicts

The great majority of moral decisions are straightforward and do not need to be subjected to critical analysis in order for us to know what is right and what is wrong. Moral decision making is such a normal part of our everyday life that we generally don't even give it a second thought. For example, we don't run over a pedestrian even though he may be annoying us by jaywalking. We don't club a student in the library and steal her class notes just because we happened to miss class that day (or for any reason short of self-defense, for that matter). Similarly, we don't need to lay out our premises and engage in logical analysis to know that, as healthcare professionals, we ought not to euthanize a patient who has just found out that she has contracted gonorrhea, a treatable disease, even though she may exclaim in dismay, "I am so embarrassed; I wish I were dead!" We don't need to struggle over whether it would be morally acceptable to kidnap and kill a fellow student in order to use his organs to save a parent's life.

Sometimes, however, we encounter a situation or issue in which the right thing to do is not so clear-cut. Most of the issues covered in this text contain moral conflicts. Issues involving conflicting values, by their very nature, demand that we sort out and take a closer look at the moral values involved and learn how to analyze the arguments on all sides of the issue. John Rawls recommends that we engage in reflective equilibrium, a process that is used in science, as a means of achieving this goal. According to him, we may want to change our judgments once the "regulative principles" are brought to light. Knowledge of these principles and of discrepancies between them and our judgment "may suggest further reflections that lead us to revise our judgments."[40] Practice in resolving moral conflicts has been found to be an effective means of improving our skill at moral reasoning, and learning how to identify fallacious reasoning is an essential component of this process.

LOGICAL FALLACIES

In constructing and analyzing a moral argument, we need to make sure it contains no **fallacies.** Several things can make an argument weak or invalid. Formal fallacies occur when the structure of a deductive argument is faulty. An argument that is psychologically or emotionally persuasive but logically incorrect contains what logicians call an informal fallacy. Fallacies can be used as a form of resistance to keep us or others from analyzing our position, or we may unwittingly use certain fallacies because of cultural conditioning. We are most likely to use fallacies when we are unsure of how to support our position. The use of fallacies may be effective in the short run, but thoughtful people will eventually begin to question faulty reasoning.

Knowing how to recognize informal fallacies makes us less likely to fall victim to them or to use them unwittingly in an argument. Discussion of some of the informal fallacies that are most likely to appear in arguments on moral issues follows.

Equivocation

Some terms have several meanings. Most often, the context in which a particular word or phrase appears tells us which definition is being used; however, this is not always the case. A particular term that has several meanings is called an ambiguous term. The fallacy of **equivocation** occurs when an ambiguous word or phrase changes meaning in the course of an argument, as in the following argument:

ABDUL: All people have a right to a minimal level of healthcare.
SAM: That's not true. Our Constitution says nothing about people having a right to healthcare; therefore, as taxpayers we have no obligation to provide it.

The term *right* is frequently the subject of equivocation, in one instance being used to mean a legal right and in another a moral right. In the above argument, Abdul and Sam are using different meanings of the term *right*. The term is notoriously ambiguous, with *Webster's Encyclopedic Unabridged Dictionary* listing sixty-two meanings! Taking a closer look at their argument, we can see that Abdul is most likely talking about rights in terms of moral or human rights, while Sam is using the term to refer to legal rights. Their first task in resolving their disagreement is to agree on which definition of *right* they will use. The fact that something is a legal or constitutional right does not logically imply that it is a moral right, because we do not live in an ideal society. The morality of certain practices, as noted in the section on the fallacy of appeal to tradition, has to be justified on other than legal grounds.

Because Abdul and Sam did not first clearly define their key terms, they have become caught up in a **verbal dispute** rather than engaging in genuine analysis of the issue at hand. In order to avoid the fallacy of equivocation, key terms should be clearly defined and used in a consistent manner throughout the argument.

Ad Hominem Fallacy

The **ad hominem fallacy** occurs when we attack an opponent rather than respond to his or her argument. There are two types of ad hominem fallacies: the abusive fallacy and the circumstantial fallacy. The **abusive fallacy** occurs when we disagree with someone's conclusion and, instead of addressing their argument, turn and attack their character. In doing so, we attempt to evoke disapproval of the person who made the argument, with the expectation that it will overflow into disapproval of that person's argument.

The abusive fallacy may take the form of mocking or putting down people whose views conflict with those of the establishment. For example, the interpretation of Christianity by black Americans has been shaped by their African heritage, in which the body is regarded as sacred in all its parts. One consequence of this is that many black Americans are reluctant to donate organs because they believe that they need all their organs in order to enter heaven. In a column in the *Washington Post*, journalist Courtland Milloy used the ad hominem fallacy to try to convince black Americans to change their view:

> It was my idea to ridicule those who are so superstitious that they would rather see a body rot in a grave than donate an organ to help save a life. Those who believe that donating eyes, for example, will cause them to miss seeing their friends in heaven should be pegged for what they are: stupid.[41]

In the above argument, the issue of organ donation has been completely sidestepped. Instead, the journalist has become caught up in slandering the character of those who hold the opposing view. The abusive fallacy can also take the form of namecalling, cutting humor, sarcastic remarks, eye rolling, or scoffing. While it may be tempting to respond in kind by attacking the character of the person who has engaged in slander, a person skilled in critical thinking knows how to calmly bring the discussion back to the subject at hand rather than fall for such diversionary tactics.

The **circumstantial fallacy** occurs when we argue that our opponent should accept a certain position because of his or her special circumstances, such as a particular lifestyle or membership in a particular group based on race, ethnicity, gender, nationality, or religion. The following argument is an example of this fallacy:

Granted, you may be opposed to the use of animals in research, but you certainly can't argue against it. After all, you use and benefit from products that are tested on animals.

Contrary to the above argument, a person can use products tested on animals and still argue against animal testing, just as people who wore clothes made from cotton grown on Southern plantations could still argue against slavery. The fact that they wore cotton clothes is irrelevant to the validity or strength of their argument against slavery. Similarly, healthcare professionals who are heavy smokers or drinkers can still give their clients sound arguments against smoking and alcohol abuse.

Also, membership in a particular group does not entail accepting all the views of that group. It might be assumed that a woman should hold certain views on women's issues or that a person who is Catholic should subscribe to the Church's views on medical issues, as in the following example of the circumstantial fallacy:

How can you argue in favor of cloning? After all, you're a Catholic, and the Church recently issued a statement calling for a ban on human cloning.

The fact that a person is a member of a particular group does not logically entail that he or she uncritically accepts the views held by the majority of people, or at least the spokespersons, in that group.

Hasty Generalization

Used properly, generalization can be a valuable tool for gathering information in both the physical and the social sciences. A generalization is valid if it is based on observations of a representative sampling of a group. The fallacy of **hasty generalization** occurs when we use only a few or only unusual or atypical cases to support our conclusion, hastily generalizing to a rule or conclusion that fits only these unusual cases rather than the whole group. For example, in the case study mentioned at the opening of this chapter, Dr. Joseph Collins concluded that "many experiences show that patients do not want the truth about their maladies, and that it is prejudicial to their well-being to know it," based on a few atypical cases in which patients later stated that they regretted learning that they had cancer. In fact, most of Collins's patients told him that they wanted to know the truth about their condition.

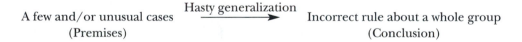

A few and/or unusual cases   Hasty generalization   →   Incorrect rule about a whole group
(Premises)   (Conclusion)

The following example is a hasty generalization that was frequently heard during the debate several years ago regarding nationalized healthcare in the United States:

Canadians are clearly dissatisfied with their nationalized healthcare system, as is demonstrated by the large number of Canadians who cross the border to get healthcare in the United States.

This fallacious argument took me by surprise when I first heard it. During the ten years I lived in Canada, I never heard of one Canadian going to the United States for medical treatment, nor have I seen any studies bearing out the claim of a mass exodus of ailing Canadians pouring into American hospitals and doctors' offices.

The following is another example of hasty generalization:

> Smoking isn't all that bad for your health. After all, my grandfather began smoking when he was thirteen, and he's ninety-three years old now and still in good health!

The fact that the grandfather's health has not been adversely affected does not mean that smoking, in general, is not unhealthy. We cannot generalize from one unusual case to a general rule that "smoking isn't all that bad for your health."

Accident

The **fallacy of accident** is the opposite of hasty generalization. Instead of going from a specific case to a general rule, this fallacy applies a general rule or principle to a particular situation that is an exception to the rule. Because the rule works in most cases, it is assumed that the rule should work for all cases.

Good general rule   <u>Accident</u> → Atypical or accidental cases
(Premises)   (Conclusion)

The following is an example of the fallacy of accident:

> Jonathan Camel just found out he has lung cancer. He is in shock and is suicidal as well as homicidal. A nonsmoker, he is also furious at his wife, Josephine, a smoker, who he believes gave him the cancer. He is in the doctor's office with his terrified wife and is ranting and waving a gun in the air, yelling that if he is going to die he is going to kill her, too. He demands that the doctor tell him his prognosis. *Since it is wrong to lie, the doctor is morally obligated to tell him that his prognosis is very poor and he will probably die within the year.*

In the above example, the person making the argument has committed the fallacy of accident by applying a good rule—"Do not lie"—to an atypical or accidental case. While "Do not lie" is a good rule in the majority of cases, the harm of telling the truth—the death of at least two people—outweighs the moral duty to tell the truth in this case.

The fact that there are exceptions to rules does not mean that we should throw out the rules and become ethical subjectivists, any more than the fact that there are exceptions to legal rules means that we should become anarchists. Consider the following example: Your toddler is critically ill after accidentally swallowing some rat poison. He is blue in the face and is having convulsions. On your way to the hospital, you run a red light at an empty intersection. A police officer pulls you over. Desperate, you explain the situation. The police officer, however, responds, "Sorry, the law is the law and you broke the law." She then detains you to check your driver's license and write you a ticket. Most of us would consider the officer to have been remiss in her duty, even though she was obeying the letter of the law. While we may agree that laws against speeding and running red lights are, in general, good, almost all of us agree that in exceptional circumstances these otherwise good laws may not apply. The same is the case with moral rules, such as "Do not lie." As with any rule, we have to use our discernment in applying moral rules and consider the context in which they are being applied.

Popular Appeal

We commit the fallacy of **popular appeal** when we use the fact that the majority of people agree with a particular position as support for the truth of that position. Also known as the bandwagon approach, it assumes that a certain conclusion is right simply because "everyone" is doing it or "everyone" believes it. Consider this example:

> Everyone (there is general consensus) agrees that humans have higher moral value than animals. Therefore, it is morally acceptable to use animals in medical experiments that benefit humans.

The fact that a consensus, or the majority of people, agrees with a certain worldview or a certain practice, such as animal experimentation, does not mean that it is right. After all, the majority of people once believed that the earth was flat, that women were morally inferior to men, and that slavery was morally acceptable. Similarly, the fact that there is a consensus within a particular culture against a certain practice, such as human cloning, doesn't mean that it is immoral.

John Stuart Mill once said that one danger of living in a democracy is the "tyranny of the majority." In 1826, historian Alexis de Tocqueville visited the United States, where he made the observation that, although democracy may have liberated us from tradition, the great democratic danger is enslavement to public opinion. In fact, studies show that the majority of Americans define morality primarily in terms of what the majority believes to be right or wrong.[42] The heavy reliance on opinion polls to appraise the morality of a particular issue, such as legalized abortion or human cloning, is a case in point. This fallacious belief that the majority opinion determines what is moral can lead to an erosion of intellectual freedom and to intolerance of ideas and people who are different. Because of the tendency to conform and go along with the majority, we need to be especially alert to the temptation to succumb to this fallacy.

Appeal to Inappropriate Authority

In discussions of moral issues, it is appropriate to use the testimony of someone who is an expert in the field. For example, it is reasonable to accept the authority of a physician or X-ray technician regarding diagnosis of a broken bone or the expertise of a nurse regarding the effects of a certain medication on a particular patient, or to consult a geneticist to learn more about the possible long-term consequences of genetic engineering. We commit the fallacy of **appeal to inappropriate authority,** however, when we appeal to an expert or authority in a field other than the one under debate.

> My priest says that genetic engineering and cloning are dangerous. Therefore, all experimentation in this field should be discontinued immediately.

In the above example, the person cited is an authority in theology rather than in the medical field. On the other hand, physicians are not necessarily experts in healthcare ethics. Medical pronouncements may be confused with value judgments because of the perception that physicians are authorities.

According to my physician, a feeding tube and ventilation for a comatose patient is considered ordinary, rather than extraordinary, treatment. Therefore, it would be immoral to remove the feeding tube or turn off the respirator.

Titles such as Reverend, Doctor, and Professor increase our perception of a person's authority. We tend to believe and obey authority figures even when they overextend their authority to the point that it would be appropriate to question their authority. This was poignantly demonstrated in the Milgram study on obedience to authority, in which two-thirds of the subjects continued to follow the orders of an authority, figure even though they thought doing so might result in the injury or death of another person.[43] Because of the high status and often uncritical acceptance of the authority of physicians in many cultures, including most Western cultures, we may commit this fallacy when we defer to the physician's authority on matters that are not matters of medical judgment.

Ignorance

The **fallacy of ignorance** does not imply that we are stupid; it simply means that we are ignorant of how to go about proving something. This fallacy occurs whenever it is argued that our conclusion is true simply because it has not been proved false or that it is false simply because it has not been proved true. For example, in defense of his position that black people are innately inferior to white people, biologist Arthur Jensen writes:

> No one has yet produced any evidence based on a properly controlled study to show that representative samples of Negro and white children can be equalized in intellectual ability through statistical control of environment and education.[44]

However, it does not logically follow from lack of evidence that "Negro and white children" *cannot* be "equalized in intellectual ability," a conclusion Jensen later draws. Similarly, we cannot conclude that life does not exist in other galaxies simply on the basis of lack of evidence of its existence. The most we can conclude in both cases is that we don't know.

Tobacco companies use this fallacy when they argue that smoking is safe because studies have not conclusively proved that smoking causes lung cancer. However, as we noted in the section on inductive arguments, scientific studies such as those on the relation between smoking and cancer offer not conclusive proof but only probable evidence of their conclusions.

We also commit the fallacy of ignorance when we dismiss someone's views on the grounds that they are based on superstition or religion. Some people, including Orthodox Jews and many Africans, are reluctant to donate their organs. The Ebira of Nigeria, for example, believe that the body is sacred in all its parts. All body organs are treated with reverence. Hair and nail cuttings are carefully disposed of because of their spiritual power. Corpses are also treated with reverence. In this worldview, body parts or organs are not interchangeable, like machine parts.[45] This worldview has been challenged on the grounds that "it is based upon superstition or myth," the implication being that it is mistaken. The often paternalistic assumption that other cultures' values are mere superstition prevents us from taking them seriously and, perhaps, learning from the other cultures. On the other hand, we also need to learn how to discern the difference

MEDIEVAL EUROPE:
Demons, Genetic Disorders, and Infanticide

Attitudes toward pregnancy and birth in medieval Europe were a blend of pagan myth, Christian beliefs, superstition, and folklore. Many people believed that the sexual behavior of the parents, especially the mother, and demonic intervention were responsible for abnormal births. Women who had a child with birth defects were sometimes accused of having had an illicit affair or even a sexual liaison with the devil. Other explanations placed the blame on forces outside the parents' control. According to the pagan changling myth, fairies who were envious of humans substituted an elf child for the real child.[46]

The changling myth was later Christianized, and it became the devil who stole the real child and substituted a demon child. With this development, blame was once again placed on the mother. God, it was believed, allowed this switch as punishment for women bearing children outside of marriage or having illicit affairs. Brutal methods were used to exorcise the devil from "illegitimate" children and children born with defects. Few infants survived these ordeals.

Laws against infanticide were passed late in the Middle Ages. However, infants born outside of marriage and infants with serious deformities were not considered persons and fell outside the protection of the law. This placed a tremendous hardship on their mothers. Unmarried women who killed their infants were often accused of being witches and were severely punished, usually by drowning, live burial, or impalement. Punishment was not so much for killing the infant, since illegitimate children fell outside the pro-

between superstition and reason, both in the worldviews of other cultures and in our own cultural views.

False Cause

In healthcare ethics, claims regarding cause and effect must be based on solid research rather than on mere opinion. The fallacy of **false cause** occurs when we mistakenly think something is the cause of an event when, in fact, it is not. The fact that one event follows another does not logically imply that the first event caused the other. For example, physicians assumed until recently that cancer patients fare better if they do not know the terrible truth about their condition. Later studies, however, revealed that withholding this information actually has a negative effect on the health of most cancer patients. Any improvement that did occur in the studies was caused not by naiveté, but by other factors such as a strong social support system.

Similarly, it has long been assumed that exposure to cold, damp weather causes people to catch colds. Despite numerous studies showing no causal relationship between being cold and wet and catching a cold, many people continue to believe in this

tection of the law, but for engaging in illicit sex.

The medical profession did little to enhance the lives of these children. Although abandonment of illegitimate children and babies with serious defects at foundling hospitals was considered less morally objectionable than infanticide, in reality most of the children in these institutions died of neglect or disease.

The beliefs that genetic defects are the fault of the parent and that children with genetic disorders have less moral value have been slow in dying. Even today, members of the family of a child with a serious genetic disorder frequently experience "cosmic guilt" and shame associated with being carriers of "bad" genes. They may also "interpret nature's machinations as punishment resulting from their own conduct."[47]

This guilt is exacerbated by the social stigma that is attached to the parents and family of children who are retarded or have genetic defects. This stigma can lead to a lack of community support and outright rejection by neighbors, as well as a lack of support from the medical profession. The message is often conveyed that these children should not have been born. In her study of families of children with genetic disorders, Rosalyn Darling found that medical professionals frequently treated the children as "things" and that the "medical treatment their children received had often been delivered in a rude and dehumanizing way."[48]

Even though we may know on an intellectual level that parents are not morally responsible for their children's genetic disorders and that children with disorders are not "bad," old myths die hard. Fallacious thinking is not morally neutral; it affects our actions as well as our reasoning processes. Discarding fallacious thinking requires constantly being aware of how easy it is to fall for fallacious reasoning and making an effort to overcome it.

false cause to this day. Another medical myth based on false cause is that reading in the dark damages your eyes.

An apparent causal connection between two events may sometimes seem so obvious that it may be years before anybody bothers to check the validity of the presumed connection. Consider the following argument:

Restrictive abortion laws lead to unwanted children. Children who are unwanted are more likely to be abused. Therefore, legalizing abortion will result in a decline in child abuse.

In fact, a controlled study at Johns Hopkins Medical Center found that having had an abortion is one of the main predictors of whether a woman will become a child abuser.[49] In addition, child abuse rates in the United States began increasing dramatically in 1974, the year abortion was legalized.[50] Further studies should be conducted to see whether this is a genuine causal relationship or simply a correlation, with the increase in child abuse due to a third factor.

Assumptions believed by the majority of people or by those in power are less likely to be subjected to critical analysis. The optimistic belief that legalizing abortion would lead to a decline in child abuse has not been borne out in studies. This does not mean that abortion is immoral, only that it cannot be justified on the grounds that it benefits children. Similarly, the fact that being damp and cold does not cause colds does not mean that we should send our children out in raw winter weather without hats and coats. There may be other compelling reasons for staying warm and dry, just as there may be other compelling reasons for legalizing abortion.

Begging the Question

Also known as circular reasoning, the fallacy of **begging the question** occurs when a premise and a conclusion are rewordings of the same proposition. In other words, in presenting our argument we assume the truth of our conclusion rather than offer proof for it. In some cases, the premise simply defines the key term in the conclusion rather than supporting it. This fallacy is often difficult to recognize because the premise and the conclusion are worded differently. At first glance, the argument may seem to be airtight because the premise seems to support the conclusion so perfectly, as in the following argument:

> Suicide is morally acceptable because people have the right to choose when and how they will end their life.

Rather than offering support for the conclusion "suicide is morally acceptable," the premise simply restates it. If we reverse the premise and the conclusion, we can see that the premise and the conclusion are the same proposition: "People have a right to choose when and how they will end their life because suicide is morally acceptable."

Irrelevant Conclusion

The fallacy of **irrelevant conclusion** occurs when we support or reject a conclusion by using premises that are directed at a different conclusion. We may try to avoid a specific topic that makes us feel uncomfortable by changing the topic to something more general or less controversial. In other words, we throw in a "red herring" in an attempt to divert attention from the real issue.

> BEN: As medical professionals, I think we have a moral obligation to provide medical services to people who are HIV positive, even if doing so puts us at a slight risk of contracting AIDS.
>
> JEN: I think AIDS is a terrible disease. I hope we find a cure for AIDS.

In this argument, Jen sidesteps the discussion of the moral obligation to treat people who are HIV positive by changing the topic to a less controversial topic—finding a cure for AIDS. When this fallacy appears in a discussion of a moral issue, we should immediately bring the discussion back to the topic at hand rather than let it go off on a tangent.

The fallacy of irrelevant conclusion is, unfortunately, all too common in discussions of political issues and often impedes rational discussion and resolution of public policy issues in healthcare. For example, in 1998, the U.S. Justice Department was considering bringing a Medicare lawsuit against the tobacco industry to recover medical expenses for treatment of smoking-related diseases, expenses footed by taxpayers.

Asked about the lawsuit, a tobacco company spokesman replied that it sounded like an effort by the administration "to find a way to cover their own failures of leadership in this matter by trying to come up with a political and public relations gesture."[51] The spokesman deflected any discussion of the legitimacy of the lawsuit or the efforts of the U.S. Justice Department by instead focusing attention on the alleged failures of the Democratic administration.

Naturalistic Fallacy

This fallacy is a special type of irrelevant conclusion. We commit the **naturalistic fallacy** when we assume that because something *is* the case then it *ought* to be that way, as illustrated in the following examples:

Euthanasia is wrong because it interferes with the natural dying process. We should wait until it is our time to die.

Cloning is morally wrong because it is unnatural for humans to reproduce asexually.

The following example is a more insidious use of the naturalistic fallacy:

Men are larger and naturally more aggressive than women. Therefore, the man ought to be the dominant partner in a relationship.

The above observation, which seems to have some basis in reality, has been used to justify a patriarchal society in which men occupy the dominant positions, such as physicians, and women play subordinate, nurturing roles, such as nurses or aides. However, the fact that men may be more dominating and aggressive and women more nurturing, if in fact this is true, does not logically imply that our social structure ought be patterned on this natural difference, nor does it mean that physicians should have a higher status than nurses. One need not deny that natural differences exist between men and women in order to argue that patriarchal social structures that privilege men are immoral.

People who use the naturalistic fallacy sometimes cite the natural activities of non-human animals. However, it does not follow logically from the fact that male mammals usually behave more aggressively and are dominant over females, or that other animals eat meat, or that they sometimes kill and eat their young, or that most animals have several sexual partners (and a few even eat their partner after mating!) that it is morally acceptable for humans to do the same. The morality of these behaviors must be evaluated on grounds other than the fact that they are natural.

Appeal to Tradition

According to psychologist Lawrence Kohlberg, the majority of American adults base their moral decisions primarily on conformity to cultural and legal norms rather than on universal moral principles.[52] In other words, most American adults are cultural relativists.

The fallacy of **appeal to tradition** occurs when we argue that a certain practice is morally justified because it is the custom or tradition. This fallacy is often accompanied

🌿 TWELVE INFORMAL FALLACIES

Informal fallacies are psychologically persuasive but incorrect arguments.

1. *Equivocation:* A key term shifts meaning during the course of an argument.

2. *Ad hominem fallacy:* We attack our opponents' character (abusive fallacy) or argue that they should accept a particular conclusion because of their life-style or group membership (circumstantial fallacy) rather than address their conclusion.

3. *Hasty generalization:* Our conclusion is based on atypical cases.

4. *Accident:* A good general rule is applied to an atypical case.

5. *Popular appeal:* The opinion of the majority is used as support for a conclusion.

6. *Appeal to inappropriate authority:* The testimony of someone who is an authority in a different field is used as support for our conclusion.

7. *Ignorance:* We argue that a certain position is true because it hasn't been proved false or that it is false because it hasn't been proved true.

8. *False cause:* We mistake something for the cause of an event when, in fact, it is not the cause.

9. *Begging the question:* The premise and the conclusion are different wordings of the same proposition.

10. *Irrelevant conclusion:* Our argument is directed at a conclusion other than the one under discussion.

11. *Naturalistic fallacy:* We argue from an "is" to an "ought."

12. *Appeal to tradition:* We argue that something is moral because it is a tradition.

by the fallacy of popular appeal, as in the following example from an article in a science journal on the use of genetically modified pigs as organ donors for humans:

> As organ donors, the only nonhuman animals that make more sense than pigs are apes, our closest relatives. But most people would question the ethics of breeding chimpanzees or gorillas or orangutans for their organs. . . . [On the other hand] raising pigs for their flesh is a venerable, 7,000-year-old tradition. With 95.7 million pigs making that one-way trip each year to the supermarket, an extra few thousand sacrificed for a nobler cause than sausage would probably not bring out the Porcine Liberation Army.[53]

Appeal to tradition may also take the form of an argument that a particular practice, such as abortion, is moral because it is constitutional. However, the U.S. Constitution is a legal document, not a moral document. Our Constitution also permitted slavery for almost a century and prevented women from voting for even longer. Like slavery, abortion has been defended as a constitutional right. However, a constitutional right is not the same as a moral right, although in a perfectly just society legal institutions would be in harmony with the moral law.

A CRITICAL ANALYSIS OF JUDITH JARVIS THOMSON'S "A DEFENSE OF ABORTION"

In this section we will apply critical thinking skills to Judith Jarvis Thomson's argument on the morality of abortion, which appears at the end of this chapter. The various parts of her argument are broken down into their premises (bracketed in the article) and main conclusions (underlined). Her arguments as well as the counterarguments (CA) are identified in the margins to assist you in the critical analysis process.

In her analysis of the abortion issue, Thomson, starts off by examining one of the basic assumptions or premises of the pro-life position: that the human fetus is a person. After examining the relevant facts about the biological and mental development of the fetus, Thomson concludes that the fetus becomes a person sometime after conception but before birth. However, she does not venture to state at what point in pregnancy this might occur.

Because she is unable to prove that the fetus is not a person, Thomson decides to give the pro-life position the benefit of the doubt. She accepts as true the premise that the human fetus is a person. Having accepted this initial premise, Thomson goes on to analyze the rest of the argument in support of the position that "abortion is immoral." The deductive argument, which is in two parts, proceeds as follows:

1. The fetus is a person.
   A person has a right to life.
   Therefore, the fetus has a right to life.

2. The fetus has a right to life.
   Abortion destroys the life of the fetus.
   Therefore, abortion is immoral.

Although Thomson accepts the premises of the pro-life argument, she disputes the final conclusion. The conclusion "abortion is immoral," she argues, does not follow from the premises. In particular, Thomson maintains that the right to life is not absolute. Therefore, even if the fetus does have a right to life, this right is not absolute. Furthermore, she continues, the right to life is a negative right, not a positive right. A negative right to life does not entail a positive right to life support by the woman.

In addition, pure deductive logic fails to take into consideration the context of pregnancy and abortion. The fetus lives inside the body of a woman. Pregnancy, especially an unwanted pregnancy, requires considerable sacrifice on the part of a woman. Instead of adopting a deductive approach, as used in the pro-life argument above, Thomson uses a primarily inductive approach, in the form of a series of analogies that illustrate the relationship between a woman and her fetus. Among the analogies she uses is her well-known analogy between being pregnant and waking up one morning to find a famous, unconscious violinist attached to your back. The analogy is presented as follows:

> You wake up in the morning and find yourself back to back in bed with an unconscious violinist. A famous unconscious violinist. He has been found to have a fatal kidney

ailment, and the Society of Music Lovers has canvassed all available medical records and found that you alone have the right blood type to help. They have therefore kidnapped you, and last night the violinist's circulatory system was plugged into yours, so that your kidneys can be used to extract poisons from his blood as well as your own. The director of the hospital now tells you, "Look, we're sorry the Society of Music Lovers did this to you—we would never have permitted it if we had known. But still, they did it, and the violinist is now plugged into you. To unplug you would be to kill him. But never mind, it's only for nine months. By then he will have recovered from his ailment, and can be safely unplugged from you.

After presenting this analogy, Thomson poses a series of questions: "Is it morally incumbent on you to accede to this situation . . . do you *have* to accede to it? What if it were not nine months, but nine years?" After asking these questions, she proceeds with her analysis by examining the different possible answers to these questions.

Thomson first considers what she calls the "extreme view" that "abortion is impermissible even to save the mother's life." This view, she points out, conflicts with the mother's right to life as well as her right to decide what happens to her own body. The generally accepted belief that people have a right to defend their own life implies that it is not wrong for a woman to perform an abortion on herself if the purpose is to save her life. Thomson uses another analogy to further illustrate her point. Suppose a child is growing so rapidly inside a tiny house that it threatens to destroy the house (the mother). Surely in this case the mother has a right to self-defense, even if it means destroying the life of an innocent child.

What about situations in which the fetus is not threatening the life of the mother? Does the mother, in this case, have a duty to allow the fetus to use her body? Thomson asks us to consider a situation in which she is dying and the only thing that will save her life is the "touch of Henry Fonda's cool hand on my fevered brow." She suggests that, while it would be awfully nice if Henry Fonda came to her bedside to soothe her fevered brow, he surely does not have a moral duty to do so. Similarly, while it would be awfully nice if a woman allowed a fetus to use her body, she does not have a moral duty to do so. "The right to life," Thomson concludes, "consists not in the right not to be killed, but rather in the right not to be killed unjustly. We do not violate another person's right to life by refusing to allow them to use our body."

In the final analysis, the strength of Thomson's argument depends on whether or not you accept her analogies. Thomson's argument depends primarily on a casuistic, inductive approach. Analogies, as we noted earlier, unlike deductive reasoning, are not true or false but simply better or worse. Casuists use representative case studies to generate solutions to moral problems. However, are the analogies used by Thomson typical of the situation of women with unwanted pregnancies? Some critics think that Thomson's analogies have too many dissimilarities. The relationship between a mother and her fetus, they maintain, is not the same as that between Henry Fonda and a stranger on her deathbed or even between the violinist and a kidnapped organ donor, although this analogy is generally thought to be the stronger of the two.

Analogies also should be checked for fallacies. For example, is Thomson's violinist analogy based on a hasty generalization regarding the burdensomeness of pregnancy that, in turn, is based on a medical model of pregnancy as a "disease" or disability? In actual fact, is even an unwanted pregnancy as burdensome as carrying an unconscious and unrelated adult (who will presumably be snatched from us at the moment of "birth") on our back for nine months?

Even if we accept the violinist analogy, it is relevant only in cases of rape, given that the person was coercively hooked up to the violinist. What about cases in which the woman consents to sexual intercourse knowing that she might become pregnant as a result? Does the act of participating in sexual intercourse entail giving tacit consent, should she become pregnant, for the fetus to use her body, even though it is an unwanted pregnancy?

Thomson uses a further analogy to deal with this question. Suppose, she argues, there are people-seeds drifting around in the air like pollen and you put screens on your windows because you don't want children. Despite the best precautions, sometimes a people-seed does get into a house. Do you have a moral obligation to allow the people-seed to take up residence in your house even though you have done everything reasonable to prevent such a scenario? Thomson says no; you are morally justified in sweeping out the people-seed, even though this destroys its chance to germinate.

Again, we need to analyze this analogy critically before accepting her conclusion. First of all, for Thomson, positive rights are created only by voluntary commitments. The fetus has a right to a woman's body only if the woman makes a voluntary commitment to let the fetus use her body. However, can an involuntary commitment also create a positive right? Furthermore, is Thomson taking the personhood of the fetus seriously in comparing him or her to a seed pod, which surely is not very personlike? To correct these dissimilarities in her analogy, we can analyze her line of reasoning using another analogy in which the fetus is compared to a being that most of us would surely agree is a person but the commitment under consideration is still involuntary. One such analogy is that of a cabin and an abandoned child. It is the middle of winter, which lasts nine months where you live. One morning you wake up to find a young child sitting just inside your door. You have no transportation to take the child to town. However, you have plenty of food for both you and the abandoned child. Given this situation, is it morally acceptable for you to put the child back outside, where she will surely freeze to death; or do you have a moral obligation to house and feed the child until spring, when you can take her to a nearby town and turn her over to someone else?

Thomson's Henry Fonda analogy has also been criticized as being weak. It can be strengthened by making it more similar to an actual pregnancy. For example, what if Fonda happened to be getting his annual checkup in the hospital where Thomson was staying and he was aware that his magic touch would save her life? Furthermore, what if Thomson was related to Fonda—perhaps his child or his younger sister or cousin? Would his refusal to comply under these circumstances still be considered morally acceptable?

Thomson tends to view people as distinct autonomous beings rather than as interdependent beings. Are we willing to accept her views of human nature and community? Or does Thomson, in her arguments, place too much weight on the principle of autonomy, in particular maternal autonomy, and neglect other principles, such as duties of beneficence and nonmaleficence toward fetuses? Good moral reasoning requires that we check our intuition against the universal moral principles. How does Thomson address moral concerns, such as community, fidelity, and self-improvement, that tend to be downplayed in Western culture?

While Americans tend to regard beneficence as a negative duty, are there in fact times when we have a positive duty to save the lives of other persons? Most people believe that we have a moral obligation to save the life of someone, even a stranger, if we can do so with only minimal risk to ourselves. We have a moral obligation to try to help, or at least summon help, for someone who has been struck by a car or is being assaulted outside our window, as in the case of Kitty Genovese, which Thomson cites. What we cannot do, morally, is simply walk away from or ignore calls for help. Similarly, we are morally obligated to pick up drowning swimmers, even though we may be far out at sea and the rescue may interfere with our romantic honeymoon cruise.

Taking this obligation into account, Thomson concludes that each person has a duty to be a *Minimally Decent Samaritan*. It would be indecent, for instance, for a seven-month-pregnant woman to request an abortion because she doesn't want to postpone a trip abroad. Conceding this, she goes on to emphasize that no one has a right to force us to be *Good Samaritans* and compel us to carry an unwanted pregnancy for the full nine months.

However, at this point Thomson shows her bias. While Thomson began by saying that she would take the personhood of the fetus seriously, her analogies, which take the personhood of the woman seriously but not the personhood of the fetus, suggest that she does not really consider the fetus to be a person. In the very last sentence of her argument she states, "A very early abortion is surely not the killing of a person." Thomson offers no support for this statement. Nowhere has she dealt with the criteria for personhood, and this is one of the biggest weaknesses of her argument. Indeed, this bias against the fetus shows up in her analogies.

In critical analysis, it is important to take a position—even if it is an unpopular position—and resist the temptation to fall into relativism or superficial tolerance. Martin Luther King, Jr., once said that "many people fear nothing more terribly than to take a position which stands out sharply and clearly from prevailing opinion. The tendency of most is to adopt a view that is so ambiguous that it will include everything, and so popular that it will include everyone."[54] If an argument is weak, we should reject it.

Even if we reject Thomson's argument, this does not mean that abortion, in general, is not morally defensible. Mary Anne Warren, whose article appears in Chapter 4, rejects Thomson's argument. However, rather than concluding that abortion is indefensible, Warren goes back to the initial premises and argues that the fetus is not a person. Now we have the task of deciding if Warren's definition of personhood, which eliminates fetuses as well as some born humans, is based on rational criteria. And so the process of moral analysis continues, as we examine moral issues and particular circumstances from different points of view and apply different facets of logic to the analysis.

JUDITH JARVIS THOMSON

A Defense of Abortion

Judith Jarvis Thomson is a professor of philosophy at the Massachusetts Institute of Technology. Her article "A Defense of Abortion," published two years before *Roe v. Wade*, has become a classic in the abortion debate. Rather than attempt to refute the premises that the fetus is a person and that every person has a right to life, Thomson argues that abortion may be morally permissible even if these premises are true. Using her now-famous violinist analogy, Thomson attempts to show that even if the fetus has a right to life, this right does not entail the right to have whatever one needs—including use of a woman's body—to stay alive.

Most opposition to abortion relies on the premise that the fetus is a human being, a person, from the moment of conception. The premise is argued for, but, as I think, not well. Take, for example, the most common argument. We are asked to notice that the development of a human being from conception through birth into childhood is continuous; then it is said that to draw a line, to choose a point in this development and say "before this point the thing is not a person, after this point it is a person" is to make an arbitrary choice, a choice for which in the nature of things no good reason can be given. It is concluded that the fetus is, or anyway that we had better say it is, a person from the moment of conception. But this conclusion does not follow. *[Similar things might be said about the development of an acorn into an oak tree, and it does not follow that acorns are oak trees, or that we had better say they are.]* Arguments of this form are sometimes called "slippery slope arguments"—the phrase is perhaps self-explanatory—and it is dismaying that opponents of abortion rely on them so heavily and uncritically.

I am inclined to agree, however, that the prospects for "drawing a line" in the development of the fetus look dim. I am inclined to think also that *[we shall have to agree that the fetus has already become a human person well before birth.]* Indeed, it comes as a surprise when one first learns how early in its life it begins to acquire human characteristics. By the tenth week, for example, it already has a face, arms and legs, fingers and toes; it has internal organs, and brain activity is detectable. On the other hand, I think that the premise is false, that the fetus is not a person from the moment of

Margin notes:

CA* 1: Fetus is a person

J. T.'s response to CA 1

Oak tree analogy

Definition of key term "person"

Premise #1: Fetus is a person

---

*CA stands for counterargument.

conception. A newly fertilized ovum, a newly implanted clump of cells, is no more a person than an acorn is an oak tree. But I shall not discuss any of this. For it seems to me to be of great interest to ask what happens if, for the sake of argument, we allow the premise. . . .

Explanation of premise #1

I propose, then, that [we grant that the fetus is a person from the moment of conception.] How does the argument go from here? Something like this, I take it. [Every person has a right to life.] So the fetus has a right to life. No doubt the [mother has a right to decide what shall happen in and to her body;] everyone would grant that. But surely a person's right to life is stronger and more stringent than the mother's right to decide what happens in and to her body, and so outweighs it. [So the fetus may not be killed; an abortion may not be performed.]

Premise #1 and premise #2: Fetus has a right to life

Premise #3: The mother has a right to life

CA 2: The fetus may not be killed

It sounds plausible. But now let me ask you to imagine this. You wake up in the morning and find yourself back to back in bed with an unconscious violinist. A famous unconscious violinist. He has been found to have a fatal kidney ailment, and the Society of Music Lovers has canvassed all available medical records and found that you alone have the right blood type to help. They have therefore kidnapped you, and last night the violinist's circulatory system was plugged into yours, so that your kidneys can be used to extract poisons from his blood as well as your own. The director of the hospital now tells you, "Look, we're sorry the Society of Music Lovers did this to you—we would have never permitted it if we had known. But still, they did it, and the violinist now is plugged into you. To unplug you would be to kill him. But never mind, it's only for nine months. By then he will have recovered from his ailment, and can be safely unplugged from you." Is it morally incumbent on you to accede to this situation? No doubt it would be very nice of you if you did, a great kindness. But do you *have* to accede to it? What if it were not nine months, but nine years? Or longer still? What if the director of the hospital says, "Tough luck, I agree, but you've now got to stay in bed, with the violinist plugged into you, for the rest of your life. Because remember this. All persons have a right to life, and violinists are persons. Granted you have a right to decide what happens in and to your body, but a person's right to life outweighs your right to decide what happens in and to your body. So you cannot ever be unplugged from him." [I imagine you would regard this as outrageous, which suggests that something really is wrong with that plausible-sounding argument I mentioned a moment ago.]

J. T.'s response to CA 2: Violinist analogy

Rejection of CA 2

In this case, of course, you were kidnapped; you didn't volunteer for the operation that plugged the violinist into your kidneys. Can those who oppose abortion on the ground I mentioned make an exception for a pregnancy due to rape? Certainly. They can say that persons have a right to life only if they didn't come into existence because of rape; or they can say that all persons have a right to life, but that some have less of a right to life than others, in particu-

Violinist analogy

Explanation

lar, that those who came into existence because of rape have less. But these statements have a rather unpleasant sound. Surely the question of whether you have a right to life at all, or how much of it you have, shouldn't turn on the question of whether or not you are the product of a rape. And in fact the people who oppose abortion on the ground I mentioned do not make this distinction, and hence do not make an exception in case of rape.

Nor do they make an exception for a case in which the mother has to spend the nine months of her pregnancy in bed. They would agree that would be a great pity, and hard on the mother; but all the same, all persons have a right to life, the fetus is a person, and so on. I suspect, in fact, that they would not make an exception for a case in which, miraculously enough, the pregnancy went on for nine years or even the rest of the mother's life.

Some won't even make an exception for a case in which continuation of the pregnancy is likely to shorten the mother's life; they regard abortion as impermissible even to save the mother's life. Such cases are nowadays very rare, and many opponents of abortion do not accept this extreme view. All the same, it is a good place to begin: a number of points of interest come out in respect to it.

CA 3: Extreme pro-life view

1. Let us call the view that abortion is impermissible even to save the mother's life "the extreme view." I want to suggest first that it does not issue from the argument I mentioned earlier without the addition of some fairly powerful premises. Suppose a woman has become pregnant, and now learns that she has a cardiac condition such that she will die if she carries the baby to term. What may be done for her? The fetus, being a person, has a right to life, but as

J. T.'s response to extreme view

the mother is a person too, so has she a right to life. Presumably they have an equal right to life. How is it supposed to come out that an abortion may not be performed? If mother and child have an equal right to life, shouldn't we perhaps flip a coin? Or should we add to the mother's right to life her right to decide what happens in and to her body, which everybody seems to be ready to grant—the sum of her rights now outweighing the fetus' right to life?

The most familiar argument here is the following. We are told that performing the abortion would be directly killing the child, whereas doing nothing would not be killing the mother, but only letting her die. Moreover, in killing the child, one would be killing an innocent person, for the child has committed no crime, and is not aiming at his mother's death. . . .

If directly killing an innocent person is murder, and thus is impermissible, then the mother's directly killing the innocent person inside her is murder, and thus is impermissible. But [it cannot seriously be thought to be murder if the mother performs an abortion on herself to save her life. It cannot seriously be said that she *must* refrain, that she *must* sit passively by and wait for her death.] Let us look again at the case of you and the violinist. There you are, in bed with the violinist, and the director of the hospital says to you, "It's all most distressing, and I deeply sympathize, but you see this is putting an additional strain on your kidneys, and you'll be dead within the month. But you *have* to stay where you are all the same. Because unplugging you would be directly killing an innocent violinist, and that's murder, and that's impermissible." If anything in the world is true, it is that you do not commit murder, you do not do what is impermissible, if you reach around to your back and unplug yourself from that violinist to save your life.

Violinist analogy explanation of premise #4

The main focus of attention in writings on abortion has been on what a third party may or may not do in answer to a request from a woman for an abortion. This is in a way understandable. Things being as they are, there isn't much a woman can safely do to abort herself. So the question asked is what a third party may do, and what the mother may do, if it is mentioned at all, is deduced, almost as an afterthought, from what is concluded that third parties may do. But it seems to me that to treat the matter in this way is to refuse to grant to the mother that very status of person which is so firmly insisted on for the fetus. For we cannot simply read off what a person may do from what a third party may do. Suppose you find yourself trapped in a tiny house with a growing child. I mean a very tiny house, and a rapidly growing child—you are already up against the wall of the house and in a few minutes you will be crushed to death. The child on the other hand won't be crushed to death; if nothing is done to stop him from growing he'll be hurt, but in the end he'll simply burst open the house and walk out a free man. Now I could well understand it if a bystander were to say, "There's nothing we can do for you. We cannot choose between your life and his, we cannot be the ones to decide who is to live, we cannot intervene." But it cannot be concluded that you too can do nothing, that you cannot attack it to save your life. However innocent the child may be, you do not have to wait passively while it crushes you to death. Perhaps a pregnant woman is vaguely felt to have the same status of house, to which we don't allow the right of self-defense. But if the woman houses the child, it should be remembered that she is a person who houses it. . . .

Explanation of rejection of CA 3: Analogy of house with growing child

Premise #5: A pregnant woman's body is her own

In sum, [a woman surely can defend her life against the threat to it posed by the unborn child, even if doing so involves its death.] And this shows not merely that the theses in (1) through (4) are false; it shows also that the extreme view of abortion is false, and so we need not canvass any other possible ways of arriving at it from the argument I mentioned at the outset.

2. The extreme view could of course be weakened to say that while abortion is permissible to save a mother's life, it may not be performed by a third party, but only by the mother herself. But this cannot be right either. For what we have to keep in mind is that the mother and the unborn child are not like two tenants in a small house which has, by an unfortunate mistake, been rented to both: the mother *owns* the house. The fact that she does adds to the offen-

J. T.'s rejection of CA 4: Smith owns the coat

Premise #4: It is not murder to perform an abortion to save your life

Rejection of CA 3: Extreme pro-life position

Sub-conclusion & Premise #6: A woman can defend herself against threats from the unborn child even if it results in child's death

CA 4: Self-defense allows only mother to perform abortion

siveness of deducing that the mother can do nothing from the supposition that third parties can do nothing. But it does more than this: it casts a bright light on the supposition that third parties can do nothing. Certainly it lets us see that a third party who says "I cannot choose between you" is fooling himself if he thinks this is impartiality. If Jones has found and fastened on a certain coat, which he needs to keep him from freezing, but which Smith also needs to keep him from freezing, then it is not impartiality that says "I cannot choose between you" when Smith owns the coat. Women have said again and again "This body is *my* body!" and they have reason to feel angry, reason to feel that it has been like shouting into the wind. . . .

We should really ask what it is that says "no one may choose" in the face of the fact that the body that houses the child is the mother's body. It may be simply a failure to appreciate this fact. But it may be something more interesting, namely the sense that one has a right to refuse to lay hands on people, even where it would be just and fair to do so, even where justice seems to require that some-

J. T.'s rejection of CA 4: Smith owns the coat

body do so. Thus justice might call for somebody to get Smith's coat back from Jones, and yet you have a right to refuse to be the one to lay hands on Jones, a right to refuse to do physical violence to him. This, I think, must be granted. But then what should be said is not "no one may choose," but only *"I cannot choose,"* and indeed not even this, but *"I will not act,"* leaving it open that somebody else can or should, and in particular that anyone in a position of authority, with the job of securing people's rights, both can and should. So this is no difficulty. I have not been arguing that any given third party must accede to the mother's request that he perform an abortion to save her life, but only that he may. . . .

CA 5: The child's right to life is stronger than the mother's rights

3. Where the mother's life is not at stake, the argument I mentioned at the outset seems to have a much stronger pull. "Everyone has a right to life, so the unborn person has a right to life." And isn't the child's right to life weightier than anything other than the mother's own right to life, which she might put forward as ground for an abortion?

This argument treats the right to life as if it were unproblematic. It is not, and this seems to me to be precisely the source of the mistake.

For we should now, at long last, ask what it comes to, to have a right to life. In some views having a right to life includes having a right to be given at least the bare minimum one needs for continued life. But suppose that what in fact *is* the bare minimum a man needs for continued life is something he has no right at all to be given? If I am sick unto death, and the only thing that will save my

J. T.'s reply to CA 5: Henry Fonda analogy

life is the touch of Henry Fonda's cool hand on my fevered brow, then all the same, I have no right to be given the touch of Henry Fonda's cool hand on my fevered brow. It would be frightfully nice of him to fly in from the West Coast to provide it. It would be less nice, though no doubt well meant, if my friends flew out to the West

Coast and carried Henry Fonda back with them. But I have no right at all against anybody that he should do this for me. Or again, to return to the story I told earlier, the fact that for continued life that violinist needs the continued use of your kidneys does not establish that he has a right to be given the continued use of your kidneys. He certainly has no right against you that *you* should give him continued use of your kidneys. For nobody has any right to use your kidneys unless you give him such a right; and nobody has the right against you that you shall give him this right—if you do allow him to go on using your kidneys, this is a kindness on your part, and not something he can claim from you as his due. Nor has he any right against anybody else that *they* should give him continued use of your kidneys. Certainly he had no right against the Society of Music Lovers that they should plug him into you in the first place. And if you now start to unplug yourself, having learned that you will otherwise have to spend nine years in bed with him, there is nobody in the world who must try to prevent you, in order to see to it that he is given something he has a right to be given. . . .

Certainly [the violinist has no right against you that *you* shall allow him to continue to use your kidneys. As I said, if you do allow him to use them, it is a kindness on your part, and not something you owe him.]

Sub-conclusion and premise #7: It is a kindness rather than an obligation to let someone else use our body

The difficulty I point to here is not peculiar to the right to life. It reappears in connection with all the other natural rights; and it is something which an adequate account of rights must deal with. For present purposes it is enough just to draw attention to it. But I would stress that I am not arguing that people do not have a right to life—quite to the contrary, it seems to me that the primary control we must place on the acceptability of an account of rights is that it should turn out in that account to be a truth that all persons have a right to life. [I am arguing only that having a right to life does not guarantee having either a right to be given the use of or a right to be allowed continued use of another person's body—even if one needs it for life itself.] So the right to life will not serve the opponents of abortion in the very simple and clear way in which they seem to have thought it would.

Premise #7 restated

4. There is another way to bring out the difficulty. In the most ordinary sort of case, [to deprive someone of what he has a right to is to treat him unjustly.] Suppose a boy and his small brother are jointly given a box of chocolates for Christmas. If the older boy takes the box and refuses to give his brother any of the chocolates, he is unjust to him, for the brother has been given a right to half of them. But suppose that, having learned that otherwise it means nine years in bed with that violinist, you unplug yourself from him. You surely are not being unjust to him, for you gave him no right to use your kidneys, and no one else can have given him any such right. But we have to notice that in unplugging yourself, you are killing him; and violinists, like everybody else, have a right to life, and thus in the

Premise #8: It is unjust to deprive someone of something to which they have a right

Explanation of premise #8

view we were considering just now, the right not to be killed. So here you do what he supposedly has a right you shall not do, but you do not act unjustly to him in doing it.

The emendation which may be made at this point is this: [the right to life consists not in the right not to be killed, but rather in the right not to be killed unjustly.] This runs a risk of circularity, but never mind: it would enable us to square the fact that the violinist has a right to life with the fact that you do not act unjustly toward him in unplugging yourself, thereby killing him. For if you do not kill him unjustly, you do not violate his right to life, and it is no wonder you do him no injustice.

Premise #9: The right to life consists only of the right not to be killed unjustly

But if this emendation is accepted, the gap in the argument against abortion stares us plainly in the face: it is by no means enough to show that the fetus is a person, and to remind us that all persons have a right to life—we need to be shown also that killing the fetus violates its right to life, i.e., that abortion is unjust killing. And is it?

I suppose we may take it as a datum that in a case of pregnancy due to rape the mother has not given the unborn person a right to the use of her body for food and shelter. Indeed, in what pregnancy could it be supposed that the mother has given the unborn person such a right? It is not as if there were unborn persons drifting about the world, to whom a woman who wants a child says "I invite you in."

But it might be argued that there are other ways one can have acquired a right to the use of another person's body than by having been invited to use it by that person. Suppose a woman voluntarily indulges in intercourse, knowing of the chance it will issue in pregnancy, and then she does become pregnant; is she not in part responsible for the presence, in fact the very existence, of the unborn person inside her? No doubt she did not invite it in. But doesn't her partial responsibility for its being there itself give it a right to the use of her body? If so, then her aborting it would be more like the boy's taking away the chocolates, and less like your unplugging yourself from the violinist—doing so would be depriving it of what it does have a right to, and thus would be doing it an injustice.

CA 6: If mother "invites" fetus to use her body, it is unjust to then kill the fetus

And then, too, it might be asked whether or not she can kill it even to save her own life: If she voluntarily called it into existence, how can she now kill it, even in self-defense?

The first thing to be said about this is that it is something new. Opponents of abortion have been so concerned to make out the independence of the fetus, in order to establish that it has a right to life, just as its mother does, that they have tended to overlook the possible support they might gain from making out that [the fetus is *dependent* on the mother, in order to establish that she has a special kind of responsibility for it,] a responsibility that gives it rights against her which are not possessed by any independent person—such as an ailing violinist who is a stranger to her.

Premise #10: The fetus is dependent on the mother

J. T.'s response to
CA 6: People
seeds analogy

On the other hand, this argument would give the unborn person a right to its mother's body only if her pregnancy resulted from a voluntary act, undertaken in full knowledge of the chance a pregnancy might result from it. It would leave out entirely the unborn person whose existence is due to rape. Pending the availability of some further argument, then, we would be left with the conclusion that unborn persons whose existence is due to rape have no right to the use of their mothers' bodies, and thus that aborting them is not depriving them of anything they have a right to and hence is not unjust killing.

And we should also notice that it is not at all plain that this argument really does go even as far as it purports to. For there are cases and cases, and the details make a difference. If the room is stuffy, and I therefore open a window to air it, and a burglar climbs in, it would be absurd to say, "Ah, now he can stay, she's given him a right to the use of her house—for she is partially responsible for his presence there, having voluntarily done what enabled him to get in, in full knowledge that there are such things as burglars, and that burglars burgle." It would be still more absurd to say this if I had had bars installed outside my windows, precisely to prevent burglars from getting in, and a burglar got in only because of a defect in the bars. It remains equally absurd if we imagine it is not a burglar who climbs in, but an innocent person who blunders or falls in. Again, suppose it were like this: people-seeds drift about in the air like pollen, and if you open your windows, one may drift in and take root in your carpets or upholstery. You don't want children, so you fix up your windows with fine mesh screens, the very best you can buy. As can happen, however, and on very, very rare occasions does happen, one of the screens is defective; and a seed drifts in and takes root. Does the person-plant who now develops have a right to the use of your house? Surely not—despite the fact that you voluntarily opened your windows, you knowingly kept carpets and upholstered furniture, and you knew that screens were sometimes defective. Someone may argue that you are responsible for its rooting, that it does have a right to your house, because after all you *could* have lived out your life with bare floors and furniture, or with sealed windows and doors. But this won't do—for by the same token anyone can avoid a pregnancy due to rape by having a hysterectomy, or anyway by never leaving home without a (reliable!) army.

Premise #11: There
are some cases
where the fetus
has a right to the
mother's body

It seems to me that the argument we are looking at can establish at most that [there are *some* cases in which the unborn person has a right to the use of its mother's body,] and therefore [*some* cases in which abortion is unjust killing.] There is room for much discussion and argument as to precisely which, if any. But I think we should sidestep this issue and leave it open, for at any rate the argument certainly does not establish that all abortion is unjust killing.

Sub-conclusion
and premise #12:
There are some
cases where
abortion is unjust
killing

5. There is room for yet another argument here, however. [We surely must all grant that there may be cases in which it would be

morally indecent to detach a person from your body at the cost of his life.] Suppose you learn that what the violinist needs is not nine years of your life, but only one hour: all you need do to save his life is to spend one hour in that bed with him. Suppose also that letting him use your kidneys for that one hour would not affect your health in the slightest. Admittedly you were kidnapped. Admittedly you did not give anyone permission to plug him into you. Nevertheless it seems to me plain you *ought* to allow him to use your kidneys for that hour—it would be indecent to refuse.

Explanation of premise #10: The violinist analogy revisited

Again, suppose pregnancy lasted only an hour, and constituted no threat to life or health. And suppose that a woman becomes pregnant as a result of rape. Admittedly she did not voluntarily do anything to bring about the existence of a child. Admittedly she did nothing at all which would give the unborn person a right to the use of her body. All the same it might well be said, as in the newly emended violinist story, that she *ought* to allow it to remain for that hour—that it would be indecent in her to refuse.

Now some people are inclined to use the term "right" in such a way that it follows from the fact that you ought to allow a person to use your body for the hour he needs, that he has a right to use your body for the hour he needs, even though he has not been given that right by any person or act. They may say that it follows also that if you refuse, you act unjustly toward him. This use of the term is perhaps so common that it cannot be called wrong; nevertheless it seems to me to be an unfortunate loosening of what we would do better to keep a tight rein on. Suppose the box of chocolates I mentioned earlier had not been given to both boys jointly, but was given only to the older boy. There he sits, stolidly eating his way through the box, his small brother watching enviously. Here we are likely to say "You ought not to be so mean. You ought to give your brother some of those chocolates." My own view is that it just does not follow from the truth of this that the brother has any right to any of the chocolates. If the boy refuses to give his brother any, he is greedy, stingy, callous—but not unjust. . . .

Premise #13: Even if there are cases in which the mother ought to allow the unborn child to use her body this does not mean the child has a right to her body

So my own view is that even though you ought to let the violinist use your kidneys for the one hour he needs, we should not conclude that he has a right to do so—we should say that if you refuse, you are, like the boy who owns all the chocolates and will give none away, self-centered and callous, indecent in fact, but not unjust. And similarly, that even supposing a case in which a woman pregnant due to rape ought to allow the unborn person to use her body for the hour he needs, we should not conclude that he has a right to do so; we should conclude that she is self-centered, callous, indecent, but not unjust, if she refuses. The complaints are no less grave; they are just different. However, there is no need to insist on this point. If anyone does wish to deduce "he has a right" from "you ought," then all the same he must surely grant that there are cases in which it is not morally required of you that you allow that violinist to use your kidneys, and in which he does not have a right to use them, and in which you do not do him an injustice if you refuse. . . .

6. We have in fact to distinguish between two kinds of Samaritan: the (Good Samaritan) and what we might call the (Minimally Decent Samaritan . . .) The Good Samaritan went out of his way, at some cost to himself, to help one in need of it. . . . [in Luke 10:30–35]

Key terms: "Good Samaritan" and "Minimally Decent Samaritan"

Explanation of two types of Samaritans

These things are a matter of degree, of course, but there is a difference, and it comes out perhaps most clearly in the story of Kitty Genovese, who, as you will remember, was murdered while thirty-eight people watched or listened, and did nothing at all to help her. A Good Samaritan would have rushed out to give direct assistance against the murderer. Or perhaps we had better allow that it would have been a Splendid Samaritan who did this, on the ground that it would have involved a risk of death for himself. But the thirty-eight not only did not do this, they did not even trouble to pick up a phone to call the police. Minimally Decent Samaritanism would call for doing at least that, and their not having done it was monstrous.

After telling the story of the Good Samaritan, Jesus said "Go, and do thou likewise." Perhaps he meant that we are morally required to act as the Good Samaritan did. Perhaps he was urging people to do more than is morally required of them. At all events it seems plain that [it was not morally required of any of the thirty-eight that he rush out to give direct assistance at the risk of his own life] and that [it is not morally required of anyone that he give long stretches of his life—nine years or nine months—to sustaining the life of a person who has no special right (we were leaving open the possibility of this) to demand it.]

Premise #14: We are morally required only to be Minimally Decent Samaritans

Premise #15: Being a Minimally Decent Samaritan does not require us to give long stretches to sustain the life of someone who has no special rights

Explanation of premises #14 and #15

Indeed, with one rather striking class of exceptions, no one in any country in the world is *legally* required to do anywhere near as much as this for anyone else. The class of exceptions is obvious. My main concern here is not the state of the law in respect to abortion, but it is worth drawing attention to the fact that in no state in this country is any man compelled by law to be even a Minimally Decent Samaritan to any person; there is no law under which charges could be brought against the thirty-eight who stood by while Kitty Genovese died. By contrast, in most states in this country women are compelled by law to be not merely Minimally Decent Samaritans, but Good Samaritans to unborn persons inside them. This doesn't by itself settle anything one way or the other, because it may well be argued that there should be laws in this country—as there are in many European countries—compelling at least Minimally Decent Samaritanism. But it does show that there is a gross injustice in the existing state of the law. And it shows also that the groups currently working against liberalization of abortion laws, in fact working toward having it declared unconstitutional for a state to permit abortion, had better start working for the adoption of Good Samaritan laws generally, or earn the charge that they are acting in bad faith.

I should think, myself, that Minimally Decent Samaritan laws would be one thing, Good Samaritan laws quite another, and in fact highly improper. But we are not here concerned with the law. What we should ask is not whether anybody should be compelled by law to be a Good Samaritan, but whether we must accede to a situation in which somebody is being compelled—by nature, perhaps—to be a Good Samaritan. We have, in other words, to look now at third-party interventions. I have been arguing that no person is morally required to make large sacrifices to sustain the life of another who has no right to demand them, and this even where the sacrifices do not include life itself; we are not morally required to be Good Samaritans or anyway Very Good Samaritans to one another. But what if a man cannot extricate himself from such a situation? What if he appeals to us to extricate him? It seems to me plain that there are cases in which we can, cases in which a Good Samaritan would extricate him. There you are, you were kidnapped, and nine years in bed with that violinist lie ahead of you. You have your own life to lead. You are sorry, but you simply cannot see giving up so much of your life to the sustaining of his. You cannot extricate yourself, and ask us to do so. I should have thought that—in light of his having no right to the use of your body—it was obvious that we do not have to accede to your being forced to give up so much. We can do what you ask. There is no injustice to the violinist in our doing so.

CA 7: The woman has a special kind of obligation toward her fetus because she is the mother

7. Following the lead of the opponents of abortion, I have throughout been speaking of the fetus merely as a person, and what I have been asking is whether or not the argument we began with, which proceeds only from the fetus' being a person, really does not establish its conclusion. I have argued that it does not.

But of course there are arguments and arguments, and it may be said that I have simply fastened on the wrong one. It may be said that what is important is not merely the fact that the fetus is a person, but that it is a person for whom the woman has a special kind of responsibility issuing from the fact that she is its mother. And it might be argued that all my analogies are therefore irrelevant—for you do not have that special kind of responsibility for that violinist, Henry Fonda does not have that special kind of responsibility for me. And our attention might be drawn to the fact that men and women both *are* compelled by law to provide support for their children.

I have in effect dealt (briefly) with this argument in section 4 above; but a (still briefer) recapitulation now may be in order.

J. T.'s response to CA 7

Surely [we do not have any such "special responsibility" for a person unless we have assumed it, explicitly or implicitly.] If a set of parents do not try to prevent pregnancy, do not obtain an abortion, and then at the time of birth of the child do not put it out for adoption, but rather take it home with them, then they have assumed responsibility for it, they have given it rights, and they cannot *now* withdraw

Premise #16: We do not have a responsibility for another person unless we have assumed it

support from it at the cost of its life because they now find it difficult to go on providing for it. But if they have taken all reasonable precautions against having a child, they do not simply by virtue of their biological relationship to the child who comes into existence have a special responsibility for it. They may wish to assume responsibility for it, or they may not wish to. And I am suggesting that if assuming responsibility for it would require large sacrifices, then they may refuse. . . .

8. My argument will be found unsatisfactory on two counts by many of those who want to regard abortion as morally permissible. First, while I do argue that abortion is not impermissible, I do not argue that it is always permissible. There may well be cases in which carrying the child to term requires only Minimally Decent Samaritanism of the mother, and this is a standard we must not fall below. I am inclined to think it a merit of my account precisely that it does *not* give a general yes or a general no. It allows for and supports our sense that, for example, a sick and desperately frightened fourteen-year-old schoolgirl, pregnant due to rape, may *of course* choose abortion, and that any law which rules this out is an insane law. And it also allows for and supports our sense that in other cases resort to abortion is even positively indecent. It would be indecent in the woman to request an abortion, and indecent in a doctor to perform it, if she is in her seventh month, and wants the abortion just to avoid the nuisance of postponing a trip abroad. The very fact that the arguments I have been drawing attention to treat all cases of abortion, or even all cases of abortion in which the mother's life is not at stake, as morally on a par ought to have made them suspect at the outset.

Secondly, while I am arguing for the permissibility of abortion in some cases, I am not arguing for the right to secure the death of the unborn child. It is easy to confuse these two things in that up to a certain point in the life of the fetus it is not able to survive outside the mother's body; hence removing if from her body guarantees its death. But they are importantly different. I have argued that you are not morally required to spend nine months in bed, sustaining the life of that violinist; but to say this is by no means to say that if, when you unplug yourself, there is a miracle and he survives, you then have a right to turn around and slit his throat. You may detach yourself even if this costs him his life; you have no right to be guaranteed his death, by some other means, if unplugging yourself does not kill him. There are some people who will feel dissatisfied by this feature of my argument. A woman may be utterly devastated by the thought of a child, a bit of herself, put out for adoption and never seen or heard of again. She may therefore want not merely that the child be detached from her, but more, that it die. Some opponents of abortion are inclined to regard this as beneath contempt—thereby showing insensitivity to what is surely a powerful source of despair. All the

Part 1 of conclusion: Abortion is permissible except in cases where it falls beneath the standard of Minimally Decent Samaritanism

Part 2 of conclusion: The woman does not have a right to secure the death of her child, but only to remove it from her body

same, I agree that the desire for the child's death is not one which anybody may gratify, should it turn out to be possible to detach the child alive.

At this place, however, it should be remembered that we have only been pretending throughout that the fetus is a human being from the moment of conception. A very early abortion is surely not the killing of a person, and so is not dealt with by anything I have said here.

QUESTIONS FOR COMPREHENSION AND REFLECTION

1. What is Thomson's position regarding the personhood of the fetus?
2. How does Thomson use the violinist analogy to illustrate the relationship between the fetus and the woman?
3. What conclusion regarding the rights of the fetus, the rights of the mother, and the moral permissibility of abortion does Thomson draw based on the violinist analogy?
4. Why does Thomson reject the "extreme" pro-life view of abortion?
5. Which position on abortion is Thomson addressing when she uses the analogy of a person being trapped in a tiny house with a rapidly growing child?
6. How does Thomson respond to the pro-life argument that if the fetus has a right to life, abortion is unjust killing?
7. What analogy does Thomson use to justify abortion in cases of contraceptive failure?
8. Are there any circumstances, according to Thomson, in which abortion is not morally permissible?
9. What is the difference between a Minimally Decent Samaritan and a Good Samaritan? What is the relevance of this distinction in the abortion debate?
10. On what grounds does Thomson draw a moral distinction between the right to have an abortion and the right to secure the death of an unborn child?

C H A P T E R   3

The Relationship Between Healthcare Professionals and Patients

It was the day before Juanita Diaz's baby girl's heart surgery. Her baby, Maria, had a heart valve obstruction. The surgeon, Dr. Merkle, met with the mother to explain the procedure and to obtain her consent. Diaz knew very little English, and, unfortunately, Merkle could barely get by in Spanish. Nevertheless, he tried his best to describe Maria's condition, even drawing a picture of a heart showing quadrants with arrows to indicate the blood flow from the valves. After a long interval, Diaz signed the consent form.

Early the next morning, just before the operation, the Diaz' family physician, Dr. Gomez, met Juanita Diaz at the hospital. She was extremely distraught and told him in Spanish that she had not slept that night. When asked whether Maria's condition had been explained to her, she nodded. Did she understand that the operation was fairly routine and that there was no serious threat to her baby's life? She again nodded. After crying for some time, she told Dr. Gomez that she had had such great faith and trust in God all her life. She could not understand why "her baby was born with a square heart."[1]

Here we face the most fundamental issue in the relationship between health professionals and patients—communication. Dr. Merkle's best attempt to convey adequate information to the distressed mother failed. In fact, it was his drawing of a squared heart that seized the mother's attention. The lesson is painfully clear: During distress, our attention is selective, yet the key ingredient in interacting with patients continues to be the degree to which healthcare professionals are not only competent in their disciplines but also skilled communicators.

PHYSICIANS AND PATIENTS

The interns clustered outside Mr. K's room while one of them presented the patient's case. Mr. K had previously been in the hospital's trauma unit after suffering multiple injuries from an automobile accident that had left him partially paralyzed. His spinal cord was nearly severed, and his kidneys and liver were badly damaged. Almost as an afterthought, the presenter also pointed out to the group a curious growth and strange coloration around Mr. K's fingertips that was incidental to the accident.

As the interns entered the patient's room, they barely greeted Mr. K. Instead, they surrounded his bed and took turns lifting up his hands and gazing at his fingertips without saying a word to him. He soon became somewhat anxious and asked what was wrong. No one answered him. After discussing his injuries from the accident, the group filed out without ever acknowledging the patient.

As this example illustrates, obvious disparities exist between physicians and patients. First is the difference in medical education. There is also economic disparity. Since American physicians usually make more money than their patients, they are higher on the scale of social status. Most important, however, is the discrepancy in vulnerability. Illness, an unwelcome reminder of our fragility, situates the patient in a more exposed and dependent state, subject to a barrage of tests and procedures and under the control of professionals—professionals who, as knowledgeable as they are, are also strangers.

Such disparity between patients and physicians can translate into a relationship of inequity if physicians remain strangers who treat patients merely as cases, that is, as objects for diagnosis and medical study. Treating patients in this way in effect desecrates the heart of medical ethics, which aims to bring some level of equity into what is already an unequal relationship so that the relationship develops into one of mutual trust and respect.

In medicine, there are three fundamentally imperative questions:

1. What is wrong with this patient?
2. What can be done about it?
3. What ought to be done about it?

The first two questions are empirical in nature, requiring the expertise and good judgment of the physician. The third question goes deeper, since what *can* be done is not necessarily what *ought* to be done. What ought to be done depends on the values and beliefs of the patient, along with the physician's sound professional judgment. What ought to be done, according to the predominant autonomy model in American healthcare ethics, must be the result of a decision-making process shared by the healer and the patient, with the patient having the final say.

It is worth bearing in mind that in America this point of view is still rather new, having come about only in the past four decades. Traditionally, physicians assumed near-total control when it came to deciding what ought to be done for their patients. In turn, patients expected their physicians to make decisions in the patients' best interests. This deference to physician authority sanctioned practices that were essentially paternalistic. In some cases, physicians overrode individual patient preferences and justified their action by appealing to the principle of beneficence.

This situation changed due to various factors. First, landmark court cases and rulings upheld the privacy of patients and censured clinical and medical invasions of patients' privacy. In 1957, in the case of *Salgo v. Leland Stanford Board of Trustees,* the court underscored the importance of respecting patients' privacy by upholding the duty of physicians to disclose all relevant information to patients so that they could make their own informed choices. In fact, this was the first case to legally coin the term *informed*

CULTURAL WINDOWS

THE HEALER IN NATIVE AMERICAN MEDICINE

In Native American traditions, the notion of healing takes on broader dimensions. Healing occurs on various levels that interact with one another: bodily, emotional, social, and spiritual. The last two levels are especially important. Illness is brought on not only by physical ailments, but also by the quality of one's interrelationships with family, friends, coworkers, and so on. Furthermore, illness is produced by an individual's state of spirituality, not in a church-going sense but in terms of one's relationship with one's own self, or spirit. An imbalance among these various levels acts as a catalyst for the development of symptoms of illness.

This interaction, in turn, affects the role of the healer, or **shaman.** In essence, the shaman must be a person of wisdom who can see through the bodily manifestations of illness and help guide the patient to recognize their source in the patient's spiritual life, that is, in how connected he or she is with the self. Both shaman and patient work together in restoring balance to the patient. Lewis Mehl-Madrona, a physician from a Native American background who has been trained in modern Western medicine, points out that healing requires that the following three questions be addressed:

1. Who are you?
2. Where did you come from?
3. Why are you here?[2]

Note the difference between these three questions and those posed in the text: What is wrong? What can be done? What ought to be done? A good shaman does more than simply provide an effective medical diagnosis and treatment. The shaman approaches healing in a holistic manner, integrating the bodily, or physical, with the spiritual. The shaman, therefore, approaches healing through the spiritual transformation of the patient. In order for healing to occur, the shaman must genuinely listen to the patient, listening not only to what is said but also to what is not said. Then, together with the patient, the shaman creates a story, or vision, of the patient as healthy. This story offers necessary hope to the patient that he or she will be healed and integrates both bodily and spiritual dimensions so that the patient's quest for health is also a spiritual journey. Shaman and patient embark on this journey together.

Healing can occur only if there is sincere, bona fide trust between the shaman and the patient. And since healing requires a spiritual transformation, the personal character of the shaman is all-important. The shaman must be a person of virtue. He or she must have integrity and modesty; there is no room for hubris or false pride. The shaman must be truly committed to spiritual self-development before he or she can act as a guide and accompany patients along their own spiritual journey to health.

consent. Second, a growing societal awareness of the personhood of patients paralleled this legal climate. The ground-breaking work by Paul Ramsey, *The Patient as Person*, proposed the notion that patients are not simply cases or objects for treatment. Instead, particularly in view of the rise of more sophisticated medical technologies that can jeopardize the relationship between physicians and patients, patients are in essence persons, possessing the full range of rights and respect that persons deserve.

The Contractual Model

In view of the increasing focus on patients' rights, Robert Veatch submitted a classic exposé of four possible models of the physician/patient relationship for analysis: the engineering model, the priestly model, the collegial model, and the contractual model.[3] He proposed that the contractual model most closely resembles the ideal ethical relationship between physician and patient.

In the **engineering model,** the physician simply presents the medical diagnosis and prognosis to the patient and refrains from suggesting a course of treatment. On the surface, this model appears to respect the patient's autonomy because it grants full decision making to the patient. Yet the physician actually morally abdicates his or her role by not offering a professional opinion. In contrast, the **priestly model** represents the traditional paternalistic role of the physician. In this model, the physician conveys little in the way of medical information to the patient and makes the final decision regarding treatment. This describes a familiar scene between many physicians and their patients. The major flaw with this model is that it diminishes the role of the patient as a decision-maker. The **collegial model** works under the naive assumption that the patient and the physician are, in a sense, colleagues and hold similar values and goals. Yet, although both physicians and patients may desire positive outcomes, they frequently differ as to what constitutes a positive outcome. Is it a few extra months, weeks, or days of life under heavy sedation? Or is it less time alive but in relative alertness?

Veatch concluded that the contractual model is what we ought to strive for, and this became the generally accepted position in American medical ethics. The **contractual model** assumes a special contract between the physician and the patient that entails a mutual respect for and acceptance of each other's role and participation. The physician not only fulfills professional obligations through diagnosis but also offers his or her own professional opinion and encourages the patient to pursue the course of treatment believed to be in the patient's best interests. At the same time, the physician respects the patient's right to make the final decision regarding his or her own treatment. The physician thus respects the patient's autonomy, and physician and patient have mutual respect for each other's rights and duties.

Criticisms of the Contractual Model

Even though the contractual model has come to be the most prominent expression of the ideal relationship between physician and patient in American healthcare ethics, it has been criticized on three grounds:

1. Focusing solely on this model as a panacea for healthcare neglects other factors. As we will later discuss, healthcare professionals work within an organization with struc-

ISLAMIC VIEWS ON PATIENTS AND HEALTHCARE PROFESSIONALS

The Islamic Code of Medical Ethics, promulgated after a 1981 conference on medical ethics in Kuwait, was the first official statement of its kind. The code is essentially Islamic in that it underscores the idea that medical ethics must be practiced within the context of Islamic religious beliefs and the devout belief in Allah. In other words, the physician should be first and foremost a devout Muslim. Sound, moral medical practice will stem from this.

The 1981 code systematized a number of long-standing Islamic beliefs regarding the nature of the proper relationship between healthcare professionals and patients that address a number of uniquely Islamic concerns.[4] Islamic teachings emphasize a rather strict segregation of the sexes when it comes to healthcare. Male physicians should not treat female patients (and vice versa) unless the circumstances are medically necessary and urgent, such as prenatal care in obstetrics. This segregation underscores the importance in Islam of respecting each sex's *'awra,* or private bodily areas. Similarly, great weight is placed on avoiding **khalwa,** or situations in which a man and a woman not married to each other are alone together. Out of respect for Muslims and Islamic teach-ings, the code urges that a spouse, family member, or friend be present, for instance, during examination of Islamic patients. However, the presence of third parties is not suitable for psychotherapeutic or psychiatric care, which requires that the nature of the relationship between the therapist and the patient be held in strict confidentiality. In this case, the therapist or psychiatrist should be a faithful Muslim, particularly when the therapist is male and the patient female.

This emphasis on segregating male and female has far-reaching consequences. For instance, it affects how nurses, who are all female in Muslim countries, are viewed. Consider the case of Hamid Sadeghi, a twenty-five-year-old affluent Iranian. In Iran, men were traditionally expected to play the more dominant role. When Sadeghi was admitted as a patient in an American hospital, he continued to exert his traditional role. He became extremely controlling, insisting on his nurses' attention whenever he felt the need and refusing medications at will. He even posted a sign outside his room demanding that everyone, including nurses, knock before entering. Sadeghi was not being deliberately mean-spirited. He felt that he was behaving

tural constraints and policies. Moreover, physicians and nurses work within the context of a team approach to healthcare delivery. Various specialists and others often become part of patient care, which may make patients' rapport with their primary physicians tenuous.

2. The language behind a contractual relationship has legalistic overtones. It can be interpreted mechanistically and could suggest a minimalist approach to treatment

according to the way things were done in his country. In any case, his behavior stirred quite a bit of indignation among the staff, particularly among the nurses who had to deal directly with him. The following description of the role of nurses in Iran may help explain, though not necessarily justify, his behavior:

Nursing is a low-level position in the Middle East because the job requires a woman to violate the laws of the Koran—she must both look at and touch the bodies of naked male strangers. The Koran stipulates extreme sexual segregation, primarily to protect the purity of women. . . . It is no wonder that Saudi Arabians pay huge salaries to foreign nurses; it is difficult to attract many Saudi women to the profession.[5]

The Muslim emphasis on segregation also reveals itself in the issue of whether or not Muslim patients are permitted to receive treatment from non-Muslim physicians. Here again, the religious context of Islam comes to light, for the Muslim is required to participate in certain strict religious practices. These specific duties, called the Five Pillars of Islam, are witnessing to the Muslim faith, praying five times daily at appointed hours, fasting during the month of Ramadan (that is, strict fasting during the daytime hours), making the once-in-a-lifetime pilgrimage to Mecca (called *hajj*), and giving alms. The primary concern for the Muslim patient, whether treated by a Muslim or not, is whether treatment will interfere with these practices.

Problems can arise when medically necessary treatment appears to intrude upon traditional cultural beliefs. For example, a young Muslim woman living in the United States was found to have tumors in her uterus. The thirty-year-old woman was a virgin. Her non-Muslim physician felt that he had to remove her hymen in order to diagnose the tumors, but the woman refused to have this done—most likely because the hymen is a sign of chastity. She evidently felt that the removal of her hymen would incur some social stigma. She eventually sought to consult a Muslim physician.[6] According to the code, every effort must be made to seek the advice of a Muslim physician; the patient can consult with a non-Muslim doctor only if a Muslim physician cannot be found.

In short, the professional duties of Muslim physicians extend beyond the purely medical realm. The practice of medicine goes hand in hand with adherence to religious beliefs and obligations. The Muslim physician must also be a devout Muslim and should do all in the physician's power to encourage patients to be faithful Muslims as well. In the Islamic tradition, therefore, the practice of medicine cannot be separated from the practice of religion.

and decision making. In other words, the relationship could be construed as simply a matter of respecting each other's legal rights and duties, in which case the moral basis of the relationship is overlooked.

3. The contractual model does not pay enough attention to the element of care, including the effect of caring on the wider community.

A Covenantal Relationship

For the reasons stated above, instead of *contractual* we suggest the term recommended by William May—*covenantal*.[7] A **covenant** denotes a consecrated, inviolable bond of trust between the physician as healer and the patient. The relationship between healer and patient is precisely a relationship in that it requires an active relating to each other, or an engaging with each other.

What does this mean? To begin with, a genuinely moral relationship between physician and patient is not simply a matter of following rules, acknowledging rights, and performing duties. A covenantal relationship is a natural expression of the character of both the physician and the patient. It is not a matter of doing the right things; it involves being good persons.

Recall that, according to Aristotle, being virtuous is a matter of cultivating good character by behaving habitually in good ways. Moses Maimonides (1135–1204), a Jewish philosopher who was especially interested in medicine and its relevance to Jewish law, stressed the importance of character. Maimonides underscored the critical importance of good character with respect to the physician. In his famous *Prayer*, he wrote:

> May neither avarice nor miserliness, nor thirst for glory, nor for great reputation engage my mind; for the enemies of truth and philanthropy could easily deceive me and make me forgetful of my lofty aim of doing good to my patients.[8]

Both Aristotle's and Maimonides' point is clear: We cannot separate our actions from our character. We cannot split apart what we do from who we are. Our deeds form our character, and our character informs our deeds. Being and doing exist in a mutually defining relationship. Of course, there is no guarantee that the virtuous physician will always make the right choices. Nonetheless, when patient and physician enter into a covenant with each other, they engage each other in a mutually trusting relationship in which the fundamental concerns become trust and respect.

NURSES AND PATIENTS

PATIENT TO NURSE: You're so smart. Did you ever think of being a doctor?

Of the various healthcare professionals—physicians, orderlies, therapists, technicians, and so on—nurses are without a doubt the most integral part of the healthcare team. Nurses are more likely than physicians to enter into their patients' world. They encounter patients in ways that make them more likely to know patients as persons. Consider their ongoing contacts with patients. They regularly handle patients in intimate bodily ways. They converse with patients as well as with patients' families. They learn about their patients' fears, hopes, values, and beliefs.

Nurses are an important part of a patient's world. Patients' remembrances of their hospital stay will no doubt include memories of certain nurses who showed either special care or a lack of care. Patients often measure the value of their care in terms of their nurses' character. Patients and nurses engage in a relationship that naturally acknowledges the other as a human person. Since the essence of nursing lies in caring for the patient, *being a nurse* and *nursing* must be congruent; that is, being and doing must correspond. Putting this ideal into practice is often difficult, because patients can be uncooperative and occasionally abusive. Also, since nurses enter into closer relationships with their patients only to see many of them grow feeble and die, nursing is taxing work. Perhaps we can more fairly appreciate the difficulties nurses face by examining nursing within some broader contexts.

Societal Context

Consider the specter of the operating room. Who holds center stage? Is it the patient who is being operated on? Look more closely. We do not actually see the patient. Instead, we catch glimpses of an exposed organ, tissue, or tumor. Our focus is riveted on the surgeon. Surrounding the surgeon, on the periphery, are the nurses—one handing the doctor surgical tools, some monitoring special equipment, others looking on—all dependably remaining in the background. In a sense, this image captures the popular view of nursing as a profession that is subordinate to the medical profession. The doctors do the "real work," the nuts and bolts of medical treatment, while the nurses are there to follow the doctors' orders and care for patients.

What accounts for this view? First, we tend to assume an association between physicians and science in that science legitimizes the practice of medicine. The physician thus represents for us a sort of scientific imprimatur. Physicians are in a relationship of authority with respect to their patients, and this authority puts physicians in the privileged position of meting out information to their patients. Due to this interplay between power and knowledge, healthcare professionals must work to establish trust between themselves and their patients. This can come about only through a sharing of knowledge and power.

Second, societal views of nursing stem from a deeper social current: our society's general reluctance to view professional women as equal to men in the workplace. Despite all the efforts to bolster women's rights and to achieve equal status, the public still defers to the authority of physicians over the authority of nurses. This deference explains why patients freely complain to their nurses even when they are reluctant to complain to their physicians. Even though more men are becoming nurses, in the mind of the general public the nursing profession is still "feminine."

Professional Context

Physicians with whom nurses work most closely also tend to view nurses in a subordinate role. This has become the source of much moral conflict, particularly in situations in which following physicians' orders conflicts with nurses' primary obligation to their patients. Suppose a physician ignores his patient's objection to a procedure because the physician believes the patient is not competent to decide for himself. The patient's primary care nurse, however, is convinced that the patient is competent enough to make his own decision and that the physician should honor his objection. The nurse is not sure how to address the matter with the physician. What strategy should the nurse use in order to avoid an unhealthy confrontation in which the physician might feel that his professional judgment is being questioned? Should the nurse be diplomatic or more direct?

Within the nursing profession, the current emphasis on obtaining a more academic background has led to a growing split between nurses with a BSN and those "in the trenches" who have been practicing for a long time since obtaining their RN diploma. Add to this the fact that traditional nursing roles have undergone changes due to cost-cutting measures in hospitals. For instance, more hospitals are hiring unlicensed nursing personnel, individuals who have not received training comparable to a formal nursing curriculum. The use of unlicensed personnel can lead to practical and ethical problems, since such individuals often perform tasks traditionally assigned to nurses—such as administering IVs—for which they may not be sufficiently qualified.

Nurses themselves may adopt the view of their own profession as essentially a service profession, ancillary to medicine. In line with the adage "If you can't beat them, join them," they actually help reinforce the views described above by "trying to be like doctors" and therefore do little to restore professional dignity to nursing as a profession. It is essential that nurses' primary moral obligation and professional responsibility center around the well-being of their patients. As Haddad points out in her article at the end of this chapter, this requires direct, honest, and nondeferential communication with physicians and all other healthcare professionals.

REALITY CHECKS

The Healthcare Organization

The relationship between patients and healthcare professionals exists within a setting that is complex, highly bureaucratic, and increasingly impersonal. Consider the following experience described by a nurse:

> I remember helping a young [woman] deal with her own bone cancer. She wanted to be a code—that is, to receive life-support measures if she stopped breathing. She was receiving morphine for pain through a continuous intravenous drip. Our current nursing policy stated that a patient couldn't have a morphine drip unless she was a no-code. When the staff found out she was a code, they discontinued the drip. They attempted to talk her into a no-code so they could start the morphine drip again. It was like saying, "We'll take care of you and give you pain medication only if you'll agree to die."[9]

This and numerous other scenarios take place in a milieu that involves nurses, physicians, technicians, anesthesiologists, radiologists, paraprofessionals, and others who are not only committed to their patients' welfare but also happen to be employed by their institution. The **Patient's Bill of Rights,** posted in various places, reflects the official position of the American Hospital Association regarding the centrality of the patient. (The Patient's Bill of Rights is included in the Additional Resources at the end of the text.) However, the reality is that, although the patient is and must remain the center of concern in healthcare practice, participants with a direct hand in caring for patients find themselves enmeshed in institutional structures and constraints that sometimes hinder their efforts. Since these same professionals are employed by the institution, they naturally feel accountable to the hospital that employs them.

From "Is" to "Ought"　What happens when nurses' primary commitment to their patients conflicts with certain administrative directives, such as the policy regarding no-code and morphine drips? Keep in mind that ethics deals primarily with what ought to be rather than with what is. Nevertheless, what ought to be cannot be divorced from what is. Ethics must have a solid footing in concrete reality; however, while what ought to be must be grounded in practical realities, it must not be defined by them. Nurses and physicians work within institutional structures that in themselves create ethical problems. Thus, resolving moral conflicts is possible only if we take into account the everyday, practical, structural realities of the institution within which the conflicts occur.

More specifically, there are two fundamental components embedded within most healthcare organizations, whether community hospitals, private hospitals, research hospitals, or nursing homes: power and politics. The two-headed beast of power and politics is most apparent when different group interests are at odds with one another, such as those of nurses and physicians. Alleged ethical conflicts may actually be disguised forms of territorialism. Dan Chambliss points out that requesting ethics consultation from ethicists and institutional ethics committees often merely provides a veneer for morality.

> In fact, such efforts at ameliorating ethical lapses may well be a distraction, fostering a public impression that something is being done. The real problems then go untouched and remain where they always were, embedded in organizational routines and structures.[10]

The typical hierarchies among hospital personnel illustrate this twin threat of politics and power. At lunch at Allegheny General Hospital, a prestigious medical research center in Pittsburgh, the hospital ethicist and other physicians present pointed out that their institutional autonomy, free from the clutches of the neighboring University of Pittsburgh Medical Center, was responsible for their more humane treatment of patients. At the same time, the difference in ambience and food between the regular eating quarters, or cafeteria, and the staff (physician's) dining room was glaring. Nurses and other hospital personnel had to eat in the cafeteria. The formal dining room, reserved mainly for physicians and their guests, was elaborate and pretentious, providing visitors with a posh image.

Consider also the hierarchies among physicians. Senior physicians often hold the highest level of prestige and control, while specialists in the various fields hold high levels of authority and defend their turf. Next in order come house staff, comprising residents and interns, the most visible group. Hierarchies in hospitals lead to a class system in that they lend themselves to inequities in the level of respect and treatment, as is often the case within the physician hierarchy.

Nursing also has its hierarchies. Nursing administrators hold the top seat and oversee nursing directors, who in turn engineer the activities within the various nursing specialties. Then come nursing supervisors, who monitor the various units. The separate units have their own head nurse, who manages the work of the staff nurses, RNs and licensed practical nurses (LPNs).

These hierarchies are strictly organizational, and it is precisely this organizational issue that lends itself to impending ethical concerns. Sociologist Daniel Chambliss puts it more bluntly:

> The hospital as an organization is not merely the setting for moral crises: *the hospital's organizational form actively generates such crises* [italics added]. Against a background of routine, structural rifts in the hospital organization—especially those between different occupational groups—emerge as "ethical differences."[11]

"Buffing the Floor"   An example of a structural rift is the common tension between nurses and administrators. The example concerning the relief of pain from bone cancer through a morphine drip illustrates the conflict between hospital policies and humane patient care. The no-code prerequisite for morphine drips clearly places unfair and cruel pressures on an already suffering patient.

Hospital administrators naturally concern themselves with the fiscal health of the institution. Besides budgetary stability, they are also interested in promoting a good public image. Thus, sizable chunks of monies are allocated to programs that are more highly visible to the public, such as organ transplantation and heart surgery. Yet such a policy can come into direct conflict with nurses' priorities. Nurses correctly perceive themselves as the people working on the front lines of patient care; however, policy is determined by administrators who operate at a precarious distance from the realities of day-to-day care. Nurses and physicians may resent that fewer funds are channeled into less visible programs such as the prevention and treatment of hypertension and prenatal care for women. The administrative concern with public image is likened to "buffing the floor":

> In the Newborn Unit at H. Hospital, janitors come in at all hours with floor buffing machines—make a lot of noise so babies can't sleep. The nurses have complained and are told that patient satisfaction surveys show that *parents* (of the infants here) are very impressed with how nice [the floor tiles] of the unit look. When nurses complained that there was too much noise from the machines (you can't even hear people talk over it), and that they need another housekeeper since the garbage cans are often full and go unemptied, they are told that the floor buffing is more important![12]

Marketing and Medicine

In 1998, nearly six thousand physicians attended the annual Transcatheter Cardiovascular Therapeutics meeting in Washington, D.C., sponsored by the Cardiology Research Foundation and devoted to the new and growing field of interventional cardiology, a specialty that deals with eliminating obstructed blood vessels. Throughout the sessions, many companies that manufacture interventional devices went out of their way to solicit physician endorsement.

> . . . [these physicians] wandered the exhibitors' hall, getting free shoe shines at one booth, entering a contest to win free golf clubs at another. They paid $1,200 to register—about four times more than the fee for similar events, like those of the American Heart Association. Included for their registration: bag of gifts from Johnson & Johnson, among them a ticket for a company-sponsored performance by John Mellencamp and a computer carrying case.[13]

Some companies spent enormous sums of money to help sponsor the meeting and to solicit sales. Boston Scientific, a company that specializes in interventional devices, spent $5 million! Furthermore, a few companies gave new meaning to the term *interventional*, even sponsoring special sessions and selecting their own speakers. The meeting breached the customary divide between marketing and science. The new devices are costly. Stents, wire devices that compress the plaque against the vessel wall, were touted as an improvement over angioplasty, the standard way of treating obstructed vessels, as companies cited the benefits of stents over the balloon compression used in angioplasty. Yet these stents cost around $8,000 per patient.

Why is this another reality check? To begin with, physicians employed by healthcare institutions find themselves under institutional pressure to be cost-effective. For instance, the establishment of **diagnostic related groups (DRGs),** which set up guidelines concerning length of hospital stay for all different categories of conditions, has forced physicians to be cost-conscious. Institutions have dispensed strong financial rewards and penalties on physicians to foster compliance with these guidelines. Cardiologists who attend the annual Transcatheter Cardiovascular Therapeutics meetings face opportunities to apply new, cutting-edge devices that may financially benefit their hospital. Throughout the meetings, cardiologists are encouraged to use these new devices on their (oftentimes unsuspecting) patients.

> Being among the first to use new devices . . . "places you at a competitive advantage," Dr. Brinker of Johns Hopkins said. It can also bring in money, he said, because companies pay $1,000 to $5,000 per patient to compensate doctors for the work of participating in the study.[14]

This "competitive advantage" appears to be good for the hospital, because it conveys to the public a positive image that the organization as a whole is committed to providing the newest and best in medical technologies, and the general public tends to equate the newest medical technologies with the best. This raises serious questions regarding the relationship between healthcare professionals and patients.

One question involves the fact that quite a few medical companies are urging physicians to use their new devices in clinical trials. When physicians do so, will they tell their patients that they are using new devices and why, or will patients be left in the dark? Will physicians view their patients as research subjects? Furthermore, these new devices have no proven track record. For instance, no long-term studies have been conducted to show the use of stents to be more effective and safer than the standard balloon angioplasty.

Despite the absence of long-term clinical studies, device manufacturers aggressively promote their devices by offering all sorts of inducements to physicians. The result is that promotional efforts and marketing may become leading factors in determining whether or not a device will be utilized for patients. (Of course, patients themselves will not be expected to know this, making it imperative for them to inquire into the device's research record.) In view of the financial inducements offered by companies, will the relationship between physician and company come to supersede the venerated covenantal relationship between physician and patient?

Acting on the basis of financial incentives grossly impedes the convenantal relationship between healthcare professionals and patients. While cost-cutting measures and "floor buffing" may be fiscally advantageous for the institution, they further erode the trust patients should have in their healthcare providers. It is not at all far-fetched to envision in the near future a time when, for instance, surgeons will appear in the operating room wearing surgical gowns that bear company logos and colors and hair bonnets that carry the logo of Boston Scientific.

Medical Technology

Without a doubt, the presence of increasingly sophisticated medical technologies affects the relationship between patients and healthcare professionals. Consider the influence of technologies in general on our personal relationships. The telephone surely enables us to "reach out and touch" family and friends, yet it has also become a technical substitute for relating on a more personal level. The television maintains its altarlike

CULTURAL WINDOWS

HEALTH AND DHARMA IN HINDU AYURVEDIC MEDICINE

Duties of the Hindu physician extend beyond the clinical context. The majority of physicians in India are family practitioners, and the family physician is often welcomed into the home as an intricate part of the Hindu family. This inclusion in the family circle entails all sorts of advice from the physician on nonmedical aspects of life. The sources for the physician's duties and obligations are delineated in the most important text in Hindu medicine, the **Carakasamhita,** written in the first century A.D. This body of literature and the system derived from it are known as **Ayurveda.**

The text is a fascinating account of the intimate connection between health; proper moral behavior, or **dharma;** and spiritual awakening. Ayurveda reflects the interaction among moral conduct, religious observance, and health. The opening scene in the Carakasamhita depicts a gathering of priests and sages in a Himalayan retreat. They seek divine guidance on how to deal with pestilences that have raged throughout the countryside and overtaken many people. They are especially concerned because these diseases have impeded the people's ability to carry out their religious observances. The sages realize that physical and mental health and moral conduct work together and affect people's capacity to attain spiritual enlightenment, known as **moksha.** As the text unfolds, it makes clear that dharma, right conduct, can provide a measure of security against disease. Right conduct involves not only proper religious observances, but also behavior conducive to good health such as proper sleep and nutrition. At the same time, right conduct refers to morally sound conduct such as refraining from dispositions such as greed and anger. This is reinforced by the teaching of karma, the principle of moral cause and effect. It states that all conduct, whether good or bad, will eventually produce its consequences— if not in this life, than in another.

position in our homes. It could become a focal point where family members physically join together, but instead it replaces family dialogue. Technologies provide all sorts of conveniences, but convenience has its price—in this case, genuine human contact. In short, the bitter irony is that our technological modes of communication actually impede the potential for real communication.

Medical technologies are pervasive in the clinical setting. Consider all the tools used in the course of an ordinary physical exam: stethoscope, otoscope, sphygmomanometer, perhaps X rays or an EKG. Such tools are extremely worthwhile, as are the more sophisticated techniques such as cardiac catheterizations. The issue is not with technologies per se, but with how technologies affect the real-life encounter with patients. Are the technologies used as a means to engage and learn about the patient, or are they a substitute for the encounter? Are the tools simply a necessary part of the patient-centered encounter, or is the encounter itself test-centered?

Despite all the progress that has been made in medical technologies, the real needs of patients remain the same, including a need to feel that the healthcare team is

Ayurvedic teachings regarding medicine and health do not assume any separation between the mind and the body. Our mental dispositions and moral attitudes affect our bodily state, and vice versa. The Ayurvedic physician, called **vaidya,** is not exempt from this connection. For example, Ayurvedic physicians can be effective only if they themselves refrain from greed and self-seeking. They must avoid the pursuit of material gain as the primary motive in helping their patients, This stress on moral conduct is clear in the Carakasamhita's Oath of Initiation. This oath was written for medical students and exhorts them to practice celibacy, to speak only the truth, to refrain from eating meat, and to practice with humility and without arrogance. Following is an excerpt from the oath:

Day and night, however thou mayest be engaged, thou shalt endeavour for the relief of patients with all thy heart and soul. Thou shalt not desert or injure thy patient for the sake of thy life or thy living. Thou shalt not commit adultery even in thought. Even so, thou shalt not covet others' possessions. Thou shalt be modest in thy attire and appearance. Thou shalt not be a drunkard or a sinful man not shouldst thou associate with the abettors of crimes. Thou shouldst speak words that are gentle, pure and righteous, pleasing, worthy, true, wholesome, and moderate. Thy behaviour must be in consideration of time and place and heedful of past experience. Thou shalt act always with a view to the acquisition of knowledge and fullness of equipment.[15]

This further means that the vaidya must behave in a morally appropriate way in order to help patients so that they not only remain healthy but also are able to seek the highest goal of spiritual enlightenment, or moksha. All activities in Hindu life are conducted with this highest goal in mind. The four aims in Hindu teachings are material comfort (artha), physical pleasure (kama), right conduct (dharma), and spiritual awakening (moksha). Maintaining bodily and mental health is a precondition for achieving any of these aims, and Ayurvedic physicians assist in the process to the best of their ability.[16]

genuinely working on their behalf. Nothing can replace the trust that must exist between the healthcare team and the patient. Yet in our fascination with technologies, we stand in danger of allowing ourselves to be bewitched by the machinery and to overlook the real need for human contact, rapport, and dialogue.

Managed Care

As stated earlier, healthcare professionals work in settings that place inordinate amounts of pressure on them to be cost-conscious, and allegiance to the institution often competes directly with allegiance to the patient. This conflict is especially evident in **managed care** health programs.[17] Managed care is particularly problematic when it comes to the physician/patient relationship. Managed care plans represent the broader area of healthcare policy known as managed competition (we will discuss this further in Chapter 10). As market-driven expressions of healthcare delivery in an increasingly competitive market, **health maintenance organizations (HMOs)** vie with one another for patients on the basis of cost, scope of services offered, and quality care. HMOs' most eloquent advocates claim that effective managed care plans are designed so that "the interests of doctors would be aligned with those of patients in providing economical care of high quality and avoiding incentives to provide care that was not in the patients' best interests, considering both quality and cost."[18]

While this description sounds appealing, the managed care system poses special difficulties regarding the quality of the relationship between healthcare professionals and patients. First, continuity of care is critical in order to maintain a mutually trusting and respectful engagement between healthcare professionals and patients, yet managed care plans by their nature tend to impede this continuity of care. According to ethicists Ezekiel Emanuel and Allan Brett, managed care plans disrupt the continuity of patient care in a variety of ways:

- A change in job status—a new employer or unemployment—may bring about a change in healthcare plans.

- Even without a job change, employers may change health plans.

- Since plans compete with one another, some plans may eventually lose out, and so do their enrollees.

- If entire families are enrolled in a plan, one single member who switches plans affects the whole family.

- The exclusion of **Medicare**, the government-funded healthcare support for the elderly, from this managed care system means that individuals lose their plan coverage on retirement.[19]

Moreover, changes in plans mean shifting to new offices and physicians, which can create bureaucratic havoc. The transfer of records for chronically ill patients can be tedious and may result in "redundant testing."

> Busy physicians find it much simpler to reorder tests than to await the arrival of outside records or search through those records for test results. Redundant testing may be efficient for the individual practitioner, but it will increase overall medical expenditures and inefficiency while providing no benefit to patients.[20]

To further illustrate managed care plans' disruption of the continuity of care, let us consider the phenomenon of the termination of a plan's contract with a physician, known as **physician deselection.** Imagine the case of Dr. Jacqueline Howard, a primary care physician in Pennsylvania who has signed on with Health USA. In the three years since she has signed on, her number of patients has grown only slightly, due in part to the increasing number of both competing managed care plans and physicians contracting with these plans. Nevertheless, she has managed to retain the same pool of patients and is quite conscientious concerning the care of her patients.

On a number of occasions, Dr. Howard has had to justify to Health USA certain referrals to specialists for patients to undergo further tests. Since these tests would incur higher costs, the plan challenged her judgment as to their medical necessity. Although Health USA has so far reluctantly approved her referrals, she has begun to feel a bit uneasy about the continued exercise of her professional autonomy. Dr. Howard is fully aware of measures taken by the plan to streamline health costs, and she fears that her professional judgment may inevitably clash with the policy of Health USA.

She is particularly apprehensive because her contract with Health USA, although it has been renewed each year, may eventually be in jeopardy of nonrenewal. Furthermore, her contract contains a clause indicating that the plan can end its contract with her without even specifying a cause for termination! Dr. Howard fears that Health USA's termination of her contract would mar her reputation among her colleagues as well as make her chances of contracting with another plan more difficult. More important, if Health USA ended her contract, her patients would stand to lose, since they would for the most part be ineligible to receive care from whatever other plan she joined.[21]

In 1986, in the early phase of managed care organizations, 43 percent of physicians in the United States had contracted with at least one managed care plan (MCP). By 1995, this number had risen to over 83 percent of physicians.[22] Thus, the number of patients to which physicians have access (their salary base) has become much more closely tied to their affiliation with managed care groups.

Physicians are under escalating pressure to cooperate in the MCPs' goal of containing costs. For instance, MCPs often extend certain perks and bonuses to physicians who are able to keep the cost of care sufficiently low. As for penalties, many MCPs retain part of the physician's salary to compensate for treatment costs in excess of an established standard set by the MCP.[23] Furthermore, quite a few MCPs have a termination-without-cause statement as part of their contract with physicians, meaning that they can close a contract with a physician without having to provide a rationale, as was the case with Dr. Howard. While MCPs may claim that medical incompetence or noncompliance is the major reason for deselection, the real rationale appears to be economic in nature.

What are the likely consequences for "deselected" physicians? Obviously, they face loss of salary as well as loss of patients. In addition, the opportunity to contract with another plan may be threatened. One commentator cites the possibility of "wayward" physicians being reported to the National Practitioner Data Bank, a database blacklist consulted by peer review boards.[24] The most important consequence of deselection, however, is its impact on patients' relationship with their healthcare provider. Given the pressures placed on physicians to comply with the cost-saving goals of MCPs and their professional obligations to their primary patients, physicians face a precarious conflict of interest. Can they serve two masters, their patients and their MCP?

The second set of difficulties posed by managed care concerns public expectations. There is an assumed, though misplaced, rubric among the public that doing more is always better than doing less, so receiving more medical treatment is thought by many to increase their chances of getting better. In promoting their plans on the grounds of quality care, breadth of coverage, new technologies, and low costs, HMOs may resort to marketing strategies that raise unreasonable expectations on the part of the public. Touting state-of-the-art medical technologies may win over many new patients who expect the same state-of-the-art treatment for their own conditions. When these expectations are not met, patients end up mistrusting the plan as well as the health profession.

The ultimate test of MCPs' true efficacy will rest not in factors having to do with cost-effectiveness but rather in whether they serve to enhance the covenantal rapport between healthcare providers and patients. This covenantal relationship hinges on trust. Without trust, factors such as the cost-containment pressures faced by healthcare professionals enter into that relationship and may end up jeopardizing the outcome of care.

THE HEBREW PHYSICIAN'S OATH

The independent state of Israel was created in 1948. It was the first time in almost two thousand years that Jewish self-rule officially existed. Four years later, in May 1952, Dr. Lipman Halpern wrote the Hebrew Physician's Oath, now the standard oath that physicians in Israel take upon graduation from medical school. Here it is in its entirety:

New Men of Medicine in Israel!
Ye stand this day all of you before your masters in the ways of medicine and its statutes.
That you should enter into covenant with medicine, to fulfil its laws with uprightness, and with all your might and mind.
That there may be established a generation of physicians worthy to do, and faithfully dedicated to succour the sick.
And this is the covenant which I maketh with you this day saying:—

You are charged night and day to be custodians at the side of the sick man at all times of his need.
You shall watch verily over the life of man even from his mother's womb and let his welfare always be your chief concern.
You shall help the sick, base or honourable, stranger or alien or citizen, because he is sick.
And you shall seek to fathom the soul of the sick, to restore his spirit, through understanding and compassion.
Do not hasten to bring forth judgement, and weigh your advice on a wise balance, tried in the crucible of experience.
Be true to him who puts his trust in you. Reveal not his secret and go not about as a talebearer.
And make wise your heart to the wellbeing of the many, to bring healing for the ailments of the people.
Give honour and esteem to your teach-

DISCLOSURE

In the 1961 study of over two hundred U.S. physicians discussed at the beginning of Chapter 2, two-thirds of the physicians indicated that they would not tell a cancer patient the true diagnosis.[27] They assumed that patients did not really want to know the truth about their condition and also felt that telling patients the truth would actually produce more harm than good. Patients might become depressed, overly anxious, and even suicidal. However, in 1979, another study revealed that most American physicians would, in fact, reveal the true diagnosis of cancer.[28] In 1999, with the increasing fear of litigation and the ubiquitous rhetoric accompanying the Patient's Bill of Rights, there seems to be a solid consensus among physicians that telling the truth is advisable in most cases.

What accounts for this remarkable transition from nondisclosure to disclosure? In short, the prior assumptions were directly refuted. Further studies revealed that most patients want to know the truth about their condition, even if it is terminal. Also, telling the truth not only shows respect for the patient but in the long run brings about more

ers who have striven to lead you in the paths of medicine.

Increase wisdom, and weaken not, for wisdom is your life and out of it are issues of life.

Be heedful of the honour of your brothers as in honouring them you will yourselves be honoured.

The words of this covenant are most right unto you. They are in your mouths and hearts that you may do them and you will all answer—

Amen!

Amen, so will we do.

May your efforts to enhance the heritage of medicine in Israel grow and multiply.[25]

This oath reflects the moral teachings within the Jewish tradition. As such, it demonstrates the interaction between cultural beliefs and traditions and attitudes toward healthcare. However, some Jewish commentators, including Amihay Levy and Abraham Ohry, raise the question of whether the oath is genuinely meaningful. Is it simply a general expression of some vague intent? Is it merely a ritualistic formula without practical merit? Or does it express the special covenantal relationship between healthcare professionals and patients?

For instance, Levy and Ohry point out what they consider to be obscurities in the Hebrew oath. To begin with, no clear guidance is given regarding how to resolve the tension between the oath's advice to serve humanity and the physician's duty to serve his or her individual patient. A similar tension exists between the physician's duty to protect and sustain life and the duty to alleviate suffering. Furthermore, the oath contains some evident idealization, for example, in the exhortation to care for the sick both "night and day" and "at all times of his need." Levy and Ohry question whether the apparently widespread skepticism regarding the Hippocratic Oath among Western physicians, due to the increasing emphasis on cost-containment measures, finds a parallel in Israel. In any case, it is worth comparing the two oaths.[26]

positive consequences. For instance, patients who know the facts can make decisions regarding their own treatment plans as well as other personal plans.

Furthermore, the patient rights movement exploded to such a degree that physicians are legally compelled to disclose relevant information to their patients. This climate of interest in patient rights, however, does not necessarily signify an increasing interest in moral matters in themselves. Instead, it exists within the all-too-familiar context of medical litigation, which healthcare professionals naturally fear for obvious reasons: its time-consuming process, emotional and financial drain, and negative professional aftermath.

There are three categories of moral reasons why, in the context of American medicine, healthcare professionals should tell the truth to patients: deontological, utilitarian, and virtue. From a deontological perspective, patients should be told the truth out of respect for them as human persons. Being honest with persons acknowledges their human dignity. Thus, Kant clearly indicates that truth telling is a universal principle. From a utilitarian point of view, telling the truth yields more favorable results for patients in the long run and enhances their well-being. Not only does it lessen the potential for liability, but it also enables patients to make relevant choices regarding the course of treatment and life plans and helps sustain a climate of trust between patients and healthcare professionals. We will look more closely at the third perspective, virtue.

The Art and Virtue of Being Honest

A person can be deceitful in two ways: by committing a lie, such as telling a spouse you were at the library when you were actually at the Dew Drop Inn, or by omitting relevant and necessary information, such as telling a patient that he or she needs to await further test results when in fact there is already sufficient data to make a proper diagnosis. The virtue of truthfulness therefore embraces two components: the information itself and our way of informing. Truthfulness concerns not only what we say but, more important, how we say it. The answer to the all-important question healthcare professionals face—How should we convey bad news?—is, therefore, with clarity, sensitivity, and compassion. Truthfulness is a critical ingredient in enhancing the necessary trust and faith the patient needs to have in the healthcare provider.

The Thin Ice of Nondisclosure: Is It Ever Justifiable?

Because each situation needs to be assessed on its own merits, there are times when nondisclosure is justified, for example, in emergencies or when patients are incapacitated due to their condition or age. More problematic are occasions when physicians invoke **therapeutic privilege**, that is, nondisclosure to otherwise competent patients because they believe telling the truth would incur more harmful effects than not telling the truth.

Morally, physicians are on thin ice unless they can provide solid indications that disclosure would in effect unduly harm the patient. The fact that certain kinds of information may bring about distress and anxiety in a patient is an unsatisfactory ground for not disclosing that information. Patients are naturally vulnerable due to their condition, and being in a hospital setting is in itself distressful. Promoting the patient's own self-determination through disclosure is one way to compensate for this vulnerability.

Under the autonomy model, the standard for determining whether paternalism is ever justifiable centers around the capacity for self-determination. Physicians ought to do whatever enhances a patient's autonomy or self-determination. Therefore, if some types of information will impede the patient's exercise of autonomy, then protecting the patient from such information might be warranted. Suppose solid evidence exists that disclosure will make the patient so emotionally distraught as to compromise his or her ability to act autonomously. In this case, withholding information is justifiable. Suppose a patient waives the right to know about his or her condition. It stands to reason that if patients possess a moral right to know the truth about their condition—and we believe that they do have this right—then they also possess the right to waive that right.

Are all patient waivers justifiable? What if a patient's waiver conflicts with the healthcare interests of others? If a patient refuses to be informed about whether he has a certain genetic disorder, such as Huntington's disease, when there is a clear possibility that he carries the disorder, his refusal could have a deleterious effect on his children. When a patient's waiver of the right to know may jeopardize others, the waiver is generally not justifiable. What if a patient refuses to be informed about her condition because she believes such knowledge to be too distressful to bear? The waiver would be

CULTURAL WINDOWS

DISCLOSURE AMONG THE GREEKS

What are medical ethics like today in the country that gave us the Hippocratic Oath? More specifically, what is the Greek attitude toward the principle of patient autonomy, a principle that people in the United States cherish? What about disclosing the truth to patients? In an interesting study using Greek subjects, researchers concluded that, in modern-day Greece, individual autonomy is not an accepted principle. The same study also revealed that physicians generally act paternalistically toward their patients, choosing not to tell them the truth because they believe that doing so would bring about dire health consequences.[29]

The researchers asked three sets of questions related to whether or not the truth should be told to patients who (1) will die rather soon, (2) will most likely die within a few years, or (3) are seriously ill but have little likelihood of dying soon. The responses among the mixed group of subjects varied and were contingent on factors such as age, occupation, educational background, residence, the role of religion in their lives, and whether any of their own parents had died. For instance, younger subjects generally felt that patients ought to be told the truth. Those who were more educated gave the conditional response "It depends." Those who lived in more rural areas tended to be opposed to disclosure. Religious persons generally rejected truth telling. Despite the variety of responses, however, it was clear to the research team that neither truth telling nor nondisclosure was universally accepted.

Particularly interesting were the reasons the subjects gave for their responses. Almost all of those who advocated truth telling did so for practical, sentimental, and utilitarian reasons. They felt that conveying the truth to a dying patient could be justified in order to allow the patient to more conscientiously follow the doctor's regimen and to allow the patient to put his or her affairs in order before death. None of the reasons for disclosure were directly related to notions of the patients' rights. There was no reference to patient autonomy and self-determination, the principles valued so highly in the United States. The authors of the study attributed this to the fact that ideas concerning patients' rights and autonomy are rather new to Greek medicine. They pointed out that Greece, the birthplace of the Hippocratic Oath, still strongly emphasizes patient beneficence, along with the principle of *primum non nocere* ("first do no harm"), or nonmaleficence. These two principles work together to support paternalism among many Greek physicians. The study revealed that, when it comes to Greek medical practice, most Greek physicians continue to claim that patients do not really desire to know the truth and that revealing the truth tends to produce more harm than good.

legitimate if there is sufficient reason to believe that disclosure will cause an excessive amount of harm and distress to that patient. But if the patient yields to the authority of her physician yet at the same time holds the physician fully accountable for the results of her treatment, she is taking no active role in her own healthcare, in which case the waiver is questionable.

CONFIDENTIALITY

When one couple visited their local Health America (HMO) office, its small waiting area filled with other patients, they perfunctorily checked in at the desk, which was located in the center of the room. In a booming voice, without any regard for discretion, the nurse-receptionist proceeded to ask the wife about the nature of her visit. Her drill-like questioning as to the wife's condition filled the room, loud enough for everyone to hear—soliciting information of a private and intimate nature. It was an embarrassing invasion of privacy. Unfortunately, all other arrivals were subjected to similar embarrassment.

Typical hospital practices—such as medical staff consultations, conversations about patients in hallways and elevators, access to patient charts and other information, routine divulging of patient data for reasons of billing, quality assurance, research, and access to computerized records—seem incompatible with the notion of patient privacy and confidentiality. Is privacy even possible today?

Patient confidentiality remains one of the sacrosanct and leading ideas in the time-honored Hippocratic Oath. As a general rule, information between healthcare professionals and the patient must remain confidential and can be shared with others only if medically necessary or legally mandated. For instance, it is legally required for physicians to report gunshot wounds and instances of child abuse. Physicians are also required to report to the proper authorities medical conditions that adversely affect the safety of society, such as the weak heart condition of a flight controller.

Despite the fact that breaches of confidentiality are commonplace within the institutional setting, maintaining patient confidentiality is a prima facie principle. It sets the tone for the ideal covenantal relationship between healthcare professional and patient; without an assurance of confidentiality there can be no grounds for trust between healthcare professionals and patients.

The Individual and the Social Nexus

In 1969, a young university student, Tatiana Tarasoff, was brutally stabbed to death by her former boyfriend, Prosenjit Poddar. Later, the family of the victim sued the University of California's medical staff. Poddar had been undergoing therapy with a university psychologist, and during the course of their sessions he informed his therapist that he desired to kill Tarasoff. The psychologist and his supervisor requested that the campus police detain Poddar. He was eventually released by the police, and two months after his release Poddar carried out his wishes. Seven years later, in 1976, the California Supreme Court ruled that the university was negligent in not acting to protect Tarasoff and ruled in favor of her family. This case remains a benchmark in cases dealing with limits to confidentiality. Even though the majority opinion in this case supported overriding the patient's privacy, there was also strong dissension. The minority opinion stated that legally mandating psychiatrists and other healthcare professionals to warn others in the case of a real and serious threat may be counterproductive. If "dangerous" individuals, those in desperate need of counseling, know that certain types of information revealed during sessions might be disclosed, they may refrain from seeking counseling in the first place.

The Tarasoff ruling set a legal precedent. What it essentially claims is that privacy takes a back seat when it comes to a conflict between the patient's privacy and the safety of another. Patients' civil and moral rights do not trump the public's civil and moral right to protection. Although the Tarasoff case was the first of its kind to stipulate a legal duty to warn, it essentially acknowledges a long-standing moral expectation: An individual's moral rights do not justify infringing upon others' moral rights.

In another case, a young woman named Sheila Norbert was admitted into emergency for a seizure disorder. She had been admitted three months earlier for the same reason. However, at that time, not even a complete neurological workup had been able to determine the cause of the seizures. Nevertheless, on her second admittance, the attending physician ordered the same barrage of tests. Norbert had earlier confided to her family doctor the real reason for her first admittance: Her husband had beaten her, and not for the first time. When she told this story to her doctor, Norbert insisted on keeping it confidential. Her family doctor assured her that he would keep matters confidential unless doing so would endanger her health and safety. At the time of her readmittance, her family physician was convinced that her husband had again beaten her. Should he share what he knows with the attending physician?[30]

The family physician, naturally concerned about his patient's safety, may understandably feel tempted to override her request. We could argue that safeguarding Norbert morally justifies breaching her privacy. Also, if her physician knows there is harm but keeps the matter secret, then he could be construed as an accomplice to her abuse. On the other hand, for whatever reasons Norbert requested her doctor's silence on the matter, she needs to know that she can trust him and can count on him to protect her in case of real harm. How should her physician deal with the tension between protecting her well-being and maintaining her trust?

One indelible truth about our lives is that we are each part of a social nexus—we each belong to a relational web. Within these social webs are two basic categories of relationships: those special relationships with family and friends and those with the broader community. This social nexus provides us with a social context for moral obligations. For instance, by virtue of my relationship with my family, I have special moral duties. At the same time, my membership in the wider community is not without its own moral duties.

When we apply this truth to the issue of confidentiality, we discern three levels of concern: self (individual patient), others, and society. These three levels furnish us with guidelines for determining legitimate exceptions to the rule of confidentiality:

- *Harm to the individual patient.* Confidentiality can be overridden if there is sufficient evidence to indicate that the patient would otherwise be seriously harmed. For instance, a psychiatrist who is fairly convinced that his or her client poses a real threat to the client's own safety can justifiably share relevant information with others who may be in a position to prevent the potential harm.

- *Harm to others.* In the case of a strong likelihood of harm or injury to a third party, confidentiality can be overridden. Suppose a husband has an affair and contracts the HIV virus. He demands that his wife not be told of his condition because he believes this would end their marriage. He is obviously putting his wife at severe risk of harm. Moreover, if she becomes pregnant, their future offspring will also be at risk. Breaching confidentiality in this situation is justifiable. Ideally, the husband himself should be clearly honest with his wife, and the physician should encourage him to proceed in this direction. However, if the husband remains adamant about keeping his condition secret, the physician has a moral duty to somehow inform his wife in the least invasive manner.

- *Harm to society.* The broadest level of concern is the welfare of society—the common good. Suppose that, in the course of a routine physical exam, a physician detects a debilitating heart condition in a patient who happens to be a bus driver. The bus driver may experience a mild or severe heart attack at any time. The physician would be morally justified in seeing that other relevant parties—namely, the driver's employer—know of the driver's condition, since the welfare of others is at stake.

The examples above reflect the inherent link between the individual and the community. "No person is an island," and the social nexus is critical—particularly when it comes to placing constraints on an individual's autonomy and privacy. Patient confidentiality is not an absolute rule, and the privacy of the patient is not an absolute right. As a prima facie rule, confidentiality must be followed as a general rule of thumb, but there are occasions that warrant its breach.

Protecting the Vulnerable

Mr. R, a man in his early forties, contracts a sexually transmitted disease (STD) while on a business trip overseas. By the time symptoms appear, he has already engaged in sexual intercourse with his wife. Both he and his wife have the same physician. When he sees his physician for treatment, he requests that his physician also treat his wife with antibiotics. He also asks his physician to fabricate a reason for her being treated with antibiotics. Mr. R insists on keeping his affair confidential.[31] Should the physician deceive Mrs. R and not interfere with this "private" matter in their marriage? How does the physician balance his duty to protect the husband's privacy with his equally serious duty to be honest with his other patient, Mrs. R?

One way to frame the discussion about confidentiality is to view it in terms of vulnerability. Patients, by virtue of their condition, are in an intrinsically vulnerable situation. One way to compensate for this vulnerability is through acknowledging patients' rights to self-determination and privacy. Yet patients are not the only vulnerable parties. In the case of a patient who poses a potential danger to others, such as a carrier of the HIV virus, the well-being of these vulnerable others must be considered.

This approach makes sound logical sense. Patients have a right to privacy in the first place not only because it may increase the prospect for successful treatment and help ensure the necessary trust between caregiver and patient, but also because the patient has a moral right to be protected against abuses due to the patient's vulnerability. In therapy sessions, patients are particularly vulnerable when they disclose personal information that they ordinarily keep concealed. Therapists, therefore, acquire a certain measure of power by possessing this private information. Respecting their patients' privacy is a way of offering them a layer of protection against possible mistreatment. In instances where other parties besides the patient are also vulnerable, they must in turn be protected.

The relevance of the vulnerability of others was made manifest in a 1983 case in California in which a male patient who had been undergoing therapy shot his lover. The victim was seriously wounded, but she was not killed. During the shooting, her son was present, and she instinctively threw herself on him to protect him from injury. She later brought suit against the therapists who had known of the patient's prior intent to harm her. The case, *Hedlund v. Superior Court of Orange County*, was decided by the California Supreme Court, and the court ruled in her favor. At the same time, the court ruled that the therapists also had a duty to warn the victim's son, since he was extremely close to his mother and at that time his own safety was in jeopardy.[32]

What is the scope of the physician's responsibility to warn? From the Hedlund ruling, we can foresee difficulties regarding the extent of the responsibility the therapist may have to warn others of potential harm. Still, the essential point is clear: Physicians and others have a prima facie duty to maintain patient confidentiality; however, when the safety and well-being of others is threatened, they must first act to safeguard these others' interests.

Whistle-Blowing

Another instance in which confidentiality can be justifiably overridden involves reporting instances of negligence and unprofessional conduct—the delicate issue of whistle-blowing. Situations arise in which the behavior of healthcare professionals may pose a serious threat to their patients and others. Suppose a male physician makes sexual advances to a female patient. She feels uncomfortable with him and changes doctors. She then confides in her new physician about her former doctor's behavior. Should her new physician maintain this revelation in strict confidence? What if her new physician hears similar reports from others? What should this physician, or any healthcare professional, do?

Sexual advances are seen by some as instances of sexual abuse. According to the Health Professional Act in Ontario, sexual abuse can involve "sexual intercourse with a patient, sexually touching a patient, and 'behavior or remarks of a sexual nature.'"[33] The Canadian Medical Association has strict guidelines, and reporting such incidents is required. However, the guidelines are less clear in the United States.

Many cases of whistle-blowing involve instances of alleged medical negligence. Healthcare professionals are understandably reluctant to report their own colleagues, since they fear negative repercussions both personally and professionally. Often there is very little institutional support for reporting negligence. Nevertheless, whistle-blowing is at times morally appropriate. Haddard and Dougherty propose the following guidelines:

- Make sure that the wrongdoing is grave.
- Document all information well.
- Look for peer support.
- Follow institutional channels of complaint, but don't expect institutional support.

- Make disclosures in good faith.
- Always assume that one's disclosure will be made public.[34]

INFORMED CONSENT

Without a doubt, **informed consent** is the leading axiom in contemporary American medical ethics. Over the past thirty years, it has become the central expression of patients' rights, for two reasons. First, it is the most concrete demonstration of patient autonomy, or self-determination. Informed consent underscores the importance placed on patients' role in their own healthcare. Second, it reinforces the necessary fiduciary and covenantal relationship between healthcare professionals and patients. It enhances trust among all parties, which is crucial in bringing about a positive health outcome.

Informed consent should be obtained for all medical procedures and interventions, whether the purpose is diagnostic, therapeutic, palliative, research, or cosmetic. The more invasive and/or serious the procedure, the more stringent are the requirements for consent. Unfortunately, all too often obtaining consent takes place in suboptimal circumstances, such as the day before the proposed surgery as in our example of Juanita Diaz, the Spanish-speaking mother of the infant with the "square heart." Patients are frequently highly anxious, thus making genuine consent problematic.

Who should request consent? It is the moral and professional obligation of the attending physician to inform the patient sufficiently in order to obtain the patient's free consent. To delegate this task to another healthcare professional, such as a nurse, is highly suspect. The physician must assume full accountability, and falling short of this standard raises ethical concerns.

Two Levels of Consent

There are essentially two levels of consent: institutional and personal. Institutional consent refers to the particular event when the patient's consent is obtained and verified in writing. (A copy of a consent form is included in the Additional Resources at the end of the text.) The problem with this view of consent is its minimalism; that is, it may fulfill the necessary institutional requirement (getting the patient's signature), but it does little beyond that. Most important, it downplays the critical need for communication with the patient.

Personal consent is a process that is the result of an ongoing discussion with the patient. This takes time and effort on the part of the physician, requiring that he or she engage more conscientiously in communicating with the patient in order to know more about the patient's preferences, values, beliefs, and fears. Physicians often object that they simply do not have the time, and to a degree this complaint is valid. The institutional pressures placed on physicians do not allow much time for discussion with every patient. Nevertheless, this particular view of the consent process is set forth as the moral ideal. It represents what genuine informed consent ought to be.

Consent's Three Hurdles

The key to understanding the ideal of informed consent lies in the two words: *informed* and *consent.* The term *informed* points to the dynamic role of the physician, who actively informs the patient. The term *consent* evokes an equally active role on the part of the patient, who has the final say about his or her healthcare. Both terms express the necessary reciprocity in the dialogue between healthcare professional and patient, so that the final decision is ultimately a shared process.

This dialogue faces three hurdles, like a race in which each hurdle counts and failure to leap over any one hurdle disqualifies the runner. Genuine informed consent requires that each of three criteria be met: information, voluntariness, and competence.

Information   The physician must provide the patient with all the relevant and sufficient information the patient will need in order to make a decision about his or her treatment. Contrary to what many physicians think, informing the patient does not mean telling him or her everything about a particular procedure. This would be both impossible and impractical. Informing a patient sufficiently means conveying all information that has a bearing on making a decision, including the following:

- The recommended procedure: its purpose, risks, and benefits. All serious risks must be conveyed to the patient, even though their likelihood may be slim. All risks that are likely must be disclosed as well.

- Any reasonable alternatives to the proposed treatment and their accompanying risks and benefits, including the alternative of no treatment and the likely results.

- The prognosis for the patient. What are likely outcomes, both with and without certain treatments?

Further considerations include pointing out **volume-sensitive procedures,** that is, procedures that are either fairly common or rare at the hospital and whose success rates reflect their frequency. Suppose a patient at Newport Hospital in Rhode Island needs to undergo coronary bypass surgery. The attending physician informs the patient that this type of operation is not commonly performed at Newport Hospital, whereas it is quite frequently performed at Deaconess Hospital in nearby Boston and the success rate at Deaconess is also higher. Informing the patient of these facts gives the patient the option of having the surgery at Newport Hospital, with the support of family and friends, or at Deaconess Hospital, farther away from such support. It now becomes the patient's choice in line with his or her own values.

Also relevant is a physician's—particularly a surgeon's—success rate with a given procedure. For instance, a new treatment for prostate cancer is the injection of radiation pellets directly into the prostate. A patient is fully justified in wanting to know more not only about this new procedure, but also about the success rate of his radiologist and of the clinic out of which the radiologist operates. This means that the patient needs to ask questions. More important, the physician should encourage any questions the patient might have. The physician's willingly encouraging questions is a good sign.

As the opening story of the baby with the "square heart" shows, how the physician conveys information is just as important as what the physician says. The physician must somehow convey information in ways the patient can comprehend, which means avoiding technical language. Body language is all-important. There is a world of difference between standing at the foot of the patient's bed and sitting down face-to-face with the patient. The physician also needs to ask the patient to repeat what was said in the pa-

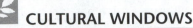

CULTURAL WINDOWS

INFORMED CONSENT IN JAPAN

Japan has an enduring tradition of deference to the authority of physicians. This respect for authority finds its roots in Confucian teachings, which became a predominant part of Japanese tradition. Japanese patients will usually entrust their care without question to their physician. The common expression *Sensei ni omakase shimasu* means "I entrust everything to you, Doctor." The primary physician, or **shujii,** will make the primary decisions. From the perspective of bioethics in the United States, with its emphasis on patient autonomy and informed consent, this appears to be a morally questionable attitude on the part of patients. However, for many Japanese, it reveals a unique vote of confidence in the physician that acknowledges a fundamental premise: Faith and trust in the healer are essential to the healing process. Therefore, the Japanese patient's respect for the authority of the physician

indicates a type of covenant between patient and physician. This covenant is signified at the foot of the patient's bed as well as on the door to the room, where the names of both the patient and his or her physician are posted.

As an example of this deference to physician authority, physicians typically will not disclose a diagnosis of terminal cancer to the patient. Many Japanese physicians believe that such disclosure could make the patient extremely and unnecessarily anxious and could depress the patient. They feel that such despondency could lead to despair and threaten to diminish the quality of life for that patient, thus violating the teaching of *Iwa jin jitsu nari*, or "Medicine is the practice of humaneness." The term *jin* comes from the Chinese *jen* and refers to the Confucian virtue of humaneness. Japanese physicians believe that they are obliged to protect their patients. They assume total re-

tient's own words. Finally, it helps to have a family member or close friend with the patient during the discussion. All of these actions convey to the patient a sincere effort to communicate, as well as a genuine interest in and respect for the patient as a person.

Voluntariness   Voluntariness means that consent must be uncoerced and free of excessive manipulation. This condition is especially difficult, though not impossible, in settings such as prisons, where some prisoners may consent to be research subjects. It is also tricky in situations in which potentially life-saving procedures are experimental as well as risky. When the first baboon-to-human liver transplant took place at Pittsburgh's Presbyterian University Hospital, the patient was informed that the procedure could save his life. Like most patients in life-threatening situations, he experienced tremendous anxiety. When does anxiety compromise free consent? What does it mean to give free consent? All of us face certain constraints, and every day we make decisions in the face of pressures. Yet we still presume our decisions to be free. When do our decisions become less free?

sponsibility for their patients—for their total well-being, not just their medical care. Disclosing a diagnosis of cancer without the likelihood of remission would place an unfair burden on the patient, a burden that the physician has agreed to assume.

Japanese patients themselves often will not insist on knowing the truth, whereas Americans may feel that all patients have a right to know the truth. In Japanese medical history, the ideas of patient's rights, patient autonomy, and informed consent are foreign notions, although this is changing in contemporary Japan due to Western influences. In fact, the Japanese term for "rights," *kenri*, is a term that came into use only during the Meiji Restoration (1868–1912) and is not the precise equivalent of what the term means for Westerners. Most Japanese still trust in the decision-making authority of their physicians.

In the case of terminal cancer, physicians in Japan will share their decision making with the family of the patient. Family members are usually told the diagnosis, yet even they may not share the information with the patient for the same reasons stated above. They will often carry the burden among themselves and continue to provide whatever care and comfort they can. This not only reflects the vote of confidence that the patient places with his or her family but also demonstrates the relational quality of the patient's identity. In other words, Japanese tend to view their identity in terms of relationships, with the most important being that within the family. When a family member enters the hospital, it becomes a family affair. All family members share in the care. They also share in the decision making along with the physician. In this respect, the kind of informed consent familiar to Americans, which assumes some individualized or private autonomy, makes little sense to many Japanese. Instead, the patient's identity is understood collectively within the relational web of the family. Therefore, patients will entrust decision making to family members as well as to their physician.

Think of a spectrum of decision making that ranges from choices that are free to those that are not free. Along this spectrum appear certain pressures that are reasonable, manipulative, or coercive. **Reasonable pressures** are pressures placed on us that appeal to our rational nature and to our sense of logic. Suppose a physician attempts to persuade a patient to undergo a recommended intervention by appealing to that patient's sense of reason and providing rational premises. In doing so, the physician respects the patient as a rational decision-maker and a self-determining agent. In such a context, the patient, if competent, freely decides.

Manipulation appeals more to a patient's emotional state than to his or her reason. Suppose a physician tries to persuade a patient to undergo a procedure by addressing the patient's fears, hopes, anxieties, and other emotive factors, using logical fallacies rather than reasoning. Such manipulative pressures are often effective with patients, since they are already in a stressful situation and, as with most of us, their hopes and fears may play a more powerful role than their reason. When patients' emotions are the sole driving force behind their decisions, these decisions are less free. If a cosmetic surgeon tells a patient that rhinoplasty (plastic surgery on the nose) will definitely make him or her much more attractive and desirable, the surgeon may be playing on the patient's emotional state in order to get the patient to comply. The physician in this case is manipulating the patient, which is morally questionable because the patient's choice is less free. There are times when appealing to emotions may be legitimate, for example, when a patient disregards all the sound reasons for not smoking. A physician may then use the strategy of appealing to the fear of dying, since the stakes are high and fear is a powerful motivator. But such manipulation may be justified only as a last resort, after all other avenues of persuasion have been exhausted.

Coercion occurs when a patient is compelled to act by being presented with an option that no rational person would refuse. Coercion is essentially a threat, whether physical or emotional. Suppose a physician is the only surgeon within a wide area who can perform a particular type of procedure. The procedure itself is experimental. The physician forewarns the patient that unless he or she agrees to undergo the experimental procedure, the physician will neither keep him or her as a patient nor refer the patient to any other physician. No rational person would desire to be abandoned by a physician under such circumstances. Whether or not the physician's posture is perceived as a threat, the posture is still coercive and therefore unjustifiable (as well as illegal if it amounts to patient abandonment without making necessary provisions). Even if the physician were to make provisions to transfer the patient to another physician, it could still amount to coercion because the posture is a threat. When patients are coerced to decide, their decision is no longer free.

The difficulty lies in ascertaining when manipulation crosses the line into coercion. Although manipulation may at times be sanctioned, the general rule of thumb is that the less free a choice is, the more problematic it becomes.

Competence   A surgeon requested that a hospital ethics committee consult concerning an eighty-year-old female patient who had gangrene spreading through her legs. The physician tried to persuade her to undergo an amputation below the knee before the gangrene could spread any further and become life-threatening. She refused. Knowing that her life was in jeopardy, she did not want the operation. When the physician asked her why she refused surgery, she responded that she was a devout Christian. She believed that God would take care of her and would cure her. Her physician concluded that she was incompetent to decide on her own behalf and requested the recommendation of ethics committee members. Should the patient be determined to be incompetent on these grounds? What do we mean by competency and incompetency?

Context Dependency   Defining competency and incompetency represents the last hurdle in arriving at sound consent. The patient must be competent in order to give consent. The first thing we need to be clear about is that both terms are **context-dependent,**[35] which means that the assessment of competency and incompetency must consider each specific situation. For instance, it is not meaningful simply to claim that a patient is incompetent. We need to be more specific. Incompetent to do what? To say what? To decide what? This distinction underscores Aristotle's important distinction between a condition and an act. For example, even though I may be a patient at Western Psychiatric Hospital and assessed as being in a condition of incompetence, I may still at times act competently. Even though a condition is the result of repeated actions, a condition of either incompetence or competence does not necessarily preclude, respectively, competent or incompetent actions and decisions. As a psychiatric patient, I could still make competent decisions, even if these might be as basic as finding my way to the rest room or feeding myself. Rather than claim that a patient is incompetent, we need to be more specific: incompetent with respect to what?

Decision-Making Capacity Not only is competency context-dependent, but it is also based on an assessment of a patient's decision-making capacity. When a person's decision-making capacity becomes questionable, a professional evaluation from at least two psychiatrists is in order. Our decision-making capacity is grounded in contextual features related to abilities and expectations. For instance, I am expected to be able to feed myself. If I cannot do so, then I am incompetent to feed myself. As a philosopher, I have a strong background in philosophical studies, yet I have no training in atomic physics. There is no expectation that I will be able to teach atomic physics. However, that I cannot teach atomic physics does not mean that I am incompetent to do so.

In determining the decision-making capacity of patients, we need to consider a number of ascending levels: comprehensive awareness, logical ordering, understanding, and appreciation. First, does the patient have a basic comprehensive awareness? In other words, does the patient know where he or she is, when he or she is there, and why? This is the most fundamental and minimal level of decision-making capacity. It is one the courts often rely on when determining the cognitive level of a person who makes a will. The next level of decision-making capacity is that of logical ordering, which involves the patient's capacity to think logically. For instance, if a patient desires to achieve D and knows that this necessitates accomplishing first B and then C, this patient possesses some degree of logical ordering. A higher level of comprehension comes with understanding. Understanding requires a comprehension of the circumstances as well as the reasons behind achieving D; it goes beyond mere rote memory. Higher than understanding is appreciation, in which the patient not only has an essential understanding of a particular subject, in this case D, but also can evaluate D in view of his or her own personal beliefs and values. Whereas understanding involves a distancing from D, appreciation incorporates an application of personal values. Obviously, evaluating competence is no easy test. Perhaps recognizing the lack of competence is easier than actually defining competence itself. Nevertheless, it constitutes the last hurdle that must be cleared in order for genuine consent to be obtained.

Proxy Consent and Minors

If a person is determined to be incompetent to make a specific healthcare decision, then a proxy decision-maker must take his or her place. **Proxy consent** can be given by a family member, a close friend, or a court-appointed surrogate. The principal purpose of the proxy decision-maker is to make the decision that the patient would most likely make if he or she could do so. This decision, referred to as **substituted judgment,** will be discussed in more detail in Chapter 8, on euthanasia. Substituted judgment requires a sound knowledge of the patient's values, preferences, and beliefs. It is extremely important that proxy decision-makers do not project their own values onto the patient, a situation called "projected judgment."

A sticky issue arises in the case of minors, children under legal age. Consider the case of a twelve-year-old Jehovah's Witness in Ontario who refused blood transfusions for her acute myeloid leukemia because of her religious beliefs. The court allowed her refusal to stand, pointing out that she possessed wisdom and maturity well beyond her years. She died a few weeks after the ruling.[36] Can minors give informed consent? As a general rule, minors do not have the cognitive and emotional ability to make the important decisions called for regarding medical interventions. Of course, there are exceptions. Age in and of itself is not the sole factor in determining competence. In the case of the twelve-year-old girl, the Canadian court recognized the possibility that some minors may have the decision-making capacity generally reserved for adults.

AMY M. HADDAD

The Nurse/Physician Relationship and Ethical Decision Making

Amy M. Haddad is an associate of the Creighton Center for Health Policy and Ethics at Creighton University and teaches at the School of Pharmacy and Allied Health Professions. Haddad points out some differences between physicians and nurses in terms of roles and power. She adds that men and women may approach ethical decision making in distinct ways as well. All this reinforces the doctor/nurse game, a communication method that is indirect and deferential. Using a case study, she concludes that a more direct approach to communication on the part of nurses is critical.

FACTORS AFFECTING THE NURSE/PHYSICIAN RELATIONSHIP

In 1967, Leonard I. Stein, MD, identified a basic communication pattern that physicians and nurses used. He called it the "Doctor-Nurse Game."[1] The game is still played daily in many surgery departments. The object of the game is for the nurse to be bold, have initiative, and be responsible for making significant recommendations while appearing to be doing none of this. It should appear that it was the physician who made the recommendations.

Both the nurse and physician need to be acutely aware of subtle nonverbal cues and verbal nuances in the conversation. The major rule of the game is that open disagreement must be avoided at all costs. Nurses learn to make suggestions and ask for recommendations in a way that sounds like they are not doing so. It is interesting that Dr Stein and his colleagues revisited the Doctor-Nurse Game in 1990.[2] Twenty-three years later, they found only minor changes in the way the game is played.

Consequences of this indirect method of communication are that it is inefficient and stifles open communication that is essential in ethical decision making. The doctor-nurse game is similar to the superior-subordinate game that occurs in almost all organizational hierarchies. Subordinates often use the passive voice to make suggestions to superiors within the organization.

Stereotypes are oversimplified, unvarying conceptions about a person or a group. Traditional gender stereotypes in nursing, both positive (eg, ministering, self-sacrificing angels, nurturing mothers) and negative (eg, sexpots, battle axes), add a new dimension to the superior-subordinate game. Positive (eg, noble, decisive leaders; captain of the ship) and negative (eg, egotistical, arrogant dictators) stereotypes in medicine have the same effect. Unfortunately, negative stereotypes in nursing and medicine tend to mirror those of women and men in society at large.

Another influencing factor in the nurse/physician relationship arises from the inherent inequity in power and authority that each discipline exercises. Physicians exercise a great deal of direct power in the health care system. Even though some reimbursement systems have begun to erode the physician's role as gatekeeper, physicians still tend to determine who is admitted and what type of treatments and procedures are to be performed. These decisions translate directly into revenue for the hospital.

Nurses are not a direct source of revenue for the hospital, but the hospital would not be able to function without them. Nurses' work is largely unseen but essential. Therefore, nurses, like others in traditionally female jobs, exercise little direct authority regarding decisions that affect their work or welfare. They generally receive little pay for the amount of responsibility associated with their work, and they receive little recognition and respect for their contribution to the enterprise as a whole.

Physicians, especially surgeons, earn more and generally are self-employed. The difference in income and employment status result in class barriers between physicians and nurses. The two groups rarely socialize with each other, which limits opportunities for informal discussions outside of the work setting. Informal discussions over coffee, at lunch, or during social activities, help individuals understand each other's values and motivations, which inevitably affect how the people work together.

Physicians and nurses also differ in educational preparation. Nurses generally have fewer years of formal education, which puts them at a disadvantage. Efforts to increase entry-level education in nursing have been strongly resisted by organized medicine. Physicians argue that increased education pulls nurses away from patient care. The more education a nurse has, however, the more she or he threatens the status quo and the authority of the physician. All of these factors influence the ability to collaborate and resolve ethical problems. The process becomes even more difficult because nurses and physicians usually do not perceive ethical problems in the same way.

APPROACHES TO ETHICAL DECISION MAKING

Carol Gilligan, PhD, noted some significant differences in how males and females reason morally.[3] One view predominant in females acknowledges that people's lives are embedded in relationships and that the relationships are central to moral decision making. People with this interdependent view are concerned about being responsible and responsive to others. They consider the specifics of a situation when making a decision. This view is most clearly reflected in the concept of mercy and commonly is used by nurses in making ethical decisions.

A counter view of moral reasoning consists of a rights and rules perspective and is directed toward justice and fair play. Males tend to use this type of moral reasoning. They seek a general rule that can be applied to specific situations. Physicians often take this approach when making ethical decisions.

These different attitudes affect ethical decision making. Nurses may appear unsure. They may seem overly concerned with details and the specifics of a situation and, therefore, slow to come to decisions. Nurses will identify interrelationships and include these as important factors when coming to a decision. They will ask how people are related and who will be affected by the decision and how. Often, nurses will consider quality of life and ability to function in ethical decision making.

Physicians, on the other hand, may have difficulty seeing the need for details and ambiguity. This is particularly true of surgeons who are rewarded, both financially and professionally, for their decisiveness and ability to act quickly under pressure. Because physicians are still trained in a reductionistic framework, they are likely to use a "rule out" approach to analyze ethical problems. Therefore, they have a tendency to break down the problem to its essential elements and dispense with all the extraneous details that nurses seem to believe are important. It is common for physicians to confuse professional expertise for moral authority. They often take it upon themselves to make ethical decisions with little or no collaboration or input.

CASE STUDY

The following case illustrates these different perspectives in action and how they affect ethical decision making. Dorothy Donahoe, RN, is assigned to complete the preoperative assessment on Wilford Cook, a 77-year-old patient in the intensive care unit. He is scheduled for spinal fusion. Dorothy reads through Wilford's clinical record and is overwhelmed at Wilford's course of treatment since he was admitted.

Wilford had no living relatives and had lived in a state institution for the mentally handicapped most of his life. With deinstitutionalization, he was placed in a group living setting in the community. To everyone's surprise, he surpassed all expectations regarding his functional abilities. Wilford learned to read and write, and he was able to work independently in the community.

Wilford had been admitted one month earlier for evaluation of chronic respiratory insufficiency and recurrent bronchitis and pneumonia. Dorothy notes that Wilford had carefully signed each permit for the various tests and procedures performed since his admission. Wilford had not, however, signed the surgical permit for removal of a mediastinal mass. On the line where his signature should have been are the words, "No, No, No." Below these words is the signature of the surgeon who had operated on Wilford and removed not only a malignant mediastinal mass but several vertebrae.

Since the surgery two weeks ago, Wilford has remained on a ventilator and in a semiconscious state. The head of the bed can be elevated only slightly because of the possibility of compressing the spinal cord. Dorothy decides to speak to the nurse in the critical care unit. He tells Dorothy the following:

> Wilford didn't want the initial surgery. I believe he understood the risks and alternatives to surgery. I guess the surgeon thought Wilford wasn't capable of giving consent. Because Wilford doesn't have any family, I guess the surgeon thought he was acting in Wilford's best interest. Wilford hasn't done well since surgery.
>
> Now the surgeon wants to put in Harrington rods to help support the spine so we can get Wilford up. If you ask me, I think that's too aggressive. However, when I suggested to Dr Anton that a tracheostomy would be easier to manage and more comfortable for Wilford, he told me that a tracheostomy was too aggressive!

Dorothy goes in to see Wilford. He has an endotracheal tube attached to the ventilator. Wilford responds to Dorothy's touch. Dorothy introduces herself and asks Wilford if he understands that the surgeon wants to take him back to the operating room and place support rods in his spine in place of the bones that were removed. Wilford nods. Dorothy asks, "Wilford, do you want to have this surgery?" Wilford shakes his head "no" slowly but purposefully.

Dorothy returns to the surgery department to speak to Dr Anton. She knows it is against hospital policy for a surgeon to sign a consent form unless it is an emergency procedure. She also thinks that Wilford needs someone to speak for him, but she is not certain how to go about finding someone. Dorothy finds Dr Anton and speaks to him. "Dr Anton, I have just been up to see Mr Cook in the critical care unit. Have you spoken to him about surgery?"

Dr Anton responds,

> I see no point in talking to him. He has a long history of mental retardation. Without the support of Harrington he'll never be able to sit up, let alone walk. He definitely needs the operation.

Dorothy has assisted with this type of procedure before. She knows it is an extremely complicated and lengthy operation that is hard on healthy adolescents, much less a terminally ill man who obviously does not want to go through the procedure. Dorothy hesitantly continues,

> When I went in to see Mr Cook, he seemed to under-stand me and responded negatively when I brought up the surgery. I also noticed that the oncologist on the case doesn't think any treatment would be helpful at this point. The prognosis is very poor.

Dr Anton responds, "Just what are you saying? Are you suggesting that this operation is not indicated?"

What is Dorothy saying? She is using indirect communication patterns of the doctor-nurse game. Dr Anton has picked up on the underlying theme of her concerns and is directly challenging her.

Dorothy and the critical care nurse have demonstrated many characteristics of the interdependent view of ethical decision making. They are concerned about honoring the patient's wishes and about his quality of life. Hence, the critical care nurse saw the need for a tracheostomy to improve Wilford's quality of life. Dorothy expressed concern about a procedure that offered little benefit but would surely increase Wilford's pain and suffering in whatever time he has left.

The surgeon is concerned about Wilford's life and may believe that quality of life applies only if there is life. The surgeon has not only made a medical decision but an ethical one. He has decided what kind of life Wilford will have during his last days. It is obvious that the surgeon will do what he thinks is necessary to help this questionably competent patient, and he is willing to override any concerns expressed by the patient.

Neither Dorothy nor Dr Anton is completely right or wrong. To come to a decision that draws on the strengths of both perspectives, some fundamental changes must occur in the way they work together. The following changes in the nurse's attitude may help improve the nurse-physician relationship.

AREAS FOR CHANGE

Nurses must learn to be credible, articulate, knowledgeable, and strong. This means anticipating arguments and heated exchanges. One place to begin is with language. Nurses must practice assertiveness and avoid over-qualifying and hesitancy. This requires direct communication and an abandonment of the doctor-nurse game.

For example, in the exchange between Dr Anton and Dorothy, Dr Anton responded, "Just what are you saying? Are you suggesting that this operation is not indicated?"

Dorothy wants to avoid a confrontation about the efficacy of the surgery so she could respond with, "No, I'm not suggesting that. I am saying that Mr Cook has clearly communicated that he does not want to undergo surgery." This response is assertive and direct. Dorothy has focused her response on Mr Cook's expressed wishes, not the appropriateness of the operation. Now the discussion revolves around Mr Cook's competency. Since there is a disagreement regarding Mr Cook's competency, Dorothy could then pursue guardianship to protect Mr Cook's interests.

Other types of language that discredit the speaker, such as, "I think this is probably wrong, but . . ." or "I know you're terribly busy and I hate to bother you, but . . ." also should be eliminated. These phrases interpret for the listener and give the listener permission to discount what follows. Nurses' observations about the specific details of a patient's life are important and should be shared with clarity and conviction. Nursing contributions to the decision-making process must not be lost in deferential language. One way to change language is to listen to peers and correct usage that undermines the speaker's intent.

In addition to direct communication, nurses should use every available opportunity to teach physicians about their roles and responsibilities within the health care system. It is ironic, but frequently true, that health care professionals who work in close proximity are not remotely aware of what the other members of the team do.

Education can occur in interdisciplinary committees, during workshops and in-service programs, and especially during one-to-one interactions. On a more formal basis, a surgery department could set up an interdisciplinary ethics committee to review particularly troublesome cases and to establish guidelines for common ethical problems in surgery. The shared authority of the group process allows for better decisions to emerge. There also is greater commitment to the decision by those involved. The establishment of such a group can be an excellent source of support for nurses and physicians.

Finally, nurses must realize that the patterns of interaction highlighted throughout this discussion are large trends and not just personal, isolated experiences. It is important for nurses to recognize the personal and structural aspects of people and situations at work. By doing this, they will learn to cut their losses and focus energy on relationships that are amenable to change. Because of their roles and expertise, nurses have access to information regarding patients' responses to health problems and the meaning patients give to the phrase *quality of life*. Both are major factors in all ethical decisions.

Because of their roles, physicians have expertise in diagnosis, prognosis, and treatment of disease and disability. Both aspects of these two essential health care professionals are necessary for humane and competent ethical decision making.

NOTES

1. L I Stein, "The doctor-nurse game," *Archives of General Psychiatry* 16 (June 1967) 699–703.

2. L I Stein, D T Watts, T Howell, "The doctor-nurse game revisited," *The New England Journal of Medicine* 322 (Feb 22, 1990) 546–549.

3. C Gilligan, *In a Different Voice: Psychological Theory and Women's Development* Cambridge, Mass.: Harvard University Press, 1982).

QUESTIONS FOR COMPREHENSION AND REFLECTION

1. According to Haddad, what factors affect the nurse/physician relationship? How do negative stereotypes influence how this relationship is perceived?

2. Do you agree with Carol Gilligan's theory that men and women tend to approach, as well as resolve, moral conflict differently? Do you agree with the author that this distinction is played out in the healthcare setting among professionals? Support your answers.

3. Do you believe that the author's recommendations do in fact lead to a more direct, assertive, and at the same time nonconfrontational strategy for nurses in dealing with physicians? Why or why not? What suggestions would you add?

4. How may cultural influences play a role in the nurse/physician relationship? Explain.

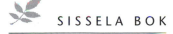

SISSELA BOK

Lies to the Sick and Dying

Sissela Bok is Distinguished Fellow at the Harvard Center for Population and Development. She examines the most prominent arguments supporting physicians' nondisclosure of the truth to their patients: total honesty is not possible; patients do not really want to know the truth; the truth will often cause more harm than good. She points out flaws in each argument and concludes that truth telling is a serious moral duty.

DECEPTION AS THERAPY

A forty-six-year-old man, coming to a clinic for a routine physical checkup needed for insurance purposes, is diagnosed as having a form of cancer likely to cause him to die within six months. No known cure exists for it. Chemotherapy may prolong life by a few extra months, but will have side effects the physician does not think warranted in this case. In addition, he believes that such therapy should be reserved for patients with a chance for recovery or remission. The patient has no symptoms giving him any reason to believe that he is not perfectly healthy. He expects to take a short vacation in a week.

For the physician, there are now several choices involving truthfulness. Ought he to tell the patient what he has learned, or conceal it? If asked, should he deny it? If he decides to reveal the diagnosis, should he delay doing so until after the patient returns from his vacation? Finally, even if he does reveal the serious nature of the diagnosis, should he mention the possibility of chemotherapy and his reasons for not recommending it in this case? Or should he encourage every last effort to postpone death?

In this particular case, the physician chose to inform the patient of his diagnosis right away. He did not, however, mention the possibility of chemotherapy. A medical student working under him disagreed; several nurses also thought that the patient should have been informed of this possibility. They tried, unsuccessfully, to persuade the physician that this was the patient's right. When persuasion had failed, the student elected to disobey the doctor by informing the patient of the alternative of chemotherapy. After consultation with family members, the patient chose to ask for the treatment.

Doctors confront such choices often and urgently. What they reveal, hold back, or distort will matter profoundly to their patients. Doctors stress with corresponding vehemence their reasons for the distortion or concealment: not to confuse a sick person needlessly, or cause what may well be unnecessary pain or discomfort, as in the case of the cancer patient; not to leave a patient without hope, as in those many cases where the dying are not told the truth about their condition; or to improve the chances of cure, as where unwarranted optimism is expressed about some form of therapy. Doctors use information as part of the therapeutic regimen; it is given out in amounts, in admixtures, and according to timing believed best for patients. Accuracy, by comparison, matters far less.

Lying to patients has, therefore, seemed an especially excusable act. Some would argue that doctors, and *only* doctors, should be granted the right to manipulate the truth in ways so undesirable for politicians, lawyers, and others.[1] Doctors are trained to help patients; their relationship to patients carries special obligations, and they know much more than laymen about what helps and hinders recovery and survival.

Even the most conscientious doctors, then, who hold themselves at a distance from the quacks and the purveyors of false remedies, hesitate to forswear all lying. Lying is usually wrong, they argue, but less so than allowing the truth to harm patients. B. C. Meyer echoes this very common view:

> [O]urs is a profession which traditionally has been guided by a precept that transcends the virtue of uttering truth for truth's sake, and that is, "so far as possible, do no harm."[2]

Truth, for Meyer, may be important, but not when it endangers the health and well-being of patients. This has seemed self-evident to many physicians in the past—so much so that we find very few mentions of veracity in the codes and oaths and writings by physicians through the centuries. This absence is all the more striking as other principles of ethics have been consistently and movingly expressed in the same documents.

The two fundamental principles of doing good and not doing harm—of beneficence and non-maleficence—are the most immediately relevant to medical practitioners, and the most frequently stressed. To preserve life and good health, to ward off illness, pain, and death—these are the perennial tasks of medicine and nursing. These principles have found powerful expression at all times in the history of medicine. In the Hippocratic Oath physicians promise to:

> use treatment to help the sick . . . but never with a view to injury and wrong-doing.[3]

And a Hindu oath of initiation says:

> Day and night, however thou mayest be engaged, thou shalt endeavor for the relief of patients with all thy heart and soul. Thou shalt not desert or injure the patient even for the sake of thy living.[4]

But there is no similar stress on veracity. It is absent from virtually all oaths, codes, and prayers. The Hippocratic Oath makes no mention of truthfulness to patients about their condition, prognosis, or treatment. Other early codes and prayers are equally silent on the subject. To be sure, they often refer to the confidentiality with which doctors should treat all that patients tell them; but there is no corresponding reference to honesty toward the patient. One of the few who appealed to such a principle was Amattis Lusitanus, a Jewish physician widely known for his skill, who, persecuted, died of the plague in 1568. He published an oath which reads in part:

> If I lie, may I incur the eternal wrath of God and of His angel Raphael, and may nothing in the medical art succeed for me according to my desires.[5]

Later codes continue to avoid the subject. Not even the Declaration of Geneva, adopted in 1948 by the World Medical Association, makes any reference to it. And the Principles of Medical Ethics of the American Medical Association[6] still leave the matter of informing patients up to the physician.

Given such freedom, a physician can decide to tell as much or as little as he wants the patient to know, so long as he breaks no law. In the case of the man mentioned at the beginning of this chapter, some physicians might feel justified in lying for the good of the patient; others might be truthful. Some may conceal alternatives to the treatment they recommend, others not. In each case, they could appeal to the AMA Principles of Ethics. A great many would choose to be able to lie. They would claim that not only can a lie avoid harm for the patient, but that it is also hard to know whether they have been right in the first place in making their pessimistic diagnosis; a "truthful" statement could therefore turn out to hurt patients unnecessarily. The concern for curing and for supporting those who cannot be cured then runs counter to the desire to be completely open. This concern is especially strong where the prognosis is bleak; even more so when patients are so affected by their illness or their medication that they are more dependent than usual, perhaps more easily depressed or irrational.

Physicians know only too well how uncertain a diagnosis or prognosis can be. They know how hard it is to give meaningful and correct answers regarding health and illness. They also know that disclosing their own uncertainty or fears can reduce those benefits that depend upon faith in recovery. They fear, too, that revealing grave risks, no matter how unlikely it is that these will come about, may exercise the pull of the "self-fulfilling prophecy." They dislike being the bearers of uncertain or bad news as much as anyone else. And last, but not least, sitting down to discuss an illness truthfully and sensitively may take much-needed time away from other patients.

These reasons help explain why nurses and physicians and relatives of the sick and dying prefer not to be bound by rules that might limit their ability to suppress, delay, or distort information. This is not to say that they necessarily plan to lie much of the time. They merely want to have the freedom to do so when they believe it wise. And the reluctance to see lying prohibited explains, in turn, the failure of the codes and oaths to come to grips with the problems of truth-telling and lying.

But sharp conflicts are now arising. Doctors no longer work alone with patients. They have to consult with others much more than before; if they choose to lie, the choice may not be met with approval by all who take part in the care of the patient. A nurse expresses the difficulty which results as follows:

> From personal experience I would say that the patients who aren't told about their terminal illness have so many verbal and mental questions unanswered that many will begin to realize that their illness is more serious than they're being told. . . .
>
> Nurses care for these patients twenty-four hours a day compared to a doctor's daily brief visit, and it is the nurse many times that the patient will relate to, once his underlying fears become overwhelming. . . . This is difficult for us nurses because being in constant contact with patients we can see the events leading up to this. The patient continually asks you, "Why isn't my pain decreasing?" or "Why isn't the radiation treatment easing the pain?" . . . We cannot legally give these patients an honest answer as a nurse (and I'm sure I wouldn't want to) yet the problem is still not resolved and the circle grows larger and larger with the patient alone in the middle.[7]

The doctor's choice to lie increasingly involves co-workers in acting a part they find neither humane nor wise. The fact that these problems have not been carefully thought through within the medical profession, nor seriously addressed in medical education, merely serves to intensify the conflicts.[8] Different doctors then respond very differently to patients in exactly similar predicaments. The friction is increased by the fact that relatives often disagree even where those giving medical care to a patient are in accord on how to approach the patient. Here again, because physicians have not worked out to common satisfaction the question of whether relatives have the right to make such requests, the problems are allowed to be haphazardly resolved by each physician as he sees fit.

THE PATIENT'S PERSPECTIVE

The turmoil in the medical profession regarding truth-telling is further augmented by the pressures that patients themselves now bring to bear and by empirical data coming to light. Challenges are growing to the three major arguments for lying to patients: that truthfulness is impossible; that patients do not want bad news; and that truthful information harms them.

The first of these arguments . . . confuses "truth" and "truthfulness" so as to clear the way for occasional lying on grounds supported by the second and third arguments. At this point, we can see more clearly that it is a strategic move intended to discourage the question of truthfulness from carrying much weight in the first place, and thus to leave the choice of what to say and how to say it up to the physician. To claim that "since telling the truth is impossible, there can be no sharp distinction between what is true and what is false"[9] is to try to defeat objections to lying before even discussing them. One need only imagine how such an argument would be received, were it made by a car salesman or a real estate dealer, to see how fallacious it is.

In medicine, however, the argument is supported by a subsidiary point: even if people might ordinarily understand what is spoken to them, pa-

tients are often not in a position to do so. This is where paternalism enters in. When we buy cars or houses, the paternalist will argue, we need to have all our wits about us; but when we are ill, we cannot always do so. We need help in making choices, even if help can be given only by keeping us in the dark. And the physician is trained and willing to provide such help.

It is certainly true that some patients cannot make the best choices for themselves when weakened by illness or drugs. But most still can. And even those who are incompetent have a right to have someone—their guardian or spouse perhaps—receive the correct information.

The paternalistic assumption of superiority to patients also carries great dangers for physicians themselves—it risks turning to contempt. The following view was recently expressed in a letter to a medical journal:

> As a radiologist who has been sued, I have reflected earnestly on advice to obtain Informed Consent but have decided to "take the risks without informing the patient" and trust to "God, judge, and jury" rather than evade responsibility through a legal gimmick. . . .
>
> [I]n a general radiologic practice many of our patients are uninformable and we would never get through the day if we had to obtain their consent to every potentially harmful study.
>
> . . . We still have patients with language problems, the uneducated and the unintelligent, the stolid and the stunned who cannot form an Informed Opinion to give an Informed Consent; we have the belligerent and the panicky who do not listen or comprehend. And then there are the Medicare patients who comprise 35 percent of general hospital admissions. The bright ones wearily plead to be left alone. . . . As for the apathetic rest, many of them were kindly described by Richard Bright as not being able to comprehend because "their brains are so poorly oxygenated."[10]

The argument which rejects informing patients because adequate truthful information is impossible in itself or because patients are lacking in understanding must itself be rejected when looked at from the point of view of patients. They know that liberties granted to the most conscientious and altruistic doctors will be exercised also in the "Medicaid Mills"; that the choices thus kept from patients will be exercised by not only competent but incompetent physicians; and that even the best doctors can make choices patients would want to make differently for themselves.

The second argument for deceiving patients refers specifically to giving them news of a frightening or depressing kind. It holds that patients do not, in fact, generally want such information. That they prefer not to have to face up to serious illness and death. On the basis of such a belief, most doctors in a number of surveys stated that they do not, as a rule, inform patients that they have an illness such as cancer.

When studies are made of what patients desire to know, on the other hand, a large majority say that they *would* like to be told of such a diagnosis.[11] All these studies need updating and should be done with larger numbers of patients and nonpatients. But they do show that there is generally a dramatic divergence between physicians and patients on the factual question of whether patients want to know what ails them in cases of serious illness such as cancer. In most of the studies, over 80 percent of the persons asked indicated that they would want to be told.

Sometimes this discrepancy is set aside by doctors who want to retain the view that patients do not want unhappy news. In reality, they claim, the fact that patients say they want it has to be discounted. The more someone asks to know, the more he suffers from fear which will lead to the denial of the information even if it is given. Informing patients is, therefore, useless; they resist and deny having been told what they cannot assimilate. According to this view, empirical studies of what patients say they want are worthless since they do not probe deeply enough to uncover this universal resistance to the contemplation of one's own death.

This view is only partially correct. For some patients, denial is indeed well established in medical experience. A number of patients (estimated at between 15 percent and 25 percent) will give evidence of denial of having been told about their illness, even when they repeatedly ask and are repeatedly informed. And nearly everyone experiences a period of denial at some point in the course of approaching death.[12] Elisabeth Kübler-Ross sees denial as resulting often from premature and abrupt information by a stranger who goes through the process quickly to "get it over with." She holds that denial functions as a buffer after unexpected shocking news, permitting individuals to collect themselves and to mobilize other defenses. She describes prolonged denial in one patient as follows:

> She was convinced that the x-rays were "mixed up"; she asked for reassurance that her pathology report could not possibly be back so soon and that another patient's report must have been marked with her name. When none of this could be confirmed, she quickly asked to leave the hospital, looking for another physician in the vain hope "to get a better explanation for my troubles." This patient went "shopping around" for many doctors, some of whom gave her reassuring answers, others of whom confirmed the previous suspicion. Whether confirmed or not, she reacted in the same manner, she asked for examination and reexamination. . . .[13]

But to say the denial is universal flies in the face of all evidence. And to take any claim to the contrary as "symptomatic" of deeper denial leaves no room for reasoned discourse. There is no way that such universal denial can be proved true or false. To believe in it is a metaphysical belief about man's condition, not a statement about what patients do and do not want. It is true that we can never completely understand the possibility of our own death, any more than being alive in the first place. But people certainly differ in the degree to which they can approach such knowledge, take it into account in their plans, and make their peace with it.

Montaigne claimed that in order to learn both to live and to die, men have to think about death and be prepared to accept it.[14] To stick one's head in the sand, or to be prevented by lies from trying to discern what is to come, hampers freedom—freedom to consider one's life as a whole, with a beginning, a duration, an end. Some may request to be deceived rather than to see their lives as thus finite; others reject the information which would require them to do so; but most say that they want to know. Their concern for knowing about their condition goes far beyond mere curiosity or the wish to make isolated personal choices in the short time left to them; their stance toward the entire life they have lived, and their ability to give it meaning and completion, are at stake.[15] In lying or withholding the facts which permit such discernment, doctors may reflect their own fears (which, according to one study,[16] are much stronger than those of laymen) of facing questions about the meaning of one's life and the inevitability of death.

Beyond the fundamental deprivation that can result from deception, we are also becoming increasingly aware of all that can befall patients in the course of their illness when information is denied or distorted. Lies place them in a position where they no longer participate in choices concerning their own health, including the choice of whether to be a "patient" in the first place. A terminally ill person who is not informed that his illness is incurable and that he is near death cannot make decisions about the end of his life; about whether or not to enter a hospital, or to have surgery; where and with whom to spend his last days; how to put his affairs in order—these most personal choices cannot be made if he is kept in the dark, or given contradictory hints and clues. . . .

The reason why even doctors who recognize a patient's right to have information might still not provide it brings us to the third argument against telling all patients the truth. It holds that the information given might hurt the patient and the concern for the right to such information is therefore a threat to proper health care. A patient, these doctors argue, may wish to commit suicide after being given discouraging news, or suffer a cardiac arrest, or simply cease to struggle, and thus not grasp the small remaining chance for recovery. And even where the outlook for a patient is very good, the disclosure of a minute risk can shock some patients or cause them to reject needed protection such as a vaccination or antibiotics.

The factual basis for this argument has been challenged from two points of view. The damages associated with the disclosure of sad news or risks are rarer than physicians believe; and the *benefits* which result from being informed are more sub-

stantial, even measurably so. Pain is tolerated more easily, recovery from surgery is quicker, and cooperation with therapy is greatly improved. The attitude that "what you don't know won't hurt you" is proving unrealistic; it is what patients do not know but vaguely suspect that causes them corrosive worry.

It is certain that no answers to this question of harm from information are the same for all patients. If we look, first, at the fear expressed by physicians that informing patients of even remote or unlikely risks connected with a drug prescription or operation might shock some and make others refuse the treatment that would have been best for them, it appears to be unfounded for the great majority of patients. Studies show that very few patients respond to being told of such risks by withdrawing their consent to the procedure and that those who do withdraw are the very ones who might well have been upset enough to sue the physician had they not been asked to consent beforehand.[17] It is possible that on even rarer occasions especially susceptible persons might manifest physical deterioration from shock; some physicians have even asked whether patients who die after giving informed consent to an operation, but before it actually takes place, somehow expire because of the information given to them.[18] While such questions are unanswerable in any one case, they certainly argue in favor of caution, a real concern for the person to whom one is recounting the risks he or she will face, and sensitivity to all signs of distress.

The situation is quite different when persons who are already ill, perhaps already quite weak and discouraged, are told of a very serious prognosis. Physicians fear that such knowledge may cause the patients to commit suicide, or to be frightened or depressed to the point that their illness takes a downward turn. The fear that great numbers of patients will commit suicide appears to be unfounded.[19] And if some do, is that a response so unreasonable, so much against the patient's best interest that physicians ought to make it a reason for concealment or lies? Many societies have allowed suicide in the past; our own has decriminalized it; and some are coming to make distinctions among the many suicides which ought to be prevented if at all possible, and those which ought to be respected.[20]

Another possible response to very bleak news is the triggering of physiological mechanisms which allow death to come more quickly—a form of giving up or of preparing for the inevitable, depending on one's outlook. Lewis Thomas, studying responses in humans and animals, holds it not unlikely that:

> . . . there is a pivotal movement at some stage in the body's reaction to injury or disease, maybe in aging as well, when the organism concedes that it is finished and the time for dying is at hand, and at this moment the events that lead to death are launched, as a coordinated mechanism. Functions are then shut off, in sequence, irreversibly, and, while this is going on, a neural mechanism, held ready for this occasion, is switched on. . . .[21]

Such a response may be appropriate, in which case it makes the moments of dying as peaceful as those who have died and been resuscitated so often testify. But it may also be brought on inappropriately, when the organism could have lived on, perhaps even induced malevolently, by external acts intended to kill. Thomas speculates that some of the deaths resulting from "hexing" are due to such responses. Levi-Strauss describes deaths from exorcism and the casting of spells in ways which suggest that the same process may then be brought on by the community.[22]

It is not inconceivable that unhappy news abruptly conveyed, or a great shock given to someone unable to tolerate it, could also bring on such a "dying response," quite unintended by the speaker. There is every reason to be cautious and to try to know ahead of time how susceptible a patient might be to the accidental triggering—however rare—of such a response. One has to assume, however, that most of those who have survived long enough to be in a situation where their informed consent is asked have a very robust resistance to such accidental triggering of processes leading to death. . . .

Apart from the possible harm from information, we are coming to learn much more about the benefits it can bring patients. People follow instructions more carefully if they know what their disease is and why they are asked to take medications; any benefits from those procedures are therefore much more likely to come about. Similarly, people recover faster from surgery and tolerate pain with less medication if they understand what ails them and what can be done for them.

RESPECT AND TRUTHFULNESS

Taken all together, the three arguments defending lies to patients stand on much shakier ground as a counterweight to the right to be informed than is often thought. The common view that many patients cannot understand, do not want, and may be harmed by, knowledge of their condition, and that lying to them is either morally neutral or even to be recommended, must be set aside. Instead, we have to make a more complex comparison. Over against the right of patients to knowledge concerning themselves, the medical and psychological benefits to them from this knowledge, the unnecessary and sometimes harmful treatment to which they can be subjected if ignorant, and the harm to physicians, their profession, and other patients from deceptive practices, we have to set a severely restricted and narrowed paternalistic view—that *some* patients cannot understand, *some* do not want, and *some* may be harmed by, knowledge of their condition, and that they ought not to have to be treated like everyone else if this is not in their best interest.

Such a view is persuasive. A few patients openly request not to be given bad news. Others give clear signals to that effect, or are demonstrably vulnerable to the shock or anguish such news might call forth. Can one not in such cases infer implied consent to being deceived?

Concealment, evasion, withholding of information may at times be necessary. But if someone contemplates lying to a patient or concealing the truth, the burden of proof must shift. It must rest, here, as with all deception, on those who advocate it in any one instance. They must show why they fear a patient may be harmed or how they know that another cannot cope with the truthful knowledge. A decision to deceive must be seen as a very unusual step, to be talked over with colleagues and others who participate in the care of the patient. Reasons must be set forth and debated, alternatives weighed carefully. At all times, the correct information must go to *someone* closely related to the patient.

The law already permits doctors to withhold information from patients where it would clearly hurt their health. But this privilege has been sharply limited by the courts. Certainly it cannot be interpreted so broadly as to permit a general practice of deceiving patients "for their own good." Nor can it be made to include cases where patients might calmly decide, upon hearing their diagnosis, not to go ahead with the therapy their doctor recommends.[23] Least of all can it justify silence or lies to large numbers of patients merely on grounds that it is not always easy to tell what a patient wants.

For the great majority of patients, on the contrary, the goal must be disclosure, and the atmosphere one of openness. But it would be wrong to assume that patients can therefore be told abruptly about a serious diagnosis—that, so long as openness exists, there are no further requirements of humane concern in such communication. Dr. Cicely Saunders, who runs the well-known St. Christopher's Hospice in England, describes the sensitivity and understanding which are needed:

> Every patient needs an explanation of his illness that will be understandable and convincing to him if he is to cooperate in his treatment or be relieved of the burden of unknown fears. This is true whether it is a question of giving a diagnosis in a hopeful situation or of confirming a poor prognosis.
>
> The fact that a patient does not ask does not mean that he has no questions. One visit or talk is rarely enough. It is only by waiting and listening that we can gain an idea of what we should be saying. Silences and gaps are often more revealing than words as we try to learn what a patient is facing as he travels along the constantly changing journey of his illness and his thoughts about it.
> . . . So much of the communication will be without words or given indirectly. This is true of all real meeting with people but especially true with those who are facing, knowingly or not,

difficult or threatening situations. It is also particularly true of the very ill.

The main argument against a policy of deliberate, invariable denial of unpleasant facts is that it makes such communication extremely difficult, if not impossible. Once the possibility of talking frankly with a patient has been admitted, it does not mean that this will always take place, but the whole atmosphere is changed. We are then free to wait quietly for clues from each patient, seeing them as individuals from whom we can expect intelligence, courage, and individual decisions. They will feel secure enough to give us these clues when they wish.[24]

Above all, truthfulness with those who are suffering does not mean that they should be deprived of all hope: hope that there is a chance of recovery, however small; nor of reassurance that they will not be abandoned when they most need help.

Much needs to be done, however, if the deceptive practices are to be eliminated, and if concealment is to be restricted to the few patients who ask for it or those who can be shown to be harmed by openness. The medical profession has to address this problem.

NOTES

1. Plato, *The Republic*, 389 b.
2. B. C. Meyer, "Truth and the Physician," *Bulletin of the New York Academy of Medicine* 45 (1969): 59–71.
3. W. H. S. Jones, trans., *Hippocrates*, Loeb Classical Library (Cambridge, Mass.: Harvard University Press, 1923), p. 164.
4. Reprinted in M. B. Etziony, *The Physician's Creed: An Anthology of Medical Prayers, Oaths and Codes of Ethics* (Springfield, Ill.: Charles C Thomas, 1973), pp. 15–18
5. See Harry Friedenwald, "The Ethics of the Practice of Medicine from the Jewish Point of View," *Johns Hopkins Hospital Bulletin*, no. 318 (August 1917), pp. 256–61.
6. "Ten Principles of Medical Ethics," *Journal of the American Medical Association* 164 (1957): 1119–20.
7. Mary Barrett, letter, *Boston Globe*, 16 November 1976, p. 1.
8. Though a minority of physicians have struggled to bring them to our attention. See Thomas Percival, *Medical Ethics,* 3d ed. (Oxford: John Henry Parker, 1849), pp. 132–41; Worthington Hooker, *Physician*

and *Patient* (New York: Baker and Scribner, 1849), pp. 357–82; Richard C. Cabot, "Teamwork of Doctor and Patient Through the Annihilation of Lying," in *Social Service and the Art of Healing* (New York: Moffat, Yard & Co., 1909), pp. 116–70; Charles C. Lund, "The Doctor, the Patient, and the Truth," *Annals of Internal Medicine* 24 (1946): 955; Edmund Davies, "The Patient's Right to Know the Truth," *Proceedings of the Royal Society of Medicine* 66 (1973): 533–36.

9. Lawrence Henderson, "Physician and Patient as a Social System," *New England Journal of Medicine* 212 (1955).

10. Nicholas Demy, Letter to the Editor, *Journal of the American Medical Association* 217 (1971): 696–97.

11. For the views of physicians, see Donald Oken, "What to Tell Cancer Patients," *Journal of the American Medical Association* 175 (1961): 1120–28; and tabulations in Robert Veatch, *Death, Dying, and the Biological Revolution* (New Haven and London: Yale University Press, 1976), pp. 229–38. For the view of patients, see Veatch, ibid; Jean Aitken-Swan and E. C. Easson, "Reactions of Cancer Patients on Being Told Their Diagnosis," *British Medical Journal*, 1959, pp. 779–83; Jim McIntosh, "Patients' Awareness and Desire for Information About Diagnosed but Undisclosed Malignant Disease," *The Lancet* 7 (1976): 300–303; William D. Kelly and Stanley R. Friesen, "Do Cancer Patients Want to Be Told?," *Surgery* 27 (1950): 822–26.

12. See Avery Weisman, *On Dying and Denying* (New York: Behavioral Publications, 1972); Elisabeth Kübler-Ross, *On Death and Dying* (New York: The Macmillan Co., 1969); Ernest Becker, *The Denial of Death* (New York: Free Press, 1973); Philippe Ariès, *Western Attitudes Toward Death*, trans. Patricia M. Ranum (Baltimore and London: Johns Hopkins University Press, 1974); and Sigmund Freud, "Negation," *Collected Papers*, ed. James Strachey (London: Hogarth Press, 1950), 5: 181–85.

13. Kübler-Ross, *On Death and Dying*, p. 34.

14. Michel de Montaigne, *Essays*, bk. 1, chap. 20.

15. It is in literature that these questions are most directly raised. Two recent works where they are taken up with striking beauty and simplicity are May Sarton, *As We Are Now* (New York: W. W. Norton & Co., 1973); and Freya Stark, *A Peak in Darien* (London: John Murray, 1976).

16. Herman Feifel *et al.*, "Physicians Consider Death," *Proceedings of the American Psychoanalytical Association*, 1967, pp. 201–2.

17. See Ralph Alfidi, "Informed Consent: A Study of Patient Reaction," *Journal of the American Medical Association* 216 (1971): 1325–29.

18. See Steven R. Kaplan, Richard A. Greenwald, and Arvey I. Rogers, Letter to the Editor, *New England Journal of Medicine* 296 (1977): 1127.

19. Oken, "What to Tell Cancer Patients"; Veatch, *Death, Dying, and the Biological Revolution*; Weisman, *On Dying and Denying*.

20. Norman L. Cantor, "A Patient's Decision to Decline Life-Saving Treatment: Bodily Integrity Versus the Preservation of Life," *Rutgers Law Review* 26: 228–64; Danielle Gourevitch, "Suicide Among the Sick in Classical Antiquity," *Bulletin of the History of Medicine* 18 (1969): 501–18; for bibliography, see Bok, "Voluntary Euthanasia."

21. Lewis Thomas, "A Meliorist View of Disease and Dying," *The Journal of Medicine and Philosophy* 1 (1976): 212–21.

22. Claude Lévi-Strauss, *Structural Anthropology* (New York: Basic Books, 1963), p. 167; see also Eric Cassell, "Permission to Die," in John Behnke and Sissela Bok, eds., *The Dilemmas of Euthanasia* (New York: Doubleday, Anchor Press, 1975), pp. 121–31.

23. See Charles Fried, *Medical Experimentation: Personal Integrity and Social Policy* (Amsterdam and Oxford: North Holland Publishing Co., 1974), pp. 20–24.

24. Cicely M. S. Saunders, "Telling Patients," in S. J. Reiser, W. J. Dyck, A. J. Curran, *Ethics in Medicine* (Cambridge, Mass.: M.I.T. Press, 1977), pp. 238–40.

QUESTIONS FOR COMPREHENSION AND REFLECTION

1. What does Bok mean by the confusion of "truth" and "truthfulness"? How does this confusion pave the way for the justification of deception of patients?

2. Bok points out that most patients do want to know the truth about their condition. How does respecting this desire to know reflect a Kantian perspective? Explain your answer.

3. How does telling the truth bring about more positive results for the patient? Could a utilitarian approach also legitimize, in some situations, not telling the truth? Explain.

4. Is truthfulness a universal principle? Japanese physicians still tend to not tell the truth to their dying patients, even though the rest of the family knows it. Would insisting on telling the truth be justified in Japanese culture, or would it in effect be a way of imposing our own morality? Explain.

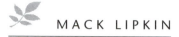

MACK LIPKIN

On Telling Patients the Truth

Mack Lipkin was a professor of internal medicine at the University of North Carolina. In direct contrast to Bok's position, Lipkin defends the practice of nondisclosure by arguing that conveying the truth completely to patients is virtually impossible. Patients simply do not know enough to understand the nature of their condition. He adds that patients often do not genuinely desire to know the truth. For Lipkin, what is critical is that the deception be intended to benefit the patient.

Should a doctor always tell his patients the truth? In recent years there has been an extraordinary increase in public discussion of the ethical problems involved in this question. But little has been heard from physicians themselves. I believe that gaps in understanding the complex interactions between doctors and patients have led many laymen astray in this debate.

It is easy to make an attractive case for always telling patients the truth. But as L. J. Henderson, the great Harvard physiologist-philosopher of decades ago, commented:

> To speak of telling the truth, the whole truth and nothing but the truth to a patient is absurd. Like absurdity in mathematics, it is absurd simply because it is impossible. . . . The notion that the truth, the whole truth, and nothing but the truth can be conveyed to the patient is a good specimen of that class of fallacies called by Whitehead "the fallacy of misplaced concreteness." It results from neglecting factors that cannot be excluded from the concrete situation and that are of an order of magnitude and relevancy that make it

imperative to consider them. Of course, another fallacy is also often involved, the belief that diagnosis and prognosis are more certain than they are. But that is another question.

Words, especially medical terms, inevitably carry different implications for different people. When these words are said in the presence of anxiety-laden illness, there is a strong tendency to hear selectively and with emphases not intended by the doctor. Thus, what the doctor means to convey is obscured.

Indeed, thoughtful physicians know that transmittal of accurate information to patients is often impossible. Patients rarely know how the body functions in health and disease, but instead have inaccurate ideas of what is going on; this hampers the attempts to "tell the truth."

Take cancer, for example. Patients seldom know that while some cancers are rapidly fatal, others never amount to much; some have a cure rate of 99 percent, others less than 1 percent; a cancer may grow rapidly for months and then stop growing for years; may remain localized for years or spread all over the body almost from the beginning; some can be arrested for long periods of time, others not. Thus, one patient thinks of cancer as curable, the next thinks it means certain death.

How many patients understand that "heart trouble" may refer to literally hundreds of different abnormalities ranging in severity from the trivial to the instantly fatal? How many know that the term "arthritis" may refer to dozens of different types of joint involvement? "Arthritis" may raise a vision of the appalling disease that made Aunt Eulalee a helpless invalid until her death years later; the next patient remembers Grandpa grumbling about the damned arthritis as he got up from his chair. Unfortunately but understandably, most people's ideas about the implications of medical terms are based on what they have heard about a few cases.

The news of serious illness drives some patients to irrational and destructive behavior; others handle it sensibly. A distinguished philosopher forestalled my telling him about his cancer by saying, "I want to know the truth. The only thing I couldn't take and wouldn't want to know about is cancer." For two years he had watched his mother die slowly of a painful form of cancer. Several of my physician patients have indicated they would not want to know if they had a fatal illness.

Most patients should be told "the truth" to the extent that they can comprehend it. Indeed, most doctors, like most other people, are uncomfortable with lies. Good physicians, aware that some may be badly damaged by being told more than they want or need to know, can usually ascertain the patient's preference and needs.

Discussions about lying often center about the use of placebos. In medical usage, a "placebo" is a treatment that has no specific physical or chemical action on the condition being treated, but is given to affect symptoms by a psychologic mechanism, rather than a purely physical one. Ethicists believe that placebos necessarily involve a partial or complete deception by the doctor, since the patient is allowed to believe that the treatment has a specific effect. They seem unaware that placebos, far from being inert (except in the rigid pharmacological sense), are among the most powerful agents known to medicine.

Placebos are a form of suggestion, which is a direct or indirect presentation of an idea, followed by an uncritical, i.e., not thought-out, acceptance. Those who have studied suggestion or looked at medical history know its almost unbelievable potency; it is involved to a greater or lesser extent in the treatment of every conscious patient. It can induce or remove almost any kind of feeling or thought. It can strengthen the weak or paralyze the strong; transform sleeping, feeding, or sexual patterns; remove or induce a vast array of symptoms; mimic or abolish the effect of very powerful drugs. It can alter the function of most organs. It can cause illness or a great sense of well-being. It can kill. In fact, doctors often add a measure of suggestion when they prescribe even potent medications for those who also need psychologic support. Like all potent agents, its proper use requires judgment based on experience and skill.

Communication between physician and the apprehensive and often confused patient is delicate and uncertain. Honesty should be evaluated not only in terms of a slavish devotion to language often misinterpreted by the patient, but also in terms of intent. *The crucial question is whether the deception was intended to benefit the patient or the doctor.*

Physicians, like most people, hope to see good results and are disappointed when patients do poorly. Their reputations and their livelihood depend on doing effective work; purely selfish reasons would dictate they do their best for their patients. Most important, all good physicians have a deep sense of responsibility toward those who have entrusted their welfare to them.

As I have explained, it is usually a practical impossibility to tell patients "the whole truth." Moreover, often enough, the ethics of the situation, the true moral responsibility, may demand that the naked facts not be revealed. The now popular complaint that doctors are too authoritarian is misguided more often than not. Some patients who insist on exercising their right to know may be doing themselves a disservice.

Judgment is often difficult and uncertain. Simplistic assertions about telling the truth may not be helpful to patients or physicians in times of trouble.

1. What are the primary reasons why Lipkin advocates withholding information from patients? In what ways does his position differ from that of Bok?
2. Why does Lipkin believe that it is impossible to tell the "whole truth" to patients? How does he support this belief with examples of patients suffering from cancer, heart problems, and arthritis? Do you agree or disagree? Explain.
3. How does he support the use of placebos in medicine? Do you agree or disagree? Explain.
4. Is Lipkin's line of reasoning more utilitarian or more deontological? Support your answer.

HILDE LINDEMANN NELSON

Knowledge at the Bedside: A Feminist View of What's Happening with This Patient

Hilde Lindemann Nelson is director of the Center for Applied and Professional Ethics at the University of Tennessee in Knoxville. She offers another perspective on the physician/patient relationship by introducing her "feminist standpoint theory" and applying it to clinical encounters. By using some vignettes as cases, Nelson concludes that the healthcare professional's judgment ought to be a collaborative effort, not one that is derived entirely from a single epistemic perspective.

Mrs. Alexandros, 78 years old and wheezing for lack of breath, is dying of lung cancer. Dr. Bishop finishes examining her chest and asks, "Do you have any questions about your illness? Do you understand how ill you are?" The old woman pulls in the corners of her thin blue lips and looks out the window. "I can't talk about this," she says. She has said this or something like it every time Dr. Bishop invites her to discuss her illness. He does not explore this with her, but drops the subject. She is still in denial, he thinks, and makes a note on her chart.

A second story.

Angie Gates, a young black woman, has just had the blood test that confirms she is pregnant. She grins when Dr. Elders gives her the news and asks what happens next. "Next," says Dr. Elders, "I'd like to test you for HIV. If you have the virus that causes AIDS, you don't want to pass it on to the baby. We know what to do to keep that from happening. Okay?" But Angie refuses. "I don't need that test," she says, "I'm fine." Dr. Elders explains in greater detail why the test is necessary. But despite the doctor's best efforts to change her patient's mind, Angie remains immovable. Finally Dr. Elders gives up—at least for the moment—and Angie leaves the office. She's hiding something, Dr. Elders thinks to herself, and moves on to her next patient.[1]

These rather commonplace clinical interactions raise a number of questions about knowledge. What counts as knowledge and how is it produced? What kinds of assumptions are physicians likely to make about patients and what they know, and how might patients' faulty assumptions about clinical knowing further complicate matters? What conception of objectivity do physicians use to ensure that their own knowledge is free from bias, and how, paradoxically, does this limit what they can know?

I am going to argue that the knowledge that gives medicine its social authority is frequently accompanied by assumptions about knowledge and knowing that can keep physicians from fully appreciating what may be going on with a patient in a given clinical encounter. I shall show how feminist standpoint theory helps to explain why physicians may too readily conclude that patients who deviate from certain epistemic standards are practicing some form of self-deception or covering up discreditable behavior. As such conclusions wrong the patient, I shall argue that the connection between epistemology and ethics is tighter than is generally suspected and that the remedy for the physician's epistemic shortcomings is an ethical one. Finally, I note that the rather mysterious conception of judgment that physicians invoke (for example, against overzealous use of practice guidelines) can form an alliance with feminist epistemology to destabilize standard theories of knowledge in interesting and productive ways.

SCIENCE AND THE NATURE OF KNOWLEDGE

Most physicians consider their profession to be both an art and a science, but it is the science, not the art, that authorizes the practice of medicine. Medicine is accorded authority because it "works,"

and it works because it rests on a scientific footing. It is training in such sciences as chemistry and microbiology that separates the doctor from the New Age crystal-healer and entitles the one, but not the other, to be licensed to practice medicine. Keeping abreast of scientific advances in one's subspecialty is a mark of medical competence, and contributing to these advances increases one's medical prestige.

But why is the scientific method itself so successful? Science succeeds, it is often thought, because the world is knowable through the laws that govern it. These laws are independent of time, place, and the characteristics of the investigator; they are in principle verifiable by anyone. Lynn Nelson has identified three assumptions implicit in this understanding of science: there is one world to discover, our sense organs can uniquely discriminate that world, and science is a process which will lead, in a finite amount of time, to a single view about what that reality is.[2]

All three assumptions have come under fire in recent years. W. V. O. Quine argued as early as 1960 that there are indefinitely many theories that allow us to explain and predict our experience of the world, that no single system can be shown to be the best (although some can be shown to be worse than others), and that we therefore have no reason to think there is one unique and comprehensive true account of the world.[3]

There is no evidence for the belief that our sense organs are exactly suited to provide us with data on everything that is the case about the universe. Our senses do tell us enough about the world so that we can organize and predict experience and so enhance our prospects of survival, but this fact does not preclude the possibility that other combinations of sense organs couldn't do this better. At minimum, we have no reason to suppose that our sense organs are uniquely matched to what goes on in nature.[4]

As for the claim that science will lead us to a single and definitive view of reality, Quine and Duhem discredited this as well.[5] Theories, they demonstrated, are always underdetermined by the data that support them, which means that other theories can always be found that will account for the same set of data. And as every statement in any theory is connected to the others like the strands of a web, no single observation can decisively refute the theory: the torn strand of web can be patched by weaving in new explanations.

Contemporary epistemologists have also emphasized the degree to which knowledge is constructed. Many facts are established by negotiations among experts who decide, on the basis of some theory, whether there is good evidence for them. These or other experts also negotiate what counts as evidence. And research agendas too are socially constructed: a combination of the research that is currently being done, political and economic pressures, and the prestige of the persons who want to know determine what investigations will be undertaken in the future to produce new knowledge.

THE OBJECT OF KNOWLEDGE AS SOCIAL CONSTRUCTION

What does all this mean for Dr. Bishop, the physician treating Mrs. Alexandros in my opening story? It means that the judgment he makes about her—that she's deceiving herself about the fact that she is dying—may be mistaken, and if it is, the mistake is likely to have arisen because Dr. Bishop has too narrow a view of the object of knowledge. He may, that is, be assuming that his patient's condition is a matter of fact that any interested knower could acquire—a piece of the "one world to discover"—and that all knowers will converge on and take in this fact in the way he himself has done. He would then interpret Mrs. Alexandros's statement, "I can't talk about this," as evidence that she has not taken in this fact that anyone could discover, and her inability to absorb the fact is in turn pathologized as "being in denial."

The "fact" of dying, however, is a fact that must be socially constructed. In medieval Europe, for example, the *Totentanz* and depictions of it, the bas-reliefs of rotting corpses carved into many sarcophagi, and the human skulls that, by literary convention at any rate, reposed on the desks of scholars—all these served to remind good Chris-

tians that their sojourn on earth was one long dying. On that understanding of dying, Mrs. Alexandros has been dying all her life.

Less floridly, the point at which Mrs. Alexandros has passed from being ill with lung cancer to dying of it is a matter of judgment, not a discoverable fact. Who wants to know? The theatrical producer who is counting on Mrs. Alexandros to back his new play? The hospice worker who cannot admit Mrs. Alexandros into hospice care unless she is within six months of death? The oncologist, pulmonologist, and other specialists in the ICU, who must determine when supporting Mrs. Alexandros on the respirator is no longer appropriate? Or Mrs. Alexandros herself, who believes that if she focuses on what she can still do and resolutely refuses to be categorized as dying, she can end her days more gracefully and positively?

Her bodily processes are, to be sure, the same no matter who is considering them—at least in the sense that her blood gases are what they are regardless of who monitors them. But that these processes mean "Mrs. Alexandros is now dying" is not something that can be known by direct observation. Dr. Bishop need only reflect on the ongoing debates over whole-brain versus heart-lung criteria of death to realize that the point in the dying process where "dead" begins is contestable and negotiable.[6] That being so, it should not strike him as odd that the point where "dying" begins is equally contestable.

SCIENCE AND THE ONE WHO KNOWS

The corollary to a unified, experientially discoverable, and uniquely specifiable set of truths as the *object* of knowledge is a knowing *subject*—a solitary individual—who takes in sense-data that are not mediated socially in any way and whose judgments are objective, free from bias, because he has purified himself of all social and personal allegiances.[7] Naomi Scheman points out that this Cartesian subject establishes its claim to cognitive authority by separating itself off from its body, which then becomes not the lived body but the object of investigation—a mechanical body best known by being dissected. This body became the paradigmatic object in an epistemology founded on a firm and unbridgeable subject-object distinction. And it became bad—because it had been once part of the self and it had to be pushed away, split off, and repudiated. So, too, with everything else from which the authorized self needed to be distinguished and distanced. The rational mind stood over and against the mechanical world of orderly explanation, while the rest—the disorderly, the passionate, the uncontrollable—was relegated to the categories of the "primitive or exotic."[8]

The objective knower is thus privileged by its estrangement from the body, other persons, and the "outside" world. The objective knower is in this sense a bodiless self: a mind.

The Cartesian knower too has frequently come under fire. Knowledge, as many contemporary theorists have begun to argue (and physicians, who typically coauthor papers, have reason to remember), is produced not primarily by individuals thinking in isolation, but by communities of knowers. Interpersonal experience is necessary for a person to have beliefs and to know: we believe and know in a language shared by others in our society, and we become proficient in wielding concepts because various people in our community train us to do this.[9] Indeed, an individual belief can only become knowledge when it is legitimated by the community to which the person belongs.[10] Moreover, the unexamined background beliefs of the community shape not only the concepts available to individual knowers, but also the kinds of thoughts they can—and cannot—have.[11] This is not to say that individuals do not know, but rather that their knowledge is derivative: as Lynn Nelson puts it, "Your knowing or mine depends on *our* knowing."[12]

THE KNOWER AS ONE WHO TRUSTS

These observations about knowers can shed some light on the second story with which I began. Dr. Elders concludes that the newly pregnant Angie Gates has something to hide because she refuses to be tested for HIV infection. In the absence of a blood assay, Dr. Elders supposes, Angie can't *know*

she is uninfected. At best, she can only *hope* she is free of the virus. At worst—and Dr. Elders believes the worst—Angie knows that her partner is infected and is hiding this knowledge from her doctor.

Like Dr. Bishop, Dr. Elders may be making a mistake about what her patient knows. This time, however, the mistake likely arises from an impoverished understanding of what it is to be a knower, rather than what counts as an object of knowledge. If knowers are embodied, socially situated, personally interconnected selves whose knowing depends on "our knowing," then much of what Angie Gates knows is a function of what other people know. I do not mean merely that she learns from others. I mean that her best evidence for something's being so is often the trust she reposes in other people. As John Hardwig puts it, "much of our knowledge rests on trust."[13]

Dr. Elders too knows most of what she knows on trust. She, for example, cannot personally verify all the knowledge claims made even in her own area of expertise, let alone in other areas: she rightly trusts other people's assertions that, if begun early in pregnancy, AZT reduces the chances of vertical HIV transmission from 20 percent to 8 percent. For that matter, she trusts other people's assertions for much of the chemistry and biology undergirding AIDS research, and for the mathematics and other bodies of knowledge that in turn undergird chemistry and biology. Her appeals to the intellectual authority of experts in these areas can be formulated as an epistemological principle, the "principle of testimony":

(T) If *A* has good reasons to believe that *B* has good reasons to believe *p*, then *A* has good reasons to believe *p*.[14]

But trust plays a role in knowledge not only because of the principle of testimony. In our story, Angie knows she is not infected with HIV, not because she trusts the testimony of, say, the lab technician who could tell her the ELISA test is negative, but because she knows she can trust *her partner*. Let us say that she has known him intimately for three years. During that time, she has observed many of his acts and utterances, his emotional and ethical responses to people and ideas, his behavior when fatigued or irritated, his tastes, his political opinions, and any number of other things about him. She has set these observations, bit by bit, into a mosaic of belief about her partner that, when considered in its entirety, warrants her judgment that he can be trusted not to infect her with a fatal disease.

Her judgment is of course fallible. Maybe her partner succumbed to a siren one night without telling her; maybe he is HIV positive without knowing it. The bare possibility that she could be mistaken, however, is insufficient reason for her to act as if she were in fact mistaken. Indeed, entertaining these suspicions when there is no warrant for them is the surest way to undermine the trust between her and her partner.

This does not mean, of course, that Dr. Elders has the same reasons to trust Angie's partner as Angie does. But then, it is not necessary that she have direct knowledge of his trustworthiness. It is Angie, not she, who is vulnerable with respect to this man. Dr. Elders, in short, need not trust Angie's partner in any strong sense of the word. All she needs is the extended version of the principle of testimony:

> A has good reasons for believing C (also D, E., . . .) has good reason for believing B has good reason for believing p,

which, Hardwig tells us, may be used when B (Angie's partner) is not personally known to A (Dr. Elders).[15]

Dr. Elders's good reasons are simply the absence of reasons to the contrary. Unless she has evidence that Angie is decisionally incapacitated, that Angie's partner is betraying her trust, or that the trust relationship between the two is a corrupt one, Dr. Elders has no reason to discredit Angie's judgment.[16] To put the principle of testimony negatively, she has no reason for not believing Angie, who has no reason for believing her partner has no reason for believing himself to be uninfected. Because there can be no epistemic community without trust, this lack of reason for not believing Angie is sufficient reason for believing her. To reverse the burden of proof by insisting on positive reasons to believe instead of lack of reason to disbelieve is not a sign of epistemic rigor, but of paranoia.

FEMINIST STANDPOINT THEORY

As a corrective to positivistic models of knowledge and the disembodied knower, epistemologists since Wittgenstein and Quine have insisted that real knowledge—judgment that tracks the truth—is at the same time socially situated knowledge. The fantasy of a disembodied Cartesian knower directly sensing the world "as it is in itself" is replaced by the more accurate image of a multiplicity of knowers engaged in a great variety of activities and occupying very diverse negotiating postures that have a direct bearing on what knowledge is available.

The special importance for feminists of these insights is that not everyone within an epistemic community has the same status or recognition, and so not everyone is granted the same cognitive authority. Feminists begin from the premise that women have been second-class citizens of the communities they inhabit, and they note that women's claims to know or justifiably believe have often been ignored, belittled, or dismissed. One reason for this is that those who are authoritatively "in a position to know" cannot easily see how the world looks from less powerful perspectives, and so are vulnerable to the temptation of supposing that their own understanding is normative. From this supposition it is only a short hop to the idea that understandings that *differ* from the dominant ones are also understandings that are *defective*. But when authoritative knowers consider judgments produced by women to be defective for the sole reason that women occupy a lower place in the social and epistemic hierarchy, they are making a factual as well as a moral mistake. And in making this mistake, they help to perpetuate the oppression of women.

Feminist standpoint theory starts from the claim that in communities stratified by gender, "the activities of those at the top both organize and set limits on what persons who perform such *activ-*

ities can understand about themselves and the world around them."[17] Important features of people's actual relations with each other and with the world are simply not visible to those high up in the hierarchy, because at that altitude there is often no reason to care about these matters, and so no incentive to understand them. In fact, at that altitude, one has a lot to lose by taking seriously the justice claims of those who occupy the rungs below.

By contrast, the activities of people at the bottom of the gender hierarchy provide a starting point for anyone's understanding of the world and the people in it, as all sorts of things about the lives of women don't neatly fit into the dominant standpoint, and this provides us all—women and men alike—with problems to be explained. The action at the bottom is, however, only a starting point. The claim I wish to defend is not that the positions at the bottom yield the best or better knowledge, as any social theory that allows you to identify a particular position as epistemologically privileged would in turn require a standpoint to justify it—and what would that be?[18] Rather, I join those who have noted that "the bottom" itself consists of multiple positions, from any of which one is able to see something different and so to correct for the biases and blind spots of one's own standpoint.[19]

Beginning from women's activities thus becomes a way of making visible certain experiences that are, from the standpoint of privileged men, invisible. And because women's lives are very different and in important respects not only opposed to each other (lesbian and heterosexual, rich and poor, European and African, religiously observant and atheist) but also internally conflicted (a fundamentalist Muslim feminist, a young mother who is a surgeon, a Latina who is lesbian), one begins from many women's lives, each of which has multiple and contradictory commitments. In this way one replaces the chimera of objectivity that sought to purify the knower of all his passions, allegiances, and personal characteristics—"the position of no position that provides a view from nowhere"[20]—with the more realistic objectivity that is attained by bringing together in a critically reflective dialogue the representatives of as many diverse positions as possible.

In the move to let a thousand standpoints bloom, however, have we done away with standpoint theory altogether? That is to say, if there is no particular women's standpoint that is epistemically privileged, shouldn't we just drop the terminology of standpoint and work out a theory of epistemic democracy? There's a reason not to do this. Although we've rejected the idea that any one position a woman might occupy produces better judgments than all others, we may nevertheless retain the idea that the standpoint of powerful men is where no knower wants to be, since the dominant standpoint is the one position that is sure to generate faulty judgments—the one position that is most to be distrusted. The weak version of feminist standpoint theory, then, is still open to us.

STANDPOINT THEORY IN THE CLINIC

There are important differences between the oppression of women in societies that favor the interests of socially privileged men, on the one hand, and the relationship of a patient to her physician, on the other. But with regard to who knows what and whose judgments are or aren't authorized, there are intriguing similarities as well. For this reason, the weak version of standpoint theory can be used to explain why Dr. Bishop and Dr. Elders may have attributed cognitive failings to their patients.

Just as privileged men have occupied the positions of dominance in their epistemic communities, so too have physicians. These observations are, of course, interrelated; many physicians *are* privileged men, and they have lent the profession its epistemic sheen.[21] What dominant men—and physicians of either gender—have wanted to investigate has been socially supported as worth investigating; what they have not regarded to be worth knowing has frequently been passed down the epistemic hierarchy, to be known by those of lesser status.

Moreover, people in both positions of epistemic privilege enjoy a defining connection to their minds rather than their bodies. As Scheman notes,

> The privileged are precisely those who are defined not by the meanings and uses of their bodies for others but by their ability either to control their bodies for their own ends or to seem to exist virtually bodilessly. They are those who have conquered the sexual, dependent, mortal, and messy parts of themselves—in part by projecting all those qualities onto others, whom they thereby earn the right to dominate and, if the occasion arises, to exploit.[22]

For women, of course, the connection to the body has been paramount. In the standard dichotomies regarding gender, "woman" has been identified with nature as opposed to science, emotion as opposed to reason, body as opposed to mind. If, as a creature of nature, woman is disorderly, passionate, and uncontrolled, it would seem to follow equally "naturally" that she "lacks deliberative authority," as Aristotle put it.[23]

The patient too possesses a defining connection to the body, and an ailing body to boot—one that is even less under the patient's control than a woman's healthy body is seen to be. Indeed, the illness, pain, or injury the patient suffers can set up its own interference with the patient's thought processes. Emotional and cognitive regression in the ill is a well-documented phenomenon, and physicians are taught to make allowances for it.

The difference between women and patients, of course, is that women have been set on the lower rungs of the cognitive hierarchy against their will and for no good reason, whereas patients defer to physicians' expertise because, with respect to the illness that occasions the clinical encounter, the physician can actually be expected to know more than the patient.[24] This difference, however, does not affect the limitations associated with being at the top of the hierarchy. The standpoint of medical privilege, like the standpoint of male privilege, is precisely the one from which important features of the lives of those below are not visible. And as it is the lives of those below with which the physician is professionally concerned, the inability to see clearly here is particularly unsatisfactory.

There is another drawback to occupying the standpoint of medical privilege. Because one powerful strategy for maintaining cognitive authority and control is to insist that only certain kinds of knowledge "count"—namely, the kinds that the authoritative knowers themselves have authorized—physicians are continually tempted to affirm the very practices that perpetuate their inability to see. That is, they are continually tempted to discount what their patients know, which then makes their own claims to knowledge appear inevitable and right. As Margaret Urban Walker points out, reducing, circumscribing, or discrediting the status of those further down the epistemic hierarchy constitutes a kind of "epistemic firewall" that insulates those in authority by allowing them to dismiss the knowledge claims of those below and "prove" their unreliability as judges.[25]

If feminist standpoint theory provides the correct account of what physicians can't see, we can sum up by observing that Dr. Bishop and Dr. Elders have been entertaining two false beliefs: (1) Mrs. Alexandros and Angie Gates are guilty of bad judgments generated by their unruly and problematic bodies, and (2) the doctor knows best.

THE ETHICS OF EPISTEMOLOGY

But, someone might object at this point, does it really matter what these doctors think, so long as they keep the thought to themselves? Dr. Bishop didn't attempt to break through what he took to be Mrs. Alexandros's denial; Dr. Elders didn't manipulate or coerce Angie Gates into having the blood test. Actions of that kind would clearly be unethical, but where's the harm in entertaining a false belief now and again?

There are, I think, two answers to this. The first is that it is wrong to hold someone in unwarranted contempt. In the absence of any real conversation with a person that could provide evidence one way or another, to conclude that she is in denial, as Dr. Bishop does, is to pathologize the person's thought processes and so to judge without warrant that the person "lacks deliberative authority." If it was disrespectful of Aristotle to make this judgment about women, it is equally disrespectful for a physician to think it about a patient, unless there are specific grounds for doing so. As for Dr. Elders, in falsely imputing base motives—whether of cowardice, deception, self-deception, or guilty knowledge—to another person, she dishonors her, even if she never lets it show. The moral wrongness of dishonoring another may be *compounded* by speaking ill of the person to others, or by acting toward her in ways that express contempt, but the unspoken thought itself robs her of the respect that is her due, and that is wrong enough.

The second answer is that a habit of disrespectful judgments about another, made solely because that person occupies a lower position in the cognitive hierarchy, is a form of oppression and oppression too is wrong. Thinking one knows more than someone else is not in itself disrespectful: a physician generally *does* have knowledge the patient lacks, and with regard to medical matters the patient would generally prefer to trust the physician's judgment over her own. In the area of medical expertise, the physician rightly commands cognitive deference from a patient. When, however, a physician attributes discreditable behavior to a patient for no other reason than that the patient is epistemically inferior, the physician's position at the top of the hierarchy loses its legitimacy and cognitive deference is no longer warranted. At this point, the doctor-patient relationship stops being merely a hierarchy and becomes an oppressive hierarchy, no different morally from that of a powerful man who discredits a woman's judgment just because she is a woman.

PHYSICIAN JUDGMENT AND THE *ART* OF MEDICINE

If the standpoint of medical privilege is the very one that causes blindness, is there nothing that can be done to restore physicians' sight? Indeed there is, and physicians themselves are the very ones to do it. In addition to correcting any positivistic assumptions they might happen to harbor about their knowledge of medical science, physicians can also cultivate a new understanding of another kind of knowledge they have traditionally relied upon: the Hippocratic notion of "judgment perilous."

Judgment, as physicians use the term, involves a nuanced and practiced attention to the specific details of a particular clinical situation. It replaces (or augments) rule-governed decision making with beliefs based on the physician's previous experience and discernment; it relies heavily on a savvy, "I've-seen-it-before" probabilism.

This sort of judgment has often been taken to be individualistic and not publicly available: it is not so much taught as acquired over the course of many years. In the hands of the novice, then, it is indeed judgment "perilous." Here, however, is where a revised understanding of the notion is in order. Judgments can be and often are formed privately by individuals, but they can also be constructed *collaboratively*. And that is what can save physicians from being hopelessly trapped within the one epistemic standpoint that is guaranteed to leave important things about their patients invisible. For if the physician begins from the standpoint of the patient, taking seriously the patient's judgments about her bodily experience, the quality of her intimate relationships, the character of her daily life, what conduces to her happiness, and other considerations that can in a broad sense be brought to bear on the patient's presenting condition, then patient and physician together can construct a joint understanding of what is going on with the patient and what constitutes an optimal medical response.

In suggesting that physicians begin from the standpoints of their patients, I do not mean that they should allow patients' judgments to supplant their own. They should argue with patients, point out mistakes of fact, challenge patients' values, question, and probe. But in turn they must also lay their own opinions open to scrutiny, by thinking out loud, in terms the patient can understand, about what they see and conclude and think appropriate to do.[26] In this way patient and physician become collaborators, together seeking the patient's good—not solely as the patient understands it, and not solely as the doctor understands it, but as they jointly learn together to understand it.

In the deepest sense, then, this is judgment perilous, for it requires physicians to trust their patients in unaccustomed ways and to unaccustomed degrees, and this necessarily involves sharing a certain amount of power. Others have already offered ethical arguments for why physicians should do this;[27] indeed, the bioethics revolution of the last 25 years has largely revolved around precisely this point.

My hope here, however, has been to buttress the ethical arguments with epistemological ones, in the belief that correct judgments and right conduct are not so separate as we often take them to be. If clinical knowledge of patients is constructed by a community of knowers rather than imbibed by a solitary observer, and if physicians have no other way of assuring objectivity except by starting from the patient's standpoint and trusting her testimony, then knowing itself requires that we be morally accountable to each other. This seems to me a thought worth considering.

ACKNOWLEDGMENTS

Thanks to John Hardwig, Erik Parens, James Lindemann Nelson, Rosemarie Tong, and Margaret Urban Walker for their collaboration in constructing these ideas.

NOTES

1. Françoise Baylis suggested these stories to me in conversation, 19 October 1995.
2. L. H. Nelson, "Epistemological Communities," in *Feminist Epistemologies*, ed. L. Alcoff and E. Potter (New York: Routledge, 1993), 131.
3. W. V. O. Quine, *Word and Object* (Cambridge, Mass.: MIT Press, 1960).
4. See note 2, p. 133.
5. See note 3 and Pierre Duhem, *La Théorie physique, son objet et sa structure*, 1906, trans. P. P. Wiener as *The Aim and Structure of Physical Theory* (Princeton: Princeton University Press, 1954).
6. For a recent overview of and creative contribution to these debates, see L. Emanuel, "Reexamining Death: The Asymptotic Model and a Bounded Zone Definition," *Hastings Center Report* 25, no. 4 (1995): 27–35.
7. Conceptualizing the knower as subject and the thing known as object is problematic, as social scientists have pointed out, because knowers can also be objects of knowledge. Nevertheless, distinguishing between the knower and what she knows can be useful, as I hope to demonstrate.
8. N. Scheman, "Though This Be Method, Yet There Is Madness in It: Paranoia and Liberal Epistemology," in *A Mind of One's Own: Feminist Essays on Reason and Objectivity,* ed. L. M. Antony and C. Witt (Boulder, Colo.: Westview Press, 1993), 159. This essay is reprinted in N. Scheman, *Engenderings: Constructions of Knowledge, Authority, and Privilege* (New York: Routledge, 1993).
9. The *locus classicus* for these observations is Ludwig Wittgenstein. See his arguments against the notion of a private language in *Philosophical Investigations* (New York: Macmillan, 1953), §§ 243–79.
10. This observation has been crucial in motivating the development of standpoint epistemologies, beginning with Marx and more recently encompassing C. A. MacKinnon, "Feminism, Marxism, Method, and the State: An Agenda for Theory," *Signs* 7, no. 3 (1982): 515–44; N. Hartsock, "The Feminist Standpoint: Developing the Ground for a Specifically Feminist Historical Materialism," in *Discovering Reality*, ed. Harding and Hintikka; S. Harding, both *The Science Question in Feminism* (Ithaca, N.Y.: Cornell University Press, 1986) and *Whose Science? Whose Knowledge? Thinking from Women's Lives* (Ithaca, N.Y.: Cornell University Press, 1991); and P. H. Collins, *Black Feminist Thought: Knowledge, Consciousness, and the Politics of Empowerment* (Boston: Unwin Hyman, 1990).
11. A. Jaggar, *Feminist Politics and Human Nature* (Totowa, N.J.: Rowman & Allenheld, 1983); N. Scheman, "Individualism and the Objects of Psychology," in *Discovering Reality: Feminist Perspectives on Epistemology, Metaphysics, Methodology, and Philosophy of Science*, ed. S. Harding and M. Hintikka (Dordrecht, The Netherlands: Reidel, 1983); L. H. Nelson, *Who Knows? From Quine to a Feminist Empiricism* (Philadelphia: Temple University Press, 1990); and L. Code, *What Can She Know? Feminist Theory and the Construction of Knowledge* (Ithaca, N.Y.: Cornell University Press, 1991) all have made this point.
12. See note 2, p. 124. See also J. Hardwig, " The Role of Trust in Knowledge," *Journal of Philosophy* 88, no. 12 (1991): 693–708, who notes that "a belief based partly on second-hand evidence will be epistemically superior to any belief based completely on direct empirical evidence whenever the relevant evidence becomes too extensive or too complex for any one person to gather it all" (p. 698).
13. Hardwig, "Role of Trust in Knowledge," 694.
14. Ibid., 697.
15. Ibid., 701.

16. For the test of a morally corrupt trust relationship, see A. C. Baier, "Trust and Antitrust," in *Moral Prejudices: Essays on Ethics* (Cambridge, Mass.: Harvard University Press, 1995), 123.

17. S. Harding, "Rethinking Standpoint Epistemology: What Is 'Strong Objectivity'?" in *Feminist Epistemologies*, 54.

18. This objection is put succinctly by Helen Longino, "Subjects, Power, and Knowledge: Description and Prescription in Feminist Philosophies of Science," in *Feminist Epistemologies*, 107.

19. Elizabeth V. Spelman eloquently urged the importance for feminist philosophy of noting differences among women in *Inessential Woman: Problems of Exclusion in Feminist Thought* (Boston: Beacon Press, 1988). For an account of how this insight can be incorporated into standpoint theory, see note 17.

20. See note 18, p. 110.

21. Within medicine itself, of course, there is a gender hierarchy wherein women occupy the bottom rungs. Nevertheless, women who work as physicians enjoy greater epistemic prestige than women who do most other forms of work. On the gender hierarchy in medicine, see B. J. Tesch, et al., "Promotion of Women Physicians in Academic Medicine: Glass Ceiling or Sticky Floor?" *Journal of the American Medical Association* 273, no. 13 (1995): 1022–25; see also, C. Eisenberg, "Medicine Is No Longer a Men's Profession; or, When the Men's Club Goes Coed, It's Time to Change the Regs," *New England Journal of Medicine* 321 (1989): 1542–44.

22. See note 8, p. 155.

23. Aristotle, *Politics*, trans. B. Jowett, in *The Complete Works of Aristotle*, ed. J. Barnes (Princeton: Princeton University Press, 1984), 1999.

24. This is true even when the patient is a physician herself. It is generally agreed that people aren't at the top of their cognitive form when they don't feel good.

25. M. U. Walker, "Made a Slave, Born a Woman: Knowing Others' Places," in *Moral Understandings* (New York: Routledge, 1997), forthcoming.

26. H. Brody, "Transparency: Informed Consent in Primary Care," *Hastings Center Report* 19, no. 5 (1989): 5–9.

27. See, *inter alia*, H. Brody, *The Healer's Power* (New Haven, Conn.: Yale University Press, 1992); see note 26, pp. 5–9.

QUESTIONS FOR COMPREHENSION AND REFLECTION

1. What does Nelson mean by the "feminist standpoint theory"? How is it intended to counter the prevailing epistemic assumptions in the clinical encounter with patients?

2. Would this "feminist standpoint theory" be applicable within other cultures, or is Nelson unfairly assuming that this theory is universal? Explain.

3. According to Nelson, what is the nature of the relationship between ethics and epistemology?

4. What does Nelson suggest be done in order to reasonably incorporate physicians' clinical judgment within a context of shared authority with the patient? Do you agree? Why or why not? Explain.

Decision in the *Tarasoff* Case

In this landmark case, the California Supreme Court ruled that therapists should have warned a woman of a threat to her life presented by a patient. The majority opinion, expressed by Justice Matthew Tobriner, provides an argument against the absolute inviolability of patient confidentiality, particularly in cases where life and well-being are seriously threatened. Such intervention extends not only to a duty to warn but even in some cases to involuntary hospitalization. In contrast, the dissenting opinion, given by Justice William Clark, gives three reasons why the confidentiality between therapist and patient should not be violated.

Justice Matthew O. Tobriner, Majority Opinion

On October 27, 1969, Prosenjit Poddar killed Tatiana Tarasoff. Plaintiffs, Tatiana's parents, allege that two months earlier Poddar confided his intention to kill Tatiana to Dr. Lawrence Moore, a psychologist employed by the Cowell Memorial Hospital at the University of California at Berkeley. They allege that on Moore's request, the campus police briefly detained Poddar, but released him when he appeared rational. They further claim that Dr. Harvey Powelson, Moore's superior, then directed that no further action be taken to detain Poddar. No one warned plaintiffs of Tatiana's peril. . . .

We shall explain that defendant therapists cannot escape liability merely because Tatiana herself was not their patient. When a therapist determines, or pursuant to the standards of his profession should determine, that his patient presents a serious danger of violence to another, he incurs an obligation to use reasonable care to protect the intended victim against such danger. The discharge of this duty may require the therapist to take one or more of various steps, depending upon the nature of the case. Thus it may call for him to warn the intended victim or others likely to apprise the victim of the danger, to notify the police, or to take whatever other steps are reasonably necessary under the circumstances. . . .

1. PLAINTIFFS' COMPLAINTS

. . . Plaintiffs' first cause of action, entitled "Failure to Detain a Dangerous Patient," alleges that on August 20, 1969, Poddar was a voluntary outpatient receiving therapy at Cowell Memorial Hospital. Poddar informed Moore, his therapist, that he was going to kill an unnamed girl, readily identifiable as Tatiana, when she returned home from spending the summer in Brazil. Moore, with the concurrence of Dr. Gold, who had initially examined Poddar, and Dr. Yandell, assistant to the director of the department of psychiatry, decided that Poddar should be committed for observation in a mental hospital. Moore orally notified Officers Atkinson and Teel of the campus police that he would request commitment. He then sent a letter to Police Chief William Beall requesting the assistance of the police department in securing Poddar's confinement.

Officers Atkinson, Brownrigg, and Halleran took Poddar into custody, but, satisfied that Poddar was rational, released him on his promise to stay away from Tatiana. Powelson, director of the department of psychiatry at Cowell Memorial Hospital, then asked the police to return Moore's letter, directed that all copies of the letter and notes that Moore had taken as therapist be destroyed, and "ordered no action to place Prosenjit Poddar in 72-hour treatment and evaluation facility."

Plaintiffs' second cause of action, entitled "Failure to Warn On a Dangerous Patient," incorporates the allegations of the first cause of action, but adds the assertion that defendants negligently permitted Poddar to be released from police custody without "notifying the parents of Tatiana Tarasoff that their daughter was in grave danger from Prosenjit Poddar." Poddar persuaded Tatiana's brother to share an apartment with him near Tatiana's residence; shortly after her return from Brazil, Poddar went to her residence and killed her. . . .

2. PLAINTIFFS CAN STATE A CAUSE OF ACTION AGAINST DEFENDANT THERAPISTS FOR NEGLIGENT FAILURE TO PROTECT TATIANA

The second cause of action can be amended to allege that Tatiana's death proximately resulted from defendants' negligent failure to warn Tatiana or others likely to apprise her of her danger. Plaintiffs contend that as amended, such allegations of negligence and proximate causation, with resulting damages, establish a cause of action. Defendants, however, contend that in the circumstances of the present case they owed no duty of care to Tatiana or her parents and that, in the absence of such duty, they were free to act in careless disregard of Tatiana's life and safety.

. . . In analyzing this issue, we bear in mind that legal duties are not discoverable facts of nature, but merely conclusory expressions that, in cases of a particular type, liability should be imposed for damage done. As stated in *Dillon* v. *Legg* (1968): . . . "The assertion that liability must . . . be denied because defendant bears no 'duty' to plaintiff 'begs the essential question—whether the plaintiff's interests are entitled to legal protection against the defendant's conduct. . . . [Duty] is not sacrosanct in itself, but only an expression of the sum total of those considerations of policy which lead the law to say that the particular plaintiff is entitled to protection.' " . . .

In the landmark case of *Rowland* v. *Christian* (1968), . . . Justice Peters recognized that liability should be imposed "for an injury occasioned to another by his want of ordinary care or skill" as expressed in section 1714 of the Civil Code. Thus, Justice Peters, quoting from *Heaven* v. *Pender* (1883) . . . stated: " 'whenever one person is by circumstances placed in such a position with regard to another . . . that if he did not use ordinary care and skill in his own conduct . . . he would cause danger of injury to the person or property of the other, a duty arises to use ordinary care and skill to avoid such danger.' "

. . . We depart from "this fundamental principle" only upon the "balancing of a number of considerations"; major ones "are the foreseeability of harm to the plaintiff, the degree of certainty that the plaintiff suffered injury, the closeness of the connection between the defendant's conduct and the injury suffered, the moral blame attached to the defendant's conduct, the policy of preventing future harm, the extent of the burden to the defendant and consequences to the community of imposing a duty to exercise care with resulting liability for breach, and the availability, cost and prevalence of insurance for the risk involved."

The most important of these considerations in establishing duty is foreseeability. As a general principle, a "defendant owes a duty of care to all persons who are foreseeably endangered by his conduct, with respect to all risks which make the conduct unreasonably dangerous." As we shall explain, however, when the avoidance of foreseeable harm requires a defendant to control the conduct of another person, or to warn of such conduct, the common law has traditionally imposed liability only if the defendant bears some special relationship to the dangerous person or to the potential victim. Since the relationship between a therapist and his patient satisfies this requirement, we need not here decide whether foreseeability alone is sufficient to create a duty to exercise reasonable care to protect a potential victim of another's conduct. . . .

. . . Although plaintiffs' pleadings assert no special relation between Tatiana and defendant therapists, they establish as between Poddar and defendant therapists the special relation that arises between a patient and his doctor or psychotherapist. Such a relationship may support affirmative duties for the benefit of third persons. Thus, for example, a hospital must exercise reasonable care to control the behavior of a patient which may endanger other persons. A doctor must also warn a patient if the patient's condition or medication renders certain conduct, such as driving a car, dangerous to others.

. . . Although the California decisions that recognize this duty have involved cases in which the defendant stood in a special relationship *both* to the victim and to the person whose conduct created the danger, we do not think that the duty should logically be constricted to such situations. Decisions of other jurisdictions hold that the single relationship of a doctor to his patient is sufficient to support the duty to exercise reasonable care to protect others against dangers emanating from the patient's illness. The courts hold that a doctor is liable to persons infected by his patient if he negligently fails to diagnose a contagious disease, . . . or, having diagnosed the illness, fails to warn members of the patient's family.

Since it involved a dangerous mental patient, the decision in *Merchants Nat. Bank & Trust Co. of Fargo* v. *United States* . . . comes closer to the issue. The Veterans Administration arranged for the patient to work on a local farm, but did not inform the farmer of the man's background. The farmer consequently permitted the patient to come and go freely during nonworking hours; the patient borrowed a car, drove to his wife's residence and killed her. Notwithstanding the lack of any "special relationship" between the Veterans Administration and the wife, the court found the Veterans Administration liable for the wrongful death of the wife.

In their summary of the relevant rulings Fleming and Maximov conclude that the "case law should dispel any notion that to impose on the therapists a duty to take precautions for the safety of persons threatened by a patient, where due care so requires, is in any way opposed to contemporary ground rules on the duty relationship. On the contrary, there now seems to be sufficient authority to support the conclusion that by entering into a doctor-patient relationship the therapist becomes sufficiently involved to assume some responsibility for the safety, not only of the patient himself, but

also of any third person whom the doctor knows to be threatened by the patient." . . .

Defendants contend, however, that imposition of a duty to exercise reasonable care to protect third persons is unworkable because therapists cannot accurately predict whether or not a patient will resort to violence. In support of this argument amicus representing the American Psychiatric Association and other professional societies cites numerous articles which indicate that therapists, in the present state of the art, are unable reliably to predict violent acts; their forecasts, amicus claims, tend consistently to overpredict violence, and indeed are more often wrong than right. . . .

. . . We recognize the difficulty that a therapist encounters in attempting to forecast whether a patient presents a serious danger of violence. Obviously we do not require that the therapist, in making that determination, render a perfect performance; the therapist need only exercise "that reasonable degree of skill, knowledge, and care ordinarily possessed and exercised by members of [that professional specialty] under similar circumstances." Within the broad range of reasonable practice and treatment in which professional opinion and judgment may differ, the therapist is free to exercise his or her own best judgment without liability; proof, aided by hindsight, that he or she judged wrongly is insufficient to establish negligence.

In the instant case, however, the pleadings do not raise any question as to failure of defendant therapists to predict that Poddar presented a serious danger of violence. On the contrary, the present complaints allege that defendant therapists did in fact predict that Poddar would kill, but were negligent in failing to warn.

. . . Amicus contends, however, that even when a therapist does in fact predict that a patient poses a serious danger of violence to others, the therapist should be absolved of any responsibility for failing to act to protect the potential victim. In our view, however, once a therapist does in fact determine, or under applicable professional standards reasonably should have determined, that a patient poses a serious danger of violence to others, he bears a duty to exercise reasonable care to protect the foreseeable victim of that danger. While the discharge of this duty of due care will necessarily vary with the facts of each case, in each instance the adequacy of the therapist's conduct must be measured against the traditional negligence standard of the rendition of reasonable care under the circumstances.... As explained in Fleming and Maximov, *The Patient or His Victim: The Therapist's Dilemma* (1974): "... the ultimate question of resolving the tension between the conflicting interests of patient and potential victim is one of social policy, not professional expertise.... In sum, the therapist owes a legal duty not only to his patient, but also to his patient's would-be victim and is subject in both respects to scrutiny by judge and jury." ...

The risk that unnecessary warnings may be given is a reasonable price to pay for the lives of possible victims that may be saved. We would hesitate to hold that the therapist who is aware that his patient expects to attempt to assassinate the President of the United States would not be obligated to warn the authorities because the therapist cannot predict with accuracy that his patient will commit the crime.

Defendants further argue that free and open communication is essential to psychotherapy; ... that "Unless a patient ... is assured that ... information [revealed by him] can and will be held in utmost confidence, he will be reluctant to make the full disclosure upon which diagnosis and treatment ... depends." ... The giving of a warning, defendants contend, constitutes a breach of trust which entails the revelation of confidential communications.

... We recognize the public interest in supporting effective treatment of mental illness and in protecting the rights of patients to privacy, ... and the consequent public importance of safeguarding the confidential character of psychotherapeutic communication. Against this interest, however, we must weigh the public interest in safety from violent assault. ...

... We realize that the open and confidential character of psychotherapeutic dialogue encourages patients to express threats of violence, few of which are ever executed. Certainly a therapist should not be encouraged routinely to reveal such threats; such disclosures could seriously disrupt the patient's relationship with his therapist and with the persons threatened. To the contrary, the therapist's obligations to his patient require that he not disclose a confidence unless such disclosure is necessary to avert danger to others, and even then that he do so discreetly, and in a fashion that would preserve the privacy of his patient to the fullest extent compatible with the prevention of the threatened danger.

The revelation of a communication under the above circumstances is not a breach of trust or a violation of professional ethics; as stated in the Principles of Medical Ethics of the American Medical Association (1957), section 9: "A physician may not reveal the confidence entrusted to him in the course of medical attendance ... *unless he is required to do so by law or unless it becomes necessary in order to protect the welfare of the individual or of the community.*" (Emphasis added.) We conclude that the public policy favoring protection of the confidential character of patient-psychotherapist communications must yield to the extent to which disclosure is essential to avert danger to others. The protective privilege ends where the public peril begins. ...

For the foregoing reasons, we find that plaintiffs' complaints can be amended to state a cause of action against defendants Moore, Powelson, Gold, and Yandell and against the Regents as their employer, for breach of a duty to exercise reasonable care to protect Tatiana.

Justice William P. Clark, Dissenting Opinion

Until today's majority opinion, both legal and medical authorities have agreed that confidentiality is essential to effectively treat the mentally ill, and that imposing a duty on doctors to disclose patient threats to potential victims would greatly impair treatment. Further, recognizing that effective treatment and society's safety are necessarily intertwined, the Legislature has already decided effective and confidential treatment is preferred over imposition of a duty to warn.

The issue whether effective treatment for the mentally ill should be sacrificed to a system of warnings is, in my opinion, properly one for the Legislature, and we are bound by its judgment. Moreover, even in the absence of clear legislative direction, we must reach the same conclusion because imposing the majority's new duty is certain to result in a net increase in violence. . . .

Overwhelming policy considerations weigh against imposing a duty on psychotherapists to warn a potential victim against harm. While offering virtually no benefit to society, such a duty will frustrate psychiatric treatment, invade fundamental patient rights and increase violence. . . .

Assurance of confidentiality is important for three reasons.

DETERRENCE FROM TREATMENT

First, without substantial assurance of confidentiality, those requiring treatment will be deterred from seeking assistance. It remains an unfortunate fact in our society that people seeking psychiatric guidance tend to become stigmatized. Apprehension of such stigma—apparently increased by the propensity of people considering treatment to see themselves in the worst possible light—creates a well-recognized reluctance to seek aid. This reluctance is alleviated by the psychiatrist's assurance of confidentiality.

FULL DISCLOSURE

Second, the guarantee of confidentiality is essential in eliciting the full disclosure necessary for effective treatment. The psychiatric patient approaches treatment with conscious and unconscious inhibitions against revealing his innermost thoughts. "Every person, however well-motivated, has to overcome resistance to therapeutic exploration. These resistances seek support from every possible source and the possibility of disclosure would easily be employed in the service of resistance." . . . Until a patient can trust his psychiatrist not to violate their confidential relationship, "the unconscious psychological control mechanism of repression will prevent the recall of past experiences." . . .

SUCCESSFUL TREATMENT

Third, even if the patient fully discloses his thoughts, assurance that the confidential relationship will not be breached is necessary to maintain his trust in his psychiatrist—the very means by which treatment is effected. "[T]he essence of much psychotherapy is the contribution of trust in the external world and ultimately in the self, modelled upon the trusting relationship established during therapy." . . . Patients will be helped only if they can form a trusting relationship with the psychiatrist. . . . All authorities appear to agree that if the trust relationship cannot be developed because of collusive communication between the psychiatrist and others, treatment will be frustrated.

Given the importance of confidentiality to the practice of psychiatry, it becomes clear the duty to warn imposed by the majority will cripple the use and effectiveness of psychiatry. Many people, potentially violent—yet susceptible to treatment—will be deterred from seeking it; those seeking it will be inhibited from making revelations necessary to effective treatment; and, forcing the psychiatrist to violate the patient's trust will destroy the interpersonal relationship by which treatment is effected.

VIOLENCE AND CIVIL COMMITMENT

By imposing a duty to warn, the majority contributes to the danger to society of violence by the mentally ill and greatly increases the risk of civil commitment—the total deprivation of liberty—of those who should not be confined. The impairment of treatment and risk of improper commitment resulting from the new duty to warn will not be limited to a few patients but will extend to a large number of the mentally ill. Although under existing psychiatric procedures only a relatively few receiving treatment will ever present a risk of violence, the number making threats is huge, and it is the latter group—not just the former—whose treatment will be impaired and whose risk of commitment will be increased.

Both the legal and psychiatric communities recognize that the process of determining potential violence in a patient is far from exact, being fraught with complexity and uncertainty. In fact precision has not even been attained in predicting who of those having already committed violent acts will again become violent, a task recognized to be of much simpler proportions. . . .

This predictive uncertainty means that the number of disclosures will necessarily be large. As noted above, psychiatric patients are encouraged to discuss all thoughts of violence, and they often express such thoughts. However, unlike this court, the psychiatrist does not enjoy the benefit of overwhelming hindsight in seeing which few, if any, of his patients will ultimately become violent. Now, confronted by the majority's new duty, the psychiatrist must instantaneously calculate potential violence from each patient on each visit. The difficulties researchers have encountered in accurately predicting violence will be heightened for the practicing psychiatrist dealing for brief periods in his office with heretofore nonviolent patients. And, given the decision not to warn or commit must always be made at the psychiatrist's civil peril, one can expect most doubts will be resolved in favor of the psychiatrist protecting himself.

Neither alternative open to the psychiatrist seeking to protect himself is in the public interest. The warning itself is an impairment of the psychia-trist's ability to treat, depriving many patients of adequate treatment. It is to be expected that after disclosing their threats, a significant number of patients, who would not become violent if treated according to existing practices, will engage in violent conduct as a result of unsuccessful treatment. In short, the majority's duty to warn will not only impair treatment of many who would never become violent but worse, will result in a net increase in violence.

The second alternative open to the psychiatrist is to commit his patient rather than to warn. Even in the absence of threat of civil liability, the doubts of psychiatrists as to the seriousness of patient threats have led psychiatrists to overcommit to mental institutions. This overcommitment has been authoritatively documented in both legal and psychiatric studies. This practice is so prevalent that it has been estimated that "as many as twenty harmless persons are incarcerated for every one who will commit a violent act." . . .

Given the incentive to commit created by the majority's duty, this already serious situation will be worsened, contrary to Chief Justice Wright's admonition "that liberty is no less precious because forfeited in a civil proceeding than when taken as a consequence of a criminal conviction."

QUESTIONS FOR COMPREHENSION AND REFLECTION

1. Discuss Justice Tobriner's ruling (the majority opinion) and his supporting arguments. Do you agree or disagree? Explain.
2. Does Tobriner's position represent more of a utilitarian or a deontological perspective? Support your answer.
3. Discuss the minority opinion represented by Justice Clark. Do you agree or disagree? Explain.
4. Does Clark's position reflect more of a utilitarian or a deontological perspective? Support your answer.

✤ CASES FOR ANALYSIS*

1. Bob Hobart's Vacation

Bob Hobart's lifelong dream has been to travel to Switzerland and see the Swiss Alps. He has finally saved up enough money for the trip and is scheduled to leave next week, hoping to spend three weeks sight-seeing and skiing. During his routine annual checkup with additional tests, his physician discovers that he has a type of cancer that is likely to be fatal within six months. Hobart has not yet developed overt symptoms, nor is he experiencing any pain or discomfort. As far as Hobart is concerned, there is no reason to think of himself as anything other than completely healthy, and he is quite excited about his coming trip. What should the physician tell him?

DISCUSSION QUESTIONS

1. Is telling the truth the right thing to do here?
2. What are some possible organizational and legal issues that his physician might face?
3. What approach in this case would reflect more of a covenantal relationship with Hobart?

2. Clara Roy[37]

After her brother committed suicide, Clara Roy began to see a psychiatrist. She was suffering from depression and suicidal tendencies. During the course of her therapy, her psychiatrist started putting pressure on her to engage in a sexual relationship. She resisted his advances for a while, but she finally gave in, believing that such a relationship might have a positive effect on her and her treatment. After this had gone on for some time and she had become rather distraught, Roy confronted her therapist, yet he forbade her to tell anyone about their relationship. Roy then devised a plan to murder him and then kill herself. However, she was hospitalized before she could put her plan into action. After her hospitalization, she sued her psychiatrist for sexual abuse. This became the first successful case of sexual abuse brought against a therapist.

DISCUSSION QUESTIONS

1. How should Roy have handled the sexual advances made to her by her psychiatrist?
2. Suppose a coworker of the psychiatrist knew of the sexual relationship. What should he or she have done?
3. How would a utilitarian address this issue? A Kantian? An Aristotelian virtue theorist?

3. Helen Robbins

Helen Robbins is a forty-year-old single woman. She has a family history of breast cancer. Her mother has recently died from it. Robbins is concerned about her chances of cancer, although she is healthy in all other respects. During her routine physical examination, she voices this concern to her physician, Dr. Gary Michael. The results of her

---

*Names and cases are fictional unless noted otherwise.

examination are normal, and since she already had a mammogram last year he declines to prescribe another one. In view of her family history, as well as her personal concern, he feels that he should recommend a mammogram. However, according to the policy of the HMO he contracts for, women are entitled to only one mammogram every other year until the age of fifty. He suspects that the policy was established in order to control unnecessary spending. What should he do?

DISCUSSION QUESTIONS

1. Should Dr. Michael make it a point to always abide by HMO policies?
2. How can the physician resolve the tension between cost-containment measures and patient beneficence?
3. How would utilitarians, Kantians, and virtue theorists deal with this issue?
4. From a feminist standpoint theory, what specific moral issues exist in this case?

4. Executions in Texas: Another Day at the Office[38]

Executions by lethal injection generally involve the participation of physicians. Consider the case of Texas. In the past, executions were scheduled for midnight, but now they take place at 6:00 P.M. This time is convenient for witnesses as well as for the physician who administers the lethal drug. The prisoner enters the death chamber, and the process itself appears almost uneventful: no blood, no screams of terror. The physician inserts a needle into the condemned prisoner's arm, and it looks as if the inmate simply falls asleep. The physician then checks for vital signs and certifies the death. After witnessing the execution of murderer Billy Joe Woods, journalist Michael Graczyk wrote, "It was bizarre to look around and see all these people just doing their job. It was just another day at the office."

DISCUSSION QUESTIONS

1. Should physicians participate in executions? Does this require physicians to go against their professional code of ethics? Support your answers.
2. Does the principle of nonmaleficence prohibit physicians from participating in any way in executions? Does this same principle forbid anyone to participate in executions? Support your answers.
3. Is the prisoner to be regarded as a patient?

5. Rosa Gutierrez[39]

Rosa Gutierrez was a twenty-six-year-old Mexican mother who brought her two-month-old baby daughter to the emergency room of a local hospital. The baby had not been nursing and was experiencing bouts of diarrhea. Upon further examination, the emergency physician on duty also found that the baby was experiencing high fever, sepsis, and dehydration. The physician felt that a spinal tap was in order and recommended this treatment to Gutierrez. He also asked for her signed permission to go ahead with the procedure. However, she refused to sign the consent form. Staff members then attempted to persuade her to sign the form, since this procedure was fairly routine and involved very little risk for the baby. Nevertheless, Gutierrez still refused. She claimed that she could not sign any form without the express permission of her husband. This was the custom in Mexican households, and she was not about to break that custom. So everything was put on hold until the husband arrived.

DISCUSSION QUESTIONS

1. Was Rosa Gutierrez right in insisting on her husband's permission to sign the consent form?
2. As a healthcare staff member, how should one seek to alleviate the possible conflict between cultural norms and patient safety—in this case, the well-being of the baby?
3. Obtaining informed consent is not a universal practice. Do you think it should be a universal rule?

6. Mustafa Said

Twenty-seven-year-old Mustafa Said, a Muslim Arab, has been admitted to a Chicago hospital for biopsies of suspicious tumors along his spine. He shares a semiprivate room with another patient. Throughout his hospital stay, he has been an extremely difficult patient for the nursing staff. He constantly issues orders to the nurses. He demands their attention for even the smallest detail. Many of the nurses feel that he has acted condescendingly toward them on a number of occasions.

Nurse Saladiak is the primary nurse in charge. The nurses on all the shifts have complained about Said. One time, she entered Said's room well after visiting hours only to find the room filled with his family members. A few times, Said refused to follow the special medical diet he had been placed on and instead was eating food given to him by family members. When she pointed this out to him, he made it clear that he would not comply with her instructions. Some of the nurses have already refused to take care of him, and Saladiak's own patience is nearing its limit. She has no idea how to deal with Said.

DISCUSSION QUESTIONS

1. How should Nurse Saladiak deal with this situation?
2. What factors need to be taken into consideration in this case, given that Said is a Muslim? How might his being a Muslim explain any of his behavior?
3. Is it ever justifiable for nurses to refuse to care for their patients? If so, when? Explain.

7. A Pig's Liver for Henry Adams

Forty-three-year-old Henry Adams had been on the waiting list for a liver transplant for over four years. During that time, he had regularly been undergoing dialysis treatments at a local clinic four times a week. Finally, his primary physician informed him that a liver was available for him. He was admitted to nearby Pittsburgh's Presbyterian University Hospital for the transplant.

Soon after he was admitted, the transplant surgeon, Richard Horst, met with Adams. Dr. Horst revealed to Adams that, with Adams's consent, he could be the recipient of a liver taken from a pig. Horst explained that pigs had for some time been bred for research purposes and had been genetically engineered so that their organs could eventually be used, after thorough testing, for transplantation into humans. He also indicated that pigs were being considered since there would be less likelihood of organ rejection by humans. After meticulous research and testing, the time was ripe to test the transplantation of a pig's liver into a human, and Adams appeared to be the closest match.

A nurse, Judy Wolfson, was present during this discussion. When Adams asked about the likelihood of success, Horst replied that the chances of success were very high, with a greater than 70 percent chance of having a good quality of life after the procedure. This reply puzzled Nurse Wolfson because the operation would amount to an experiment, with no prior experiments having been done on humans. However, she did not raise the issue with the surgeon. Adams seemed satisfied with Horst's explanation and, later that day, signed the consent form. Nurse Wolfson is not at all sure that the patient was adequately informed, nor is she convinced that the patient may not have been subtly coerced. She believes she ought to bring up the issue with her supervisor.

DISCUSSION QUESTIONS

1. Given what you know about his case, do you believe Adams was sufficiently informed regarding the procedure? Explain your response.
2. Do you believe there was any coercion? Any manipulation? Explain in detail.
3. Applying Haddad's analysis, how should Nurse Wolfson address this issue? Should she deal directly with the surgeon? Explain.
4. If Nurse Wolfson deals first with Dr. Horst, how should she present her concerns to him? Explain your response.

8. The Bus Driver

Roy Eckhert had been a New York City Transit Authority bus driver for over twenty-one years. When his physician, Tom Coster, gave him his annual physical exam, Coster noted that Eckhert's heart experienced occasional premature ventricular contractions. In other words, his heart was beating irregularly, and there was a possibility of ventricular damage. This could lead to a myocardial infarction, or a heart attack.

In Coster's opinion, the irregularities did not appear that serious, although they could become worse. He shared his concern with Eckhert. Eckhert, wanting to stay with the company and obtain his generous pension benefits upon retirement, pleaded with Coster not to divulge this information to anyone else. Coster complied with his patient's request.

DISCUSSION QUESTIONS

1. Is Dr. Coster justified in agreeing to keep this information about his patient confidential? Give reasons for your response.
2. If you were Eckhert's physician, how would you deal with his request?
3. Provide deontological support both for maintaining confidentiality in this case and for infringing upon it.
4. What would be utilitarian grounds for maintaining confidentiality in this case? For violating it?

C H A P T E R   4

Abortion and Maternal-Fetal Conflicts

In 1962, Sherri Finkbine, star of a popular Arizona children's show and pregnant mother of four, discovered to her horror that the drug thalidomide, which she had taken early in her pregnancy to help her sleep, could cause birth defects such as missing limbs or seal-like flippers, paralysis, and malformed internal organs. After much tortured soul-searching, the Finkbines decided that the best course of action was an abortion. Her husband had picked up the drug during a business trip to Europe, where it was readily available. Because it was not sold in the United States, the devastating effects of thalidomide on unborn children had not received as much coverage in the American press as in the European press. Shortly before the scheduled day for her abortion, Sherri Finkbine decided to go public in order to warn other women about the dangers of thalidomide. Although she requested that her name not be used by the press, the newspaper article made her identity easy to figure out. As a result of the ensuing publicity, the hospital, fearful of legal prosecution, withdrew its consent to perform the abortion. Sherri Finkbine eventually obtained an abortion in Sweden. The fetus was severely deformed.

The thalidomide tragedy sparked international public interest in overhauling restrictive abortion legislation and rethinking the moral status of abortion. Prior to the early 1960s, there had been little public debate over the morality of abortion or support for reform of the restrictive abortion laws that had been on the books in the United States since the turn of the century. Despite the legalization of abortion in the United States by the 1973 U.S. Supreme Court *Roe v. Wade* decision, abortion remains one of the most controversial issues in healthcare ethics, touching many lives.

About 43 percent of American women will have an abortion by age forty-five. While the abortion rate has been dropping in the United States, it is increasing worldwide. According to the World Health Organization, 45 million abortions were performed worldwide in 1995, up from 25 million in 1990. This increase raises serious moral questions. When, if ever, is abortion morally justified? What moral principles and considerations are relevant in discussions of the morality of abortion? When does personhood begin? Is the fetus a person? If the fetus is a person, how should the fetus's rights be balanced against the mother's autonomy? Should medical professionals have input in an abortion decision, or should it be solely a woman's choice? Are the reasons why a woman wants an abortion morally relevant?

THE DEFINITION OF ABORTION

Spontaneous and Induced Abortions

The term *abortion* will be used to refer to induced abortion, which is defined for the purposes of this book as the intentional termination of a pregnancy at any stage in the pregnancy. This definition excludes spontaneous abortions (known as miscarriages), the unintentional or accidental loss of a pregnancy prior to viability (about twenty-four weeks). Losses after viability are referred to as preterm deliveries. Because spontaneous abortions occur on their own, independent of human intervention or intention, they are not usually considered morally problematic. Unlike some definitions of abortion, the one we use in this book also includes induced abortions after viability, such as partial-birth abortions, since they are considered as such under laws that permit abortion in the United States and many other countries.

Selective and Elective Abortions

There are two types of induced abortion: selective and elective. Like Sherri Finkbine, some women seek an abortion not because they don't want the pregnancy, but because of the risk of fetal abnormalities or because the fetus[1] is of the "wrong" gender. An abortion in which the particular fetus, rather than the pregnancy, is unwanted is known as a **selective abortion.** Selective abortion accounts for less than 2 percent of abortions in the United States. In countries such as India and China, where sex selection is widely practiced, the percentage is much higher. **Therapeutic abortions,** which are performed to save the life of the mother, are even rarer, although some people include abortions for severe fetal abnormalities, rape, and incest in the category of therapeutic abortions. Most women, however, choose to have an abortion because they do not want the pregnancy. Such abortions are known as **elective abortions.**

METHODS OF ABORTION

There are three primary types of abortion: medical abortion, surgical abortion, and medical induction of uterine contractions. The method used depends primarily on the time of gestation. About 85–90 percent of abortions in the United States are performed in the first twelve weeks of pregnancy,[2] 5–10 percent between twelve and sixteen weeks, 4 percent between sixteen and twenty weeks, and 1.5 percent after twenty-one weeks. Younger women are more likely to have abortions after 16 weeks.[3]

Medical Abortions

Medical abortions include the morning-after pill and mifepristone, popularly known as RU-486. They are used only early in pregnancy.

The Morning-After Pill   The morning-after pill is actually a high dose of birth control pills taken at two intervals in the three days following intercourse. The doses prevent the blastocyst from implanting in the uterine wall. This method is 75 percent successful at preventing implantation.

Mifepristone (RU-486)   Mifepristone, or RU-486, was developed in France and approved for use by the U.S. Food and Drug Administration in 1997. Mifepristone induces menstruation, thus expelling the implanted embryo. It is more than 90 percent effective in terminating pregnancies of less than seven weeks gestation.[4]

Surgical Abortions

Most abortions are performed surgically. The 98–99 percent success rate of surgical abortion is much higher than that of medical abortion.

Dilation and Curettage (D&C)   D&C used to be one of the most popular methods of abortion. The cervix of the uterus is expanded, and a curette is inserted to scrape the surface of the uterine wall. This method has fallen out of favor because of the risk of puncturing the uterus, which can cause maternal hemorrhaging and even death.

Vacuum Aspiration (D&E)   The development in China in the early 1960s of the safer vacuum aspiration method was accompanied by a sharp decline in the death rate from abortions. Also known as dilation and evacuation (D&E), it was first used in the United States in the late 1960s. This method is similar to D&C, except that the fetus is suctioned rather than scraped out of the uterus. In 1999, over 90 percent of abortions in the United States involved vacuum aspiration.

Partial-Birth Abortion   Also less commonly known as intact dilation and evacuation (IDE), **partial-birth abortion** is used only in late abortions. After partially delivering an intact fetus feet-first, the doctor punctures the fetus's skull, suctions out the brain, and then crushes the skull so the fetus fits easily through the birth canal. An estimated 3,000 to 5,000 partial-birth abortions are performed annually in the United States.[5]

Hysterectomy and Hysterontomy   Surgical removal of the fetus is generally reserved for late-term abortions. A hysterectomy entails the surgical removal of the whole uterus; a hysterontomy is the removal of the fetus through an incision in the uterus. Because of the high number of fetuses who survive and the high incidence of maternal complications, this method is rarely used except in emergencies.

Medical Induction of Uterine Contractions

Abortions between sixteen and twenty weeks can be carried out by either surgical removal of the fetus or medical induction of uterine contractions.

Saline Solution   In this method, about 200 ml of amniotic fluid is withdrawn from the amniotic sac and replaced with a similar amount of saline solution. The fetus's heartbeat usually stops within one to one and a half hours after the injection, and the fetus is expelled from the womb within seventy-two hours. Although the saline solution is meant to kill the fetus, this method occasionally results in a live birth.

Prostaglandins   This method involves an intramuscular or intravaginal injection of prostaglandins to induce labor. The use of prostaglandins, or a combination of prostaglandins and saline solution, is associated with fewer live births than the use of saline solution alone and has replaced saline abortions in many hospitals and clinics.

THE LEGAL STATUS OF ABORTION

On a cool December day in 1969, Linda Coffee, a young lawyer, and Norma McCorvey, a twenty-one-year-old single mother, sat down together at a pizza parlor in Dallas, Texas. A few minutes later, they were joined by another lawyer, Sarah Weddington. Weddington was interested in challenging the constitutionality of an 1854 Texas law that outlawed abortion except to save the life of the mother. As the two lawyers listened, McCorvey told them that she had been traveling during the summer with a carnival, where she had a job selling tickets to an animal sideshow. According to McCorvey, one evening while returning with some friends to her motel room, she had been raped and left in a ditch. When McCorvey began experiencing nausea, she went to a physician, who confirmed her pregnancy. She tried without success to find an abortionist. Coffee and Weddington were both deeply touched by McCorvey's story. They had been looking for a woman to be a plaintiff in an abortion suit and asked McCorvey if she would be willing to sue the state of Texas. McCorvey agreed to sue. To protect her privacy, McCorvey was given the name Jane Roe in the lawsuit. The case of *Roe v. Wade*, which ended up going to the U.S. Supreme Court, dramatically altered prevailing abortion practices in the United States.

Abortion Laws Worldwide

Few countries had laws regulating abortion prior to the late nineteenth century. However, during the early twentieth century, many countries passed laws restricting abortion. Abortion remained a taboo topic in much of the world until the 1960s. As late as 1965, abortion was legal only in Japan, China, and parts of Scandinavia and Eastern Europe. During the 1960s and 1970s, restrictions on abortion were eased in many countries.

The former Soviet Union, in 1920, was the first country to legalize abortion at the request of the woman. In 1939, both Sweden and Denmark liberalized their abortion laws. Czechoslovakia followed suit in the 1950s. In Japan, abortion was legalized under the 1948 Eugenic Protection laws, which were designed to protect women's health and to discourage the birth of children with genetic disorders, although in actual practice abortion in Japan is available on demand.

In 1967, Great Britain passed a law permitting abortion if two doctors certified that continuation of the pregnancy would have a more adverse effect on the health of the woman or her existing children than would termination of the pregnancy of if there was a substantial risk that the child would have serious handicaps. Several other governments, including those of Zambia, Hong Kong, and Australia, modeled their laws on Great Britain's.

Canada is one of the few countries where abortion is a criminal act. Its 1969 abortion law retains criminal penalties for both abortion providers and women who seek abortions. The law, however, permits abortion under three conditions: (1) The abortion must be performed by a qualified medical practitioner in an approved hospital, (2) it must be approved by a therapeutic abortion committee of the hospital, and (3) it must

CULTURAL WINDOWS

CHINA:
Abortion as a Means of Population Control

One-fifth of the world's population lives in China. With more than 1.2 billion people, China has the highest population of any country in the world.[6] In 1953, China adopted a "planned birth" policy that, through a system of rewards and punishment, aggressively promoted abortion as a means of limiting family size. The goal of the program was to ensure that the population of China did not exceed 1.2 billion by the year 2000. Under the Chinese constitution, both the government and the individual are held responsible for adhering to the abortion policy. This goal conflicts with traditional Chinese and Confucian values, which emphasize family and filial piety. Unlike families in most Western nations, Chinese families depend on their children to care for them in old age.

In 1974, the policy was amended to limit couples to two children. In 1979, the limit was changed to one child per couple, and then only with government authorization. To enforce this policy, abortion is offered at no cost. As a result of this policy, the abortion rate in China is one of the highest in the world. As an added incentive, women who have abortions are given a two-week paid leave from their jobs. Women who agree to be sterilized or have an intrauterine device (IUD) inserted at the time of the abortion are given additional paid leave. In many villages, to ensure compliance, local officials keep records of women's marital status, number of children, and even menstrual cycles. Violators of the one-child policy may be subject to forced abortions, even in the last trimester of pregnancy.[7] Some have been jailed or have lost their homes.

Because of the one-child policy, many Chinese families resort to selective abortion, or female infanticide, to ensure that their child will be male. Ninety percent of female fetuses identified by prenatal diagnosis are aborted.[8] Female infants may be turned over to orphanages or abandoned to die. The preference for sons is tied to a patriarchal society in which women have few economic opportunities and daughters are perceived as economic burdens. The majority of Chinese people do not appear to be concerned about the shortage of wives for their sons. The parents' immediate concern is to have sons who can help out in the fields, carry on the family name, and provide them with security in their old age.[9]

There is considerable opposition to the official program of forced sterilization and abortion, both internationally and among the Chinese people. As a result, the Chinese government began relaxing enforcement of the policy in the late 1990s.[10]

be shown that continuation of the pregnancy would be likely to endanger the life or health of the woman seeking the abortion. Opponents of abortion protest that the Canadian law is too liberal, while libertarians argue that it is too restrictive. Legislative attempts to revise the law have been unsuccessful.

India's 1971 Medical Termination Law permits abortion primarily as a means of population control. In 1996, alarmed by the high rate of selective abortion in some areas, India enacted a law banning the abortion of healthy female fetuses.

China, which also encourages abortion for population control, has one of the highest abortion rates in the world. Each year about one in ten Chinese women has an abortion.[11] Abortion was also prevalent in ancient Confucian culture.[12] While contemporary Buddhists are, for the most part, opposed to abortion because it violates the principle of ahimsa (no harm), the influence of Confucianism and the pressures of overpopulation have ameliorated the influence of Buddhism in China, where abortion is legal and even mandatory under some circumstances.

Although Buddhists are opposed to any intentional destruction of life, they are divided on the role the state should play in prohibiting abortion. In Taiwan and Thailand, where Buddhism is very strong, abortion is legally restricted. In Japan, on the other hand, where abortion was legalized after World War II, abortion is tolerated as a regrettable but necessary evil.

The abortion rate in West Germany is among the lowest in Europe. Following World War II, West Germany vowed that it would never again declare a group of humans to be worthless or legally sanction the "destruction of life unworthy of life," as happened during the Nazi regime. The constitution of the Federal Republic of Germany states that "everyone has a right to life." This right includes a constitutional obligation to protect prenatal human life. In 1975, in response to the growing international movement to liberalize abortion laws, the Fifth Statute was passed, which criminalized abortion after the thirteenth day of conception (the time when the fertilized egg implants in the wall of the uterus) except when the pregnancy was considered a danger to the mother's life or health or if the fetus was malformed. This law has since been challenged.

Abortion laws are most restrictive in the Arab world, Latin America, Central Asia, and sub-Saharan Africa.[13] The highly restrictive abortion laws in many poorer Latin American countries and the lack of access by women to economic opportunities have been accompanied by a high maternal death rate from illegal abortions.

Because of the high infant mortality rate in many parts of Africa, most Africans attach a high value to having children and have an abhorrence of abortion.[14] Although South Africa liberalized its laws in 1975, most South Africans are opposed to elective abortion. In 1996, despite public opposition, the South African legislature passed the Choice of Termination of Pregnancy Bill permitting abortion-on-demand up to the twelfth week of pregnancy. Following the passage of the bill, 82 percent of South African doctors and several hospitals stated that they would refuse to comply with requests for abortion-on-demand.[15]

Abortion is illegal in most Catholic countries. Five countries—El Salvador, Malta, Andorra, Vatican City, and Chile—forbid abortion even to save the life of the mother. In Spain, abortion is permitted only in cases of rape, fetal deformity, or danger to the physical or mental life of the mother.[16] In Argentina, Ireland, and Italy, abortion is illegal except to save the life of the mother. The British abortion act does not apply to Northern Ireland, where there is strong opposition to abortion. In 1983, the eighth

CULTURAL WINDOWS

JAPAN:
Mizuko Rituals for Aborted Children

Japanese attitudes toward abortion are influenced by both its Buddhist and its Shinto heritage. Unlike Buddhism in some Southeast Asian nations where abortion is illegal or heavily restricted, Japanese Buddhism is an amalgamation of traditional Buddhist beliefs and Japanese religious beliefs and traditions that permit the taking of human life under certain circumstances. In addition, women in Japan, unlike women in most developed countries, do not have access to low-dose contraception pills. Consequently, abortion is the principal means of birth control, with approximately half of all pregnancies in Japan ending in abortion.[17]

In Japan, it is believed that the aborted fetus, or *mizuko* (meaning "unseeing child"), returns to the Buddha to await birth at a later time. These children are very sad beings, since they have been denied the bliss of coming into this world and have been abandoned by those who were to be their parents. Mizuko rituals, memorial services for the aborted child, are performed to placate the unhappy spirit lest he or she seek retaliation. As part of the service, small statues of the Buddhist god Jizo, who watches over aborted spirits, are erected. Some Buddhist temples in Japan house thousands of these small statues.

Mizuko rituals also provide an opportunity for the woman to deal with her anguish and grief. In his book *The Forgotten Child*, Japanese Buddhist priest Miura Domyo writes of how the mizuko service and praying for the spirit of the aborted child help women who have had abortions overcome some of the problems that arise in their lives.[18]

The demand for mizuko services has increased dramatically since 1975, leading to the development of large commercialized mizuko temples that charge high fees for their services. Prices for mizuko services, which generally last about an hour, can be as high as $2,100. Many Japanese are critical of these temples, claiming that their primary purpose is to extort money from naive people by playing on their fear of retribution.[19]

Mizuko services are also related to the high importance given to ancestors and the extended family in Japan. People attending mizuko services include women who have had miscarriages as well as men and women with relatives who have had miscarriages or abortions. Some participants come because they hope that the lost child will be reborn into their family.

---

amendment to the Irish constitution gave "the unborn" the same right to life as other citizens.

In contrast to regulations in most countries, which require a physician's approval for abortion, French regulations enacted in 1975 allow a woman to make the decision about whether she is entitled to an abortion on the grounds of hardship. In this respect, French law more closely resembles the 1973 U.S. Supreme Court *Roe v. Wade* decision.

The History of Abortion Law in the United States

Abortion was not uncommon in America from the colonial period until the late 1800s. When abortion was mentioned, it was not the abortion itself that was usually condemned but rather the violation of other social taboos, such as sexual relations outside of marriage, that led to the abortion.[20]

During the early 1820s, American physicians began taking an interest in medical law and the legal regulation of abortion.[21] In 1821, Connecticut passed the country's first antiabortion law. Antiabortion laws in the early nineteenth century, for the most part, applied only to women "quick with child." Quickening is the moment when a woman first feels the movement of her fetus, generally between sixteen and eighteen weeks. Despite laws against abortion, folk remedies and patent medicines continued to be widely available.

In the mid-nineteenth century, the newly founded American Medical Association (AMA) spearheaded a movement to outlaw abortion. In 1859, it passed a resolution condemning abortion as an "unwarranted destruction of human life," calling on state legislators to pass antiabortion laws or toughen existing laws.[22]

Although many people, including physicians, blamed the prevalence of abortion on feminist ideas, the early feminists disapproved of abortion, which they considered to be "a revolting outrage against . . . our common humanity" and a form of infanticide.[23] Elizabeth Cady Stanton regarded abortion as just one more result of the degradation of woman.[24] However, unlike the physicians, the early feminists did not think that outlawing abortion without dealing with the root cause of abortion—the oppression of women—would have the desired effect, believing instead that the need for abortion should be eliminated. "We want prevention, not merely punishment," Susan B. Anthony wrote in 1869. "We must reach the root of the evil, and destroy it."[25] The early feminist argument against abortion is reiterated by Sidney Callahan in her article at the end of this chapter.

Between 1855 and 1880, most states that did not have laws on abortion passed antiabortion laws. By 1900, every state had laws prohibiting or restricting abortion; all but six included a "therapeutic exception" in their abortion laws. These laws remained virtually unchanged until the 1960s, when several events led to increased dissatisfaction with the restrictive abortion laws. These events included an increase in the number of women in the work force, a desire for smaller families, increased publicity about the dangers of illegal abortion, improvements in the safety of surgical abortion, and increasing public pressure to permit therapeutic abortion in the case of fetal deformity.

The thalidomide tragedy was closely followed by an outbreak of rubella (German measles). If a woman contracts German measles during the first three months of pregnancy, there's a fifty percent chance that some organs of her embryo will not form properly. Many pregnant women who came down with German measles were unable to obtain legal abortions in the United States. Between 1963 and 1966, 15,000 babies were born with birth defects, including blindness, mental retardation, and heart problems. Newspapers and magazines ran front-page stories chronicling the desperate circumstances of women, such as Sherri Finkbine, who were denied legal therapeutic abortions.

Fueled by the publicity generated by the thalidomide and German measles tragedies, the push for legal reform came primarily from the medical and legal professions. Although most people supported more liberal laws regarding therapeutic abor-

CULTURAL WINDOWS

UNITED STATES:
Roe v. Wade (1973)

It is ... apparent that at common law, at the time of the adoption of our Constitution, and throughout the major portion of the nineteenth century, abortion was viewed with less disfavor than under most American statutes currently in effect. . . .

Three reasons have been advanced to explain historically the enactment of criminal abortion laws in the nineteenth century and to justify their continued existence.

[First] It has been argued occasionally that these laws were the product of a Victorian special concern to discourage illicit sexual conduct. . . .

A second reason is concerned with abortion as a medical procedure. When most criminal abortion laws were first enacted, the procedure was a hazardous one for the woman. . . . Modern medical techniques have altered this situation. . . .

The third reason is the state's interest—some phrase it in terms of duty—in protecting prenatal life. . . . Only when the life of the pregnant mother herself is at stake, balanced against the life she carries within her, should the interest of the embryo or fetus not prevail. . . . A legitimate state interest in this area need not stand or fall on acceptance of the belief that life begins at conception or at some other point prior to live birth. In assessing the state's interest, recognition may be given to the less rigid claim that as long as at least *potential* life is involved, the state may assert interests beyond the protection of the pregnant woman alone. . . .

The Constitution does not explicitly mention any right of privacy. . . . [Earlier Supreme Court] decisions make it clear that only personal rights that can be deemed "fundamental" or "implicit in the concept of ordered liberty" . . . are included in this guarantee of personal privacy. They also make it clear that the right has some extension to ac-

tion, there was little public support in the late 1960s for nontherapeutic abortion, or abortion-on-demand—what later became known as the pro-choice position.[26]

In 1969, Planned Parenthood, which under the leadership of Margaret Sanger had been opposed to abortion, reversed its position and called for the repeal of all antiabortion laws. The following year, the AMA followed suit, voting to support a physician's right to perform abortions if the woman's social and economic circumstances made it difficult for her to have a baby. These changes, together with the first legal acknowledgment of a constitutional "right to privacy" in the 1965 U.S. Supreme Court case *Griswold v. Connecticut*, provided lawyers with the grist they needed to turn the wheels of reform by challenging the constitutionality of existing antiabortion laws. Between 1967 and 1970, twelve states, including California, Hawaii, New York, Alaska, and Washington, repealed their restrictive abortion laws.

tivities relating to marriage ... [and] procreation. ...

We therefore conclude that the right of personal privacy includes the abortion decision, but that this right is not unqualified and must be considered against important state interests in regulation.

... no case could be cited that holds that a fetus is a person within the meaning of the Fourteenth Amendment. ... All this, together with our observation, *supra*, that throughout the majority portion of the nineteenth century prevailing legal abortion practices were far freer than they are today, persuades us that the word "person," as used in the Fourteenth Amendment, does not include the unborn. ...

There has always been strong support for the view that life does not begin until live birth. ... Physicians and their scientific colleagues have ... tended to focus either upon conception or upon live birth or upon the interim point at which the fetus becomes "viable," that is, potentially able to live outside the mother's womb, albeit with artificial aid. Viability is usually placed at about seven months (28 weeks) but may occur earlier. ...

With respect to the state's important and legitimate interest in the health of the mother, the compelling point, in the light of present medical knowledge, is at approximately the end of the first trimester. This is so because of the now established medical fact ... that until the end of the first trimester mortality in abortion is less than mortality in normal childbirth. It follows that, from and after this point, a state may regulate the abortion procedure to the extent that the regulation reasonably relates to the preservation and protection of maternal health. Examples ... are requirements as to the qualifications of the person who is to perform the abortion. ...

State regulations protective of fetal life after viability have both logical and biological justifications. If the state is interested in protecting fetal life after viability, it may go so far as to proscribe abortion during that period except when it is necessary to preserve the life or health of the mother. ...

Roe v. Wade

A major turning point in the reform movement came when the battleground moved from the states into the federal courts. In January 1973, the U.S. Supreme Court ruled in *Roe v. Wade* that the Texas antiabortion law violated women's fundamental constitutional right to privacy as implied in the Fourteenth Amendment. The effect of this ruling was to legalize abortion throughout the United States, at least prior to **viability,** when the fetus can survive outside the womb. Because it is based on a right to privacy rather than on a First Amendment guarantee of freedom, *Roe v. Wade* does not grant women procreative freedom or the right to control their own bodies, nor does it permit abortion-on-demand.

Since 1973, several states have passed legislation that places restrictions on abortion. Thirty-seven states enacted laws restricting abortion in 1997 alone. Restrictions include parental and spousal notification requirements, mandatory waiting periods, bans on federal funding for abortions, and laws prohibiting partial-birth abortions. Several bills for a constitutional amendment that would overturn *Roe v. Wade* have been introduced, including the Human Life Amendment, which would extend personhood or legal protection to "all human beings." Despite a highly vocal pro-life movement, the United States has one of the highest abortion rates in North America and Europe—perhaps in part because of the lack of universal healthcare and adequate family support services, such as maternity leave and inexpensive day care, in the United States.

The Law and Morality

Many people confuse the legal and moral issues in the abortion debate, thus committing the fallacy of appeal to tradition. This confusion is most evident in talk of rights. The fact that women may have a legal right to abortion does not mean that they also have a moral right. In addition, believing abortion is immoral does not necessarily imply that it ought to be illegal, especially in cultures where women have few options. Some people who are morally opposed to abortion still support the legalization of abortion on utilitarian grounds because of the greater harm to women of making it illegal. Worldwide, thousands of women die each year from complications due to unsafe illegal abortions; the vast majority of these deaths occur in poorer nations in sub-Saharan Africa and South Asia.

The use of abortion depends on a number of factors, including access to contraception, the status of women, fertility preferences, and abortion laws. In Japan, abortion rates have been dropping in direct proportion to access to effective contraception. The lowest abortion rates are found in the Netherlands, which has one of the world's most liberal abortion laws but also protects equal opportunities for women. Illegal abortion is one of the main causes of maternal mortality in some countries. In Chile, in contrast, a patriarchal culture in which abortion is illegal under all circumstances, about one in three pregnancies is terminated by an illegal abortion. Chile's abortion rate is the highest in Latin America and slightly higher than that in the United States.[27]

While social and economic factors affect abortion rates, there seems to be a correlation between legalized abortion and the abortion rate in some countries. The former Soviet Union, the first country to legalize abortion, has one of the highest abortion rates in the world. In part because of lack of access to effective contraception, abortion is often used as a means of birth control, and a Russian woman may have as many as ten abortions in her lifetime. In the United States between 1973, when 760,000 abortions were performed, and 1988, the abortion rate increased every year, reaching a peak of 1,600,000 in 1988. The same phenomenon occurred in Canada, where the number of women seeking legal abortions increased almost sevenfold between 1970 and 1982. The drop in abortion rates in the United States during the 1990s has been attributed to a combination of factors, including changes in contraceptive and sexual practices; reduced access to abortion services, with fewer doctors and medical centers willing to perform abortions; changes in attitudes toward abortion, with more people trying to avoid it; greater acceptance of unmarried mothers; and a decline in the number of pregnancies.[28]

Does legalizing abortion make women more likely to seek abortions? If so, is this situation morally problematic? Should the decision of abortion be left up to the individual woman, or do fetuses have rights that ought to be protected by society? If fetuses do have moral value, how should we weigh protecting their rights, by enacting laws

ISLAMIC CULTURES:
Islamic Law and Abortion

In some, though not all, Islamic nations, there is no separation between law and religion. The physician's duty is to provide medical advice and recommendations based on medical expertise as well as the requirements of Islamic law.

The majority of Muslims believe that life begins at conception. Islamic medical scholars have a high regard for medical science and the study of embryology, which in their view confirms the Islamic position on the human status of the fetus. Since human life is sacred and created in the image of God, the protection of human life is one of the fundamental goals of Islamic law. Abortion, therefore, is wrong at any stage of pregnancy. The Quran teaches:

We [God and his cosmic agents] have created man out of an extraction of clay; then we turn it into semen and settle it in a firm receptacle. We then turn semen into a clot which we then fashion into a lump of chewed flesh. Then we fashion the chewed flesh into bones and we clothe the bones with intact flesh. Then we develop out of it another creature. So blessed be God, the best of creators. (23:12–14)

Abortion is permitted, however, if the pregnancy poses a serious threat to the life of the mother. According to revealed Islamic law (Shari'a), "the mother is the root and the fetus the offshoot, and it is lawful to sacrifice the latter if it is the only way to save the former."[29]

Some Arab countries permit abortion under other circumstances as well. Because family honor is highly valued, an abortion may be permitted in order to avoid tarnishing the family name in the case of the pregnancy of a single woman. Tunisia also permits abortion after the third child as a means of family planning. Selective abortion of girls, on the other hand, is considered especially heinous in Arab countries, since it not only destroys the life of the fetus but discriminates against women as well. There is also fear that upsetting the gender ratio may have grave social consequences.[30]

against abortion, against the suffering that some women are forced to endure because of lack of access to safe abortions?

Abortion and Religion

The majority of religious groups oppose abortion.[31] For example, Muslims believe that human life is sacred and that the fetus is a person with rights under the law from the moment of **ensoulment,** when the soul enters the body. However, this belief is tempered by practical concerns, and Islamic law generally permits early abortions on medical grounds.[32]

Traditional Hinduism, like Islam, accepts the premise that the fetus is a person. In Hinduism, the killing of a conscious fetus carries the same penalty as the murder of a learned Brahman. The current emphasis on having sons in many Asian countries, however, has led to a high rate of selective abortion for gender, despite laws in some Asian countries specifically prohibiting abortion for sex selection.

There is little mention of abortion in the Bible, and what mention there is is ambiguous. Orthodox Jews emphasize passages in Genesis that teach that, because we are created in the image of God, all human life is inviolable and sacred. Thus, abortion is prohibited except to save the life of the mother. Liberal and Reform Jews, on the other hand, point out that Adam did not become a living human being until God breathed life into him. Likewise, infants do not become a "nephesh," that is, a person with a soul, until they take their first breath of air. Abortion, therefore, is permissible at any time during the pregnancy.

The position of the early Christian Church was similar to that of Orthodox Jews. The Didache, written no later than A.D. 100, contains a prohibition against abortion, calling those who procure abortions "destroyers of God's image." The only exception to the prohibition was abortion to save the life of the mother.

In contrast to the early Church, Thomas Aquinas set the time of ensoulment at forty days for males and eighty days for females. Based on this distinction, for centuries the Roman Catholic Church regarded late abortions as more sinful than early ones, a belief still common. In the nineteenth century, the Church changed its position, returning to the early Christian prohibition against abortion at any time. In his 1995 papal encyclical *Evangelium Vitae*, Pope John Paul II urged people not to support laws that permit abortion because they contradict God's (natural) law.

The reaction of modern Protestants to abortion is varied. Most fundamentalist, evangelical, and African-American Protestant churches are opposed to abortion, while most "mainstream" Protestant churches take a moderate stand, supporting abortion prior to viability. Some Protestant churches support a woman's right to choose an abortion throughout her pregnancy.

Given the diversity of religious views on the morality of abortion, what should we do when they come into conflict, especially in a pluralistic society? Isn't it wrong for someone to force his or her religious views on someone else? Natural law ethicists maintain that, while religious teachings may support morality, morality also exists independent of religion. Roman Catholic healthcare ethicists, for example, do not regard Catholic teachings on morality as binding only on Catholics, since the teachings are based on a universal moral law that is binding on everyone. Nor do Muslims and Hindus believe that only Muslim and Hindu fetuses have moral value; all fetuses have moral value, no matter what the religious views of their parents or the culture may be. If a law is inconsistent with natural law, then it is an unjust, immoral law. On the other hand, not all natural law ethicists accept the conclusion that abortion is unjust under all or even most circumstances. In addition, we need to examine the validity of the premise that fetuses have moral value.

In debating moral issues that impact several realms, such as law, religion, and morality, we need to sort out our reasoning. The moral controversy over abortion cannot be resolved simply by accepting religious dogma uncritically, any more than we can assume that a law or a court ruling such as *Roe v. Wade* will resolve the abortion issue once and for all. At the same time, the arguments used by the different religions should not be dismissed offhand, since they are generally based on philosophical as well as theological arguments. Nor should we fall prey to the fallacy of hasty generalization and assume that opposition to abortion comes only, or even primarily, from the religious right. Indeed, public polls show that the greatest decline in support for abortion in the United States since 1994 has been among those who state that religion is not important in their life. Good ethical analysis, while eschewing arguments based purely on faith, subjects to critical analysis the moral arguments put forth by the various religions as well as the nonreligious arguments on both sides of the issue.

THE ABORTION CONTROVERSY: TAKING SIDES

A billboard in a private garden in California proclaims: "Women who have abortions are Whores." Other antiabortion billboards and literature include graphic pictures of aborted fetuses. Protesters also gather outside clinics where abortions are performed. Over one hundred abortion clinics have been bombed or torched since 1973, and several physicians who perform abortions have been killed or injured.

Two days after the *Roe v. Wade* decision, the *New York Times* pronounced that the landmark ruling had at last brought a "final and reasonable resolution" to the debate over abortion. Their optimistic prognosis could not have been more off the mark. Rather than settling the abortion question once and for all, laws and court rulings such as *Roe v. Wade* have left people—including medical professionals—deeply divided.

Positions on the morality of abortion range from the "pro-life," or abolitionist, view that all abortions are wrong except to save the life of the mother to the "pro-choice" libertarian view that abortion is morally acceptable at any time during the pregnancy. The majority of people are moderates who fall somewhere in between these two extremes. The challenge to *Roe v. Wade* comes not only from the pro-life movement, but also from the pro-choice groups who would like to see all restrictions on abortion removed.

The Libertarian Position

According to libertarians, abortion is morally acceptable for any reason throughout pregnancy. Libertarians emphasize the rights and autonomy of the mother and downplay or deny the personhood of the fetus. A woman's right to control her body overrides any rights the fetus may have or any interests the father may have in the child.

Libertarians, however, do not base their arguments solely on a woman's right to control her own body. They argue that access to legal abortion is necessary for the safety and well-being of women. Decisions regarding abortion should be made by those who are most affected by them. What takes place in women's bodies can have profound effects on their lives, particularly in societies where women bear the primary responsibility for birth and child rearing.

Furthermore, women cannot rely on contraception alone, since no form is foolproof and without side effects. Feminists such as Alison M. Jaggar, professor of philosophy at the University of Colorado, also point out that women's sexual encounters are "frequently manipulated and coerced."[33] It is unjust for an oppressed group to be required to make sacrifices that will exacerbate this oppression.[34] Refusing to allow a woman to have an abortion is tantamount to coerced pregnancy and childbirth.

Abolitionists

Abolitionists, in contrast, believe that abortion is never morally acceptable, except to save the life of the mother. They stress the personhood of the fetus over a woman's right to control her body. The fetus, or preborn child, is a person and deserves the same protection as a born child. Like libertarians, most abolitionists recognize that women are more likely to have an abortion when they lack other viable options. However, they argue that abortion is not a solution to the injustices suffered by women, since the burden of having to raise a child can be avoided through adoption.

Feminist abolitionists, such as Sidney Callahan, maintain that pitting women's rights against fetal rights has prevented women from fully developing, because the rights of women and children are linked. According to these feminists, permissive abortion policies, rather than contributing to the liberation of women, have held women back. We need to move from focusing on the rights of women to control their own bodies to a more inclusive ideal of justice that gives all persons, including unborn children, equal consideration. If abortion remains legal, they argue, we run the risk that access to abortion will be used as a substitute for social reform. Instead, we need to seek alternatives to abortion for empowering women.

Moderates

Moderates occupy the large gap between the libertarian and abolitionist extremes. Some moderates believe that abortion is acceptable only in the first trimester or in cases of rape or fetal abnormalities. Other moderates oppose only late or partial-birth abortions. Despite disagreement among moderates regarding the conditions under which abortion is morally acceptable, they agree that it is morally justifiable in some cases.

Public Polls: Shifting Sides

Public views on abortion in the United States remained relatively stable between 1975 and 1995. Although the percentage of Americans who identify themselves as moderates has remained relatively stable, there has been a nationwide trend since 1995 toward wanting more restrictions placed on abortion, particularly abortions after the first trimester and abortions for social or economic reasons.[35]

A 1996 Gallup poll found that 25 percent of Americans thought abortion should be legal under all circumstances, while 15 percent thought abortion should be illegal under all circumstances. Another 56 percent were moderates, with 13 percent stating that abortion should be legal under most circumstances and 43 percent stating that it should be legal only under a few circumstances, such as rape or to save the life of the mother.[36] In a 1998 *New York Times*/CBS News poll, 61 percent of the respondents supported abortion during the first trimester (the first three months of pregnancy). Support plunged to 15 percent for second-trimester abortion and 7 percent for third-trimester abortion.[37]

This shift away from support for abortion has been due, in part, to the publicity surrounding partial-birth abortions and to advances in prenatal technology, such as real-time, three-dimensional ultrasound, which allows users to visualize the fetus. The rise in violence against abortion clinics and abortion providers and the reluctance of younger doctors to perform abortions (one-third of abortion providers are now over the age of sixty-five)[38] have also contributed to a decline in the number of facilities providing abortions and the number of doctors willing to perform them. In 1995, only 33 percent of obstetrician-gynecologists were performing abortions, compared to 42 percent in 1983.[39]

THE MORAL STATUS OF THE FETUS

Pregnancy is the only situation in which one living being is totally dependent on another for life support. Abortion, therefore, raises unique moral issues regarding the moral status and personhood of the fetus. Libertarians like Mary Anne Warren argue that even the fully developed fetus is not sufficiently personlike to have any right to life. Abolitionists, in contrast, generally see the fetus as a person separate from the mother, with all the rights of a born human. Inquiry into the moral status of the fetus is important, because persons by definition have intrinsic moral value and hence have rights that we ought to respect.[40] If the fetus is a person, then the woman may have a moral obligation to provide life support. If the fetus is not a person, then the fetus may have no more right to the woman's body than a tumor.

Is the fetus ever a person? If so, on what basis is the fetus a person or a nonperson? Is there a distinct point in time when embryos or fetuses achieve personhood, or do they gradually achieve this status based on developmental criteria? In this section, we will examine and critically analyze some of the various definitions of personhood.

All Human Life Has Moral Value

Most, though not all, abolitionists maintain that the fetus is a person from the moment of conception and, as such, has a right to life.

Ensoulment Roman Catholics, Muslims, and Orthodox Jews believe that human life is sacred because it is a special creation of God. Only humans are ensouled; therefore, all and only human life has moral value. There is no distinction between biological humanhood and personhood. We, as humans, have moral value simply because we have a human genotype, no matter what our age or stage of development. Hence, abortion is murder. One problem with using a theological criterion, such as ensoulment, for personhood is that medicine, let alone religion, has never been able to agree on exactly when ensoulment takes place. Indeed, ensoulment is a notoriously vague concept that continues to elude measurement.

Ahimsa Some abolitionists, including many Buddhists, Hindus, and pacifists, reject the notion of ensoulment and the special creation of humans. Instead, they cite the principle of ahimsa, which states that all violence against living beings, including abortion, is wrong.

Potentiality Another criterion used by both abolitionists and moderates is potentiality. According to this criterion, the potential to develop into a full-fledged adult confers personhood on a fertilized egg. Law professor John Noonan, whose article is included in the readings at the end of this chapter, defines personhood on this basis. Judith

CULTURAL WINDOWS

INDIA:
The Hindu Prohibition of Abortion

The Hindu view on abortion is shaped by both the principle of ahimsa and the belief in karma and reincarnation. Nonviolence is the most important endowment of those born with the divine nature. Because abortion entails inflicting violence on the unborn human, it violates the Hindu reverence for life.

Furthermore, the womb is revered as the creative center of the universe, where human and divine activity intersect. It is the manifestation of the divine "as a continuous process, repeated from birth to birth, and encompassing the past, present, and future."[41] Because the fetus, as a reincarnated being, has a karmic inheritance, he or she has moral standing throughout pregnancy. Rather than the embryo being a potential human or merely a collection of cells, Hindus believe that a specific human, with a past, enters the womb at conception.

Early Hindu Vedic and Upanishad literature states that the embryo deserves protection and that abortion is morally intolerable and one of the most deplorable evils. The Sanskrit word for abortion (*hatya*) implies that it is a morally reprehensible killing.[42] The prohibition against abortion is repeated in the *Susruta Samhita*, an an-cient medical treatise. In the *Satapatha Brahmana*, the abortionist is destined to go to hell for violating a sacred prohibition.

In traditional Hindu teachings, abortion can be used only as a last resort if the life of the mother is in danger or if the fetus is severely damaged and in all likelihood will not survive a normal birth. Because of the important role women play in bringing sons into the world, pregnant women, regardless of their caste, are treated with great deference.

The principle of nonviolence, or ahimsa, has never had the incontestable status in Hinduism that it enjoys in Buddhism and Jainism. In modern India, the ancient moral codes are often manipulated in the name of patriarchy and population control. While male fetuses are still held in high regard, the higher value accorded to sons and the availability of prenatal diagnosis to determine the gender of the fetus have contributed to a weakening of the prohibition against aborting female fetuses. Although abortion for sex selection is illegal in some states of India, it is widely practiced in these areas.

Jarvis Thomson, on the other hand, rejects the criterion of potentiality in her analogy between human development and the development of an acorn into an oak tree. She claims that the fact that a being has the potential to develop into another being with greater value does not confer the same moral value on the potential being. The potentiality argument is also used by moderates who look to certain developmental milestones in fetal development at which the potential for personhood becomes an actuality.

Some abolitionists concede that they cannot be sure if the fetus is a person. However, they argue, since we do not know whether the fetus is a person, it is better to err on the side of caution. Noonan uses the analogy of a hunter seeing a movement in the bushes. If we are not sure that the movement is a human being, we still refrain from shooting because it *might* be a person. Similarly, if we are uncertain of the personal status of the fetus, it is best to refrain from performing abortions.

The Fetus Is Never a Person

Some libertarians argue that at no stage of fetal development is the fetus a person. Thus, abortion is permissible at any time during a pregnancy. Mary Anne Warren's argument represents this view. According to Warren, a human does not become a person until sometime after birth, when the infant becomes a "socially responsive member of a human community." She argues that five traits are most central to the concept of personhood: consciousness, complex reasoning, self-motivated activity, intelligent communication, and self-concept.

One implication of this argument, according to opponents of abortion-on-demand, is that it also eliminates some born humans. In order to build trust as a society, we need to know we are special by virtue of being human. The social contract forms a protective armor around the human community. Under the social contract, our instinct for self-preservation becomes a duty to protect all members of the community. Devaluing some humans makes us afraid that we, too, may be devalued. This fear, in turn, weakens the trust that holds society together. Whether abortion in fact weakens this trust and the social contract that binds us together as a society is up for debate. Since we will never again become fetuses (unless we believe in reincarnation), we need not fear that we will be aborted in the future.

Developmental Criteria: Some Fetuses Are Persons

Other definitions of personhood fall between these extremes. Most moderates look to developmental criteria in assessing fetal personhood, granting an adult human with normal cognitive functioning the most moral status and hence the most rights.

Sentience According to utilitarians, all and only sentient beings need to be given moral consideration. Abortion, therefore, becomes a moral issue only after the fetus is able to experience pain. While there is considerable controversy over whether the older embryo and young fetus are able to feel pain, some physicians maintain that the fetus can experience pain by thirteen weeks.[43] Thus, abortion is permissible only in the first trimester. Other physicians place the emergence of sentience later in the second trimester.

Brain Waves A related milestone is the presence of brain waves, which occurs as early as six weeks.[44] This definition of personhood has the advantage of being symmetrical with definitions of the end of personhood at death, when brain waves cease. On the other hand, an adult whose brain waves have ceased is no longer alive and developing, whereas an embryo, despite lack of brain activity, is.

🌿 STAGES OF FETAL DEVELOPMENT

Discussions on the morality of abortion often focus on the level of development of the fetus. Following are some of the milestones in prenatal human development:

Day 1:	*Conception.* The egg and sperm, each containing twenty-three chromosomes, unite to form one cell with forty-six chromosomes. The newly fertilized egg is known as a zygote.
Day 2 to week 2:	*Blastocyst.* The fertilized egg, or blastocyst, travels down the fallopian tubes and implants in the uterus. The blastocyst is composed of an embryonic disk, which will develop into the embryo after implantation, and two cavities, an amniotic cavity and a yolk sac.
Weeks 2 to 8:	*Embryo.* The germ layers of the embryonic disk develop into the principal organ systems. At this stage of development, the cells are rapidly dividing and "transforming" into specialized cells such as eye, skin, and muscle cells. Brain waves are detectable between six and eight weeks. By eight weeks, the embryo is 23 mm long.
Week 8 to birth:	*Fetus.* By eight weeks, all organs and structural features are in place and the fetus resembles a very small newborn child. Between twenty and twenty-four weeks, the fetus becomes viable and is able to survive outside the womb.
Week 40:	*Birth.*

Viability Viability, "the capacity to survive disconnection from the placenta,"[45] replaced quickening as the most widely accepted point for granting the fetus moral rights after the 1973 *Roe v. Wade* decision. However, viability is problematic as a criterion because it makes personhood dependent on medical technology rather than on any fetal characteristic. In other words, it is a moving standard. When the *Roe v. Wade* decision was handed down, viability was set at twenty-eight weeks. Medical technology has since advanced to the point where half of babies born at twenty-four weeks (six months) and some as young as twenty-one weeks survive. Partial **ectogenesis,** the gestation of an infant outside the body of a female, has already been achieved with the gestation of embryos in vitro and the use of incubators for premature babies. If an artificial womb or another means for the young fetus to breathe and survive outside the womb were created, viability could occur much earlier, making *Roe v. Wade* a pro-life ruling.

Implications of Using Developmental Criteria The use of operational criteria to define personhood, while eliminating all unborn and some born humans, also extends the possibility of personhood to members of other species who meet these criteria. This could imply that the abortion of a human fetus, even a fully developed human fetus, may be less morally questionable than the killing of a full-grown chicken or pig, if these creatures are more "personlike" than a fetus.

Some people, frustrated with the lack of consensus on a definition of personhood, argue that it is better left to personal or religious opinion. However, to claim that one's definition of personhood is but a matter of opinion is to mire the debate in ethical subjectivism. If in one's opinion the fetus is not a person, it is possible to argue that not only abortion is morally permissible, but so are infanticide, slavery, and genocide—as long as the perpetrators of these practices believe that their victims are not persons. Also, arguments that focus on the rights and welfare of the woman maintain that even if the fetus is a person abortion is still morally permissible.

THE RIGHTS AND AUTONOMY OF WOMEN

People in the United States are split over which is the more important issue: "a woman's ability to control her body" or "the life of the fetus."[46] Libertarians, in particular, think that the emphasis in the abortion debate on the personhood of the fetus has been made at the expense of concerns about the rights and autonomy of women.

Abortion as a Liberty Right

According to libertarians, the autonomy of the pregnant woman overrides any rights the fetus may have, even if the fetus is a person. The extent to which women have a right to control their own bodies is an issue not just in abortion. It is also relevant in deciding whether women should refrain from certain prenatal behaviors, such as drug and alcohol use, that may harm their fetuses. Warren maintains that to deny women the right to control their bodies is to treat them as a means only. Interference entails paternalism, and women have too often had their interests overridden by men in power.

Opponents of abortion-on-demand reply that autonomy is not an absolute right. They argue that, while women have a moral right to control their bodies, this right does not extend to abortion, since abortion involves destroying the body of an unborn child. Furthermore, tying abortion rights to women's continuing subordination runs the risk that legal access to abortion will be used as a substitute for social reform, thus diminishing women's overall autonomy. They also point out that the father has, or should have, rights and responsibilities. Placing childbearing decisions entirely in the hands of women can further burden women by taking parental responsibility out of the hands of fathers, thereby allowing men to abdicate their responsibility as parents. In light of this, it should come as no surprise that many polls show men to be more in favor of legalized abortion-on-demand than women.[47]

On the other hand, an unwanted pregnancy can deprive a woman of the ability to participate fully in society. She, not the father of the child, must carry the pregnancy to term. Is it fair for an individual woman's autonomy to be restricted when it comes to her own body and childbearing decisions because of wider social concerns or problems that other women may encounter?

Abortion as a Welfare Right

Legal scholars generally agree that *Roe v. Wade* grants women a negative, or liberty, right to abortion—that is, a right to seek an abortion without interference from the state. However, it does not provide a welfare right to abortion. The state does not have to pay for abortions or provide access to abortion facilities.

Some people argue that abortion should also be a welfare right because abortion is a public health issue rather than simply a private choice.[48] Restrictive abortion laws, lack of money to pay for an abortion, and unavailability of a clinic in one's area contribute to situations in which some women do not have equal access to abortion and hence lack genuine choice. Lack of access, they point out, has the greatest impact on poor women and women of color.

However, people at the bottom of the socioeconomic ladder are those most often opposed to legalized abortion. Some African Americans regard abortion as genocide, especially in light of affluent libertarians' eagerness to make abortion services more available and free for people who cannot afford to pay for the services. They fear that abortion rights are being offered as a substitute for racial equality.

In contrast to the rights-based framework in which the abortion debate is typically cast in the United States, in many countries the primary issue is the consequences of prohibiting or permitting abortion. The high maternal death rate due to illegal abortions, overpopulation, the burden on women of mandatory motherhood, and the burden on society when unwanted children are neglected and abandoned are often cited in favor of liberalized abortion laws. On the other hand, studies suggest that permissive abortion policies may be contributing to an increase in child abuse and that we need to consider the possible harmful consequences of abortion on children.[49]

Severance Rights and the Principle of Double Effect

According to most abortion rights advocates, a woman has a **severance right** to terminate her pregnancy by disconnecting the fetus. However, this right does not grant her the right to ensure the death of her fetus. Thomson's violinist analogy is an example of severance theory. Under the usual definition of abortion, the intention is to terminate the pregnancy rather than to cause the death of the fetus. Abortion is not murder because the death of the fetus is an unintended, and unavoidable, side effect of abortion. It is simply bad luck that the fetus is attached to a woman. However, if a woman can end her pregnancy without killing the fetus, then she ought to do so.

According to the **principle of double effect,** "where some course of action is likely to have two quite different effects, one licit or mandatory and the other illicit, it may be permissible to take that course intending the one but not the other."[50] An example of this principle is the use of morphine to relieve pain in a terminally ill patient knowing that it might also shorten the life of the patient. The use of morphine is not usually considered a form of euthanasia, since the intended effect is to relieve pain, not kill the patient.

In Roman Catholic teaching, the principle of double effect permits therapeutic abortion for tubal pregnancies and invasive cancer of the cervix. In both instances, the intent is to save the life of the mother; fetal death is clearly unintended. Libertarians take the principle even further. They argue that in elective abortion the woman does not intend to kill the fetus, but only to rid herself of the pregnancy. The death of the fetus is an unfortunate consequence of the primary intention.

This argument, however, leaves open the question of the morality of abortions in cases where the death of the fetus is intended. In both selective abortion and partial-birth abortion, the intention is not only to terminate the pregnancy, but also to kill the

ZAMBIA:
Resorting to Illegal Abortions

Legalizing abortion is not sufficient to ensure that women will have access to legal abortion. Despite the fact that Zambia has one of the most liberal abortion laws in sub-Saharan Africa, most women still resort to dangerous, illegal abortions. For every legal abortion, there are about twenty-five incomplete abortions that require medical treatment. In 1988, 15 percent of all maternal deaths resulted from illegal abortions. More than half the deaths were schoolgirls.[51]

Why do women in Zambia resort to illegal abortions when legal abortion is available? The 1972 Abortion Act states that abortion must be performed in a hospital and that three physicians must sign the consent form. However, most women live far from a hospital. The cost of a hospital abortion is also exorbitant—more than the monthly salary of an average government worker. In addition, many physicians, for moral or religious reasons, refuse to perform abortions.

There are also social reasons why so many Zambian women resort to illegal abortions. Girls are expected to be virgins at the time of marriage; however, this expectation is not consistent with reality. About 60 percent of girls in grades 10 to 12 have had sex. Their partners are not schoolboys but businessmen, teachers, drivers, and other men who provide them with money, rides, and higher grades in school in exchange for sexual favors. Girls may engage in risky behavior because of their dependence on these men. Schools are unsympathetic to the girls' plight, and it is customary to expel pregnant girls. Some schools even perform pregnancy tests on students. About one in four girls who enter grade 8 drops out because of pregnancy before grade 12. Most schoolgirls who suspect they may be pregnant attempt an abortion before they are found out. Because of the stigma surrounding abortion, about one-third attempt a self-abortion on their own in secret. One-quarter of attempted abortions are unsuccessful and result in a live birth. Many more result in complications that require medical treatment.

Furthermore, most girls and young women are poorly informed about sexuality. Only 14 percent of women report using contraception. Schools do not have sexual education programs, and parents traditionally do not discuss sex with their children because to do so is considered insulting. Girls who are pregnant generally refrain from informing their parents because of fear. In areas of Zambia where there is a bride-price, a woman with a child fetches a lower price and is referred to as "cheap second-hand."[52]

Thus, enhancing a woman's autonomy is not simply a matter of liberalizing abortion laws. Social factors, combined with lack of access to medical care and information, can restrict a woman's reproductive choices and access to legal abortion.

fetus. Are these types of abortion morally justified? The next sections address this question.

SELECTIVE ABORTION[53]

As the rain pounds down on the rice paddies surrounding their village, a small group of barefoot peasants—pregnant women and their husbands—wait in line for ultrasounds. One of the men, Y. H. Chen, explains in a tone of awe, "Last year we had only one girl born in the village—everyone else had boys." Although it is illegal in China for doctors to tell parents the gender of their fetus, doctors will usually bend the rules for a carton of cigarettes or a monetary bribe. "Then if it's a girl," Chen says, "you get an abortion."[54]

Unlike in elective abortion, in which the pregnancy is unwanted, in selective abortion the particular fetus is unwanted. The Chens want the pregnancy, but only if the fetus is a male. What are the limits, if any, of parental autonomy? Does the right to have an abortion also give women a moral right to target a particular fetus for destruction?

Sex Selection

In many cultures, there is a preference for sons as first-born and only children, and selective abortion is used to dispose of unwanted female fetuses. Approval of abortion for sex selection is highest in the United States, India, and China. In the United States, approval is based primarily on respect for parental autonomy. In India and China, social considerations such as the mistreatment of unwanted girls, discrimination against women, and population control are more often given as reasons for support of selective abortion.

The gender of a child is determined by the father's sperm. Women have two X chromosomes; men have one X and one Y chromosome. Since Y chromosomes have only 29 genes, compared to 433 for an X chromosome, sperm carrying the male XY chromosome pair are lighter and travel faster. Consequently, more males are conceived. At birth, the ratio of males to females, based on chance alone, is 105:100.

Prenatal diagnosis provides direct information about the gender of the fetus and the presence of certain genetic and chromosomal disorders. Prenatal diagnosis using amniocentesis is generally performed during the second trimester. However, a new method known as chorionic villus sampling (CVS) can be carried out as early as eight or ten weeks' gestation. Innovations such as sophisticated three-dimensional ultrasound equipment, which makes it possible to detect most fetal abnormalities during the first trimester, should become more widely available in the early 2000s.[55] The greater social acceptability and privacy of first-trimester abortion, however, may lead to an increase in abortion for sex selection and minor defects. A study of 2,278 American women who had had CVS found that CVS was being used more often than amniocentesis for sex selection.[56]

Sex selection can also, at least theoretically, be carried out prior to conception. In September 1998, researchers at the Genetics and IVF Institute in Virginia announced that they had developed a technique that will allow parents to choose the sex of their future children prior to conception. This technique sorts the prospective father's sperm into "girl sperm" and "boy sperm." The sperm of the desired gender are then

INDIA, CHINA, AND THE UNITED STATES:
Selective Abortion and Public Opinion

Cultural relativists assume that there is agreement on moral norms within a culture. However, there can be a wide discrepancy between public opinion, medical opinion, and what is legal in a particular situation. In northern India and China, the birth of a female is often regarded as a great tragedy. Many women undergo amniocentesis or ultrasound to determine the gender of their fetus.

In China, there is general agreement that selective abortion of females is morally acceptable. Given its one-child policy and limited economic opportunities for women, almost all parents in China want a son because of the greater financial security and status associated with having a son. Because they can, at least officially, have only one child, Chinese parents will often abort a female fetus in hopes of later having a son.

While the Chinese government encourages selective abortion as a means of birth control, the Indian government is generally opposed to abortion for sex selection. However, opposition to sex selection is not universally shared in India, especially among physicians and prospective parents. Until 1983, when prenatal diagnosis for sex selection was banned in government hospitals, sex selection accounted for the majority of prenatal diagnoses in Bombay.

Despite the legal restrictions placed on sex selection in parts of India, it continues to be a common practice in India as in China. In areas of India and China where sex selection is widely practiced, the ratio of boys to girls is as high as $120 : 100$.[57]

In the United States, on the other hand, the selective abortion of females is legal, yet the majority of Americans consider amniocentesis for sex selection to be immoral.[58] Although health-care ethicists Dorothy Wertz and John Fletcher, in their reading at the end of this chapter, maintain that sex selection is not a problem in the United States, in fact the newborn gender ratio in the United States is also skewed toward males. Between 1980 and 1992, it remained relatively stable at about 110 boys born for every 100 girls.[59]

Although most Americans have misgivings about using abortion for sex selection, they generally have few qualms about using amniocentesis to detect Down syndrome or spina bifida in fetuses so that they can be aborted. The majority of American geneticists, as well as Indian physicians, believe that selective abortion should be permitted for both sex selection and genetic disorders.[60]

used to impregnate the woman. While this new technique overcomes objections regarding the use of abortion for sex selection, it does not resolve the problem of sex discrimination.

Genetic Disorders

About 7 percent of infants are born with physical and/or mental disorders of varying degrees of severity. Many disorders can be detected using prenatal diagnosis. The overwhelming majority of pregnancies in the United States in which the fetus is diagnosed as having a genetic disorder are terminated by selective abortion. Indeed, most Americans who take a moderate position on abortion believe that the moral justification for the abortion of a fetus with a genetic disorder overrides the prohibition against taking the life of a fetus.

The belief that a genetic disorder justifies abortion is not shared worldwide, particularly in countries where socialized medicine removes the burden on the family of the high costs often associated with a genetic disorder. A 1998 study of British students, for example, found that three-quarters disapproved of abortion on the grounds that the fetus had a deformity.[61] Prenatal diagnosis is also rarely used in African countries, either for sex selection or for genetic disorders. African cultures generally have more tolerance for people with disabilities.

Justice and Discrimination

The principle of nondiscrimination states that humans should not be denied benefits or equal treatment for morally irrelevant reasons, such as sex, skin color, or physical ability. Does selective abortion discriminate against females, people with disabilities, and other "socially unacceptable" people? Dorothy Wertz and John Fletcher answer yes in their article, but only in the case of sex selection given the negative societal effects of gender discrimination. Selective abortion for genetic disorders, they argue, does not encourage discrimination since society tends to view older people with disabilities differently than children born with disabilities. Their optimism is not shared by many members of the "disability community," who claim that selective abortion reinforces negative stereotypes and discrimination against people with disabilities.

One argument used for sex selection is the desire to balance the family. Selective abortion to achieve this goal does not constitute gender bias, it is argued, because the goal is not to destroy girls but to have a balanced number of girls and boys in a family. However, the ideal "balanced" two-child family, at least in the United States, is a boy first and then a girl.[62] Some parents may use selective abortion to achieve this ideal. With prenatal sex selection, this ideal will be even easier to achieve. Given the characteristics of older and younger children, this practice could further exacerbate sexism and the stereotype of the male as having the dominant, leadership role.

Quality of Life

The quality-of-life argument states that selective abortion in the case of fetal abnormalities can, and in some cases ought to, be done for the sake of the fetus. This argument developed primarily in the debate over the euthanasia of newborns with genetic disorders, rather than in the context of selective abortion. Unlike libertarian arguments, which focus on maternal autonomy, the quality-of-life argument focuses on the principle of nonmaleficence and the best interests of the fetus. According to this argument, life is a relative good and is precious only conditionally, based on other values. Therefore, the duty to preserve life is a limited one. The normal conceptual connection between *life* and *good* is shattered in the presence of a profoundly damaged fetus or child. A severe genetic disorder creates so much suffering and hardship that it threatens the very possibility of a meaningful life and meaningful human relationships.

When the good of the fetus is the primary concern, selective abortion is sometimes referred to as *therapeutic abortion* or *fetal euthanasia*.[63] Abortion becomes a type of preventive medicine performed to spare a fetus the greater harm of a life of meaningless suffering. This argument is most compelling in cases in which a disorder is incompatible with life outside the womb—such as **anencephaly,** in which the fetus has no brain, and serious chromosomal disorders such as Patua syndrome and Edward's syndrome, which are associated with severe congenital anomalies such as microcephaly (an abnormally small head), heart and kidney disease, facial and limb deformities, and extreme retardation—and in which, with a few exceptions, death results in the first months of life.

Some ethicists take the quality-of-life argument even further, arguing that it is not merely preferable that such a fetus not be born but "wrong to [knowingly] cause a person to be born" under such circumstances. According to the concept of "wrongful birth," parents who knowingly give birth to a child with severe genetic disorders are morally liable for the pain and suffering of their child."[64] In *Curlender v. Bio-Science Laboratories* (1980), a California court concluded that a child with a genetic disorder could bring a suit against her parents for not undergoing prenatal diagnosis and aborting her.[65]

Opponents of the quality-of-life argument maintain that it is based on a misuse of the principle of nonmaleficence. They point out that in healthcare the principle of "do no harm" focuses on the person, not the condition. Selective abortion, however, in order to eliminate the condition, eliminates those who suffer or might suffer in the future. In no other disease does preventive medicine consist of eliminating, without his or her consent, the patient at risk.

Another problem is assessing quality of life. How are we to calculate future suffering, especially when the early prognosis for most genetic disorders is notoriously unreliable? A fetus diagnosed with Down syndrome or spina bifida, for example, may live a relatively normal life or may be severely retarded and/or paralyzed. The quality-of-life argument can also be used to justify selective abortion of females in countries where the life of an unwanted daughter can involve suffering and neglect and even early death.[66]

In addition, the widespread belief that a person with a genetic disorder would rather not have been born has not been shown to be true. According to French geneticist Jerome Lejeune, while the majority of patients with a severe genetic disorder (if they can express their feelings) regret the affliction, they "do not regret being themselves and being alive."[67] A study in the United States of 222 successive suicides found that people with genetic disorders are much less likely to commit suicide than people without such disabilities. The only exception to this finding are people with Huntington's disease, a genetic disorder that does not generally manifest itself until the person is middle-aged.[68] Also, this study did not include, for obvious reasons, infants whose genetic disorders were incompatible with life.

We must therefore ask what constitutes a genetic disorder that is incompatible with a meaningful life, in particular with regard to those not fatal at or shortly after birth. Physicians and other healthcare professionals tend to define a meaningful life according to their own achievement-oriented standards. While life for a person with a severe genetic disorder might be viewed by a nondisabled person as being burdensomely boring or meaningless because of the limitations it imposes on that person, this does not mean it is meaningless for the person with the disorder. On the other hand, caring for a child with a severe genetic disorder can place tremendous stress on a family, both financially and emotionally, and in many cases can lead to the breakdown of the family.

It may not be long before prenatal diagnosis is available for identifying tendencies toward homosexuality, obesity, depression, cancer, and alcoholism.[69] Are these predispositions also incompatible with a meaningful life in a society that discriminates against people with these characteristics? Where should we draw the line? Healthcare ethicist John Fletcher once warned, "Whenever a strong group argues on behalf of a weaker group that their removal would be better than their survival, we should not be duly impressed."[70]

MATERNAL-FETAL CONFLICTS

When twenty-three-year-old Jennifer Johnson arrived to give birth to her fourth child, hospital drug tests found traces of cocaine in her blood. It was later revealed that her other children had all been "cocaine-affected" babies. In 1989, Johnson was arrested in a crack house. A Florida judge found her guilty of delivery (through the umbilical cord) of a controlled substance to a child. The judge ruled that "a child has a right to begin life with a sound mind and a sound body." He also noted that there is no fundamental right or liberty right to use psychoactive drugs; the fact that a woman is pregnant does not give her a right that other people lack. Johnson was sentenced to fifteen years' probation, drug treatment, random drug testing, and educational and vocational training. She was also ordered to participate in an intensive prenatal care program if she should become pregnant again.[71] The decision was overturned by the Florida Supreme Court in *Johnson v. State* (1992).

Most pregnant women who are planning to carry their pregnancy to term willingly adjust their behavior to protect their fetus. But what if a woman acts in ways that harm her fetus? If children have a right to be well born, as some ethicists claim, does this right confer the duty on mothers to not engage in behavior that will cause the fetus serious harm?

Prenatal Drug and Alcohol Use

A 1988 survey of hospitals in the United States found that as many as 375,000 infants are adversely affected every year by maternal drug use. In some hospitals, almost half of all newborns have been exposed to drugs in the womb. Also, despite warnings from the surgeon general, the number of pregnant women drinking at levels that put the fetus at risk increased between 1990 and 1995.[72] Up to five thousand babies a year are born with fetal alcohol syndrome (FAS), currently one of the leading causes of mental retardation. FAS is also associated with other physical and mental birth defects, including facial deformities, heart defects, seizures, unusually short stature, learning disabilities, and behavioral problems.

The human costs in terms of pain, suffering, and death due to maternal drug and alcohol use are incalculable. The cost of medical treatment for a baby exposed to drugs can run as high as $150,000.[73] This cost has grown enormously as more and more hospitals struggle with the problem of "boarder babies," crack-cocaine babies who are addicted because of their mother's drug use and who are abandoned by their mother after birth. In addition, it is estimated that the annual nationwide medical costs associated with fetal alcohol syndrome are about $300 million.[74]. The increasing number of children with fetal alcohol syndrome and problems stemming from maternal drug use is also putting a strain on the public education system.

In response, several states have passed civil child abuse and neglect laws under which illicit drug or alcohol use during pregnancy constitutes child abuse. Although criminal prosecution on these grounds has been largely unsuccessful, thousands of women have lost custody of their children because of prenatal drug abuse.[75] Some drug-addicted pregnant women have even been jailed because they would not stop using illegal drugs. Since 1989, South Carolina has convicted hundreds of pregnant women who use crack cocaine or other illegal drugs under the child abuse law. Cornelia Whitner, who is currently serving a jail sentence for using crack during her pregnancy, brought a case against the state charging that the law was unconstitutional. In 1999, the U.S. Supreme Court declined to hear the case of *Whitner v. South Carolina.*

Should women such as Johnson and Whitner be held liable for harm done to their fetuses because of maternal use of drugs, tobacco, and alcohol? Is paternalistic interference justified in such cases, or does a woman's autonomy override any rights the fetus may have now or in the future? How should maternal autonomy be balanced against the economic costs to society and the suffering that result from prenatal drug use?

Those who believe that the fetus has all the rights of a born child regard maternal drug use as similar to parents' giving their young children harmful drugs. Even if the fetus is not a person, it does not follow that the woman is free to engage in behavior that will irrevocably harm the fetus if she is planning to carry the pregnancy to term, because her behavior will harm the future born child.

Many libertarians disagree. According to them, a pregnant woman's right to privacy is absolute. What she does to her body during pregnancy is her own business. Hospitals that routinely perform drug tests on any pregnant woman suspected of being a drug user are violating the privacy rights of these women. Furthermore, it is argued, holding women legally liable for prenatal behavior that might harm the fetus stems from the mistaken "image of the fetus as separate from the mother-to-be" and from a patriarchal world-view in which women are reduced to "passive receptacle[s] in reproduction."[76]

The above line of reasoning puts us in the strange predicament of viewing the fetus or unborn child as separate from the born child. However, physically at least, the fetus and the born child are one and the same being; thus, harm to the fetus is harm to the child. Consequently, many healthcare ethicists maintain that the intention to carry a pregnancy to term rather than have an abortion entails the moral obligation to protect the fetus from risk of substantial harm. Children have a right to be protected from harm whether that harm be inflicted prenatally or after birth. Even though it may be difficult, pregnant women who have drug or alcohol problems have a duty of nonmaleficence to their unborn child. What if a woman is too weak-willed to change her behavior or is disinterested in the welfare of her unborn child? Should she be legally penalized or forced into treatment? Unlike child abuse after birth, when the woman who wishes to use drugs can remove herself from the child, drug use prior to birth involves the woman's body in protection of the child.

Most people agree that it is morally wrong for pregnant women to use drugs, but some of these same people also maintain that the use of criminal and civil prosecution to punish these women is counterproductive. Some utilitarians, while acknowledging that the suffering caused by maternal drug use is a moral evil, nevertheless oppose holding mothers legally responsible for prenatal behavior. Punishing pregnant drug users, they argue, will not change their behavior or help babies. Many of these women, like Johnson, come from families with a long history of drug and alcohol abuse, as well as sexual abuse and domestic violence. Instead of suffering punishment, they need to be empowered through counseling, low-cost housing, and residential treatment facilities.

The Fetus as Patient

Maternal-fetal conflicts may occur despite the woman's most conscientious efforts. The development of new fetal therapies and surgeries raises new issues, since the only way to treat the fetal patient is through the woman's body. While the great majority of mothers want what is best for their fetus and are willing to cooperate with therapeutic interventions on behalf of their fetus, this is not always the case. A woman may refuse to cooperate out of concern for her own health, for religious reasons, or because she believes that the physician's prognosis doesn't warrant surgical intervention.

Courts in the United States are increasingly willing to impose a duty of care on pregnant women to undergo medical procedures for the benefit of their fetuses. Appeals courts in both New Jersey and Georgia have overridden religious objections on the part of pregnant women and authorized forced blood transfusions for fetuses. In Illinois, a court appointed a temporary guardian for the fetus of a woman who refused a blood transfusion. As fetal surgery becomes more practical, more pregnant women may be required to submit to surgery for the sake of the fetus. The future possibility of surgically removing a fetus from the woman and continuing the gestation process outside the womb under medical supervision (ectogenesis) may also increase the pressure on women to undergo cesareans to rescue a distressed fetus or, in the case of selective abortion, a fetus that is unwanted by the mother.

Should a woman be forced to submit to therapeutic intervention on behalf of her fetus? Frank Chervenak and Laurence McCullough, in their reading at the end of this chapter, argue that paternalism based on beneficence may override a woman's refusal of medical intervention in cases in which a cesarean will in all likelihood benefit both the fetus and the woman. If persuasion fails, they suggest that a more coercive approach, such as a court order, may be morally justified. What constitutes sufficient reason to resort to legal coercion? Most healthcare ethicists maintain that the duty of care has limits. For instance, a woman does not have a moral obligation to risk her own life and health for the sake of the health of her fetus.

Libertarians such as Mary Anne Warren argue that women *never* have a moral obligation to submit to medical intervention to benefit their fetus. Even though we may think poorly of a woman who is unwilling to cooperate, especially if it is for a trivial reason such as not wanting a scar from a cesarean section, to compel her to "do the right thing" is morally wrong. We cannot use the body of one person to save another.

Will ectogenesis render the abortion debate passé? Probably not. The question of whether a woman has a right to a dead fetus or only a right to end her pregnancy is most poignant in the debate on partial-birth abortion, which involves the death of a fetus that in most cases could survive outside the womb with the assistance of technology.

PARTIAL-BIRTH ABORTION[77]

The family immigrated from India to a suburb of Detroit, Michigan, in 1997 and moved into a two-bedroom apartment, where the sixteen-year-old son and eleven-year-old daughter shared a bedroom. The following spring, the girl, now twelve, began complaining of abdominal pains. At first her physician passed them off as digestion problems. However, the pains were not in her stomach; instead, it turned out she was twenty-seven weeks pregnant. Furthermore, the father of the baby was the girl's brother. The family requested an abortion. After an anguished court battle, the girl finally obtained a partial-birth abortion at a Wichita clinic, even though Kansas bans the procedure.

An ultrasound in Vikki Stella's thirty-second week of pregnancy revealed that something was very wrong with her baby. More tests revealed that the fetus had several abnormalities, including a fluid-filled cranium with no brain tissue at all. Since she was a diabetic, Stella's pregnancy put a strain on her health, and she did not wish to continue carrying a fetus with no chance of survival after birth. She too had a partial-birth abortion.

The Procedure

According to Ron Fitzsimmons, head of the National Coalition of Abortion Providers, about 3,000 to 5,000 partial-birth abortions are performed annually.[78] Dr. Martin Haskell, who has performed over 1,000 partial-birth abortions, indicated in 1995 testimony before the U.S. Senate Judiciary Committee that about 80 percent of partial-birth abortions are purely elective and are performed on a healthy woman with a healthy fetus.

In 1997, the AMA issued a report disapproving of third-trimester abortions even in the case of life-threatening fetal abnormalities or danger to the health or life of the mother. The procedure, it was argued, results in a painful death for the baby and can pose a serious threat to the woman's health and future fertility.[79]

According to the American College of Obstetricians and Gynecologists (ACOG), after viability, partial-birth abortion is rarely if ever necessary to save the health and life of the mother. Nevertheless, unlike the AMA, it opposes a ban on the procedure, arguing that the decision regarding a third-trimester abortion should be made within the context of the patient/physician relationship, not by legislators.

In recent years, more than half of the states in the United States have passed laws banning partial-birth abortions. In June 1995, a bill (HR 1833) was introduced in Congress to ban partial-birth abortions throughout the United States. Both the Senate and the House of Representatives passed the bill; however, it was vetoed by President Clinton. The bill was revised and passed again by Congress. In October 1997, President Clinton vetoed the revised bill.

Abortion or Infanticide?

Because the fetus is viable in the majority of cases and the pregnancy could just as easily be ended by induced labor, some ethicists consider partial-birth abortion infanticide, or at least well down the slippery slope toward infanticide. The partially born child, they maintain, is a person. This view is consistent with a California Supreme Court ruling that stated that "a viable fetus 'in the process of being born' is a human being within the meaning of the homicide statutes."[80] The U.S. Supreme Court, in *Planned Parenthood v. Casey* (1992), also ruled that a woman who carries a pregnancy to viability and gives birth to most of the baby consents to state intervention to protect the child.[81]

Opponents of the procedure argue that the right to an abortion provides only for the termination of a pregnancy, not for a dead child. Abortion is a right because of the burden of being pregnant, not because having a living child is a burden (since adoption is an option after birth). The most a woman can claim is a severance right, that is, the right to be freed from the excessive burdens of pregnancy, not a right to have someone else kill her child. After viability, a woman can be freed of the burden of pregnancy without the death of the child.

Supporters of partial-birth abortion claim that the child enters the realm of personhood only when the head of the fetus crosses the magical border—set at the birth canal. And even if the fetus is a person, a woman's autonomy rights override any rights that even a viable fetus may have. Other supporters, such as Warren, claim that neither the viable fetus nor for the newborn meets the criteria for personhood. Dr. James McMahon, who performed thousands of partial-birth abortions and whose statement in a 1993 edition of *American Medical News* set off the conflict, explained how he justifies the procedure:

> After 20 weeks where it frankly is a child to me, I really agonize over it because the potential is so imminently there. I think, gee, it's too bad that this child couldn't be adopted. On the other hand I have another position, which I think is superior in the hierarchy of questions, and that is: Who owns the child? It's got to be the mother.[82]

McMahon's justification of partial-birth abortion on the grounds that the mother "owns the child" is also reflected in a 1995 study that found that most women who support abortion rights are opposed to adoption and ectogenesis as a solution to unwanted pregnancies. Participants in the study felt that any fetus they create is theirs and it would be irresponsible of them to bring into the world a child they are not willing to raise. The most moral solution in order for them to be absolved of this burden is to terminate the life of the fetus.[83]

Late Abortions, Adolescents, and Incest

Many late abortions are performed on youngsters who do not recognize the signs of pregnancy until they are well into the second trimester. Can a twelve-year-old, such as the daughter in the case described above, give informed consent to an abortion? Families often put pressure on a pregnant youngster to have an abortion because of the disgrace associated with it and the frustration of seeing a daughter's future restricted by having to care for a child. Is the fact that the pregnancy came about as the result of incest or rape morally relevant? Pro-choice advocates argue that, in this case, the girl's well-being and the reported incest outweigh moral arguments against partial-birth abortion. To further burden pregnant minors and rape victims with the stigma of an unwanted pregnancy is unjust.

Abolitionists, in contrast, argue that the circumstances of the conception are irrelevant to the moral value of the fetus and the immorality of abortion. In addition, they maintain that the girl's well-being would have been served best by delivering the fetus, which was viable, and putting the baby up for adoption.

ABORTION AND HEALTHCARE PROFESSIONALS

Abortion raises several moral issues for healthcare professionals. What if a healthcare provider is morally opposed to abortion? Should a nurse who is opposed to abortion refuse to tend to women in a recovery room following an abortion? Should a pro-life physician continue to work in a hospital that performs abortions? Should physicians, even if they support abortion rights, perform nontherapeutic abortions at all?

Physicians' Rights and Autonomy

Obstetricians and gynecologists are deeply divided over abortion. A 1995 survey found that the proportion of Ob/Gyn residency programs in the United States that routinely teach first-trimester abortion procedures dropped from 23 percent in 1985 to 12 percent in 1992.[84] A growing number of medical students are opposed to abortion. As medical student Ashley Ferdinanes explains, "When medical students learn about the development of the embryo, they don't want to commit themselves to taking life."[85] Residents who were strong supporters of *Roe v. Wade* in the 1970s are now older; currently, more than half of all abortion providers are over fifty.

Should respect for autonomy encompass respecting healthcare professionals' moral objections to abortion? Thirty-one states in the United States allow physicians to refuse to participate in abortions. However, in all but seven states, the physician is required to either counsel a patient seeking an abortion or refer her to someone who will perform the abortion. British medical ethics recognizes physicians' and nurses' right to conscientious objection and to refuse to perform an abortion. However, they are expected to advise their patients as to where they can seek assistance. Healthcare professionals are thus compelled to be indirectly complicit in an activity they find immoral.

Some abortion rights advocates maintain that doctors who can't or won't "provide the full range of Ob/Gyn service,"[86] including abortions, should not be permitted to be Ob/Gyns. In response, the Council on Resident Education in Obstetrics and Gynecology (CREOG) has recommended that training in abortion services be required in all accredited Ob/Gyn programs. However, because conscience clauses protect physicians from having to perform procedures that violate their moral principles, abortion training has remained an elective program. Abortion rights advocates fear that the number of providers will dwindle even further if training is not mandatory.

Even if a healthcare professional believes that a woman has a right to an abortion, is performing nontherapeutic abortions a suitable activity for physicians? Is it consistent with the ethics of healing? After all, physicians are supposed to be healers, not judges of quality of life or technicians whose job is to facilitate the nonmedical goals of some patients. Because of the nontherapeutic nature of elective abortions, some healthcare ethicists suggest that elective abortions be carried out by a separate group of professionals who make no pretense of being healers.[87] Indeed, some abortion advocates and women's clinics would like to remove the control of abortion from the hands of physicians and give more control to women trained in the procedure.

Violence Against Abortion Providers

The autonomy of physicians who perform abortions may be compromised by fear of violence. In several countries, such as the United States, Canada, and Britain, antiabortion protesters gather outside abortion clinics to publicize their cause and to try to dissuade women from having abortions. Others carry their protest even further by resorting to violence. The decline in the number of physicians willing to perform abortions has been, in part, a response to this violence.

Violence aimed at clinics where abortions are performed has occurred in at least twenty-eight states. Between 1977 and 1991, over a hundred abortion clinics in the United States were burned or bombed.[88] During 1995 and 1996, abortion-related crime at abortion clinics declined somewhat, only to rise again in 1997. During 1997 alone, there were six bombings, sixty-five acts of vandalism, and sixty-two cases of stalking.[89] In Florida, protesters reportedly threw acid at the facilities and the workers. Three abortion doctors were killed in the United States between 1993 and 1998, and many more were wounded. In April 1998, a U.S. district court ruled that antiabortion protesters violated federal racketeering laws.

Fetal Tissue Transplants (FTT)

The use of fetal tissue transplants (FTT) as a treatment for devastating neurological disorders such as Parkinson's disease is still in the experimental stage.[90] The fetal tissue for transplants comes primarily from aborted fetuses. Should physicians and researchers use tissue obtained from aborted fetuses?

Those who believe that the fetus is the property of the woman argue that a woman has the right to dispose of the fetal tissue as she wishes, including giving consent for the tissue of her aborted fetus to be used for FTT. Others fear that participation in FTT makes the researchers complicit in the abortion. The National Institutes of Health (NIH) disagrees, maintaining that abortion and the harvesting of fetal tissue are two distinct acts and that FTT does not imply acceptance of elective abortion. The NIH points out that the use of organs from the victim of a drunk-driving accident does not imply complicity in or approval of the act of drunk driving.

Some healthcare ethicists fear that the possibility of FTT may act as an incentive for women to have abortions, especially if it involves profit or if the tissue will be used to save the life of a loved one. Women who have mixed feelings about having an abortion may be swayed to have one by the thought that at least some good will come out of it. They may also be encouraged to time the abortion to ensure that the desired fetal tissue is at the optimal stage of development. For these reasons, some people believe that only tissue from spontaneous abortions or miscarriages, and not fetal tissue from elective abortions, should be used in FTT.

CAN THE ABORTION CONTROVERSY EVER BE RESOLVED?

As members of a pluralistic society, can we ever arrive at a resolution to the current abortion debate? Should we even bother to try? Perhaps we should just be tolerant of other people's views: "If you don't believe in abortion, don't have one." Unfortunately, the hands-off approach doesn't work because those who are opposed to abortion are not merely expressing a personal opinion about abortion but rather are saying that abortion is wrong because it goes against universal moral principles binding on everyone. Furthermore, to claim that we should be tolerant of other people's moral opinions is to advocate tolerance not only of abortion but also of other practices. Few of us would be willing to carry a bumper sticker sporting the slogan "If you don't believe in slavery, don't own slaves." Nor are those who advocate abortion rights claiming that the morality of abortion should be left to personal opinion. Rather, they are arguing that the rights of the woman outweigh the interests and rights, if any, of the fetus and that women's rights should be protected by law.

In most cultures, women's interests are perceived as less important than those of men, including the interest of women to be free from the burden of unwanted childbearing. Resolution of a moral issue such as abortion involves not simply discerning right from wrong, but determining how best to embody moral wisdom in a just public policy. Abortion is a highly political issue that must be examined in the larger societal context, since it occurs within a social context of oppression of women. Concerns about abortion must be balanced against concerns such as equal economic rights for women. As both Confucius and Aristotle taught, good laws and public policy are important because they make it easier for people to be virtuous.

Ethical analysis is not a matter of personal opinion or majority consensus. It should be logical and consistent, as well as universal in its application. Until we can approach the moral issue of abortion rationally, the issue is unlikely to be resolved. The readings at the end of this chapter invite us to rethink the abortion issue with an open and analytical mind.

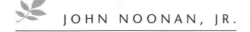

JOHN NOONAN, JR.

An Almost Absolute Value in History

John Noonan is professor of law at the University of California in Berkeley. Like Thomson's article (Chapter 2), his article on abortion, which was published in 1970, remains one of the classics in the abortion debate. Noonan and Thomson both begin with the presumption that the fetus is a person with moral standing. However, unlike Thomson, Noonan draws the conclusion that abortion is rarely, if ever, morally justified. After rejecting the various criteria of personhood used by defenders of abortion, he concludes that anyone conceived by human parents is a person.

. . . The most fundamental question involved in the long history of thought on abortion is: How do you determine the humanity of a being? To phrase the question that way is to put in comprehensive humanistic terms what the theologians either dealt with as an explicitly theological question under the heading of "ensoulment" or dealt with implicitly in their treatment of abortion. The Christian position as it originated did not depend on a narrow theological or philosophical concept. . . . [T]he theological notion of ensoulment could easily be translated into humanistic language by substituting "human" for "rational soul"; the problem of knowing when a man is a man is common to theology and humanism.

If one steps outside the specific categories used by the theologians, the answer they gave can be analyzed as a refusal to discriminate among human beings on the basis of their varying potentialities. Once conceived, the being was recognized as man because he had man's potential. The criterion for humanity, thus, was simple and all-embracing: if you are conceived by human parents, you are human.

The strength of this position may be tested by a review of some of the other distinctions offered in the contemporary controversy over legalizing abortion. Perhaps the most popular distinction is in terms of viability. Before an age of so many months, the fetus is not viable, that is, it cannot be removed from the mother's womb and live apart

from her. To that extent, the life of the fetus is absolutely dependent on the life of the mother. This dependence is made the basis of denying recognition to its humanity.

There are difficulties with this distinction. One is that the perfection of artificial incubation may make the fetus viable at any time: it may be removed and artificially sustained. Experiments with animals already show that such a procedure is possible. This hypothetical extreme case relates to an actual difficulty: there is considerable elasticity to the idea of viability. Mere length of life is not an exact measure. The viability of the fetus depends on the extent of its anatomical and functional development. . . .

The most important objection to this approach is that dependence is not ended by viability. The fetus is still absolutely dependent on someone's care in order to continue existence; indeed a child of one or three or even five years of age is absolutely dependent on another's care for existence; uncared for, the older fetus or the younger child will die as surely as the early fetus detached from the mother. The unsubstantial lessening in dependence at viability does not seem to signify any special acquisition of humanity.

A second distinction has been attempted in terms of experience. A being who has had experience, has lived and suffered, who possesses memories, is more human than one who has not. Humanity depends on formation by experience.

The fetus is thus "unformed" in the most basic human sense.

This distinction is not serviceable for the embryo which is already experiencing and reacting. The embryo is responsive to touch after eight weeks and at least at that point is experiencing. At an earlier stage the zygote is certainly alive and responding to its environment. . . . More fundamentally, this distinction leaves even the older fetus or the younger child to be treated as an unformed inhuman thing. Finally, it is not clear why experience as such confers humanity. It could be argued that certain central experiences such as loving or learning are necessary to make a man human. But then human beings who have failed to love or to learn might be excluded from the class called man.

A third distinction is made by appeal to the sentiments of adults. If a fetus dies, the grief of the parents is not the grief they would have for a living child. The fetus is an unnamed "it" till birth, and is not perceived as personality until at least the fourth month of existence when movements in the womb manifest a vigorous presence demanding joyful recognition by the parents.

Yet feeling is notoriously an unsure guide to the humanity of others. Many groups of humans have had difficulty in feeling that persons of another tongue, color, religion, sex, are as human as they. Apart from reactions to alien groups, we mourn the loss of a ten-year-old boy more than the loss of his one-day-old brother or his 90-year-old grandfather. The difference felt and the grief expressed vary with the potentialities extinguished, or the experience wiped out; they do not seem to point to any substantial difference in the humanity of baby, boy, or grandfather.

Distinctions are also made in terms of sensation by the parents. The embryo is felt within the womb only after about the fourth month. The embryo is seen only at birth. What can be neither seen nor felt is different from what is tangible. If the fetus cannot be seen or touched at all, it cannot be perceived as man.

Yet experience shows that sight is even more untrustworthy than feeling in determining humanity. By sight, color became an appropriate index for saying who was a man, and the evil of racial discrimination was given foundation. Nor can touch provide the test; a being confined by sickness, "out of touch" with others, does not thereby seem to lose his humanity. . . .

Finally, a distinction is sought in social visibility. The fetus is not socially perceived as human. It cannot communicate with others. Thus, both subjectively and objectively, it is not a member of society. As moral rules are rules for the behavior of members of society to each other, they cannot be made for behavior toward what is not yet a member. Excluded from the society of men, the fetus is excluded from the humanity of men.

By force of the argument from the consequences, this distinction is to be rejected. It is more subtle than that founded on an appeal to physical sensation, but it is equally dangerous in its implications. If humanity depends on social recognition, individuals or whole groups may be dehumanized by being denied any status in their society. Such a fate is fictionally portrayed in *1984* and has actually been the lot of many men in many societies. In the Roman empire, for example, condemnation to slavery meant the practical denial of most human rights; in the Chinese Communist world, landlords have been classified as enemies of the people and so treated as nonpersons by the state. Humanity does not depend on social recognition, though often the failure of society to recognize the prisoner, the alien, the heterodox as human has led to the destruction of human beings. Anyone conceived by a man and a woman is human. . . . Any attempt to limit humanity to exclude some group runs the risk of furnishing authority and precedent for excluding other groups in the name of the consciousness or perception of the controlling group in the society.

A philosopher may reject the appeal to the humanity of the fetus because he views "humanity" as a secular view of the soul and because he doubts the existence of anything real and objective which can be identified as humanity. One answer to such a philosopher is to ask how he reasons about moral questions without supposing that there is a sense in which he and the others of whom he speaks are human. Whatever group is taken as the society which determines who may be killed is thereby taken as human. A second answer is to ask if he does not believe that there is a right and wrong way of deciding moral questions. If there is such a difference, experience may be appealed to: to decide who is human on the basis of the sentiment of a given society has led to consequences which rational men would characterize as monstrous.

. . . There is a kind of continuity in all life, but the earlier stages of the elements of human life possess tiny probabilities of development. . . . [O]nce spermatozoon and ovum meet and the conceptus is formed, such studies as have been made show that roughly in only 20 percent of the cases will spontaneous abortion occur. In other words, the chances are about 4 out of 5 that this new being will develop. At this stage in the life of the being there is a sharp shift in probabilities, an immense jump in potentialities. . . .

It may be asked, What does a change in biological probabilities have to do with establishing humanity? The argument from probabilities is not aimed at establishing humanity but at establishing an objective discontinuity which may be taken into account in moral discourse. As life itself is a matter of probabilities, as most moral reasoning is an estimate of probabilities, so it seems in accord with the structure of reality and the nature of moral thought to found a moral judgment on the change in probabilities at conception. The appeal to probabilities is the most commonsensical of arguments; to a greater or smaller degree all of us base our actions on probabilities, and in morals, as in law, prudence and negligence are often measured by the account one has taken of the probabilities. If the chance is 200,000,000 to 1 that the movement in the bushes into which you shoot is a man's, I doubt if many persons would hold you careless in shooting; but if the chances are 4 out of 5 that the movement is a human being's, few would acquit you of blame. Would the argument be different if only one out of ten children conceived came to term? Of course this argument would be different. This argument is an appeal to probabilities that actually exist, not to any and all states of affairs which may be imagined.

The probabilities as they do exist do not show the humanity of the embryo in the sense of a demonstration in logic any more than the probabilities of the movement in the bush being a man demonstrate beyond all doubt that the being is a man. The appeal is a "buttressing" consideration, showing the plausibility of the standard adopted. The argument focuses on the decisional factor in any moral judgment and assumes that part of the business of a moralist is drawing lines. One evidence of the nonarbitrary character of the line drawn is the difference of probabilities on either side of it. If a spermatozoon is destroyed, one destroys a being which had a chance of far less than 1 in 200 million of developing into a reasoning being, possessed of the genetic code, a heart and other organs, and capable of pain. If a fetus is destroyed, one destroys a being already possessed of the genetic code, organs, and sensitivity to pain, and one which had an 80 percent chance of developing further into a baby outside the womb who, in time, would reason.

The positive argument for conception as the decisive moment of humanization is that at conception the new being receives the genetic code. It is this genetic information which determines his characteristics, which is the biological carrier of the possibility of human wisdom, which makes him a self-evolving being. A being with a human genetic code is man. . . .

Even with the fetus weighed as human, one interest could be weighed as equal or superior: that of the mother in her own life. . . . As the balance was once struck in favor of the mother whenever her life was endangered, it could be so struck again. The balance reached between 1895 and 1930 attempted prudentially and pastorally to forestall a multitude of exceptions for interests less than life.

The perception of the humanity of the fetus and the weighing of fetal rights against other human rights constituted the work of the moral analysts. But what spirit animated their abstract judgments? For the Christian community it was the injunction of Scripture to love your neighbor as yourself. The fetus as human was a neighbor; his life had parity with one's own. The commandment gave life to what otherwise would have been only rational calculation.

The commandment could be put in humanistic as well as theological terms: Do not injure your fellow man without reason. In these terms, once the humanity of the fetus is perceived, abortion is never right except in self-defense. When life must be taken to save life, reason alone cannot say that a mother must prefer a child's life to her own. With this exception, now of great rarity, abortion violates the rational humanist tenet of the equality of human lives.

QUESTIONS FOR COMPREHENSION AND REFLECTION

1. Noonan argues that parents' feelings toward their fetus are morally irrelevant. Do you agree with Noonan? Support your answer.
2. According to Noonan, "Anyone conceived by a man and a woman is human [a person]." Do you agree with Noonan? Critically evaluate the premises that Noonan offers in support of this definition of personhood.
3. While Noonan supports the Catholic position on abortion, he points out that this position can be supported on rational philosophical or humanistic premises. Has Noonan done an adequate job in supporting his position on abortion using only philosophical premises? Support your answer.

MARY ANNE WARREN

The Moral Significance of Birth

Mary Anne Warren is professor of philosophy at San Francisco State University. Warren defends a liberal pro-choice position on abortion: Women have a fundamental right to make their own decision about their bodies. After rejecting the traditional criteria of personhood, including that used by Noonan, Warren goes on to argue that personhood does not begin until after birth. Because the fetus is not a person, abortion can be justified under any circumstances. Her definition of *personhood* also permits infanticide under some circumstances.

English common law treats the moment of live birth as the point at which a legal person comes into existence. Although abortion has often been prohibited, it has almost never been classified as homicide. In contrast, infanticide generally is classified as a form of homicide, even where (as in England) there are statutes designed to mitigate the severity of the crime in certain cases. But many people—including some feminists—now favor the extension of equal legal rights to some or all fetuses. The extension of legal personhood to fetuses would not only threaten women's right to choose abortion, but also undermine other fundamental rights. I will argue that because of these dangers, birth remains the most appropriate place to mark the existence of a new legal person. . . .

THE DENIAL OF THE MORAL SIGNIFICANCE OF BIRTH

The view that birth is irrelevant to moral rights is shared by philosophers on all points of the spectrum of moral views about abortion. For the most conservative, birth adds nothing to the infant's moral rights, since all of those rights have been present since conception. Moderates hold that the fetus acquires an equal right to life at some point after conception but before birth. The most popular candidates for this point of moral demarcation are (1) the stage at which the fetus becomes viable (i.e., capable of surviving outside the womb, with or without medical assistance), and (2) the stage at which it becomes sentient (i.e., capable of having experiences, including that of pain). For those who hold a view of this sort, both infanticide and abortion at any time past the critical stage are forms of homicide, and there is little reason to distinguish between them either morally or legally.

Finally, liberals hold that even relatively late abortion is sometimes morally acceptable, and that at no time is abortion the moral equivalent of homicide. However, few liberals wish to hold that infanticide is not—at least sometimes—morally comparable to homicide. Consequently, the presumption that being born makes no difference to one's moral rights creates problems for the liberal view of abortion. Unless the liberal can establish some grounds for a general moral distinction between late abortion and early infanticide, she must either retreat to a moderate position on abortion, or else conclude that infanticide is not so bad after all.

To those who accept the intrinsic-properties assumption, birth can make little difference to the moral standing of the fetus/infant. For birth does not seem to alter any intrinsic property that could reasonably be linked to the possession of a strong right to life. Newborn infants have very nearly the same intrinsic properties as do fetuses shortly before birth. . . .

THE SENTIENCE CRITERION

Both newborn infants and late-term fetuses show clear signs of sentience. For instance, they are apparently capable of having visual experiences. Infants will often turn away from bright lights, and those who have done intrauterine photography have sometimes observed a similar reaction in the late-term fetus when bright lights are introduced in its vicinity. Both may respond to loud noises, voices, or other sounds, so both can probably have auditory experiences. They are evidently also responsive to touch, taste, motion, and other kinds of sensory stimulation.

The sentience of infants and late-term fetuses makes a difference to how they should be treated, by contrast with fertilized ova or first-trimester fetuses. Sentient beings are usually capable of experiencing painful as well as pleasurable or affectively neutral sensations. While the capacity to experience pain is valuable to an organism, pain is by definition an intrinsically unpleasant experience. Thus, sentient beings may plausibly be said to have a moral right not to be deliberately subjected to pain in the absence of any compelling reason. For those who prefer not to speak of rights, it is still plausible that a capacity for sentience gives an entity some moral standing. It may, for instance, require that its interests be given some consideration in utilitarian calculations, or that it be treated as an end and never merely as a means.

But it is not clear that sentience is a sufficient condition for moral equality, since there are many clearly-sentient creatures (e.g., mice) to which most of us would not be prepared to ascribe equal moral standing. . . . [L. W.] Sumner examines the implications of the sentience criterion primarily in the context of abortion. Given his belief that some compromise is essential between the conservative and liberal viewpoints on abortion, the sentience criterion recommends itself as a means of drawing a moral distinction between early abortion and late abortion. It is, in some ways, a more defensible criterion than fetal viability.

The 1973 *Roe v. Wade* decision treats the presumed viability of third-trimester fetuses as a basis for permitting states to restrict abortion rights in order to protect fetal life in the third trimester, but not earlier. Yet viability is relative, among other things, to the medical care available to the pregnant woman and her infant. Increasingly sophisticated neonatal intensive care has made it possible to save many more premature infants than before, thus altering the average age of viability. Someday it may be possible to keep even first-trimester fetuses alive and developing normally outside the womb. The viability criterion seems to imply that the advent of total ectogenesis (artificial gestation from conception to birth) would automatically eliminate women's right to abortion, even in the earliest stages of pregnancy. . . .

. . . At the very least, it must imply that as many aborted fetuses as possible should be kept alive through artificial gestation. But the mere technological possibility of providing artificial wombs for huge numbers of human fetuses could not establish such a moral obligation. A massive commitment to ectogenesis would probably be ruinously expensive, and might prove contrary to the interests of parents and children. The viability criterion forces us to make a hazardous leap from the technologically possible to the morally mandatory.

The sentience criterion at first appears more promising as a means of defending a moderate view of abortion. It provides an intuitively plausible distinction between early and late abortion. Unlike the viability criterion, it is unlikely to be undermined by new biomedical technologies. Further investigation of fetal neurophysiology and behavior might refute the presumption that fetuses begin to be capable of sentience *at some point in the second trimester*. Perhaps this development occurs slightly earlier or slightly later than present evidence suggests. . . .

. . . The strong version of the sentience criterion treats sentience as a sufficient condition for having full and equal moral standing. The weak version treats sentience as sufficient for having some moral standing, but not necessarily full and equal moral standing.

. . . [According to the stronger version] any being which has even minimal capacities for sensory experience is the moral equal of any person. If we accept this theory, then we must conclude that not only is late abortion the moral equivalent of homicide, but so is the killing of such sentient nonhuman beings as mice. . . . [A]ll sentient beings have some moral standing, but beings that are more highly sentient have greater moral standing

than do less highly sentient beings. This weaker version of the sentience criterion leaves room for a distinction between the moral standing of mice and that of sentient humans—provided, that is, that mice can be shown to be less highly sentient. However, it will not support the moral equality of late-term fetuses, since the relatively undeveloped condition of fetal brains almost certainly means that fetuses are less highly sentient than older human beings. . . .

THE SELF-AWARENESS CRITERION

Although newborn infants are regarded as persons in both law and common moral conviction, they lack certain mental capacities that are typical of persons. They have sensory experiences, but . . . they probably do not yet think, or have a sense of who they are, or a desire to continue to exist. It is not unreasonable to suppose that these facts make some difference to their moral standing. Other things being equal, it is surely worse to kill a self-aware being that wants to go on living than one that has never been self-aware and that has no such preference. If this is true, then it is hard to avoid the conclusion that neither abortion nor infanticide is quite as bad as the killing of older human beings. And indeed many human societies seem to have accepted that conclusion. . . .

. . . [I]nfanticide must sometimes have been the most humane resolution of a tragic dilemma. In the absence of effective contraception or abortion, abandoning a newborn can sometimes be the only alternative to the infant's later death from starvation. Women of nomadic gatherer-hunter societies, for instance, are sometimes unable to raise an infant born too soon after the last one, because they can neither nurse nor carry two small children.

But if infanticide is to be considered, it is better that it be done immediately after birth, before the bonds of love and care between the infant and the mother (and other persons) have grown any stronger than they may already be. Postponing the question of the infant's acceptance for weeks or months would be cruel to all concerned. Although an infant may be little more sentient or self-aware at two weeks of age than at birth, its death is apt to be a greater tragedy—not for it, but for those who have come to love it. I suspect that this is why, where infanticide is tolerated, the decision to kill or abandon an infant must usually be made rather quickly. If this consideration is morally relevant—and I think it is—then the self-awareness criterion fails to illuminate some of the morally salient aspects of infanticide.

PROTECTING NONPERSONS

If we are to justify a general moral distinction between abortion and infanticide, we must answer two questions. First, why should infanticide be discouraged, rather than treated as a matter for individual decision? And second, why should sentient fetuses not be given the same protections that law and common sense morality accord to infants? But before turning to these two questions, it is necessary to make a more general point.

Persons have sound reasons for treating one another as moral equals. These reasons derive from both self-interest and altruistic concern for others—which, because of our social nature, are often very difficult to distinguish. Human persons—and perhaps all persons—normally come into existence only in and through social relationships. Sentience may begin to emerge without much direct social interaction, but it is doubtful that a child reared in total isolation from human or other sentient (or apparently sentient) beings could develop the capacities for self-awareness and social interaction that are essential to personhood. The recognition of the fundamentally social nature of persons can only strengthen the case for moral equality, since social relationships are undermined and distorted by inequalities that are perceived as unjust. . . .

. . . [T]o deny that infants have equal basic moral rights is to risk being thought to condone infanticide and the neglect and abuse of infants. Here too, effective communication about human moral responsibilities seems to demand the ascription of rights to beings that lack certain properties that are typical of persons. But, of course, that

does not explain why we have these responsibilities towards infants in the first place.

WHY PROTECT INFANTS?

I have already mentioned some of the reasons for protecting human infants more carefully than we protect most comparably-sentient nonhuman beings. Most people care deeply about infants, particularly—but not exclusively—their own. Normal human adults (and children) are probably "programmed" by their biological nature to respond to human infants with care and concern. For the mother, in particular, that response is apt to begin well before the infant is born. But even for her it is likely to become more intense after the infant's birth. The infant at birth enters the human social world, where, if it lives, it becomes involved in social relationships with others, of kinds that can only be dimly foreshadowed before birth. It begins to be known and cared for, not just as a potential member of the family or community, but as a socially present and responsive individual. . . . The newborn is not yet self-aware, but it is already (rapidly becoming) a social being.

Thus, although the human newborn may have no intrinsic properties that can ground a moral right to life stronger than that of a fetus just before birth, its emergence into the social world makes it appropriate to treat it as if it had such a stronger right. This, in effect, is what the law has done, through the doctrine that a person begins to exist at birth. . . . If the line were not drawn at birth, then I think we would have to draw it at some point rather soon thereafter, as many other societies have done.

Another reason for condemning infanticide is that, at least in relatively privileged nations like our own, infants whose parents cannot raise them can usually be placed with people who will love them and take good care of them. This means that infanticide is rarely in the infant's own best interests, and would often deprive some potential adoptive individual or family of a great benefit. . . .

Some might wonder whether adoption is really preferable to infanticide, at least from the parent's point of view. Judith Thomson notes that, "A woman may be utterly devastated by the thought of a child, a bit of herself, put out for adoption and never seen or heard of again." From the standpoint of narrow self-interest, it might not be irrational to prefer the death of the child to such a future. Yet few would wish to resolve this problem by legalizing infanticide. The evolution of more open adoption procedures which permit more contact between the adopted child and the biological parent(s) might lessen the psychological pain often associated with adoption. But that would be at best a partial solution. More basic is the provision of better social support for child-rearers, so that parents are not forced by economic necessity to surrender their children for adoption. . . .

But have I not left the door open to the claim that infanticide may still be justified in some places, e.g., where there is severe poverty and a lack of accessible adoption agencies or where women face exceptionally harsh penalties for "illegitimate" births? I have, and deliberately. The moral case against the toleration of infanticide is contingent upon the existence of morally preferable options. Where economic hardship, the lack of contraception and abortion, and other forms of sexual and political oppression have eliminated all such options, there will be instances in which infanticide is the least tragic of a tragic set of choices. In such circumstances, the enforcement of extreme sanctions against infanticide can constitute an additional injustice.

WHY BIRTH MATTERS

I have defended what most regard as needing no defense, i.e., the ascription of an equal right to life to human infants. Under reasonably favorable conditions that policy can protect the rights and interests of all concerned, including infants, biological parents, and potential adoptive parents.

But if protecting infants is such a good idea, then why is it not a good idea to extend the same strong protections to sentient fetuses? The question is not whether sentient fetuses ought to be protected: of course they should. Most women readily accept the responsibility for doing whatever

they can to ensure that their (voluntarily continued) pregnancies are successful, and that no avoidable harm comes to the fetus. Negligent or malevolent actions by third parties which result in death or injury to pregnant women or their potential children should be subject to moral censure and legal prosecution. A just and caring society would do much more than ours does to protect the health of all its members, including pregnant women. The question is whether the law should accord to late-term fetuses *exactly the same* protections as are accorded to infants and older human beings.

The case for doing so might seem quite strong. . . .

But there is one crucial consideration which this argument leaves out. It is impossible to treat fetuses *in utero* as if they were persons without treating women as if they were something less than persons. The extension of equal rights to sentient fetuses would inevitably license severe violations of women's basic rights to personal autonomy and physical security. In the first place, it would rule out most second-trimester abortions performed to protect the woman's life or health. Such abortions might sometimes be construed as a form of self-defense. But the right to self-defense is not usually taken to mean that one may kill innocent persons just because their continued existence poses some threat to one's own life or health. If abortion must be justified as self-defense, then it will rarely be performed until the woman is already in extreme danger, and perhaps not even then. Such a policy would cost some women their lives, while others would be subjected to needless suffering and permanent physical harm.

Other alarming consequences of the drive to extend more equal rights to fetuses are already apparent in the United States. In the past decade it has become increasingly common for hospitals or physicians to obtain court orders requiring women in labor to undergo Caesarean sections, against their will, for what is thought to be the good of the fetus. Such an extreme infringement of the woman's right to security against physical assault would be almost unthinkable once the infant has been born. No parent or relative can legally be forced to undergo any surgical procedure, even possibly to save the life of a child, once it is born. But pregnant women can sometimes be forced to undergo major surgery, for the supposed benefit of the fetus. As George Annas points out, forced Caesareans threaten to reduce women to the status of inanimate objects—containers which may be opened at the will of others in order to get at their contents.

Perhaps the most troubling illustration of this trend is the case of Angie Carder, who died at George Washington University Medical Center in June 1987, two days after a court-ordered Caesarean section. Ms. Carder had suffered a recurrence of an earlier cancer, and was not expected to live much longer. Her physicians agreed that the fetus was too undeveloped to be viable, and that Carder herself was probably too weak to survive the surgery. Although she, her family, and the physicians were all opposed to a Caesarean delivery, the hospital administration—evidently believing it had a legal obligation to try to save the fetus—sought and obtained a court order to have it done. As predicted, both Carder and her infant died soon after the operation. This woman's rights to autonomy, physical integrity, and life itself were forfeit—not just because of her illness, but because of her pregnancy.

Such precedents are doubly alarming in the light of the development of new techniques of fetal therapy. As fetuses come to be regarded as patients, with rights that may be in direct conflict with those of their mothers, and as the *in utero* treatment of fetuses becomes more feasible, more and more pregnant women may be subjected against their will to dangerous and invasive medical interventions. If so, then we may be sure that there will be other Angie Carders.

Another danger in extending equal legal protections to sentient fetuses is that women will increasingly be blamed, and sometimes legally prosecuted, when they miscarry or give birth to premature, sick, or abnormal infants. It is reasonable to hold the caretakers of infants legally responsible if their charges are harmed because of their avoidable negligence. But when a woman miscarries or gives birth to an abnormal infant, the cause of the harm might be traced to any of an enormous number of actions or circumstances which would not normally constitute any legal offense. She might have gotten too much exercise or too little, eaten the wrong foods or the wrong quantity of the right ones, or taken or failed to take certain drugs. She might have smoked, consumed alcohol, or gotten too little sleep. She might have "permitted" her health to be damaged by hard work, by unsafe employment conditions, by the lack of affordable medical care, by living near a source of industrial pollution, by a physically or mentally abusive partner, or in any number of other ways.

Are such supposed failures on the part of pregnant women potentially to be construed as child abuse or negligent homicide? If sentient fetuses are entitled to the same legal protections as infants, then it would seem so. The danger is not a merely theoretical one. Two years ago in San Diego, a woman whose son was born with brain damage and died several weeks later was charged with felony child neglect. It was said that she had been advised by her physician to avoid sex and illicit drugs, and to go to the hospital immediately if she noticed any bleeding. Instead, she had allegedly had sex with her husband, taken some inappropriate drug, and delayed getting to the hospital for what might have been several hours after the onset of bleeding.

In this case, the charges were eventually dismissed on the grounds that the child protection law invoked had not been intended to apply to cases of this kind. But the multiplication of such cases is inevitable if the strong legal protections accorded to infants are extended to sentient fetuses. A bill recently introduced in the Australian state of New South Wales would make women liable to criminal prosecution if they are found to have smoked during pregnancy, eaten unhealthful foods, or taken any other action which can be shown to have adversely affected the development of the fetus. Such an approach to the protection of fetuses authorizes the legal regulation of virtually every aspect of women's public and private lives, and thus is incompatible with even the most minimal right to autonomy. Moreover, such laws are apt to prove counterproductive, since the fear of prosecution may deter poor or otherwise vulnerable women from seeking needed medical care during pregnancy. I am not suggesting that women whose apparent negligence causes prenatal harm to their infants should always be immune from criticism. However, if we want to improve the health of infants we would do better to provide the services women need to protect their health, rather than seeking to use the law to punish those whose prenatal care has been less than ideal.

There is yet another problem, which may prove temporary but which remains significant at this time. The extension of legal personhood to sentient fetuses would rule out most abortions performed because of severe fetal abnormalities, such as Down's Syndrome or spina bifida. Abortions performed following amniocentesis are usually done in the latter part of the second trimester, since it is usually not possible to obtain test results earlier. Methods of detecting fetal abnormalities at earlier stages, such as chorion biopsy, may eventually make late abortion for reasons of fetal abnormality unnecessary; but at present the safety of these methods is unproven.

The elimination of most such abortions might be a consequence that could be accepted, were the society willing to provide adequate support for the handicapped children and adults who would come into being as a result of this policy. However, our society is not prepared to do this. In the absence of adequate communally-funded care for the handicapped, the prohibition of such abortions is exploitative of women. Of course, the male relatives of severely handicapped persons may also bear heavy burdens. Yet the heaviest portion of the daily responsibility generally falls upon mothers and other female relatives. If fetuses are not yet persons (and women are), then a respect for the equality of persons should lead to support for the availability of abortion in cases of severe fetal abnormality.

Such arguments will not persuade those who deeply believe that fetuses are already persons, with equal moral rights. How, they will ask, is denying legal equality to sentient fetuses different from denying it to any other powerless group of human beings? If some human beings are more equal than others, then how can any of us feel safe? The answer is twofold.

First, pregnancy is a relationship different from any other, including that between parents and already-born children. It is not just one of innumerable situations in which the rights of one individual may come into conflict with those of another; it is probably the *only* case in which the legal personhood of one human being is necessarily incompatible with that of another. Only in pregnancy is the organic functioning of one human individual biologically inseparable from that of another. This organic unity makes it impossible for others to provide the fetus with medical care or any other presumed benefit, except by doing something to or for the woman. To try to "protect" the fetus other than through her cooperation and consent is effectively to nullify her right to autonomy, and potentially to expose her to violent physical assaults such as would not be legally condoned in any other type of case. The uniqueness of pregnancy helps to explain why the toleration of abortion does not lead to the disenfranchisement of other groups of human beings, as opponents of abortion often claim. . . .

But, granting the uniqueness of pregnancy, why is it *women's* rights that should be privileged? If women and fetuses cannot both be legal persons then why not favor fetuses, e.g., on the grounds that they are more helpless, or more innocent, or have a longer life expectancy? It is difficult to justify this apparent bias towards women without appealing to the empirical fact that women are already persons in the usual, nonlegal sense—already thinking, self-aware, fully social beings—and fetuses are not. Regardless of whether we stress the intrinsic properties of persons, or the social and relational dimensions of personhood, this distinction remains. Even sentient fetuses do not yet have either the cognitive capacities or the richly interactive social involvements typical of persons.

This "not yet" is morally decisive. It is wrong to treat persons as if they do not have equal basic rights. Other things being equal, it is worse to deprive persons of their most basic moral and legal rights than to refrain from extending such rights to beings that are not persons. This is one important element of truth in the self-awareness criterion. If fetuses were already thinking, self-aware, socially responsive members of communities, then nothing could justify refusing them the equal protection of the law. In that case, we would sometimes be forced to balance the rights of the fetus against those of the woman, and sometimes the scales might be almost equally weighted. However, if women are persons and fetuses are not, then the balance must swing towards women's rights.

CONCLUSION

Birth is morally significant because it marks the end of one relationship and the beginning of others. It marks the end of pregnancy, a relationship so intimate that it is impossible to extend the equal protection of the law to fetuses without severely infringing women's most basic rights. Birth also marks the beginning of the infant's existence as a socially responsive member of a human community. Although the infant is not instantly transformed into a person at the moment of birth, it does become a biologically separate human being. As such, it can be known and cared for as a particular individual. It can also be vigorously protected

without negating the basic rights of women. There are circumstances in which infanticide may be the best of a bad set of options. But our own society has both the ability and the desire to protect infants, and there is no reason why we should not do so.

We should not, however, seek to extend the same degree of protection to fetuses. Both late-term fetuses and newborn infants are probably capable of sentience. Both are precious to those who want children; and both need to be protected from a variety of possible harms. All of these factors contribute to the moral standing of the late-term fetus, which is substantial. However, to extend equal legal rights to fetuses is necessarily to deprive pregnant women of the rights to personal autonomy, physical integrity, and sometimes life itself. *There is room for only one person with full and equal rights inside a single human skin.* That is why it is birth, rather than sentience, viability, or some other prenatal milestone that must mark the beginning of legal personhood.

QUESTIONS FOR COMPREHENSION AND REFLECTION

1. Does Warren confuse cultural norms and legal rights with moral rights, or can she defend her position without reference to cultural norms and legal rights? Use specific examples to support your answer.
2. Discuss Warren's claim that deontology, rights ethics, and care ethics all support abortion and early infanticide. Would a utilitarian also agree with Warren's position on abortion? How would a Buddhist respond to Warren's argument? Support your answers.
3. Do you agree with Warren that self-concept is sufficient for personhood? How can we determine whether a being has a self-concept and a desire for a future? Support your answers. What are the implications of accepting this criterion for the moral standing of infants and brain-damaged, senile, or comatose humans? Would Warren permit euthanasia for these groups of humans? What are the implications of her criterion for how we should treat adult nonhuman animals?
4. Warren accepts selective abortion for genetic disorders. Discuss whether she would also accept, as morally permissible, abortion for sex selection, especially in countries where women are denied equal rights.
5. Warren favors earlier prenatal diagnosis. It is now possible to perform prenatal diagnosis on fetal tissue in the first trimester using a relatively new method known as chorionic villus sampling (CVS). However, the new procedure has a lower accuracy rate and results in fetal loss in 3.2 percent of the procedures (compared to a rate of less than 1 percent for amniocentesis). In addition, it is estimated that the majority of fetuses with chromosomal disorders spontaneously miscarry during the first trimester. Given these facts, apply a utilitarian calculus to decide whether CVS is preferable to amniocentesis.

SIDNEY CALLAHAN

Abortion and the Sexual Agenda

Sidney Callahan is associate professor of psychology at Mercy College in New York. Callahan offers a critique of contemporary pro-choice feminist arguments on the morality of abortion. She maintains that the modern feminist movement, rather than rejecting patriarchal values, has bought into them by adopting a male-oriented model of sexuality without commitment and the disease model of pregnancy. Instead, we need to expand our vision of what it means to be a feminist to include a vision of a social order that supports childbearing, education, and careers as well as better access to contraception.

The abortion debate continues. In the latest and perhaps most crucial development, pro-life feminists are contesting pro-choice feminist claims that abortion rights are prerequisites for women's full development and social equality. The outcome of this debate may be decisive for the culture as a whole. Pro-life feminists, like myself, argue on good feminist principles that women can never achieve the fulfillment of feminist goals in a society permissive toward abortion.

These new arguments over abortion take place within liberal political circles. This round of intense intra-feminist conflict has spiraled beyond earlier right-versus-left abortion debates, which focused on "tragic choices," medical judgments, and legal compromises. Feminist theorists of the pro-choice position now put forth the demand for unrestricted abortion rights as a *moral imperative* and insist upon women's right to complete reproductive freedom. . . .

. . . Pro-life feminists grant the good intentions of their pro-choice counterparts but protest that the pro-choice position is flawed, morally inadequate, and inconsistent with feminism's basic demands for justice. Pro-life feminists champion a more encompassing moral ideal. They recognize the claims of fetal life and offer a different perspective on what is good for women. The feminist vision is expanded and refocused.

1. From the moral right to control one's own body to a more inclusive ideal of justice. The moral right to control one's own body does apply to cases of organ transplants, mastectomies, contraception, and sterilization; but it is not a conceptualization adequate for abortion. The abortion dilemma is caused by the fact that 266 days following a conception in one body, another body will emerge. One's own body no longer exists as a single unit but is engendering another organism's life. This dynamic passage from conception to birth is genetically ordered and universally found in the human species. Pregnancy is not like the growth of cancer or infestation by a biological parasite; it is the way every human being enters the world. Strained philosophical analogies fail to apply: having a baby is not like rescuing a drowning person, being hooked up to a famous violinist's artificial life-support system, donating organs for transplant—or anything else.

As embryology and fetology advance, it becomes clear that human development is a continuum. Just as astronomers are studying the first three minutes in the genesis of the universe, so the first moments, days, and weeks at the beginning of human life are the subject of increasing scientific attention. While neonatology pushes the definition of viability ever earlier, ultrasound and fetology expand the concept of the patient in utero. Within such a continuous growth process, it is hard to defend logically any demarcation point after conception as the point at which an immature form of human life is so different from the day before or the day after, that it can be morally or legally discounted as a non-person. Even the moment of birth can hardly differentiate a nine-month fetus from a newborn. It is not surprising that those who countenance late abortions are logically led to endorse selective infanticide.

The same legal tradition which in our society guarantees the right to control one's own body firmly recognizes the wrongfulness of harming other bodies, however immature, dependent, different looking, or powerless. The handicapped, the retarded, and newborns are legally protected from deliberate harm. Pro-life feminists reject the suppositions that would except the unborn from this protection.

After all, debates similar to those about the fetus were once conducted about feminine personhood. Just as women, or blacks, were considered too different, too underdeveloped, too "biological," to have souls or to possess legal rights, so the fetus is now seen as "merely" biological life, subsidiary to a person. A woman was once viewed as incorporated into the "one flesh" of her husband's person; she too was a form of bodily property. In all patriarchal unjust systems, lesser orders of human life are granted rights only when wanted, chosen, or invested with value by the powerful.

Fortunately, in the course of civilization there has been a gradual realization that justice demands the powerless and dependent be protected against the uses of power wielded unilaterally. No human can be treated as a means to an end without consent. The fetus is an immature, dependent form of human life which only needs time and protection to develop. Surely, immaturity and dependence are not crimes.

In an effort to think about the essential requirements of a just society, philosophers like John Rawls recommend imagining yourself in an "original position," in which your position in the society to be created is hidden by a "veil of ignorance." You will have to weigh the possibility that any inequalities inherent in that society's practices may rebound upon you in the worst, as well as in the best, conceivable way. This thought experiment helps ensure justice for all.

Beverly Harrison argues that in such an envisioning of society everyone would institute abortion rights in order to guarantee that if one turned out to be a woman one would have reproductive freedom. But surely in the original position and behind the "veil of ignorance," you would have to contemplate the possibility of being the particular fetus to be aborted. Since everyone has passed through the fetal stage of development, it is false to refuse to imagine oneself in this state when thinking about a potential world in which justice would govern. Would it be just that an embryonic life—in half the cases, of course, a female life—be sacrificed to the right of a woman's control over her own body? A woman may be pregnant without consent and experience a great many penalties, but a fetus killed without consent pays the ultimate penalty.

It does not matter (*The Silent Scream* notwithstanding) whether the fetus being killed is fully conscious or feels pain. We do not sanction killing the innocent if it can be done painlessly or without the victim's awareness. Consciousness becomes important to the abortion debate because it is used as a criterion for the "personhood" so often seen as the prerequisite for legal protection. Yet certain philosophers set the standard of personhood so high that half the human race could not meet the criteria during most of their waking hours (let alone their sleeping ones). Sentience, self-consciousness, rational decision-making, social participation? Surely no infant, or child under two, could qualify. Either our idea of person must be expanded or another criterion, such as human life itself, be employed to protect the weak in a just society. Pro-life feminists who defend the fetus empathetically identify with an immature state of growth passed through by themselves, their children, and everyone now alive.

It also seems a travesty of just procedures that a pregnant woman now, in effect, acts as sole judge of her own case, under the most stressful conditions. Yes, one can acknowledge that the pregnant woman will be subject to the potential burdens arising from a pregnancy, but it has never been thought right to have an interested party, especially the more powerful party, decide his or her own case when there may be a conflict of interest.

If one considers the matter as a case of a powerful versus a powerless, silenced claimant, the pro-choice feminist argument can rightly be inverted: since hers is the body, hers the risk, and hers the greater burden, then how in fairness can a woman be the sole judge of the fetal right to life?

Human ambivalence, a bias toward self-interest, and emotional stress have always been recognized as endangering judgment. Freud declared that love and hate are so entwined that if instant thoughts could kill, we would all be dead in the bosom of our families. In the case of a woman's involuntary pregnancy, a complex, long-term solution requiring effort and energy has to compete with the immediate solution offered by a morning's visit to an abortion clinic. On the simple, perceptual plane, with imagination and thinking curtailed, the speed, ease, and privacy of abortion, combined with the small size of the embryo, tend to make early abortions seem less morally serious—even though speed, size, technical ease, and the private nature of an act have no moral standing.

As the most recent immigrants from non-personhood, feminists have traditionally fought for justice for themselves and the world. Women rally to feminism as a new and better way to live. Rejecting male aggression and destruction, feminists seek alternative, peaceful, ecologically sensitive means to resolve conflicts while respecting human potentiality. It is a chilling inconsistency to see pro-choice feminists demanding continued access to assembly-line, technological methods of fetal killing—the vacuum aspirator, prostaglandins, and dilation and evacuation. It is a betrayal of feminism, which has built the struggle for justice on the bedrock of women's empathy. After all, "maternal thinking" receives its name from a mother's unconditional acceptance and nurture of dependent, immature life. It is difficult to develop concern for women, children, the poor and the dispossessed—and to care about peace—and at the same time ignore fetal life.

2. From the necessity of autonomy and choice in personal responsibility to an expanded sense of responsibility. A distorted idea of morality overemphasizes individual autonomy and active choice. Morality has often been viewed too exclusively as a matter of human agency and decisive action. In moral behavior persons must explicitly choose and aggressively exert their wills to intervene in the natural and social environments. The human will dominates the body, overcomes the given, breaks out of the material limits of nature. Thus if one does not choose to be pregnant or cannot rear a child, who must be given up for adoption, then better to abort the pregnancy. Willing, planning, choosing one's moral commitments through the contracting of one's individual resources becomes the premier model of moral responsibility.

But morality also consists of the good and worthy acceptance of the unexpected events that life presents. Responsiveness and response-ability to things unchosen are also instances of the highest human moral capacity. Morality is not confined to contracted agreements of isolated individuals. Yes, one is obligated by explicit contracts freely initiated, but human beings are also obligated by implicit compacts and involuntary relationships in which persons simply find themselves. To be embedded in a family, a neighborhood, a social system, brings moral obligations which were never entered into with informed consent.

Parent-child relationships are one instance of implicit moral obligations arising by virtue of our being part of the interdependent human community. A woman, involuntarily pregnant, has a moral obligation to the now-existing dependent fetus whether she explicitly consented to its existence or not. No pro-life feminist would dispute the forceful observations of pro-choice feminists about the extreme difficulties that bearing an unwanted child in our society can entail. But the stronger force of the fetal claim presses a woman to accept these burdens; the fetus possesses rights arising from its extreme need and the interdependency and unity of humankind. The woman's moral obligation arises both from her status as a human being embedded in the interdependent human community and her unique lifegiving female reproductive power. To follow the pro-choice feminist ideology of insistent individualistic autonomy and control is to betray a fundamental basis of the moral life.

3. From the moral claim of the contingent value of fetal life to the moral claim for the intrinsic

value of human life. The feminist pro-choice position which claims that the value of the fetus is contingent upon the pregnant woman's bestowal—or willed, conscious "construction"—of humanhood is seriously flawed. The inadequacies of this position flow from the erroneous premises (1) that human value and rights can be granted by individual will; (2) that the individual woman's consciousness can exist and operate in an *a priori* isolated fashion; and (3) that "mere" biological, genetic human life has little meaning. Pro-life feminism takes a very different stance to life and nature.

Human life from the beginning to the end of development *has* intrinsic value, which does not depend on meeting the selective criteria or tests set up by powerful others. A fundamental humanist assumption is at stake here. Either we are going to value embodied human life and humanity as a good thing, or take some variant of the nihilist position that assumes human life is just one more random occurrence in the universe such that each instance of human life must explicitly be justified to prove itself worthy to continue. When faced with a new life, or an involuntary pregnancy, there is a world of difference in whether one first asks, "Why continue?" or "Why not?" Where is the burden of proof going to rest? The concept of "compulsory pregnancy" is as distorted as labeling life "compulsory aging."

In a sound moral tradition, human rights arise from human needs, and it is the very nature of a right, or valid claim upon another, that it cannot be denied, conditionally delayed, or rescinded by more powerful others at their behest. It seems fallacious to hold that in the case of the fetus it is the pregnant woman alone who gives or removes its right to life and human status solely through her subjective conscious investment or "humanization." Surely no pregnant woman (or any other individual member of the species) has created her own human nature by an individually willed act of consciousness, nor for that matter been able to guarantee her own human rights. An individual woman and the unique individual embryonic life within her can only exist because of their participation in the genetic inheritance of the human species as a whole. Biological life should never be discounted. Membership in the species, or collec-

tive human family, is the basis for human solidarity, equality, and natural human rights.

4. The moral right of women to full social equality from a pro-life feminist perspective. Pro-life feminists and pro-choice feminists are totally agreed on the moral right of women to the full social equality so far denied them. The disagreement between them concerns the definition of the desired goal and the best means to get there. Permissive abortion laws do not bring women reproductive freedom, social equality, sexual fulfillment, or full personal development.

Pragmatic failures of a pro-choice feminist position combined with a lack of moral vision are, in fact, causing disaffection among young women. Middle-aged pro-choice feminists blamed the "big chill" on the general conservative backlash. But they should look rather to their own elitist acceptance of male models of sex and to the sad picture they present of women's lives. Pitting women against their own offspring is not only morally offensive, it is psychologically and politically destructive. Women will never climb to equality and social empowerment over mounds of dead fetuses, numbering now in the millions. As long as most women choose to bear children, they stand to gain from the same constellation of attitudes and institutions that will also protect the fetus in the woman's womb—and they stand to lose from the cultural assumptions that support permissive abortion. Despite temporary conflicts of interest, feminine and fetal liberation are ultimately one and the same cause.

Women's rights and liberation are pragmatically linked to fetal rights because to obtain true equality, women need (1) more social support and changes in the structure of society, and (2) increased self-confidence, self-expectations, and self-esteem. Society in general, and men in particular, have to provide women more support in rearing the next generation, or our devastating feminization of poverty will continue. But if a woman claims the right to decide by herself whether the fetus becomes a child or not, what does this do to paternal and communal responsibility? Why should men share responsibility for child support or childrearing if they cannot share in what is asserted to be the woman's sole decision? Furthermore, if explicit intentions and consciously accepted contracts are necessary for moral obligations, why should men be held responsible for what *they* do not voluntarily choose to happen? By pro-choice reasoning, a man who does not want to have a child, or whose contraceptive fails, can be exempted from the responsibilities of fatherhood and child support. Traditionally, many men have been laggards in assuming parental responsibility and support for their children; ironically, ready abortion, often advocated as a response to male dereliction, legitimizes male irresponsibility and paves the way for even more male detachment and lack of commitment.

For that matter, why should the state provide a system of day-care or child support, or require workplaces to accommodate women's maternity and the needs of childrearing? Permissive abortion, granted in the name of women's privacy and reproductive freedom, ratifies the view that pregnancies and children are a woman's private individual responsibility. More and more frequently, we hear some version of this old rationalization: if she refuses to get rid of it, it's her problem. A child becomes a product of the individual woman's freely chosen investment, a form of private property resulting from her own cost-benefit calculation. The larger community is relieved of moral responsibility.

With legal abortion freely available, a clear cultural message is given: conception and pregnancy are no longer serious moral matters. With abortion as an acceptable alternative, contraception is not as responsibly used; women take risks, often at the urging of male sexual partners. Repeat abortions increase, with all their psychological and medical repercussions. With more abortion there is more abortion. Behavior shapes thought as well as the other way round. One tends to justify morally what one has done; what becomes commonplace and institutionalized seems harmless. Habituation is a powerful psychological force. Psychologically it is also true that whatever is avoided becomes more threatening; in phobias it is the retreat from anxiety-producing events which reinforces future avoidance. Women begin to see themselves as too weak to cope with involuntary pregnancies. Finally, through the potency of social pressure and the force of inertia, it becomes more and more difficult, in fact almost unthinkable, *not* to use abortion to solve problem pregnancies. Abortion becomes no longer a choice but a "necessity."

But "necessity," beyond the organic failure and death of the body, is a dynamic social construction open to interpretation. The thrust of present feminist pro-choice arguments can only increase the justifiable indications for "necessary" abortion; every unwanted fetal handicap becomes more and more unacceptable. Repeatedly assured that in the name of reproductive freedom, women have a right to specify which pregnancies and which children they will accept, women justify sex selection, and abort unwanted females. Female infanticide, after all, is probably as old a custom as the human species possesses. Indeed, all kinds of selection of the fit and the favored for the good of the family and the tribe have always existed. Selective extinction is no new program.

There are far better goals for feminists to pursue. Pro-life feminists seek to expand and deepen the more communitarian, maternal elements of feminism—and move society from its male-dominated course. First and foremost, women have to insist upon a different, woman-centered approach to sex and reproduction. While Margaret Mead stressed the "womb envy" of males in other societies, it has been more or less repressed in our own. In our male-dominated world, what men don't do, doesn't count. Pregnancy, childbirth, and nursing have been characterized as passive, debilitating, animal-like. The disease model of pregnancy and birth has been entrenched. This female disease or impairment, with its attendant "female troubles," naturally handicaps women in the "real" world of hunting, war, and the corporate fast track. Many pro-choice feminists, deliberately childless, adopt the male perspective when they cite the "basic injustice that women have to bear the babies," instead of seeing the injustice in the fact that men cannot. Women's biologically unique capacity and privilege has been denied, despised, and suppressed under male domination; unfortunately, many women have fallen for the phallic fallacy. . . .

Of course . . . feminine sexual ideals always coexisted in competition with another view. A more male-oriented model of erotic or amative sexuality endorses sexual permissiveness without long-term commitment or reproductive focus. Erotic sexuality emphasizes pleasure, play, passion, individual self-expression, and romantic games of courtship and conquest. It is assumed that a variety of partners and sexual experiences are necessary to stimulate romantic passion. This erotic model of the sexual life has often worked satisfactorily for men, both heterosexual and gay, and for certain cultural elites. But for the average woman, it is quite destructive. Women can only play the erotic game successfully when, like the "*Cosmopolitan* woman," they are young, physically attractive, economically powerful, and fulfilled enough in a career to be willing to sacrifice family life. Abortion is also required. As our society increasingly endorses this male-oriented, permissive view of sexuality, it is all too ready to give women abortion on demand. Abortion helps a woman's body be more like a man's. It has been observed that *Roe v. Wade* removed the last defense women possessed against male sexual demands.

Unfortunately, the modern feminist movement made a mistaken move at a critical juncture. Rightly rebelling against patriarchy, unequal education, restricted work opportunities, and women's downtrodden political status, feminists also rejected the nineteenth-century feminine sexual ethic. Amative, erotic, permissive sexuality (along with abortion rights) became symbolically identified with other struggles for social equality in education, work, and politics. This feminist mistake also turned off many potential recruits among women who could not deny the positive dimensions of their own traditional feminine roles, nor their allegiance to the older feminine sexual ethic of love and fidelity.

An ironic situation then arose in which many pro-choice feminists preach their own double standard. In the world of work and career, women are urged to grow up, to display mature self-discipline and self-control; they are told to persevere in long-term commitments, to cope with unexpected obstacles by learning to tough out the inevitable sufferings and setbacks entailed in life and work. But this mature ethic of commitment and self-discipline, recommended as the only way to pro-gress in the world of work and personal achievement, is discounted in the domain of sexuality.

In pro-choice feminism, a permissive, erotic view of sexuality is assumed to be the only option. Sexual intercourse with a variety of partners is seen as "inevitable" from a young age and as a positive growth experience to be managed by access to contraception and abortion. Unfortunately, the pervasive cultural conviction that adolescents, or their elders, cannot exercise sexual self-control, undermines the responsible use of contraception. When a pregnancy occurs, the first abortion is viewed in some pro-choice circles as a *rite de passage*. Responsibly choosing an abortion supposedly ensures that a young woman will take charge of her own life, make her own decisions, and carefully practice contraception. But the social dynamics of a permissive, erotic model of sexuality, coupled with permissive laws, work toward repeat abortions. Instead of being empowered by their abortion choices, young women having abortions are confronting the debilitating reality of *not* bringing a baby into the world; *not* being able to count on a committed male partner; *not* accounting oneself strong enough, or the master of enough resources, to avoid killing the fetus. Young women are hardly going to develop the self-esteem, self-discipline, and self-confidence necessary to confront a male-dominated society through abortion.

The male-oriented sexual orientation has been harmful to women and children. It has helped bring us epidemics of venereal disease, infertility, pornography, sexual abuse, adolescent pregnancy, divorce, displaced older women, and abortion. Will these signals of something amiss stimulate pro-choice feminists to rethink what kind of sex ideal really serves women's best interests? While the erotic model cannot encompass commitment, the committed model can—happily—encompass and encourage romance, passion, and playfulness. In fact, within the security of long-term commitments, women may be more likely to experience sexual pleasure and fulfillment.

The pro-life feminist position is not a return to the old feminine mystique. That espousal of "the eternal feminine" erred by viewing sexuality as so sacred that it cannot be humanly shaped at all.

Woman's *whole* nature was supposed to be opposite to man's, necessitating complementary and radically different social roles. Followed to its logical conclusion, such a view presumes that reproductive and sexual experience is necessary for human fulfillment. But as the early feminists insisted, no woman has to marry or engage in sexual intercourse to be fulfilled, nor does a woman have to give birth and raise children to be complete, nor must she stay home and function as an earth mother. But female sexuality does need to be deeply respected as a unique potential and trust. Since most contraceptives and sterilization procedures really do involve only the woman's body rather than destroying new life, they can be an acceptable and responsible moral option.

. . . For women to get what they need in order to combine childbearing, education, and careers, society has to recognize that female bodies come with wombs. Women and their reproductive power, and the children women have, must be supported in new ways. Another and different round of feminist consciousness-raising is needed in which all of women's potential is accorded respect. This time, instead of humbly buying entrée by conforming to male lifestyles, women will demand that society accommodate to them.

New feminist efforts to rethink the meaning of sexuality, femininity, and reproduction are all the more vital as new techniques for artificial reproduction, surrogate motherhood, and the like present a whole new set of dilemmas. In the long run, the very long run, the abortion debate may be merely the opening round in a series of far-reaching struggles over the role of human sexuality and the ethics of reproduction. Significant changes in the culture, both positive and negative in outcome, may begin as local storms of controversy. We may be at one of those vaguely realized thresholds when we had best come to full attention. What kind of people are we going to be? Pro-life feminists pursue a vision for their sisters, daughters, and granddaughters. Will their great-granddaughters be grateful?

QUESTIONS FOR COMPREHENSION AND REFLECTION

1. Discuss Callahan's claim that fetuses should be given the same protection enjoyed by other marginalized and powerless groups of humans. Do you agree that fetuses are currently marginalized and should be given equal rights under the law? Is the denial of fetal personhood by most pro-choice advocates comparable, as Callahan argues, to the past denials of rights to women, blacks, and other marginalized groups of people? Support your answers.

2. Callahan cites the categorical imperative, which prohibits us from using another person as a means only, to support her position. Do you agree with her that the categorical imperative would lead us to outlaw abortion?

3. How would Callahan respond to Warren's argument that "there is room for only one person with full and equal rights inside a single human skin"? Compare and contrast Callahan's argument that feminine and fetal rights are linked with Warren's claim that extension of legal personhood to the fetus would threaten a woman's right to choose and undermine other important rights. Which person presents the most compelling argument? Support your answer.

4. Discuss Callahan's claim that pro-choice feminism legitimates a patriarchal, male-oriented sexuality.

DOROTHY C. WERTZ AND JOHN C. FLETCHER

Ethical and Social Issues in Prenatal Sex Selection: A Survey of Geneticists in 37 Nations

Dorothy C. Wertz is a research professor at the School of Public Health at Boston University. John C. Fletcher is director of the Center for Biomedical Ethics at the University of Virginia. Wertz and Fletcher describe the justifications of selective abortion given in different cultures. After examining these justifications, they conclude that, while it is morally permissible to use prenatal diagnosis and selective abortion for "severe and untreatable" genetic disease, it is not morally permissible to use it for sex selection.

INTRODUCTION

Prenatal sex selection to satisfy parental desires is an ethically and socially troubling problem. The possibility of harm is great, not only in cultures that prefer males, but also in cultures that prefer gender-balanced families, because it can perpetuate gender stereotypes.

New technologies have made sex selection a reality. As yet, there is no accurate and reliable method of selecting a child's sex before conception. Sex selection before birth is possible through prenatal diagnosis (PND), including amniocentesis, chorionic villus sampling, or ultrasound, followed by selective abortion. Ultrasound, although not definitive, may show the male genitals; its major use is for parents who desire a son and who are willing to abort a fetus that is not clearly male.

The major use of prenatal diagnosis for sex selection occurs in those developing nations where there is a strong preference for sons. In some nations, such as India and China, the majority of prenatal diagnostic procedures were performed for sex selection rather than detection of fetal abnormalities until sex selection was forbidden by law under the Law on Maternal and Infant Health Care of January, 1995, which says that "sex identification of a fetus by technical means shall be strictly

banned." In Turkey, the problem reached such proportions that the Ministry of Health has restricted clinical application of sex selection methods when there is no medical indication. Ultrasound, although not always accurate, is affordable even to villagers and poses no risk to the mother. In many nations of Asia, sex selection contributes to an already unbalanced sex ratio occasioned by neglect of female children. An estimated 60,000,000–100,000,000 women are missing from the world's population (Sen, 1990), including 20,000,000 in China and 23,000,000 in India. Whereas in the United States, United Kingdom, and France, there are 105 women to every 100 men, and in Africa and Latin America the proportions of women and men are roughly equal, in much of Asia, including Pakistan, Afghanistan, Turkey, Bangladesh, India, and China, there are fewer than 95 women for every 100 men (United Nations, 1991). Families desire sons for economic reasons. In these nations, where most people have no social security or retirement pensions, sons are responsible for caring for parents in their old age. Daughters usually leave the parental family to live with their husbands and help care for their parents-in-law. Even if a daughter stays in the parental home, she seldom has the earning power to support her parents. In some nations, a daughter represents a considerable economic burden because her family must pay a dowry to her husband's family in order to arrange a marriage. . . .

. . . In China, families may abandon a daughter so that they can conceive again, under the one-child policy, in the hope that the next child will be a son. Nevertheless, the existence of prebirth technologies for sex selection presents a temptation in many countries, including those where it is illegal. . . .

The numbers of requests for prenatal diagnosis for sex selection cannot be documented in Western nations, because few parents make open requests. Medical professionals in the United States appear increasingly willing to perform prenatal diagnosis for those making such requests, however. According to a 1975 survey of 149 clinically oriented geneticists and counselors, 15% would recommend amniocentesis for sex selection in general and 28% would do so for a couple with one girl who wanted to have only two children and who wanted to be sure that their final child would be a son who could carry on the family name (Fraser and Pressor, 1977). In 1985, 62% of 295 doctoral-level geneticists in the United States would either perform prenatal diagnosis (34%) or offer a referral (28%) for a couple with four daughters who desired a son and who would abort a female fetus (Wertz and Fletcher, 1989; Wertz *et al.,* 1990). A 1990 survey, using the same question, found that 85% of Master's-level genetic counselors in the United States would either arrange for prenatal diagnosis or offer a referral (Pencarinha *et al.,* 1992).

In giving reasons for acceding to parents' requests, many geneticists in the 1985 Wertz and Fletcher survey said that sex selection was a logical extension of parents' acknowledged rights to choose the number, timing, spacing, and genetic health of their children. These geneticists regarded withholding any service, including sex selection, as medical paternalism and an infringement on patient autonomy. Those who would refuse prenatal diagnosis said that it was a misuse of scarce medical resources designed to look for serious genetic abnormalities, that sex was not a disease, or that they disapproved of the abortion of a normal fetus. Most regarded sex selection

as a private matter between doctor and patient. Few, except for geneticists in India, mentioned the societal implications of sex selection. . . .

Most requests for sex selection in developed nations are probably covert, with women requesting prenatal diagnosis on the basis of anxiety about the health of the fetus. In the 1985 survey, most geneticists in the United States (89%) and around the world (73%) would perform prenatal diagnosis for an anxious woman aged 25 with no medical or genetic indications for its use. Information about fetal sex is usually communicated to parents if they wish to know, though some clinics do not provide the information unless specifically requested. In effect, sex selection by prenatal diagnosis is therefore available to most families.

Results of the 1985 geneticist survey led to considerable discussion among bioethicists and genetics professionals. These discussions generally opposed sex selection and might be expected to decrease the willingness of professionals to comply with client requests.

In order to find out whether geneticists' views had changed between 1985 and 1994, we surveyed geneticists in 37 nations, using a mailed, anonymous questionnaire. The study included all nations known to have 10 or more medical genetics specialists as of 1993. Of 4609 persons asked to participate, 2903 (63%) responded. . . .

The questionnaires included a series of sociodemographic questions about the respondent, and 50 questions about ethical problems occurring in the practice of medical genetics. Most questions, including those on sex selection, appeared as case vignettes describing a possible situation in medical practice. We used case vignettes because these enabled us to describe the most difficult and ethically controversial situations that may challenge a respondent's general opinion. For example, if we had asked simply, "Do you approve of using prenatal diagnosis for sex selection?" most would probably have said no. However, when we described the case of a woman from another culture whose husband threatens to discard her if she does not have a son, many respondents would make exceptions. As in medicine each case in different, and therefore potentially "exceptional," we posed a variety of five cases in which couples or individuals might make open requests for prenatal diagnosis for sex selection. In addition, we posed a case where a couple's actions in requesting prenatal diagnosis are strongly indicative of a veiled request for sex selection. Finally, we asked a series of questions about an as yet hypothetical method of selecting sex before conception. (No accurate method now exists.) The sex selection questions were dispersed among questions about other ethical issues related to genetics.

After each question, respondents were given a checklist of possible actions (e.g. perform prenatal diagnosis, refuse to perform prenatal diagnosis, or refer, including out of country). Then they were asked to describe, in their own words, why they had chosen this answer. . . .

RESULTS

Almost half (47%) of all geneticist respondents reported that they had had outright requests for prenatal diagnosis solely to select the sex desired by the parents. In 10 countries, majorities reported such requests: Egypt (100%), China (79%), Sweden (75%), India (70%), Australia (67%), Hungary (67 %), Israel (62%), the U.S. (62%), Russia (56%), and Turkey (55%). In four of these countries (Egypt, China, India, and Turkey) preference for males and an actual or potentially unbalanced sex ratio are acknowledged social problems. . . .

Half of all respondents had had cases where they suspected that the patient's real reason for having prenatal diagnosis was sex selection, even though the patient gave another reason, such as a family history of genetic disorders. These included 100% in Egypt, 87% in Australia and Israel, 75% in Sweden and the U.S., 73% in China, 67% in Switzerland, 61% in India, 58% in Canada and 53% in France. In China and India, use of prenatal diagnosis for sex selection has been made illegal within the past few years. France forbids prenatal diagnosis except for the detection of disease or for forensic purposes. Canadian professional guidelines (Canadian College of Medical Geneticists, 1986) have long opposed sex selection. Therefore, we might expect high percents of covert rather

than overt requests in some of these countries. In the U.S., public opinion does not support use of abortion to select sex. Also, a prenatal diagnosis solely for this purpose would probably not be reimbursed by private insurance and certainly not by Medicaid (publicly supported care for the poor). Therefore many clients will hide their requests behind "acceptable" reasons, such as a falsified family or personal history.

CASE STUDIES

. . .

For each of the five cases, we asked respondents how they would counsel the client. In North America, genetic counseling (whether by an M.D. or Ph.D. geneticist or a Master's-level genetic counselor) is based on the premise of "non-directiveness." The counselor is supposed to provide information in an objective (unbiased) manner, and to help clients work through to the decision that the clients think is best for them in view of their own values and parenting goals. The counselor is supposed to offer emotional support, even if the counselor disagrees personally with a client's decision. Sex selection tests the limits of non-directiveness. It poses the premise of absolute client autonomy over against prevention of harm to the fetus, child (if born), family, and society. To attempt to dissuade a client from having prenatal diagnosis contravenes the non-directive approach. Not to try to dissuade the client may contravene the principle of non-maleficence ("do no harm"), at least in many people's eyes.

In Cases 1–4, 44% would attempt to dissuade the client, with no significant differences between cases, with majorities in 19 countries (including the United Kingdom, where counselors generally espouse non-directiveness). Some respondents considered this an ethically justifiable form of paternalism. The United States . . . had one of the lowest percentages who would try to dissuade (24%). In all, 35% would "provide information only," which may be considered one form of non-directiveness, though it includes no counseling aspect and implies no relationship with the client. A total of 21% would follow the classic non-directive counseling approach set forth by Fraser (1974) to "tell patients that decisions are theirs alone and that you will support whatever decisions they make," including 4% who would "help them achieve their parenting goals." In the United States, this is part of the counseling ethos, at least for some respondents. . . .

Responses to Case 5 (the professional couple in their 40s) were somewhat different from responses to Cases 1–4, with fewer (33%) saying they would dissuade, more (39%) who would offer information only, and more (28%) who would support the clients' decisions. . . . Prenatal diagnosis is, after all, medically indicated by reason of the clients' ages, and respondents said that they did not want to be responsible for the birth of a child with a chromosomal aberration. . . .

. . . In the first four cases, respondents appeared to have the least sympathy for the single woman who wishes to become a mother (Case 1), though this was not uniformly so in all countries. Some respondents thought that she should not become a mother at all because she was unmarried and the child would not have full social advantages; others thought that she was wrong in her expectations and that a girl could be harder to raise than a boy. Respondents appeared to have the most sympathy for the non-Western couple, partly because the woman was being coerced by her husband, and they feared what might happen to her if they did not perform PND.

Case 5 should be considered separately from the others, as PND is medically indicated in spite of the parents' stated reasons. In the United States and some other countries, a professional would be legally liable if a child with a chromosomal disorder were born after denial of PND. This explains the high percentage in the United States (85%) and Canada (67%) who would perform PND or offer a referral in Case 5. . . .

Some geneticists saw a clear ethical difference between performing PND and offering a referral. By refusing PND, they cleared their own consciences, and by simultaneously offering a referral, they fulfilled what they presumed to be a duty to respect the "patient's right to referral." In some

countries, they perhaps thought that the center to which they offered a referral would also refuse sex selection, or that the client would become exhausted after several failed referrals. . . .

After the cases . . . we included a checklist of possible reasons for answers. . . . For each item, respondents were asked whether they considered it extremely, very, moderately, somewhat, or not at all important in answering the questions about sex selection. "Ethical status of the profession" topped the list in importance in most of the world except the U.S., where it was second. "Maintaining my own integrity" came next. The U.S. emphasis on personal integrity may stem in part from the National Society of Genetic Counselors Code of Ethics, 1992, which places a high value on one's relationship with oneself. "Preventing a trend toward parental choices for reasons unrelated to health" (the "slippery slope" toward cosmetic choices for height, weight, hair and eye color) ranked third. "Preventing the abortion of a normal fetus" ranked fourth. . . .

Preventing harm to a child of the unwanted sex, if born (i.e. by preventing the birth of this child) ranked fifth. . . . In India, mistreatment of unwanted girls is a known problem. In Latin America, Portugal, Spain, and Thailand, there is no known social problem of this sort. . . .

Respect for parental autonomy was next in order of overall importance, ranking third for the United States and sixth elsewhere. In eleven countries, Argentina (57%), Brazil (63%), Colombia (64%), Cuba (54%), Greece (50%), Hungary (66%), Israel (91%), Mexico (73%), Portugal (64%), Russia (70%), and the United States (52%), 50% or more ranked autonomy as important. On the other hand, in eleven countries, Egypt (0%), Finland (25%), France (11%), Germany (11%), India (20%), the Netherlands (20%), Norway (11%), Sweden (17%), Switzerland (20%), Turkey (9%), and United Kingdom (24%), 25% or fewer thought that autonomy was an important consideration. The contrast between the United States and the United Kingdom in this regard is particularly interesting. Respondents in the U.K., as in much of Western Europe, apparently believed in limits to autonomy.

The position of women in society ranked seventh of nine items in importance. Only in China (71%) and India (61%) did majorities consider this important. In both nations, respondents were aware that sex selection has weighed heavily against women. . . .

Only in China (72%) and India (39%) did sizeable percentages regard lowering the birth rate (presumably by aborting female fetuses so that couples would not have "extra" children in the attempt to have a son) as important.

ATTITUDES EXPRESSED
IN FREE RESPONSES

. . .

In general, reasons in Western nations concentrated on questions of individual autonomy, the professional's own role and personal integrity, the moral status of the fetus, and family psychodynamics. In China and India, reasons focused on societal effects, limiting the birth rate, and the status of women. Many reasons appeared widely distributed across cultures. The most common reason for not doing PND was simply "sex is not a disease" (43%), alluding to the "medically indicated" use of PND to detect genetic disorders.

Respondents who opposed sex selection said that it was a misuse of genetic services, that they "use disease as the only indication for such tests" (United Kingdom) and that "being male is not a disease, nor is being a female" (the Netherlands).

Others said there should be "limits to parental autonomy" (Denmark), or that "geneticists should not become involved in non-health related testing" (Australia), or that PND "is not intended to eliminate children who do not fit in with preconceived schemes" (France). The second most frequent comment by those who would not perform PND was that the respondent opposed abortion of a normal fetus. Some said that this amounted to infanticide (United Kingdom, Mexico, Turkey). A few said procedures for sex selection were a waste of scarce resources. "Resources for prenatal diagnosis are finite, so this use would mean other patients with medical indications would be denied the test" (Canada).

About 7% saw sex selection as sex discrimination, although they approved of abortion for social reasons. "For me, specific selection against a female fetus is unacceptable—far worse than random selection against an uncharacterized unwanted fetus" (United Kingdom). Others thought that prohibiting sex selection had important symbolic value for the status of women. "Equality between the sexes will never be real if abortion because of sex is possible" (Denmark). Many Chinese geneticists said it was important to "destroy the old ideas which say men are superior to women" and that "women's self-respect and medical science should not be insulted."

Another 7% of respondents pointed out that a professional has a right to refuse a service that is unnecessary or may cause harm. This is "medical paternalism" in the ethically acceptable sense. . . .

Only 3% spoke of maintaining a balanced sex ratio. Although some of these comments came from developed nations such as France, Canada, and Japan, most came from India and China, where the sex ratio is already unbalanced. In China especially, geneticists wrote that "the aim of prenatal diagnosis is for well bearing [eugenics] and well-raising." "In our country, especially rural and remote areas, many people have the idea of favoring son, looking down on daughter. Telling the fetus' sex to the parents or family members will destroy the sexual ecological balance."

Some respondents disapproved of PND for sex selection because they considered it "eugenics," manipulation of nature, or parental irresponsibility. They did not regard elimination of fetuses with genetic disorders as "eugenic," although many critics of PND would consider it so, but instead regarded parental choices, in the absence of fetal abnormality, as eugenic. Respondents from the Netherlands and Brazil went so far as to compare sex selection with Nazi practices of eliminating the "unfit." "Eugenics" is probably not the correct term to describe what respondents meant. What most were apparently trying to say is that parents who would use sex selection are irresponsible. Such parents regard a child as "something you choose in the supermarket" (Italy) or "get from a gumball machine and then reject" (France), or are just plain selfish (Canada, Japan, South Africa). A French respondent, apparently fearing a "slippery slope" toward other kinds of selections, said "this is Huxley's *Brave New World.*" A Turkish respondent, fearing for the place of medicine as a whole, said "medicine should not be made a tool of social anxiety." Others said that sex selection would harm the moral fabric of society because it violated human dignity (Germany, China, U.S.A., Japan, U.K.).

A few said that sex selection harmed the parents, who "would potentially suffer major psychological repercussions" (United Kingdom) or would "forever mourn the therapeutic abortion of a normal child" (Canada).

The major reason given (29%) for performing sex selection was respect for parental autonomy. Variations on this theme appeared in comments from every country. . . . Many in North America referred to their "professional ethic of non-directiveness." One Danish professional said "I don't consider myself a guardian of the fetus but a service to the parents." Others, around the world, said that the professional's responsibility was only to inform, not to guide parents in their decisions. As one Mexican respondent put it, "the use they make of the information is their responsibility, not mine."

Some pointed to the wider social context of PND. "In a society where there is family planning it seems logical to fulfill the couple's wishes or expectations if it is possible" (Israel). Some stated that since abortion for social reasons was already legal in their countries, there was no reason to deny abortion for sex selection. As one U.S. geneticist said, "If I'm pro-choice, I'm pro-choice!" even if I feel uncomfortable about sex selection. Many felt that as long as "abortion on demand is also available, why withhold information?" (South Africa), or saw "no difference between termination of pregnancy based on fetal sex, and terminating for other social reasons" (U.S.A.).

Reflecting on multiculturalism, some in the U.S. said that "I don't believe we can be a gatekeeper to prenatal diagnosis," "I can't sit in judgement on other people's cultures or behaviors," or "I should refer to a geneticist who shares similar cultural values to clients" if I find myself unable to accede to patient autonomy.

Many drew the moral line at insurance payment, insisting that patients pay out of their own pockets. To some respondents, this was an acceptable limit on autonomy, especially in nations with national health insurance, where many families would, in effect, be unable to obtain sex selection privately. . . .

Some Chinese respondents thought that people who were too poor to pay for the test should not be having children at all.

A scattering of comments mentioned preventing harm to a potential child of the "unwanted" sex. Respondents from around the world reiterated the belief that "every child has the right to be born into a family in which he/she will be accepted." Some went so far as to say that "if a baby of a given sex is unwanted in a family it is better for it not to be born at all" (Russia). Geneticists in India and China said that "females are always maltreated," and that PND may avoid this.

Only 3%, mostly in developing nations, mentioned family planning or limiting the population. In China, many mentioned the "one-child" policy. . . . Some Chinese and Indian respondents thought that sex selection could help control population. "Especially in rural areas, people want to have a son. I think in a country with advanced technology we should give these families happiness so that they won't have to have many girls." Respondents in China said that the single woman in Case 1 should have an abortion, because her child will never be accepted by society and will therefore never become a full human being. . . .

DISCUSSION

In most of the world, geneticists appear unwilling to act as gatekeepers to prenatal diagnosis for sex selection. This does not mean that they approve or support sex selection, however. Most feel a conflict between maintaining their own integrity and serving what they believe to be clients' needs. The typical response presents a compromise and reads as follows: "I don't approve of sex selection, but they have the right to make their own decisions and I owe the client a referral; I don't think a national health plan should pay for this, but they should be able to have it if they're willing to pay for it themselves." Some say, "I'll do the test but I won't do the abortion" or [in countries that require a doctor's signature] "I won't sign the papers for the abortion." . . . By leaving it to someone else—real or hypothetical—to say "no," professionals can maintain the self-image of respecting client autonomy. Our questionnaire purposely described exceptional or "hard luck" cases in order to try to pierce self-illusions about opposing sex selection. Sometimes it is the exceptional case that sets the rule, for each case in medicine is unique and therefore possibly exceptional. The professional who claims to oppose sex selection may make so many exceptions that the claim of opposition becomes a mere private opinion that is irrelevant to practice.

Acceding to the requests of "special" families for sex selection reflects the general fragmentation of universal views and the rise of special interests that are part of postmodernism (Harvey, 1990). In reproduction generally, a broad, coherent view that placed all women under a general rubric of care has been replaced by intensified attention to serving the needs of special interest groups such as infertile women or women over 35. In sex selection, providers in Western nations have definitely lost a sense of the whole. They are responding not only to individual autonomy, but to the interests of ethnic groups or other "special" groups (single mothers, families with children of only one sex), which prevail over universal standards.

Comparison between the 1985 and 1994 survey results points to a clear trend in most of the world toward greater willingness to perform or refer for sex selection, with the greatest increase in the referral category. India and Turkey, the two countries in the 1985 survey where sex selection was recognized as a social problem, were exceptions to this trend.

The basic reason why geneticists in many Western nations can compromise their personal views in favor of client autonomy is that they do not regard sex selection as a social problem. Sex selection in the West is unlikely to unbalance the sex ratio. Although there is some evidence that in the United States families would prefer that the first-born be a boy or that they would prefer to have two sons and a daughter if they are to have three children, there is no evidence that families would use selective abortion in order to achieve a particular birth order.

In the absence of imminent social problems arising from sex selection, many professionals see such requests in the light of a woman's right to choose abortion for her own personal reasons. Sex selection becomes an extension of a family's rights to choose the number and spacing of their children.

Yet there are strong ethical arguments against sex selection, even for a balanced family. Sex selection is based on gender stereotyping, the belief that only members of one sex are capable of certain actions, such as inheriting property, carrying on the family name, holding well-paying jobs, or caring for elderly parents. Sex selection helps to perpetuate gender stereotyping by providing parents with a child whom they consider capable of performing these actions. A "selected" child who does not fulfill the gender stereotype could suffer. Ultimately persons of both genders may suffer because society, with the aid of sex selection technologies, forces people into rigid gender roles. In most societies, sexual stereotyping has placed greater restrictions on women than on men, and has contributed to gender inequality.

Sex selection has the potential to harm society by leading to selection on cosmetic grounds, such as height, weight, or eye, hair or skin color, if these selections are ever technically possible. Some parents would select for such purposes, especially for weight. New discoveries in behavioral genetics may lead to parental selections for personality traits such as risk-taking or risk-avoidance. Although many geneticists in the 1994 survey were aware that sex selection could be the initial step on the road to such choices, they were reluctant to infringe on clients' autonomy.

Some authors from the disability community argue that if prenatal diagnosis is ethically permissible for disabilities, it should also be permissible for characteristics such as sex and sexual orientation (Asch and Geller, 1996). Their argument goes as follows: disability is a social construction that can be overcome with adequate social support for those with disabilities and appropriate education for the general public about life with disabilities. Prenatal diagnosis discriminates against potential people with disabilities and also perpetuates existing unfair social discrimination against persons with disabilities who are already born. Female sex is a social disability in many countries; women may be prohibited from inheriting property, from education, from many kinds of jobs, and from making personal decisions about their own bodies. Female gender, like other kinds of disabilities, circumscribes lives and limits fulfillment of individuals' deeply held goals. Therefore, sex selection (against females) is not ethically different from selecting against fetuses with genetic disorders. . . . According to this argument, the social outcomes of sex selection and disability selection will not differ ethically; in both cases, fewer persons will be born who differ from the socially desired norm and the remaining people who are "different" will suffer from greater discrimination and receive fewer services. At the very least, prenatal diagnosis will support existing systems of discrimination, whether against women or people with disabilities. The same argument could be made about prenatal diagnosis for sexual orientation. In conclusion, the authors express fear that prenatal diagnosis will lead to social and familial decisions that only people with certain types of characteristics should be allowed to enter the world, and make a plea for a more open, loving, caring approach both to disability and gender. At the same time, they uphold women's rights to choose, including choices about the children's sex, on the grounds that "people deserve to choose whatever they can about the children they raise so that they and their children will receive the benefits of chosen companionship" (Asch and Geller, 1996, p. 342).

The major problem with this line of argument is that in claiming that all disability is socially constructed, it denies the physical, mental, and interpersonal reality of genetic disorders. To be sure, disability is in part socially constructed, some disabilities to greater extent than others, but the "social constructionist" view of disease overlooks some hard realities (Kitcher, 1996, pp. 205–219). The lives of some people with genetic disorders will be

severely limited no matter what is provided in the way of support; furthermore, their lives will limit the lives of others around them. Kitcher (1996) argues that there is "a moral gulf" between aborting a fetus because of sex and aborting for most genetic disorders. He bases his argument, not on medically "objective" notions of disease, but on value judgements about the quality of human lives. According to this argument, we should not condemn families in northern India who seek sex selection because they think that the life of an unwanted girl will be so hard she is better off not being born. We should, however, condemn the social system that discriminates against women (and the medical practitioners who provide prenatal diagnosis as an answer). Women's lives are limited by society, not by inborn characteristics. Sex is not in the same logical category even with genetic disorders that most people may consider minor. We are not arguing in favor of prenatal diagnosis for all genetic disorders, only pointing out that because sex imposes no inherent limitations on ordinary life, it does not belong in the same category with information about the fetus's health. The same can be said about cosmetic variations, such as eye color. . . .

Some authors from the disability community argue that the societal effects of selective abortion for fetuses with disabilities may be comparable to the societal effects of sex selection, by enforcing stereotypes about people with disabilities and discrimination against them. They believe that in the future, developed nations will have millions of "missing people with disabilities," just as some Asian nations now have millions of missing women. This is highly unlikely. As developed societies age, there will be more, rather than fewer, people with disabilities, and societies will have to accommodate themselves further to disability. It can be argued, however, that society regards older people with disabilities differently from people who are disabled from birth. It is also likely that increased use of prenatal diagnosis will lead to the births of fewer children with particular types of disabilities that cause severe retardation or physical disability. A reduction in some disabilities will not have a negative effect on society or lead to discrimination. Societies do not need to worry about a loss of diversity. Enough children undergo sufficient trauma and malnutrition, before and after birth, to ensure that there will be plenty with disabilities. Society does not, and should not, mourn the disappearance of conditions that restrict life. Children no longer have rickets, because milk contains vitamin D; infants are no longer born with rubella syndrome (a major cause of deafness) because their mothers have been vaccinated. Developed societies do not regard themselves as having lost something valuable because these conditions have virtually disappeared. A society with only eight or nine women to every 10 men, however, is affected by this imbalance in most aspects of economic and social life. Even if there is no gender imbalance, children growing up with the knowledge that they or their peers may have been selected on the basis of sex may feel pressured to conform to the gender stereotypes for which they were selected.

McCullough and Chervenak (1994) claim that all arguments against sex selection are based on the assumption that the fetus is a person or has "independent moral status" (p. 210). None of the arguments above, whether for or against sex selection, requires this assumption. The societal effect, not the status of the fetus, is the strongest argument against sex selection. Although McCullough and Chervenak regard societal effects as "purely speculative," declining sex ratios of women to men in many parts of the world (Sen, 1990) have hindered, rather than helped, women's advancement. These authors claim that withholding prenatal diagnosis for sex selection ignores parental autonomy and denies the possibility that there may be ethically justifiable reasons for sex selection, reasons which they do not elaborate. Like some authors from the disability rights community, they deny a distinction between abortion for fetal disease or anomaly and abortion for sex, but they appear to base their reasoning totally on individual autonomy, like many of the survey respondents who would perform prenatal diagnosis for sex selection. We have dealt with some of these arguments above. In doing so, we also reaffirm that the goal of genetic medicine is to ameliorate or prevent circumscription of lives. It is difficult to understand how sex selection fulfills this goal. This is

perhaps what respondents meant when they said "sex is not a disease."

It is time to reconsider whether there should be limits to client autonomy and professional nondirectiveness. Many genetics professionals would like to draw a line against sex selection but find it difficult to act as gatekeepers on their own in an autonomy-based climate. The majority in most nations (except the United States) thought that there should be laws against sex selection. Laws would presumably help them act as gatekeepers without appearing paternalistic in the professional–patient relationship.

The benefits and harms of law depend on the cultural situation. In nations where sex selection against female fetuses is a social problem, such as China and India, law has at least the symbolic virtue of reaffirming the equality of women, even if the law is not always enforced. Sex selection laws are not the answer to the problem of the millions of missing women in such nations, however, or to the equality of women in general.

In nations where sex selection is not regarded as a social problem, the harms and benefits of laws will depend upon the legal and cultural approaches to abortion in general. In nations where abortion is already forbidden except to save the mother's life or for rape, as in most of Latin America, laws against sex selection could be redundant, and also ineffective. The widespread practice of (illegal) abortion in many such countries has led to disregard of overly restrictive laws. On the other hand, in nations where abortion on request is permitted and anti-abortion groups are not a political force (as in some parts of Europe), laws against sex selection, although limiting freedom of choice, would not necessarily lead to other restrictions on abortion. In countries where abortion rights are threatened, such as the United States, laws against sex selection could be an opening wedge for anti-abortion forces and could lead to laws restricting abortions for some genetic disorders or to laws against abortion in general. Overall, law could be a dangerous solution in most nations.

An alternative solution would be for professionals to review their perspective on paternalism. Although the word has earned negative connotations, especially among feminists, in bioethics paternalism may also have the positive meaning of exercising care and of withholding services that may be harmful. Professionals do not have to honor patient requests that are unnecessary (e.g. a request for penicillin for a cold) or harmful (e.g. a parent's request to test a child for a genetic disorder that may occur in later life but cannot be prevented). Sex selection is not a medical service, and physicians do not have to honor requests or offer referrals.

In the long run, however, the best approach would be to work toward equality of the sexes and against gender stereotyping, including the stereotyping of fetuses, and to establish a moral climate against sex selection of any kind. In those developing nations where sex selection has become a social problem, long-range solutions are education for women and equality in the workforce. Societies generally place a higher value on women if their work is recognized as productive, which usually means work outside the home, if they have some economic rights, including rights to inherit property, and if there is an awareness of the social changes necessary to overcome inequalities (Sen, 1990). In developing nations, women's longevity and the ratio of women to men are in direct parallel with women's participation in the workforce.

REFERENCES

Asch, A. and Geller, G. (1996) Feminism, bioethics, and genetics. In *Feminism and Bioethics: Beyond Reproduc-tion*, ed. Susan M. Wolf, pp. 318–350. Oxford University Press, New York.

Canadian College of Medical Geneticists (1986) *Professional and Ethical Guidelines.* Canadian College, Ottawa, Canada.

Fraser, F. C. and Pressor, C. (1977) Attitudes of counselors in relation to prenatal sex determination for choice of sex. In *Genetic Counseling*, eds H. A. Lubs and F. de la Cruz, pp. 109–120. Raven Press, New York.

Harvey, D. (1990) *The Condition of Postmodernity.* Blackwell, Cambridge, MA.

Kitcher, P. (1996) *The Lives to Come: The Genetic Revolution and Human Possibilities.* Simon and Schuster, New York.

McCullough, L. B. and Chervenak, F. A. (1994) *Ethics in Obstetrics and Gynecology.* Oxford University Press, New York.

National Society of Genetic Counselors (1992) *Code of ethics. Journal of Genetic Counseling* 1(1), 41–44.

Pencarinha, D. F., Bell, N. K., Edwards, J. G. and Best, R. G. (1992) Ethical issues in genetic counseling: a comparison of M. S. counselor and medical geneticist perspectives regarding ethical issues in medical genetics. *Journal of Genetic Counseling* 1(1), 19–30.

Sen, A. (1990) More than 100 million women are missing. *New York Review of Books* 20, 61–66.

United Nations (1991) *The World's Women, 1970–1990: Trends and Statistics.* United Nations, New York.

Wertz, D. C. and Fletcher, J. C. (1989) *Ethics and Human Genetics: A Cross-Cultural Perspective.* Springer, Heidelberg.

Wertz, D. C., Fletcher, J. C. and Mulvihill, J. J. (1990) Medical geneticists confront ethical dilemmas: cross-cultural comparisons among 18 nations. *American Journal of Human Genetics* 46, 1200–1213.

QUESTIONS FOR COMPREHENSION AND REFLECTION

1. Compare and contrast the moral issues raised by elective abortion with those raised by selective abortion. Can one rationally oppose abortion for sex selection while supporting abortion on demand? Explain.
2. Wertz and Fletcher argue that the principle of relief or prevention of suffering justifies prenatal diagnosis for genetic disease, but not for sex selection. However, according to the United Nations, in many countries unwanted girls suffer terribly from neglect and abuse. In contrast, studies show that the widespread belief that people with genetic disorders would rather never have been born is false. Discuss the impact of these findings on Wertz and Fletcher's argument.
3. Wertz and Fletcher argue that, unlike genetic diseases, "sex is not a disease." What

do they mean by this? Using examples such as being mentally retarded, nearsighted, blind, obese, prone to depression, confined to a wheelchair, or gay, discuss what is meant by "disease." What is the relation between being abnormal and being diseased? Is genius a disease because it is abnormal? Discuss what role, if any, social discrimination plays in our definition of what is and what is not a disease. Relate your answer to the moral permissibility of using selective abortion to weed out fetuses with socially undesirable characteristics, including physical and mental disabilities.

FRANK A. CHERVENAK
AND LAURENCE B. McCULLOUGH

Justified Limits on Refusing Intervention

Frank Chervenak is a professor and director of the Division of Maternal-Fetal Medicine at New York Presbyterian Hospital, Cornell Medical College. Laurence B. McCullough is a professor at the Center for Ethics, Medicine, and Public Issues at Baylor College of Medicine in Houston, Texas. Chervenak and McCullough argue that autonomy gives a person a negative right to noninterference if no one else is harmed by the decision. However, in the case of fetal therapy, if a cesarean section will in all likelihood benefit both the fetus and the woman, paternalism based on beneficence may override a woman's refusal of medical intervention.

Respect for the autonomy of the patient is a dominant ethical principle in the literature on biomedical ethics, particularly in the literature on refusal of medical intervention by competent or apparently competent patients. There seems to be a near uniform consensus that refusal of surgical management of a gangrenous toe, religiously based refusal of blood products to manage shock, and refusal of cesarean delivery to manage complete placenta previa should always be respected. This consensus rests on the underlying view that refusal of medical intervention is simply an instance of the general negative right to be left alone, i.e., a negative right to noninterference in the autonomous management of the affairs of one's life when no else is being harmed. We challenge this assumption and argue that "refusal" of medical intervention, in cases where the individual is not refusing any longer to be a patient, is not simply refusal, but refusal that is necessarily combined with an implicit demand for alternative medical management. That is, refusal of medical intervention is a complex moral phenomenon because it involves both a negative right to noninterference and a positive right to alternative treatment. Because a positive right is involved, the issue of ethically justified limits on patients' refusal of medical intervention must be addressed. We undertake that task in this paper, focusing on the example of well-documented, complete placenta previa.*

NEGATIVE AND POSITIVE RIGHTS

Refusal of medical intervention is a negative right *simpliciter* when the refusal of medical intervention takes the form of refusing any longer to be a patient. In such cases, to respect the patient's refusal, that individual's physician need only do nothing. Thus, when the competent patient, for example, discharges him- or herself from the hospital against medical advice, he or she is asserting the negative right to be left alone by his or her hospital physician.

When a patient refuses medical intervention, but does not withdraw from the role of being a patient, matters are more complex. . . . A pregnant woman who in the intrapartum period refuses cesarean delivery for a well-documented, complete placenta previa in favor of vaginal delivery is exercising a negative right not to have surgery and a positive right to medical management of the only other alternative, vaginal delivery. Finally, a patient with terminal disease who refuses aggressive management of the disease process but wants aggressive management of pain and suffering while he or she is dying is also exercising a combination of negative and positive rights.

A negative right is usually understood in ethics as a right of noninterference in decisionmaking and behavior. A negative right therefore generates duties on the part of others to leave the individual in question alone. In law, the rights to privacy and to self-determination, both pertinent to medical decisionmaking by patients, are negative rights not to be subject to nonconsensual bodily invasion. By

*By well-documented, complete placenta previa we mean the following: transabdominal or transvaginal ultrasound examination is performed by individuals competent in the technique and interpretation of its results and the placenta is clearly visualized on ultrasound examination to cover the cervical os completely. To maximize reliability, ultrasound examination should be performed shortly before delivery.

contrast, positive rights involve a claim on the resources of others to have some need, desire, or want met. Such rights obligate others to act in specified ways in response, as illustrated in the above examples. As a rule, positive rights are in all cases understood to be liable to limits by their very nature. This feature of positive rights contrasts sharply with negative rights, for which the burden of proof is on others to establish limits (for example, on the basis of preventing serious harm to innocent others). In most cases there is no need to place limits on refusal of medical intervention that involves both negative and positive rights, because the alternative demanded by the positive right is reasonable from a clinical perspective. This will be the case when that alternative is consistent with promoting the interests of the patient construed on a beneficence model.

THE BENEFICENCE MODEL

The beneficence model makes a peculiar claim: to interpret reliably the interests of any patient from medicine's perspective. This perspective is provided by accumulated scientific research, clinical experience, and reasoned responses to uncertainty. It is thus not a perspective peculiar or idiosyncratic to any particular physician.

On the basis of this perspective, the beneficence model identifies the goods relevant to the application of the principle of beneficence in clinical practice. These goods are those, among the many valued by human beings, that medicine is competent to seek on our behalf: the prevention of unnecessary death (death that can be prevented at reasonable rates of morbidity), and the prevention, cure, or at least management of morbidity, which can take the form of disease, injury, handicap, or unnecessary pain and suffering. Pain and suffering become unnecessary when they do not result in achievement of the other goods of the beneficence model. . . .

Rarely, the positive right for an alternative medical intervention is justifiably understood to be unreasonable because it is altogether inconsistent with promoting the interests of the patient as construed in the beneficence model. This occurs when the positive right is exercised on behalf of an alternative that, in Joel Feinberg's terms, "dooms" or virtually "dooms" the patient's medical interests and there is some reasonable, ready-to-hand alternative that promotes those interests. . . .

This would seem the case for refusal of cesarean delivery for well-documented, complete placenta previa. Vaginal delivery, with its staggering mortality rate for the fetus and very high mortality rate for the pregnant woman, would appear to doom or virtually doom the interests of both, while cesarean delivery, by contrast, unambiguously advances those interests. Vaginal delivery is therefore unreasonable from the perspective of a beneficence model.

CLINICAL JUDGMENT

This conclusion can be immediately challenged, given alleged uncertainty regarding the outcome of complete placenta previa. George J. Annas, among others, has argued that clinical prognostic judgment regarding complete placenta previa is subject to uncertainty, because there apparently have been a few exceptions to the prognosis for complete placenta previa. In two legal cases, complete placenta previa would appear either to have been misdiagnosed (in our view the most likely explanation) or to have spontaneously resolved. Neither of these, we want to emphasize, fits the definition of well-documented, complete placenta previa.

Those who plead uncertainty make a fundamental mistake. They hold clinical prognostic judgment to a standard of truth that it can never satisfy, namely, that it never turns out to be false in an individual case. On such a standard of truth, before the outcome actually occurs, all clinical prognostic judgments must be judged possibly false and therefore disabled by uncertainty. . . .

In our view, reliability of clinical judgment involves both the process of reaching a particular clinical judgment and the data upon which that judgment is based. In the first respect, a clinical judgment is reliable when it would most likely be made again by a second competent, rigorous judger given the same data as the original judger. In the second respect, a clinical judgment is reliable when the data upon which it is based do not vary and are not expected to vary. . . .

. . . [T]he clinician needs to realize that prognostic clinical judgment is not about individual cases but about the natural history of a particular disease under different management strategies. Thus, if an outcome of very rare incidence happens to occur, this does not mean that the prior prognostic judgment that the most common event would be the most likely outcome was wrong. In particular, given that spontaneous resolution of well-documented, complete placenta previa diagnosed in the intrapartum period is at best an extremely rare event, the clinician who makes a recommendation for cesarean delivery on this basis is making a reliable clinical judgment. He or she is not wrong if an extremely unlikely spontaneous resolution happens to occur.

. . . [T]o say nonetheless that clinicians can be and often are wrong in their clinical prognostic judgments only makes sense if one is employing the clinical instrument medical students fondly dub the "retrospectroscope." It has a wonderful feature: it is always crystal clear. It also has an unfortunate feature: its findings always come too late. . . .

This analysis of the reliability of prognostic clinical judgment is crucial for our example of well-documented, complete placenta previa. First, spontaneous resolution of the condition or an erroneous diagnosis are highly unlikely. Second, the outcome of vaginal delivery for the fetus is that there is a very substantial risk, approaching certainty, of death. Third, the outcome of cesarean delivery for the pregnant woman vis-à-vis vaginal delivery is a dramatic reduction of risk of mortality.

Can the clinician say unconditionally that the fetus will not survive vaginal delivery? No. However, the issue for prognostic clinical judgment is its reliability, not its truth. The ethical issue regarding reliability here is this: Can any clinician competently claim to have documented evidence of a significant rate of fetal survival from vaginal delivery? No. Indeed, such a claim would properly be regarded as an irrational basis for obstetric management. Moreover, to study the question via a randomized clinical trial would be judged unethical by any IRB asked to review such a proposal, given the grave risk to fetuses in the vaginal delivery arm of such a clinical trial. The clinician is correct to conclude that the only obstetric management strategy consistent with promoting the interests of the fetus is cesarean delivery, because vaginal delivery dooms the beneficence-based interests of the fetus, while cesarean delivery does the opposite.

With regard to the pregnant woman's interests, the reliability of prognostic clinical judgment here means that any clinical judgment that well-documented, complete placenta previa is most likely self-limiting and most likely to resolve spontaneously is unfounded and probably irrational. The only rational assumption to make is that vaginal delivery places the pregnant woman at grave risk for exsanguination. . . .

Should bleeding occur, massive blood replacement may save some women. However, this intervention may not be sufficient to prevent maternal death. In addition, there are significant risks of morbidity and mortality associated with massive blood transfusion, risks that greatly exceed those of cesarean delivery. Here again, no one would seriously propose that studying this issue via a clinical trial is ethically justified, because the maternal risks are so well defined.

The upshot of this analysis of reliability is that vaginal delivery carries grave risks of maternal mortality that can only infrequently be managed successfully. By comparison, cesarean delivery, despite its morbidity and mortality risks for the woman and despite its invasiveness, unequivocally produces net medical benefit for the pregnant woman. Any clinical judgment to the contrary borders on the irrational and cannot, therefore, be consistent with promoting the beneficence-based interests of the woman. The clinician who recommends cesarean delivery to protect the pregnant woman is making a recommendation with the highest reliability that can be applied to clinical judgment: No competent, rigorous clinician will undertake her management on the basis of a clinical judgment of expected spontaneous resolution, because doing so will virtually doom the pregnant woman's beneficence-based interests.

The ethical implications of this level of reliability of clinical judgment and of refusal of cesarean delivery are the following: (1) no physician is justified in accepting such a refusal because doing so would be based on unreliable clinical judgment; and (2) the physician is justified in resisting a patient's exercise of a positive right when fulfilling that positive right contradicts the most highly reliable clinical judgment, dooms the beneficence-based interests of the fetus, and virtually dooms the beneficence-based interests of the pregnant woman. Patients do not have a positive ethical right to obligate physicians to practice medicine in ways that are patently inconsistent with the most reliable clinical judgment.

PREVENTIVE ETHICS

The primary response to unreasonable assertions of positive rights that are embedded in refusals of medical intervention should be the strategies of preventive ethics. The goal of these strategies is to explain to the patient why the positive right is unreasonable from a clinical perspective. This is best accomplished by informed consent as an ongoing dialogue with the patient, with special attention to adequate disclosure and to the values the physician and the pregnant woman hold in common for her pregnancy. . . . The informed consent process should also invite the pregnant woman to assess this information in terms of her values and beliefs. These values in turn serve as the basis for negotiation with the pregnant woman, as well as for respectful persuasion, which takes the form of showing how a beneficence-based clinical perspective on her interests and those of her fetus is consistent with the pregnant woman's values. This process should be open to the possibility that the pregnant woman may want to seek second opinions or even consider switching physicians. In short, informed consent as an ongoing process is a crucial autonomy-enhancing clinical tool within the strategy of preventive ethics. Provided that they are utilized in a noncoercive fashion, ethics committees can also play a useful role in conflict resolution.

COURT-ORDERED INTERVENTION

Strategies of preventive ethics will sometimes fail. Is it ever justified to seek court orders to override a patient's negative right not to be subjected to non-consensual bodily invasion when this negative right is exercised in conjunction with an unreasonable positive right? Consider again the example of well-documented, complete placenta previa.

... First, we consider [the] claim that court-ordered cesarean delivery necessarily treats the pregnant woman solely as an instrument or means by which the fetus is benefitted, but by which she is not benefitted at all, being instead only placed at risk. ... court orders treat the pregnant woman as a "mere means" to benefit her fetus. To defeat this objection, we must show that forced cesarean delivery does indeed benefit the pregnant woman.

Cesarean delivery produces significant benefit for the pregnant woman (the dramatic reduction in maternal mortality risks), and significant benefit for the fetus (essentially complete elimination of risks of fetal mortality). Cesarean delivery for well-documented, complete placenta previa produces two *causally independent* effects: benefit for the pregnant woman and benefit for the fetus. Both of these promote beneficence-based interests. Thus, the pregnant woman is not a "mere means" to the benefit of the fetus, in the sense that benefit to her is not considered relevant. Instead, she is an end and is in no way whatever reduced to being simply a "fetal container." ... The pregnant woman is, and remains throughout the procedure, a patient in her own right, a status that is never compromised, because her medical interests are promoted.

The preceding is not meant to imply that cesarean delivery is risk-free. To the contrary, because it is major abdominal surgery, it does entail risks (albeit small and usually manageable) of morbidity and rare incidence of mortality. The key feature in the present context of cesarean delivery for well-documented, complete placenta previa is that its *net effect* for the pregnant woman is to produce

benefit. Because the risks involved in cesarean delivery are a means to benefit the pregnant woman, while at the same time benefiting the fetus, the pregnant woman is not a "mere means" for benefiting the fetus. ...

[The] next objection is that forced cesarean delivery treats pregnant women as a "means merely." That is, her autonomy, her negative right against bodily invasion, is violated without sufficient justification. This objection can be defeated by establishing that the pregnant woman is ethically obligated to accept cesarean delivery for the management of well-documented, complete placenta previa. If this is the case, her autonomy is already constrained and no new constraint is introduced by forced cesarean delivery.

We have argued elsewhere that the pregnant woman, in a pregnancy being taken to term, is ethically obligated to accept reasonable risks on behalf of the fetus in the management of her pregnancy. ... If this view is reasonable in obstetric ethics, then it is all the more reasonable to hold that the pregnant woman is ethically obligated to accept obstetric interventions that benefit the fetus *while also benefiting her*. If she is obligated to accept reasonable risks, she is surely obligated to accept well-documented benefits for herself. That is, her negative right is inherently subject to the limitation imposed by this obligation. This is different from the situation in which an unconditional negative right against nonconsensual bodily invasion exists.

The harm principle provides another justification for constraining autonomy in these cases. It is a well-understood tenet of ethical theory that an individual's exercise of rights, negative and positive, can justifiably be limited to prevent virtually certain, preventable, serious, and far-reaching harm to innocent others. This justification becomes even stronger when imposing such limits also benefits the individual subject to them.

On the basis of the above analysis, it can be shown that another ... objection fails, namely, that based on analogies to forced donation of tissue, such as bone marrow or one of a matched pair of solid organs. Just as courts have refused to order family members (more precisely, distant family members—namely, cousins) to donate tissue or organs, so too, . . . courts should not order cesarean deliveries.

At first glance, these analogies possess a powerful intuitive appeal. On closer examination, the appeal fails in the case of well-documented, complete placenta previa. In cases of tissue and organ transplantation, the donor is subject to significant harms: the risks of morbidity and mortality of the medical procedures, of hospitalization, and—in the case of organ donation—subsequent life without the donated organ, though he or she may derive some psychological benefits from being a donor. . . .

In contrast to organ donation and transplantation, cesarean delivery for well-documented, complete placenta previa produces clear-cut benefit for the pregnant woman (the posited analogue of the tissue or organ donor) and clear-cut benefit for the fetus (the posited analogue of the pediatric recipient of tissue or an organ). Indeed, there is no analogy in pediatric transplantation to cesarean delivery for well-documented, complete placenta previa. Hence, [the] objection to interference with the pregnant woman's negative right on this score fails.

. . . In the present context a belief on the part of the pregnant woman that vaginal delivery would be more beneficial for her or for her fetus than cesarean delivery is a matter of empirically very poorly founded belief, not a difference between two equally empirically valid opinions. . . . Fear of the cesarean delivery is, therefore, in all likelihood, an irrational fear. False beliefs and irrational fears are properly understood in bioethics not to be an expression of autonomy, but a factor that can significantly disable autonomy. Thus, neither demonstrably false belief nor irrational fear should be treated as expressions of autonomy. Rather, they should be addressed as obstacles to the exercise of autonomy via the strategies of preventive ethics. . . .

[There are] also . . . religious objections to forced cesarean delivery. Here we believe that there is an analogy that defeats [this objection]: parents' refusal, on religious grounds, of well-documented life-saving interventions for children who are patients. . . . [O]ne reason the courts are correct to protect patients from parental religious constraints is that no physical burden is imposed on the parents by a court order to treat their child. To be sure, cesarean delivery is invasive, major abdominal surgery. Yet in the case of well-documented, complete placenta previa invasiveness should not be the sole criterion for assessing physical burdens, because invasiveness in this case is not associated with net harm. To the contrary, it is associated with net benefit, because it dramatically reduces the risk of maternal mortality. . . .

We conclude with considerable trepidation that court orders are not unjustified when strategies for preventive ethics fail to alter refusal of cesarean delivery for well-documented, complete placenta previa. We want immediately to caution that our conclusions about this clinical example should not be extended to other clinical examples of unreasonable refusal without very careful analysis and argument, especially cases in which there is only one patient. These matters are beyond the scope of this paper, the purpose of which is to put forward for serious consideration a more nuanced analysis of refusal of medical intervention and the ethical obligations of physicians in response to them. . . .

QUESTIONS FOR COMPREHENSION AND REFLECTION

1. According to Chervenak and McCullough, under what conditions is medical intervention permitted on behalf of the fetus and the pregnant woman? Discuss the relative importance of negative and positive rights and the duty of beneficence in establishing the justifiable limits of intervention.
2. Compare and contrast the positions of Warren and of Chervenak and McCullough regarding the right of a pregnant woman to refuse intervention. How would Chervenak and McCullough most likely respond to the example in Warren's article on page 215–216? Who presents the stronger arguments? Support your answers.

3. Discuss what Chervenak and McCullough would most likely think about the morality of using court orders to restrain or mandate treatment for pregnant women who abuse drugs and alcohol.

CASES FOR ANALYSIS*

1. The Unwanted Daughters

Chandra and Ramdas Malik are poor farmers who live in a village outside Bombay. They have one son and one daughter. While they would welcome another son, they do not want another daughter because raising a dowry for her future husband's family would be financially crippling for them. In India, minivans carrying ultrasound equipment cruise the countryside providing prenatal diagnosis of the sex of fetuses. Although the price is high, it is worth it to the Maliks.[91] "Better 800 rupees now for an abortion," Ramdas Malik explains, "than tens of thousands of rupees later for a dowry." The ultrasound operator tells them that the child is a boy. They let out a sigh of relief.

Chandra Malik's cousin Indira migrated in 1979 to Canada, where she met and married a successful engineer, John Sarava, whose grandparents had immigrated to Canada from India. With her son and daughter in high school, Indira Sarava returns to college for an MBA. In her first semester, she finds out she is pregnant. Because she is forty, she has amniocentesis at sixteen weeks to test for genetic disorders. The following week Dr. Lee calls her and says, "Congratulations. You're going to have a healthy baby girl!" Two weeks later, Indira Sarava calls Dr. Lee back and asks him to perform an abortion. She explains that she would have continued the pregnancy had the fetus been a boy; however, she is not interested in having another daughter. Her husband is opposed to the abortion. Having another daughter would not be a financial burden for the family, and because he is semiretired he is willing to do most of the child care.

DISCUSSION QUESTIONS

1. While the Maliks did not seek an abortion, they intended to do so if the fetus was a girl. What is the role of intention in moral responsibility? Is the use of prenatal diagnosis for sex selection morally justified? If it is morally irresponsible to obtain prenatal diagnosis for sex selection, does this create a moral obligation on the part of physicians administering prenatal diagnosis to withhold information about the gender of the fetus? Support your answers.
2. Would it have made a difference if the Maliks or Indira Sarava had requested an abortion because the amniocentesis revealed that their child had Down syndrome? What if the fetus had anencephaly or Patau syndrome? Support your answers.
3. Does the father have any rights when it comes to deciding whether or not a pregnancy should be terminated? Support your answer using the Sarava case.
4. Sometimes, because of the position of the fetus or material floating in the amniotic fluid, an ultrasound misdiagnoses the sex of the fetus. Much to the Maliks' dismay,

*Names and cases are fictional unless noted otherwise.

their much wanted son turns out to be a girl. They wrap the newborn in a rag and abandon her in a ditch beside the road. Is their action morally acceptable? Would your answer be different if the Saravas had done the same? Support your answers.

2. Selective Abortion and "The Criminal Gene"

Helen and Mark Fulman are overjoyed. After over seven years of trying, including two years of fertility treatments, Helen is pregnant with her first child. At four months, she undergoes a routine amniocentesis, since she is thirty-eight. The Fulmans' joy turns to consternation, however, when the tests reveal that the fetus, a boy, has an extra Y chromosome. Their physician suggests that, before making a decision about continuing or terminating the pregnancy, they talk to a geneticist and read about the syndrome.

The geneticist tells the Fulmans that symptoms of XYY syndrome tend to be mild and often go undiagnosed. Indeed, the frequency of XYY syndrome is about 1 in every 1,000 newborns. XYY males, she explains, are usually taller than average and have acne during adolescence. They may or may not have learning disabilities, lower-than-average intelligence, and behavior problems. They also tend to be easily frustrated and impulsive—traits that can lead to violent behavior. However, the geneticist points out, any violent behavior is usually aimed at objects and rarely results in bloodshed. After the interview, the Fulmans feel relieved and certain that they want to continue the pregnancy.

A few days later, Mark Fulman visits the city library, where he finds a series of articles on XYY syndrome in some medical journals and magazines from the late 1960s. According to one of these articles, aggressive criminals have a significantly higher incidence of XYY syndrome than the general population.[92] Other articles speculate that a "criminal gene" may be associated with XYY syndrome and recommend prenatal diagnosis and selective abortion to weed out "violent criminals." One of the Fulmans' best friends tells them about the science fiction movie *Alien*[3]. The Fulmans rent the video, which is about a decommissioned maximum-security correction facility on the planet Fiorina 161 for "double Y chromosome offenders." The movie depicts the men as violent, obscene, extremely dangerous, and not fit to live in human society. The Fulmans are alarmed and angry. They feel that the geneticist misled them, since she did not mention these studies. The following day, rather than risk giving birth to a violent criminal, Helen Fulman obtains an abortion.

DISCUSSION QUESTIONS

1. For a short period in the late 1960s, infant boys were tested after birth for XYY syndrome. Testing was stopped, however, because parents who knew that their sons had XYY syndrome came to expect aggressive behavior and to interpret any acts of aggression on the part of their sons as pathological, thus creating a self-fulfilling prophecy. Should testing be recontinued? Do parents have a right to know if their son has an extra Y chromosome? Support your answers, using both utilitarian theory and rights ethics in your analysis.
2. The geneticist correctly portrayed XYY syndrome. However, she did not mention the earlier studies, which have since been shown to be misleading. Should she have mentioned these earlier studies to the Fulmans? How should the geneticist have handled her disclosure of information to the Fulmans? Support your answers.

3. Discuss whether physicians and medical organizations have a moral responsibility to issue disclaimers when a stereotype is initially perpetuated by the medical profession itself. If so, how should they carry out this moral responsibility? Did the producers of *Alien*[3] act morally irresponsible in making the movie? How should the medical profession have responded to the film *Alien*[3]? Support your answers.

4. Imagine that you are the physician in this case and the Fulmers have told you they would have an abortion only if the child had a severe and debilitating disorder. Clearly, XYY syndrome does not fall into this category. Should you tell them about your finding? Discuss your answer in light of the principles of autonomy and nonmaleficence.

5. Would abortion be justified in this case if the fetus had Down syndrome instead of XYY syndrome? Support your answer.

3. Date Rape and Abortion

Lisa, an eighteen-year-old high school honor student, attends a fraternity party with her nineteen-year-old boyfriend, Derek, a college sophomore. Derek and his roommate have already started drinking when Lisa arrives. Lisa says she is not interested in drinking. "Come on," her boyfriend chides her, "don't be such a baby." Lisa reluctantly agrees to join them. After a few drinks, she becomes tipsy and lies down on Derek's bed. Derek's roommate winks and tells him "Go for it." Then he leaves the room. Shortly after, Derek has sex with Lisa. Drunk as she is, Lisa neither consents nor protests.

The next morning, Lisa deeply regrets what has happened. She tells her boyfriend that she is worried she might be pregnant. He gives her the name of an out-of-town doctor and assures her that the doctor "will take care of everything." Lisa goes to the doctor, who gives her a "morning-after pill" and also suggests, because of the circumstances, that she consider seeing a rape crisis counselor. Lisa, however, doesn't tell anyone else what has happened, nor does she keep her follow-up appointment to determine if the morning-after pill has been successful.

When her periods don't return and she begins putting on weight, she dismisses the changes as the effects of stress and the morning-after pill. After all, she reassures herself, she couldn't be pregnant, since she took the morning-after pill and hasn't had sex since the fraternity party. Six months after the incident, she goes to the doctor for what she thinks are stomach problems or possibly a tumor. After examining her, the doctor tells her that she is six months pregnant.

DISCUSSION QUESTIONS

1. A disproportionate number of late abortions are performed on teenagers, since many teens do not recognize the early signs of pregnancy. Would a late-term, partial-birth abortion be morally justified in Lisa's case? State why or why not.

2. Is this a case of rape? Is the answer to this question relevant to whether or not the abortion is morally permissible? Support your answers.

3. Discuss the morality of abortion in this case in light of the arguments presented by Judith Jarvis Thomson in Chapter 2.

4. Discuss the responsibility, if any, of the other people involved in this case. Was the fact that Lisa's boyfriend was also drunk morally relevant? Should he have to pay for

or share Lisa's medical expenses? Should he be compelled to provide support for the child if Lisa decides not to have a late-term abortion? To what extent is the college or fraternity responsible for what happened? Does either owe Lisa a duty of reparation? Support your answers.

5. Discuss the responsibility of the physician in this case. Did the physician have a moral obligation to follow up on Lisa after giving her the morning-after pill? What if Lisa had refused to keep the follow-up appointment? Should the doctor recommend a partial-birth abortion? What if the doctor is opposed to late-term abortions? If Lisa were under eighteen, should the physician contact her parents?

4. Aborting for Fetal Tissue

Fran and Luigi DiLuca and their three children, ages two months, four years, and six years, were coming home from a play at their daughter's school when they were struck by a drunk driver running a red light. Baby Tony, whose car seat was on the side of the car that was struck, suffered severe internal damage. Although death was not imminent, Tony would eventually need organ transplants if he was to survive. However, because he had a rare blood type, no organs were available that matched his profile and it seemed unlikely that any would be available anytime soon. After reading about the use of fetal organs for transplants, the DiLucas approached the doctor with the suggestion that they attempt to get pregnant with a fetus with a compatible blood type so the needed organs could be harvested from the fetus. If early prenatal diagnosis revealed that the fetus's blood type was incompatible, they would abort it and try again.

DISCUSSION QUESTIONS

1. If you were the physician, how would you respond to the DiLucas' request? Support your answer.
2. The first two pregnancies resulted in fetuses with incompatible blood types. By now, baby Tony's chances of surviving the next six months are less than 50 percent. Should they try again? Support your answer.
3. According to a study at the University of Toronto's Centre for Bioethics, there is a 17 percent higher likelihood that women will have an abortion if they think it will derive an altruistic benefit from the donation of fetal tissue to research.[93] Discuss the moral relevance of this finding for legalizing fetal tissue donation.

5. Fetal Alcohol Syndrome

Sue Egert of Altamonte Springs, Florida, has two adopted sons with fetal alcohol syndrome (FAS). Her fourteen-year-old son, Sam, has had fifty-five surgeries to repair damage related to FAS, including a heart defect, digestive problems, seizures, and a cleft palate. He is also mentally retarded. "It's a tough row to hoe," says Egert. "This is a very hard disability to live with. . . . If you're going to drink and be pregnant, you'd better be ready for a lifetime of this."[94]

Sam's biological mother comes from a family of alcoholics. She began drinking at the age of nine and gave birth to ten children, all of whom had severe disabilities stemming from exposure to alcohol in the womb. Only two of the children, including Sam, were still alive at the time of their mother's death at the age of thirty-four.

DISCUSSION QUESTIONS

1. Should pregnant women who continue drinking, like Sam's mother, be restricted or monitored? Should child abuse laws be extended to cover the same type of abuses to fetuses? For example, parents who coerce their children into drinking alcohol on a regular basis can be penalized under child abuse laws. Support your answers.

2. Does the fetus have a right not to be harmed, or does the same autonomy that gives women the right to have an abortion give them the right to use alcohol? Do other citizens have a moral obligation to support children like Sam through taxes if their mother refuses support? What are Sam's rights in this case?

3. Should women who have already had children and continue to drink be sterilized or put on contraceptives, such as a five-year implant, until they change their behavior? Support your answer.

4. Does the quality-of-life argument create a moral obligation for Sam's mother to have an abortion? Should alcoholic or drug-addicted women who have no intention of keeping their children be compelled to have abortions? If not, does the state have a right to take their children from them after birth? Should the mother be held responsible for the harms done to Sam, even though she decides not to raise him? Support your answers.

6. Partial-Birth Abortion[95]

Carla, a sixteen-year-old high school sophomore, had been dating Jack, a junior, for several months. When she became pregnant, she considered an abortion. She had already had an abortion when she was fourteen. However, Jack encouraged her to continue the pregnancy and boasted to his friends about his virility. Carla was flattered by the attention and assumed that they would get married once he completed high school and found a job. Carla's parents agreed to help take care of the baby while Carla finished school and, in fact, had already built an addition onto their house for the baby's room. However, when Carla was seven months pregnant, she discovered that Jack had been cheating on her and was seeing another girl in school. Distraught and angry, Carla went to a clinic, where she obtained a partial-birth abortion. Within three months, Carla had another boyfriend and was pregnant with his baby. Carla explained to her friends that she became pregnant with another man's baby in order to make Jack jealous and did not intend to actually have the baby.

DISCUSSION QUESTIONS

1. Many, if not most, of the women who have partial-birth abortions are teenagers. Most of the abortions, as in Carla's case, are elective.[96] Was the partial-birth abortion justified in Carla's case? Is the timing of the abortion morally relevant? Would the abortion have been justified if it had been obtained in the first trimester? Support your answers.

2. Examine the morality of abortion in this case in light of the various arguments, both for and against abortion, put forth in the chapter. Which arguments are strongest?

3. Should Carla's parents have been informed of her decision to have an abortion? Should they have had a say in whether or not she should have an abortion? Support your answers.

4. Many teenagers use abortion as a means of birth control. Is this morally acceptable? Why or why not? Is the fact that Carla was not using contraception when she got pregnant, and indeed did not intend to continue the latest pregnancy, morally relevant?

7. Religious Objections to Fetal Therapy

Amniocentesis reveals that Rachel's fetus has a rare metabolic disease. According to her doctor, there is a new form of genetic therapy available in which a gene can be introduced that will override the defective gene so the fetus will begin producing the missing enzyme. The therapy has been shown to be effective in more than 60 percent of cases. Without the therapy, the doctor informs her, the child will in all likelihood be born seriously mentally retarded. However, as a Christian Scientist, Rachel is opposed to surgical intervention as well as genetic tampering. She refuses to give permission for the surgery and instead decides to pray for the baby's well-being. The hospital decides to take the case to court.

DISCUSSION QUESTIONS

1. Discuss whether Rachel is morally justified in refusing the surgery. Under what circumstances are pregnant women justified in refusing surgical intervention to benefit their fetus? Does the fetus have any rights if the mother is planning to carry the pregnancy to term? Support your answers.
2. Discuss how you would respond if you were Rachel's physician. Should the hospital take the case to court? Support your answers.
3. Discuss how you would rule if you were the judge hearing this case. What morally relevant criteria are involved in your decision? Are religious beliefs morally relevant? Support your answers.
4. The hospital loses the case, and the child is born severely retarded. The hospital decides to take Rachel to court for wrongful birth, arguing that it is wrong to knowingly give birth to a child with a bleak prognosis and poor quality of life. According to the hospital, Rachel should have aborted the child if she was unwilling to have surgery performed. Rachel disagrees. She argues that it is God's will that the baby be mentally retarded and that she accepts and loves the baby the way he is. Is there such a thing as a life not worth living? Are there times when women ought to get an abortion? Discuss the merits of each side of the argument.

8. The Limits of Protest: Killing Abortion Providers and Bombing Clinics

In October 1998, obstetrician Dr. Barnett Slepain was killed in his home by a sniper's bullet. Dr. Slepain was one of only a handful of physicians in the Buffalo area who performed abortions. He was also the third abortion doctor killed in the United States since 1993. Several more have been wounded in the United States and Canada, often as the result of bomb attacks.

On January 16, 1997, for example, a bomb blast ripped through a family planning clinic in Atlanta, Georgia, sending terrified people scattering. An hour later another bomb went off in the building. Six people were injured. Windows in nearby buildings were blown out, and the clinic was left in ruins. President Clinton condemned the bombing as "a vile and malevolent act" of terrorism. "No one has the right to use violence in America to advance their own convictions over the rights of others."[97]

In 1999, a federal jury found that an antiabortion Internet site that posted "wanted" posters of physicians who performed abortions amounted to a hit list for terrorists. The Web site contained a list of abortion providers; those that had been killed were crossed out, while those who had been wounded were highlighted in gray. The defendants, who had defended their activities on First Amendment grounds, were ordered to pay damages of more than $100 million.[98]

DISCUSSION QUESTIONS

1. What are the limits of protest against what is seen as an unjust law? Discuss the morality of vandalism, harassment, stalking, the bombing of clinics, and causing injury to abortion providers as forms of protest.
2. Some of the protesters at the clinics compare abortion clinics to the Nazi death camps. Is this analogy accurate? If so, do we have a moral obligation to try to kill or incapacitate physicians who kill in the name of medicine? Support your answers.
3. Discuss Clinton's response to the Atlanta clinic bombing. Is violence ever justified as a means of achieving an end? Discuss how both a utilitarian and a Buddhist might answer this question.
4. In February 1997, the Supreme Court upheld a New York State law that established abortion clinic buffer zones banning antiabortion protesters from staging demonstrations within 15 feet of abortion clinic entrances. Antiabortion activists argue that this law restricts their freedom of speech, since it prevents them from having a one-on-one conversation or passing out leaflets to women entering the clinics. Discuss how a rights ethicist might respond to this argument.
5. Does the ruling against the owners of the antiabortion Internet site violate the defendants' right to freedom of speech? Compare and contrast this ruling with the case mentioned in question 4.

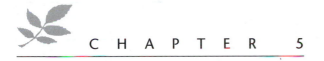

C H A P T E R 5

Genetic Engineering, Reproductive Technologies, and Cloning

It was one of the most controversial and startling birth announcements in history. On February 23, 1997, Ian Wilmut and a team of scientists at the Roslin Institute in Edinburgh, Scotland, announced to the world that they had created the first genetic clone of an adult mammal. The new arrival was a lamb called Dolly, reportedly named after Dolly Parton. To the untrained eye, Dolly looked like any other frolicking lamb. However, unlike any other mammal ever born, Dolly was created asexually from a single cell from her mother's udder. Dolly's genetic makeup was, for all practical purposes, identical to her mother's. Dolly's birth set off a flurry of debate over the morality of cloning humans. Unlike other types of reproductive technology, which require both an egg and a sperm, cloning would allow humans not only to reproduce asexually, but also to produce several identical copies of one **genotype,** the particular genetic makeup of an individual.

THE HISTORY OF EUGENICS

Until recently, humans created new offspring in the old-fashioned way. Our children may not have been perfect, but we accepted them, for the most part, as they were. However, the desire to improve humans through **genetic engineering,** the alteration of genetic material by artificial means, goes back at least to the time of Plato, who in his *Republic* proposed the use of selective breeding as a means of improving society.[1]

Eugenics

The term *eugenics* (from the Greek words for "good" and "birth") was coined in 1883 by scientist Francis Galton, a cousin of Charles Darwin, to describe the study of human improvement by genetic means. The purpose of **eugenics** programs is to systematically change the genetic makeup of a population. Positive eugenics attempts to maximize desirable genes through gene therapy or by encouraging "genetically superior" people

THE U.S. SUPREME COURT:
Buck v. Bell (1927)

In 1927, the Supreme Court in *Buck v. Bell* ruled, by a vote of eight to one, that the forced sterilization of Carrie Buck, a young woman in a Virginia mental hospital who was supposedly mentally retarded, was constitutional. Buck had been pregnant at the time of her commitment and had given birth to a daughter. Buck's mother was also deemed retarded. Justice Oliver Wendell Holmes wrote in the majority opinion: "Three generations of imbeciles are enough. . . . The principle that sustains compulsory vaccination is broad enough to cover the Fallopian tubes." The public good, he emphasized, outweighs the individual rights of the retarded to procreate.

to have children. Negative eugenics attempts to minimize what are considered undesirable genes through programs such as sterilization and prenatal diagnosis.

Positive eugenics, in the form of selective breeding, has been used for centuries for the improvement of agricultural crops and the creation of new breeds of domesticated animals. However, human genetic engineering has had a more checkered history, primarily because of its association with racist ideologies. This unfortunate development in the history of human eugenics has left the public suspicious of genetic engineering.

During the late nineteenth century, scientists and politicians in the United States became concerned that the Anglo-Saxon heritage of the United States, which was regarded as the genetic ideal, was being compromised because of increased immigration from southern and eastern Europe. The U.S. government used this concern to justify exclusionary immigration laws and compulsory sterilization laws. The Johnson Immigration Restriction Act of 1924 became the basis for refusing entry to thousands of Jewish refugees slated for extermination in Nazi concentration camps.

Mandatory Sterilization Laws

Some eugenicists encouraged sterilization of "genetically inferior" people, including criminals. Mandatory sterilization laws were established in the early twentieth century in several countries, including Sweden, Switzerland, Norway, Denmark, Germany, and the United States. These laws were justified primarily on utilitarian grounds. The Catholic Church, in contrast, forbids direct sterilization.[2]

In 1907, Indiana passed the first mandatory sterilization law in the United States. Over the next three decades, thirty-one other states enacted similar eugenic sterilization laws aimed mainly at habitual criminals, epileptics, the insane, and other groups of people deemed genetically defective.[3] During this time, up to 100,000 people were involuntarily sterilized in the United States.[4] About 25,000 Native American women were also sterilized, without their consent, at Indian Health Service clinics in a program that has been described as "a genocidal campaign waged by the U.S. government to rid itself of native people."[5] Hitler, an admirer of American eugenics, went one step further and undertook the eradication, rather than merely the sterilization, of "genetically defective" people.

Eugenics' Fall from Grace

Negative eugenics fell out of favor in the mid-twentieth century because of public reaction to the horrors of Nazism. Although the eugenics programs in the United States never reached the level of coerciveness and the magnitude of those in Nazi Germany, memories of the state-run programs of involuntary sterilization left Americans feeling uneasy when confronted by talk of genetic engineering. The goals of state-run programs of eugenics also conflicted with the emerging autonomy model in healthcare ethics and the belief in reproductive freedom and privacy. On the other hand, eugenics, properly used, has the potential to increase autonomy and reproductive freedom. In this chapter, we will use *eugenics* in the broader sense of the use of science and technology to improve the genetic quality of offspring.

THE RESURGENCE OF EUGENICS AND GENETIC ENGINEERING

While the term *eugenics* is rarely used nowadays, prenatal diagnosis, genetic screening, genetic therapy, and genetic enhancement are all examples of modern eugenics programs. Although the primary reason given for the use of many current technologies, especially prenatal diagnosis and genetic screening, is to prevent the birth of a child with serious genetic anomalies, this goal, considered in a wider social context, is eugenic. After what happened in the first half of the twentieth century, why is eugenics still alive and well?

In his 1970 landmark book *Fabricated Man: The Ethics of Genetic Control*, theologian Paul Ramsey suggested two primary reasons for the resurgence of interest in eugenics. First is the fear that the human gene pool is rapidly degenerating under the conditions of modern life. Second, scientific developments in genetics and reproductive technologies have vastly increased our ability to control our genetic future. Indeed, it is now possible to insert human genes into other species in order to create transgenic animals whose organs can be used for organ transplantation in humans.

The Deterioration of the Human Gene Pool

In addition to inherited deleterious genes, about 20 percent of people carry a deleterious mutation that can be passed on to offspring. Modern technology and medicine have done away with the natural selection process by keeping people who would otherwise have died in childhood alive through the age of reproduction. While we like to think that medicine is conquering disease, in fact, it is also making us weaker and more sickly as a species, since a greater number of deleterious genes are being passed on to future generations. For example, diabetics used to die at a young age; now that insulin can control diabetes, diabetics are living long enough to pass the gene for diabetes on to their children. We may also soon be able to correct congenital heart defects, one of the major causes of early death, simply by injecting a new gene into the heart. The new

INDIA:
Hinduism and Eugenics

In India, many marriages are still arranged by the parents on the basis of social, economic, and reproductive suitability. For example, prospective brides traditionally are closely inspected for ominous body markings. However, while the basis of Hindu marriage is, strictly speaking, eugenics, the Hindu concept of eugenics is very different from that in Western science. Members of lower, as well as higher, castes are encouraged to marry and procreate as long as they marry within their caste. The purpose of marriage and procreation is to ensure continuation of the family line and to retain caste separation, not to eliminate inferior castes.

Hinduism does not subscribe to a teleological Western view of progress toward a particular goal of evolutionary perfection. Creation instead occurs from moment to moment. Unlike Western eugenics, which seeks the elimination of what are considered in-ferior groups of humans in order to protect or enhance the integrity of the gene pool, Hinduism considers all castes necessary, with each occupying its place in the cosmos. Genes, as part of our karma, are passed down from generation to generation and from life to life. If a child with Down syndrome is aborted, the same individual, with the same affliction, will simply be reincarnated later.

On the other hand, karma has been used in the context of the Hindu caste system to justify appalling social injustices. For this reason, both Buddha and, later, Hindu philosopher Mahatma Gandhi, while accepting the concept of karma, rejected the Hindu caste system and taught that all humans deserve equal respect. The proper response to a person with a genetic disorder or a weak physical constitution is compassion rather than blame.

gene, however, will not be passed on to future generations. Some geneticists fear that someday the gene pool may degrade to such a point that the human race will not be able to survive without the support of technology. To avoid a genetic apocalypse, they argue, we need to take positive steps to prevent further deterioration of the gene pool.

Scientific Developments in Genetics and Reproductive Technologies

Scientific developments since World War II have vastly increased our ability to manipulate our genetic heritage. The impact of the genetic revolution, termed the second Copernican revolution, may be as great as that of the invention of written language.

One event that helped spark the genetic revolution was the 1953 discovery by James Watson and Francis Crick of the molecular structure of deoxyribonucleic acid (DNA), the key substance for transmitting genetic information. **DNA** is a double-helix molecule made up of four bases: adenosine (A), thymine (T), guanine (G), and cytosine (C). Each human cell, with the exception of germ (reproductive) cells, contains twenty-three pairs of **chromosomes** made up of about 6 billion base pairs of nucleotides that can be divided into roughly 100,000 sequences known as **genes.** There are also intervening sequences that have no known purpose. The first human genes were identified in the early 1970s. In 1985 and 1986, a series of scientific conferences regarding the feasibility of mapping the entire human genetic blueprint, or **genome,** led to the creation of the Human Genome Project (HGP).

Advances in reproductive technology have extended our capacity to manipulate the human genome. During the latter part of the twentieth century, reproductive technology focused primarily on the problems of infertility and on the prenatal diagnosis of birth defects. The development of amniocentesis in 1966 provided a method for diagnosing chromosomal and genetic disorders in the fetus. The birth of Louise Brown, the first "test-tube baby," in England in 1978 heralded a new era of reproductive technology and a paradigm shift in perspectives on human reproduction and genetics. The technique known as **in vitro fertilization** ("fertilization in glass") soon became a popular means of overcoming the problem of infertility and permitted couples who were unable to have children under normal conditions to become parents. Conception was no longer limited to the bedroom; it could now take place in a petri dish in a laboratory without the presence of either parent. The ability to control conception and early embryonic development in the laboratory makes it easier to genetically engineer children prior to conception or in the first few weeks after conception, and cloning technology has opened up the possibility of mass-producing desirable human genomes.

The Genetic Revolution and the Biotech Century

According to Jeremy Rifkin, economist and author of *The Biotech Century* (1998), we are entering a new age in which the biotechnology industries will reshape all aspects of our life. He predicts that genes will become the "green gold" of the biotech century as corporations, capitalizing on findings derived from the Human Genome Project, vie to gain control over and commercialize the gene pool. The genetic revolution will force us to rethink our very sense of self and what it means to be human, as well as our ideas about equality and society. The very concept of what we mean by life is being challenged. Gene pioneer J. Craig Venter hopes in the next few years to create the first synthetic life out of inanimate chemicals.[6] While this life-form will be a microbe, the success of this project will pave the way for the creation of more complex life, thus raising the question of whether scientists are usurping what some believe is God's role as creator of life.

International skittishness about genetic engineering is not limited to futuristic visions of synthetic life and genetically altered humans. In 1999, more than half of all the corn, soybean, and cotton acreage in the United States was planted with genetically engineered crops. The production of "Frankenstein foods" in the United States has caused an outcry in other countries. In Europe, regulators have blocked most shipments of genetically engineered food from the United States.[7]

THE HUMAN GENOME PROJECT (HGP)

The Guaymi Indians, a remote tribe in Panama, carry unique DNA material that stimulates the production of an antibody that scientists believe may be useful in research on AIDS and leukemia. In 1993, a researcher from the National Institutes of Health

(NIH), the primary funder of the Human Genome Project in the United States, developed a cell line from a blood sample taken from a Guaymi Indian woman. When the U.S. government sought both a U.S. and an international patent on the cell line, the Guaymi General Congress in Panama protested the patents. They argued that the NIH had violated their tribe's genetic privacy by trying to profit from their biological inheritance without advising the Guaymi of its intentions. Isidro Acosto, president of the congress, stated: "I never imagined people would patent plants and animals. It's fundamentally immoral, contrary to the Guaymi view of nature, and our place in it."[8]

An Overview of the HGP

Much of the current explosion in knowledge about genetics comes from the Human Genome Project, a fifteen-year international project to map the entire human genetic makeup. Mapping entails the assignment of genes to their specific location on a chromosome. The HGP officially got under way in the United States in 1990 under the direction of James Watson. Although France, Japan, and Germany are involved in the project, the bulk of the HGP is being carried out in the United States (over 60 percent of the work) and Great Britain (about 30 percent of the work).

As of April 6, 2000, 83 percent of the human genome has been completed. The project is ahead of schedule, and it is expected that the entire human genome will be mapped by 2003, if not earlier.[9] Although 5 percent of the money allocated to the Human Genome Project has been set aside for the study of the ethical, legal, and social implications (ELSI) of genome research and the new genetic technologies spawned by it, the rate of scientific progress has far exceeded that of progress in dealing with the ethical implications. How should the findings of the HGP be used? What do the research findings say about who we are as humans? What role do genes play in explaining our actions? Is there still room for free will?

The Human Genome Diversity Project (HGDP)

Although all humans have 99.9 percent of their DNA in common, almost all the work in human genome research has been done on people of European descent, thus ignoring genetic variations in the other 85 percent of the world population. The Human Genome Diversity Project (HGDP), an offshoot of the HGP, was established to expand the scope of genome research by collecting blood samples representing groups of isolated indigenous people. Scientists and biotech companies are scouting the world looking for rare genetic traits that may have future market potential.

The HGDP has created considerable controversy. Critics of the project dub it the "vampire project" because the researchers fly in, take blood, and then leave. Declarations against the project have been issued by indigenous communities in North America, Central and South America, Southeast Asia, and the South Pacific. In 1993, representatives of indigenous people from Japan, Australia, New Zealand, the Cook Islands, Fiji, India, Panama, Peru, the Philippines, Suriname, and the United States came together to produce the Mataatua Declaration on Cultural and Intellectual Property Rights of Indigenous People. The real purpose of the HGDP, they charge, is not inclusion of all people in the model human genome but the discovery of unique genetic traits, such as the gene from the Guaymi Indian woman in Panama, that might be medically and commercially useful.

THE MATAATUA DECLARATION ON CULTURAL AND INTELLECTUAL PROPERTY RIGHTS OF INDIGENOUS PEOPLES (1993)[10]

We

Declare that Indigenous Peoples of the world have the right to self-determination; and in exercising that right must be recognized as the exclusive owners of their cultural and intellectual property.

Acknowledge that Indigenous Peoples have a commonality of experiences relating to the exploitation of their cultural and intellectual property;

Affirm that the knowledge of the Indigenous Peoples of the world is of benefit to all humanity;

Recognize that Indigenous Peoples are capable of managing their traditional knowledge themselves, but are willing to offer it to all humanity provided their fundamental rights to define and control this knowledge are protected by the international community;

Insist that the first beneficiaries of indigenous knowledge (cultural and intellectual property rights) must be the direct indigenous descendants of such knowledge.

Declare that all forms of discrimination and exploitation of Indigenous Peoples, indigenous knowledge and indigenous cultural and intellectual property rights must cease . . .

Recommendations to Indigenous Peoples:

. . . A moratorium on any further commercialization of indigenous medicinal plants and human genetic material must be declared until indigenous communities have developed appropriate protective mechanisms.

Recommendations to the United Nations in Respect for the Rights of Indigenous Peoples; the United Nations Should:

. . . Call for an immediate halt to the ongoing Human Genome Diversity Project (HUGO) until its moral, ethical, socio-economic, physical and political implications have been thoroughly discussed, understood and approved by Indigenous Peoples.

Some indigenous people regard the HGDP as an extension of white colonialism that treats the bodies of indigenous people as commodities to be exploited. Feminists have criticized the HGDP as just another patriarchal project for dominating and exploiting the passive "other" (nature and humans who are not white males) for man's convenience, a dream of domination exemplified in the movie *Jurassic Park*.[11]

Supporters of the HGDP disagree. They maintain that the rights of indigenous people are being respected and that researchers have their informed consent. According to researchers, any genetic material they acquire as a result of their research has been freely offered as a gift.[12] They also claim that the patents resulting from applications of this genetic material have nothing to do with the actual research of the HGP or HGDP and that results of the research may be used someday to benefit indigenous people. Despite these arguments, there is little doubt that some scientists reap handsome profits as a result of their participation in the HGDP.

COMMERCIALIZATION OF THE HUMAN GENOME

In 1984, Alaskan businessman John Moore sued the University of California after he discovered that parts of his body had been patented, without his permission, and licensed to the Sandoz Pharmaceutical Corporation. A UCLA researcher and one of Moore's physicians, who was treating him for a rare form of cancer, discovered that Moore's spleen produced a blood protein that facilitates the growth of white blood cells, which could be valuable in developing a treatment for cancer. The university created a cell line from the cells produced by Moore's spleen and obtained a patent for their "invention." Moore sued, arguing that only he had a property right over his own body tissue. In 1990, the California Supreme Court, in a precedent-setting case, ruled against Moore, stating that people do not have a property right over their body tissues.

Gene Patents

The increasing corporate control over the human genome is a major contemporary moral issue. Gene patents give the holder a legal grant or the exclusive right to make, use, or sell particular sequences of DNA that form all or part of a gene or to sell that grant to others. Is it morally acceptable for private companies and individuals to patent segments of the human genome? Should human life be treated as a commodity or intellectual property?[13]

Religious leaders have called for a moratorium on gene patents on the grounds that genes are the creation of God and cannot be owned by humans. A similar philosophical argument states that human life, because it has intrinsic worth, cannot be reduced to a commodity to be sold and traded on the world market. Are gene patents, in fact, a violation of the sacredness or intrinsic worth of human life? Or is genetic material similar to bodily tissues such as blood and spleen cells, which already can be donated, sold, or claimed as property by researchers?

Some healthcare ethicists argue that gene patents violate the principle of autonomy, which requires that persons be free from unwanted interference by others. The patenting of genes, as in the Moore case, also violates individuals' privacy rights by claiming ownership over a part of another person's body.

On the other hand, it is not clear whether ownership of a process for manipulating a disembodied part of the human body is the same as ownership of a person. Moore, for example, initially was not even aware that a cell line had been created from his cells. Unlike practices such as mandatory sterilization, patenting a cell line from a person's cells does not, at least in any obvious way, interfere with the person's autonomy, since it does not impinge on future choices. Furthermore, it is not the person's body part that is being patented, but rather the cell line developed from it. Gene patents, however, may have the potential to dehumanize humans. Patents on lines of genetically engineered humans, for example, may be incompatible with respect for human autonomy.

Collective privacy, it has been argued, may also be violated by gene patenting, since patents give an individual or company ownership over what collectively belongs to all humans—the human genome, or, in the case of groups such as the Guaymi Indians, the genome of a particular community of people. Scientists cannot own what is already owned in common by people.

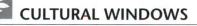

CULTURAL WINDOWS

NATIVE AMERICANS AND THE HGDP

There are approximately 2.5 million Native Americans from 515 different tribes. Despite their differences, Native Americans share a common and increasingly vocal opposition to the HGDP and gene patenting—an opposition rooted in a holistic worldview of "Mother Earth" and a belief in the sanctity of life. The biotechnological presumption that a person, or any part of a person, can be owned is inconsistent with this worldview.

In addition, many Native Americans see the HGDP as a continuation of the exploitation of Native Americans by the descendants of European colonists, "a history filled with deception and annihilation."[14] This sentiment is echoed by indigenous people throughout the world. Aroha Te Pareake Mead, a member of the Ngati Awa tribe in New Zealand, argues that the HGDP is an extension of white colonialism that treats the bodies of indigenous people as commodities to be exploited.

The removal of genetic material from a person for research into cell line development is also a serious violation of that person's dignity. ". . . many Indians believe that when they pass on, they must be buried whole. If any portion of their body is immortalized through cell lines, they will wander for-ever."[15] In many tribes, this belief extends to the person's favorite personal possessions.

Several Indian tribes have responded to the HGDP's 1997 Proposed Model Ethical Protocol for Collecting DNA Samples—which from their perspective is "the Whiteman's way of doing research in Indian communities"—with model protocols of their own.[16] The Akwesasne Model (also known as the Mohawk model), for example, addresses some of the same issues that were touched on in the 1993 Mataatua Declaration, such as empowerment of indigenous people, intellectual property rights, and disposition of the research data (see p. 255). The Navaho Nation, the Montana tribes, the Shoshone-Bannock in Idaho, and the Canadian First Nations are also in the process of developing protocols for genetic research.

The response of Native Americans to the HGDP underscores how important it is that both the HGP and the HGDP clearly communicate their objectives to indigenous people and obtain their informed consent and cooperation. Otherwise, the HGDP, rather than benefiting diverse groups, could further alienate indigenous people.

Informed Consent

John Moore's case also raises the issue of patient/physician confidentiality and informed consent. Did Moore's attending physician violate the physician/patient relationship by collaborating with researchers without Moore's informed consent? Questions about informed consent are also pertinent to the patenting of genes from isolated groups of indigenous people unfamiliar with Western medical science and economics as well as the English language.

In 1996, in another hotly controversial move, the United States issued a patent on the genetic code of a man from the remote Hagahai people in New Guinea whose DNA renders him immune to the HTLV virus that causes leukemia, thus making his DNA a veritable gold mine. Aroha Te Pareake Mead, a New Zealand Maori and spokesperson for indigenous groups, argues that this action was immoral because the Hagahai people were not able to understand the circumstances and thus were unable to give genuine informed consent for the use of their genetic material. What does informed consent require in situations in which there is a wide cultural and linguistic gap between the researchers and the subjects of the research?

Fairness and Distributive Justice

Gene patenting also raises questions of justice. Is it fair for the right to use certain gene sequences to be restricted to the patent holder, or is gene patenting a violation of distributive justice? Currently, over 90 percent of the research for the HGP is being carried out in the United States and Great Britain. Should rich nations, which can afford to finance this research, be allowed to control the benefits of the research, or should genetic information accrued from human genetic research be available to everyone, since it involves our collective genetic makeup? Is it fair to deny patents to researchers who have discovered and developed cell lines from these DNA segments? The United States is a staunch advocate of gene patenting. Other nations, including the countries of the European Union, take a more cautious stance. Allen Howard, Great Britain's science minister, has suggested that gene patenting should be replaced by an international agreement to govern rights in genome research.

Defenders of gene patents point out that scientists in virtually every other field of scientific research can patent their inventions or discoveries. From a utilitarian perspective, patents encourage initiative and progress by rewarding researchers for the time, effort, and risk they put into their work. Companies engaged in biotechnological research and development also rely on patents to protect their investments. Investors would not invest in genome research without the guarantee of patent protection and an expectation of profitable returns on their investment. Efficiency and the benefits derived from genetic research might also be sacrificed if patents are not allowed. Allowing scientists to patent the cell line from Moore's blood cells, for example, may in turn save many lives.

On the other hand, while patents protect global competitiveness in the marketplace, they inhibit the dissemination of information and stifle international collaboration on projects involving genome research. Can global competitiveness and international collaboration be reconciled, or are they incompatible goals? If they are incompatible, which goal is more important? How can these goals best be harmonized with respect for the rights and autonomy of both individuals and human communities?

GENETIC TESTING AND SCREENING

Congress funded the Human Genome Project in the United States with the hope that it would lead to cures for genetic diseases. Genetic disease extracts a high toll in terms of suffering and death and is the second leading cause of death among one- to four-year-olds in the United States. Between 25 and 30 percent of acute care hospital admissions

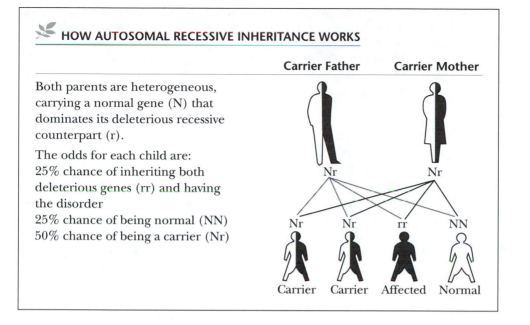

HOW AUTOSOMAL RECESSIVE INHERITANCE WORKS

Carrier Father　　**Carrier Mother**

Both parents are heterogeneous, carrying a normal gene (N) that dominates its deleterious recessive counterpart (r).

The odds for each child are:
25% chance of inheriting both deleterious genes (rr) and having the disorder
25% chance of being normal (NN)
50% chance of being a carrier (Nr)

Nr　　Nr

Nr　　Nr　　rr　　NN

Carrier　Carrier　Affected　Normal

for people eighteen and under are due to genetic disease.[17] While a plethora of new genetic tests have been developed as a result of the Human Genome Project, for most genetic diseases that can be identified the only intervention is abortion of an affected fetus.

Genetic Inheritance Patterns

Genetic disorders can be diagnosed either through direct observation of physical symptoms or through examination of the person's genotype, or particular combination of genes. Genes come in pairs, with one gene located in the same site on each of two corresponding chromosomes. Children receive one set of chromosomes, and thus genes, from each parent. If one gene of the pair is dominant and the other recessive, the dominant gene will generally be expressed in the **phenotype,** the physical appearance and makeup of an individual. Our phenotype is determined by both heredity and environmental factors. In some cases, a gene will be expressed only if environmental conditions are right. For example, the genetic contribution to schizophrenia is 50 to 70 percent, but the genetic contribution to bulimia is only 5 percent.[18]

Mendelian, or monogenic (one-gene), disorders are the most common type of inherited disorder. Genetic disorders can be divided into three categories: autosomal dominant disorders, autosomal recessive disorders, and X-linked disorders. The twenty-two pairs of chromosomes that males and females have in common are called autosomal chromosomes. Many genetic disorders, such as sickle cell disease, cystic fibrosis, and Tay-Sachs disease, are autosomal recessive disorders. The disorder will be expressed in the phenotype only if a child inherits the deleterious recessive gene from both parents—that is, if the child is homogeneous for the gene. Children who inherit only one recessive deleterious gene are known as carriers; they have a normal phenotype.

Some genetic disorders, such as Huntington's disease, are carried on dominant genes. In dominant autosomal disorders, people who are either heterogeneous (have two different genes) or homogeneous for the gene will manifest the disease in their phenotype. X- or sex-linked genetic disorders, such as hemophilia and Duchenne muscular dystrophy, are caused by genes on the X-chromosome. Because males have only one X-chromosome, genes on this chromosome will be expressed in their phenotype.

Reasons for Genetic Testing and Screening

Genetic testing is used to diagnose the presence of deleterious genes. The time may come when it will also be used to identify highly desirable genes, such as genes for musical or mathematical genius—assuming these are monogenic traits. Genetic testing is currently being used to diagnose (1) genes that will inevitably lead to disease, (2) genes that contribute to susceptibility to certain diseases, and (3) carrier status, in the case of deleterious recessive genes. Genetic screening involves testing groups or entire populations of people who are deemed to be at risk for a genetic disorder. Screening for carrier status is used primarily to inform prospective parents about the probability of their passing on deleterious genes to their children.

Multiplex genetic testing, or testing for several conditions simultaneously, is becoming increasingly common, in part because of the lucrative profits it provides to the biotech industry. Biotech companies are already offering testing by mail for cystic fibrosis and a few other disorders. Many healthcare ethicists are apprehensive about the deluge of genetic tests currently on the market.[19] While some genetic tests are more than 99 percent accurate, others yield high rates of false results, a problem compounded by multiplex genetic testing. Furthermore, many primary-care doctors are not knowledgeable in the field of genetics. In the United States, only 54 percent of physicians have had even a basic course in genetics.[20] People who receive positive results from genetic tests might suffer needless anxiety because of inaccurate results or misunderstandings about the test results. Counseling by trained geneticists, though desirable, is very costly and time-consuming, and the demand for their services currently far exceeds the availability.

Prenatal Genetic Testing

A private infertility clinic in Toronto offers embryo screening for twenty-seven genetic disorders, including Huntington's disease, cystic fibrosis, and sickle cell disease, for couples undergoing in vitro fertilization (IVF). For an additional $500 to $2,800, parents can have their preembryos screened for one or all of these disorders prior to implantation. "Defective" preembryos are killed, usually by washing them down a sink. Dr. Perry Phillips, director of the clinic, explains, "It is the job of medicine to alleviate suffering. The body makes mistakes and, with this screening, bad, bad things can be avoided. Parents who don't want to inflict this suffering on their children no longer need to." He compares the use of genetic testing to eliminate defective embryos to the use of antibiotics to eliminate bacterial disease. "The genetically-defective," he predicts, "may soon be regarded as relics of a barbarous age."[21]

Prenatal diagnosis is the most commonly used type of genetic testing. About 7 percent of infants in North America are born with physical and/or mental disorders of varying degrees of severity. Prenatal diagnosis provides direct information about many of these disorders, thus enabling prospective parents to make informed choices. Prenatal diagnosis can be used for individual at-risk fetuses or for screening. The Catholic Church permits prenatal diagnosis only if it is used to help the parents in "preparing to care for a child with genetic defects."[22]

In some states, newborn screening is mandatory for hereditary disorders such as phenylketonuria (PKU), congenital hypothyroidism, and sickle cell disease. In California, physicians are required to offer pregnant women screening tests for Down syndrome and neural tube defects. These mandatory programs are usually justified under paternalism as a means of saving children from future disease. On the other hand, the availability of prenatal genetic testing may result in parents being held responsible for the birth of a child with a genetic disorder. Some health insurance companies refuse to cover infants for genetic disorders, such as cystic fibrosis, that could have been diagnosed prenatally.

What Constitutes a Serious Genetic Disorder?

While many people assume that it is desirable to eliminate genetic disorders as a means of alleviating suffering, just what constitutes a serious genetic disorder is unclear. An international survey asked geneticists to place particular disorders in one of three categories: lethal, serious but not lethal, and not serious. The survey revealed that the same disorder could appear in any of the categories.[23]

What constitutes a disorder may become more broadly defined as more genetic tests become available. *Normality* is increasingly being defined in terms of genotype. Parents may soon be able to have their fetuses tested for genes that incline them to obesity, shortness, asthma, migraine headaches, alcoholism, depression, aggressiveness, Alzheimer's disease, dyslexia, and sexual orientation.

Research on the genetic origins of sexual orientation, in particular, has received much attention in the past few years. People who regard this research as unethical argue that the motivation to identify a "gay gene" betrays a homophobic bias, especially in light of continuing attempts to use therapy to change homosexuals' sexual orientation. If a test for prenatally diagnosing a predisposition toward homosexuality becomes available, should parents be allowed to use it as a prelude to selective abortion? Do geneticists have a moral obligation to withhold certain information from parents that they feel might be misused, such as the sex of a fetus or a genetic predisposition toward homosexuality?

When should genetic screening be used? Is it morally justified in cases of adoption or when donor sperm and eggs are used in infertility treatment? While screening will provide both parents and children with information that may be useful, it can also lead to discrimination against children who have certain genes. This discrimination may not be limited to genetic disease. In a homophobic society, infants and children who carry the "gay gene" may become unadoptable. What boundaries on individual autonomy do we want to set in the genetic age?

Nondirective Counseling and Eugenics

According to a study of 682 geneticists in nineteen nations, more than 92 percent of genetic counselors regard patient autonomy and nondirective counseling as a moral ideal. The primary purpose of genetic counseling is not eugenic but rather to inform patients of their options so they can make an informed choice. The counselor should not make decisions for patients or try to influence their decisions. At the same time, there is a tacit assumption that nondirective counseling and patient autonomy are consistent with a eugenic goal. Seventy-four percent of the geneticists surveyed also stated that "the improvement of the general health and vigor of the population is important," and 54 percent supported the eugenic goal of "reducing the number of carriers of genetic disorders in the population."[24] Is nondirective genetic counseling compatible with eugenics and public health?

Faith in nondirective counseling stems, in part, from the widely held belief that leaving the choice regarding genetic testing to the individual will have a positive impact on the gene pool, since its aim is to eliminate disease. While this conclusion may seem intuitively true, what if current genetics testing programs actually can be shown to have a negative effect on the gene pool?

Reproductive Compensation

While prenatal genetic testing may enhance patient autonomy, it is not necessarily eugenically neutral or beneficial. The present program of voluntary prenatal diagnosis and selective abortion is directly contrary to the eugenic goal and, in fact, has the effect of "polluting" the gene pool rather than improving it. Before the advent of prenatal diagnosis, most parents who gave birth to a child with a serious disorder refrained from having more children. The availability of prenatal genetic testing encourages parents to take risks they would not have taken previously.[25]

The term *reproductive compensation* describes the situation when a woman has another child to replace a fetus lost through selective abortion. When both parents carry a deleterious recessive gene, an average of one-quarter of their children will manifest the disorder, one-half will be carriers, and one-quarter will be normal (see the diagram on page 259). Reproductive compensation for the selective abortion of fetuses who are homogeneous for the deleterious gene results in two-thirds of the children who are born to the family being carriers, thus increasing by 33 percent the number of deleterious genes in the gene pool. Since people with serious genetic disorders do not usually have children, it is the carriers who generally pass on the genes. From a eugenics point of view, the so-called "replacement children," whose numbers are growing as a direct result of voluntary programs of prenatal genetic testing and selective abortion, are the "Typhoid Marys" spreading the disease to future generations.

The implementation of a eugenically sound prenatal testing program would require mandatory selective abortion of all carriers or sterilization of carriers before they reach childbearing age. The only way to implement such a program, however, would be to subordinate parental autonomy to the goals of eugenics and introduce mandatory prenatal genetic screening.

Prenatal testing raises the question of how to best resolve the conflict between respect for individual autonomy and nonmaleficence. Should the right to privacy override the need to protect the public and future generations from the burdens of genetic disease, or would the social benefits of prenatal testing programs outweigh the coercion and disregard for individual autonomy involved? Do physicians have a duty, based on nonmaleficence, to refrain from performing prenatal diagnosis and selective abortion if the goal is reproductive compensation, which results in an increase in children who are carriers of genetic diseases?

Genetic Screening and Discrimination

Sickle cell disease is an inherited autosomal recessive genetic disorder found mainly in people of West African descent that affects the ability of the iron-containing pigment in the blood to carry oxygen. Under certain conditions, the red blood cells become distorted and trapped in small blood vessels. This, in turn, precipitates a sickle cell crisis characterized by severe pain, blood clots, and even stroke or heart attack. Affected individuals usually die in childhood. However, because of improved treatment, more affected individuals are living healthy lives into early adulthood and finding themselves discriminated against in employment and insurance.

In 1972, the U.S. government decided that sickle cell disease was a public health hazard. The National Sickle Cell Anemia Control Act created a national screening program. In some states, African-American schoolchildren, athletes, and military cadets were compelled to undergo screening. There was no accompanying education regarding the disorder. African-American leaders charged that the mandatory screening programs were racially motivated and discriminatory. As a result of the state-sponsored programs, many individuals, including carriers who were quite healthy, found themselves faced with discrimination in employment and insurance. The program has been discontinued.

While screening programs for sickle cell disease were required in the United States by law, there have never been mandatory national screening programs for cystic fibrosis, a debilitating genetic disorder of the exocrine glands found primarily in people of Northern European origin. Genetic screening of adults for the Tay-Sachs gene, which is found primarily in Ashkenazi Jews of Eastern European descent, has also never been mandated by law. Instead, screening programs for carrier status have been voluntary and, for the most part, organized by the Jewish community. Tay-Sachs disease is a genetic disorder of the brain and nervous system. Unlike sickle cell disease and cystic fibrosis, Tay-Sachs disease almost always results in death by the age of five.

Many people fear that information gained from genetic tests will be used by insurance companies and employers to discriminate against people who test positive for a particular genetic trait. A 1996 study, funded by the HGP, of 332 members of genetic disease support groups found that 25 percent had experienced discrimination, including job discrimination (13 percent) or denial of health insurance (22 percent), as a result of knowledge of their condition.[26] Concerns about discrimination and losing medical insurance may partially explain why the rates of genetic testing for some diseases are lower in the United States than in countries, such as England, that have socialized medicine.[27] If a woman in the United States is diagnosed as having a gene that predisposes her to breast cancer, she could lose the insurance she may need later in her life.

Some states have laws that prohibit employers from performing genetic tests or discriminating against employees based on their genetic status. The only exception is when the genetic trait has a direct impact on employees' ability to perform their job. However, employers claim that they should have access to employees' genetic information not just because of possible effects on work performance but also because of the high costs of disability benefits and sick leave.

Over half the states have laws preventing insurance companies from requiring genetic testing or using the results of testing to deny coverage or raise premiums. On the other hand, it is accepted policy for insurance companies to exclude people with pre-existing disorders. Insurers argue that genetic tests are warranted and that genetic testing is simply an extension of the old-fashioned physical checkup. They also protest the laws, arguing that they force them either to raise everyone's premiums or to go out of business. While denying people healthcare coverage for conditions that are not their fault may be unjust, is it fair to force others to pay higher premiums to cover the healthcare costs for people with disorders that can be prenatally diagnosed or who knew of their carrier status? Higher premiums also price some people out of the healthcare market. Thirty percent of Americans did not have healthcare insurance in 1999.

The potential harms of mandatory screening need to be weighed against the benefits. Do public health concerns and costs, such as increased health insurance premiums, justify mandatory genetic screening programs? Do people have a moral obligation to seek testing if they suspect they might have a gene that could affect their job performance or that they might pass on to their children? Do insurers have a right to information about applicants' genotypes, given that everyone's premium rates might rise if coverage is granted to those with predispositions to genetic disorders? Or do people have a right not to know their genetic status? Does fear of losing one's insurance or discrimination justify ignorance about one's genetic status?

The "Right Not to Know"

Huntington's disease is a debilitating neurological disorder that does not usually manifest itself until a person is between the ages of thirty and fifty, often after the person has already had children. Because it is carried on a dominant gene, about half the children of a parent with Huntington's disease will eventually manifest symptoms of the disease, including progressive loss of motor coordination and of emotional and intellectual functions. Death results, on average, fifteen years after the onset of symptoms. Although a test for the gene that causes the disease is available, fewer than 15 percent of people who are at risk choose to be tested for it.[28] In addition, many people who know they have the disease prefer that the information be kept confidential.

This raises several moral questions. Do people with Huntington's disease have a moral obligation to inform other members of their family? Do other members of the family have a right to know? Do physicians who are privy to genetic information have a duty to inform other members of their patients' families as well as patients who don't want to know? Do young people who have a relative with Huntington's disease or another genetic disorder have a moral obligation to get tested? Should people be forced to gaze into their genetic crystal ball, or do they have a "right not to know" their genetic future?

Genetic information is deeply personal and has profound personal implications. On the other hand, genes are shared by families. If one person has a deleterious gene, chances are good that other people in the family also have the gene. This situation creates a conflict between a patient's right to autonomy and privacy and relatives' right to know important information about themselves.

Some healthcare ethicists maintain that autonomy and the right to privacy, including a right not to know, are the overriding moral concerns. They point out that the duty of nonmaleficence also supports the right not to know our genetic status. Many at-risk people refrain from getting tested because of concerns about the negative effects such knowledge might have on them and on their families. However, predictions that people who learn they have a gene for Huntington's disease or breast cancer will have catastrophic reactions, including suicide, have not been borne out by studies.[29] People with positive results do not become more distressed as a result of the news. Instead, learning that one does have a deleterious gene is actually accompanied by a decrease in the anxiety that accompanies uncertainty about one's status. The duty of nonmaleficence, therefore, does not clearly support an alleged right not to know in the case of genetic knowledge. In addition, not knowing can have adverse effects on our relatives because we share our genetic heritage with them.

In her article at the end of this chapter, Rosamond Rhodes argues that there is no right to genetic ignorance. A duty to inform our family of our genetic status stems from kinship bonds and a duty of fidelity to our family, as well as from the duty of nonmaleficence. Our genetic status is pertinent to major life decisions that affect our family, such as whether to have children, where to live, what job to take, and what type of insurance to purchase. Indeed, Austrian law requires a physician to advise a patient who has been diagnosed as having or carrying a gene for a genetic disorder to inform relatives of the test results if there is a perceived threat to the relatives.

Rhodes also argues that, rather than following from respect for autonomy, a right not to know in cases such as Huntington's disease is incompatible with autonomy. Using the analogy of a person who prefers to drive blindfolded, she argues that autonomy does not give us a right to remain ignorant about conditions that can harm us as well as others. Correct information is essential for making rational and autonomous choices. To act from ignorance is to relinquish our autonomy, which, according to Kant, is to fail to treat ourselves with respect.

GENETIC ENGINEERING

David, known in the media simply as the "bubble boy," had a rare genetic immunodeficiency disease caused by the lack of the enzyme adenosine deaminase (ADA), making him an easy target for chronic infections and cancer. Most people with ADA deficiency die in their first few months of life. David beat the odds by living in a sterile, plastic bubble before dying at the age of twelve in 1984. The gene responsible for producing ADA was identified in the early 1980s. Gene therapy was first used in 1990, when a culture containing normal ADA genes was introduced into a four-year-old girl with ADA deficiency by using genetically engineered viral vectors. Much to the geneticists' delight, the introduced genes overrode the information on the deficient genes, and the genetically altered cells began producing ADA.

Gene Therapy

Genetic engineering, which involves the alteration of genetic material by artificial means, includes both gene therapy and genetic enhancement. There are two types of gene therapy: somatic cell therapy and germ line therapy.

In **somatic cell therapy,** normal genes are introduced to produce something, such as an enzyme or a protein, that is lacking because of a genetic defect. This type of gene therapy was used in the ADA-deficiency case. Somatic cell therapy is a treatment; it does not eliminate the defective gene, nor does it change a person's genotype. Therefore, the defective gene can be passed on to future generations. Most healthcare ethicists regard this type of genetic engineering as a morally acceptable form of medical treatment. Receiving a foreign gene is comparable to receiving an organ transplant.

Germ line therapy actually alters the genetic structure of germ line cells—the sperm and the ova—so that the genotype of future generations is also altered. Germ line therapy is usually performed at the two- or four-cell stage of development. The ultimate goal is to direct a gene to a specific location on a chromosome where it will replace a deleterious or undesired gene. This goal has been accomplished with limited success in mice through the injection of the desired gene into the egg cells. Another technique being developed for use on zygotes is the insertion of retroviral vectors that probe for the deleterious DNA and then replace that piece of DNA with the desired gene(s).

In the future, germ line therapy may be available for protecting offspring against AIDS or certain types of cancer. Someday it may even be possible to synthesize completely new genes, thus overriding the human genetic code itself. If parents can afford to have a gene inserted into their child that will protect that child against AIDS or certain types of cancer, should they be allowed to do so? Indeed, would they have a moral obligation to do so, just as parents now have a moral obligation to have their children immunized against certain diseases?

One drawback of germ line therapy is the risk of inadvertently introducing genetic errors that will be passed on to future generations. Advocates of germ line therapy reply that genetic errors already occur naturally in the form of deleterious mutations. Therefore, they argue, the risk of passing on errors is not sufficient reason to prohibit germ line engineering. There may also be cases in which parents are opposed to abortion or both parents carry a gene defect that precludes the chance of having a "normal" child and germ line therapy is desired. Although the couple could turn to somatic cell therapy to ensure a "normal" child, using germ line therapy would be more cost-effective than performing somatic cell therapy on each subsequent generation.

Some healthcare ethicists oppose germ line therapy as a means of eradicating genetic disease because it involves tampering with a person's genetic inheritance. They claim that people have a "right to a genetic inheritance that has not been artificially interfered with."[30] With germ line engineering, there is no informed consent on the part of the person being altered. We need assurance that future generations would give informed consent to the alterations—a tall order given the uncertainty of what the future holds. On the other hand, if we have the technology to replace certain genes, future generations could replace the altered genes with the original ones if they desired. It is also unclear whether a person has a "right to a genetic inheritance that has not been artificially interfered with" and, if so, what the basis of such a right might be. The argument that germ line genetic engineering will change the personality of a person is based on the questionable assumption that inviolable personal identities exist prior to embodiment.

Some geneticists fear that, in using gene therapy to clean up the gene pool, we are throwing out the baby with the bath water. By getting rid of genes that may be harmful today, we become less flexible genetically. This, in turn, makes us less capable as a species to adapt to sudden climate changes or resist new diseases. A case in point is the gene for sickle cell disease. While inheriting two genes for this disease can be debilitating, carrying a gene for sickle cell disease also provides a measure of immunity against malaria—a potentially deadly disease. Although malaria is no longer a threat in most parts of the world, the deletion of this gene from the human gene pool could make us less resistant to future diseases like malaria.

Ethicists have also expressed concerns that fetal gene therapy will lead down the slippery slope to genetic enhancement, in which parents choose the genetic traits they want in their children. Few people oppose the use of gene therapy, particularly somatic gene therapy, to spare a child from a fatal or debilitating genetic disease. However, what about less obviously debilitating traits such as aggressiveness, lower-than-average intelligence, or a tendency toward alcoholism? Where do we cross the line between genetic therapy and genetic enhancement?

Genetic Enhancement

Genetic enhancement, the manipulation of genes in order to improve the genetic code, has been used since the late 1980s, when scientists began genetically altering food to improve its quality. The genetic enhancement of humans is more controversial. A Gallup poll of British parents found that 18 percent of them would be willing to use genetic enhancement on their children to alter level of aggression or disposition toward alcoholism, 10 percent to prevent homosexuality, and 5 percent to improve physical attractiveness. More than 40 percent of parents in the United States think it is acceptable to use genetic engineering to make their children more intelligent or more attractive.[31] The quest for the perfect child, combined with an emphasis on patient autonomy, has drawn the medical profession into the use of genetic enhancement to achieve this goal. Advocates of genetic enhancement argue that it is simply an extension of already accepted medical practices, such as cosmetic surgery or the use of mood-enhancing drugs.

Geneticists are also searching the gene pool for that illusive fountain of youth. Scientists at CalTech have discovered a gene that allows fruit flies to live an average of 35 percent longer and makes them resistant to heat, starvation, and even poison. This gene, named Methuselah after the biblical centenarian, holds out hope that gene therapy can be used in humans to slow down or stop the aging process. Immortality may be within our genetically enhanced reach.

If genetic engineering becomes commonplace, what is considered enhancement today might be considered therapy in the future. The question will then be not whether it is morally acceptable to use genetic engineering to enhance intelligence, beauty, or longevity, but rather whether it is morally acceptable *not* to give our children competitive social advantages.

Creating Designer Children

Biotechnology has created a connection in many people's minds between "responsible parenthood" and the "perfect baby." Some people fear that the availability of genetic engineering may turn children into commodities, with designer babies becoming a sign of success to be marketed much as cars are today. Biotechnology also raises the question of what a "perfect" human is. Should we define *perfect* in terms of the consequences for the wider community and the human species, or is perfection in children a private decision that should be left up to parents?

The flip side of perfection is rejection. What will happen to those who do not meet certain standards of perfection? Genetic engineering might give children who are products of the technology an unfair advantage. Very likely, only the wealthy will be able to afford genetically engineered designer children. The ability of those with more money to genetically engineer their children to be healthier and more intelligent, beautiful, and athletic may create a greater gap between the haves and the have-nots.

At the same time, the availability of genetic engineering technology also nullifies the need to have "inferior" children. Policymakers may become less sympathetic to the disadvantaged, and parents who have a less-than-perfect child in a society full of designer children could put their child at risk for failure and discrimination. Medical care and social services might be withheld from families that do not avail themselves of the new genetic technologies—a trend that has already begun with medical insurance companies. Thus, what began as a reproductive right could turn into a duty to have "perfect" children.

In *Curlender v. Bio-Science Laboratories* (1980), mentioned in Chapter 4, a California court ruled that a child with a genetic defect could bring a "wrongful life" suit against her parents for not undergoing prenatal screening and aborting her. This case could set a precedent for children who do not meet certain social and physical standards to sue their parents because they did not choose to have their child's genome genetically engineered to remove flaws.

Glenn McGee, in his article at the end of this chapter, opposes the use of genetic engineering. He argues that genetic engineering, because its aim is to fulfill parents' wishes for children with perfect genomes, harms children's right to an open future and to decide who they are. By imposing its concept of perfection on offspring, the parent generation will control the destiny of subsequent generations. This could lead to unfortunate consequences. Talents that may be appropriate today may be passé in years to come. The "reject" of today may be the "genius" of tomorrow.

REPRODUCTIVE TECHNOLOGY

Gaby and Bruce Vernoff's plans for having a family were thwarted when the car driven by Bruce Vernoff collided with a Honda. He was given painkillers for his injuries and later prescription mood-elevating drugs to help wean him off the painkillers. In 1995, Gaby found her husband dead in their TV room from an accidental overdose of the prescription medication. Following the tragedy, Gaby Vernoff decided to fulfill their dream of having a family. She paid fertility specialist Dr. Cappy Rothman $35,000 to harvest sperm from her dead husband. Using in vitro fertilization, Rothman injected a single sperm into one of Vernoff's eggs. In the spring of 1999, thirty-two-year-old Gaby Vernoff gave birth to a healthy baby girl, Brandalynn Danielle—the first known child in the United States conceived with the sperm of a dead man.[32] Brandalynn, however, was not the first child conceived using reproductive technology.

An estimated 10–16 percent of couples have problems conceiving a child.[33] About one-fourth of these couples turn to reproductive technology for help.[34] Each year in the United States, up to 800,000 people attend fertility clinics.[35] Fertility clinics are "the wild card in genetic engineering."[36] These for-profit, highly advanced biotech businesses are not subject to federal government regulations that prohibit germ line genetic research. Also, new reproductive technologies have greatly increased opportunities to use genetic testing and engineering, opening the door to gamete swapping and surrogacy.

Types of Reproductive Technology

There are more than a dozen ways to make babies—in addition to the old-fashioned way—including artificial insemination, in vitro fertilization, and, a relative newcomer to the field, cloning. Because cloning, unlike the types of assisted reproduction already in use, involves asexual reproduction, we will discuss it in a separate section of this chapter. It is now possible for a couple to have a child using a donated egg fertilized by a donated sperm and carried by a gestational mother with no genetic relationship to the child she carries. Using the new technologies, a dead man can father a child, an aborted fetus can be a mother, and post-menopausal women can have babies using cryogenically preserved eggs. The following box lists some of the different types of assisted reproduction. In vitro fertilization and the use of donor gametes will be discussed in greater detail in the next two sections.

In Vitro Fertilization In vitro fertilization (IVF), the foundation of infertility treatment, is often used in conjunction with the other reproductive technologies. IVF is an expensive and time-consuming procedure that involves the use of superovulation (fertility) drugs that may have adverse effects on women. In addition, IVF fails in about 80 percent of treatment cycles.[37] Some couples go through more than a dozen treatment cycles, at a cost of over $10,000 per cycle.

IVF can result in multiple births, which put both the mother and the babies at increased risk. Some countries, such as England, do not permit more than three embryos to be transferred to the uterus. In the United States, however, up to eight embryos have been transplanted in order to increase the chances of the birth of a child. In November 1997, an Iowa woman gave birth to seven children weighing between 10.3 and 28.6 ounces. In December 1998, Nkem Chukwu of Texas gave birth to octuplets. While these events have been treated by the press as joyous miracles, some healthcare ethicists are concerned about the costs of these miracles. All the children were born prematurely. The seven surviving very low birth weight octuplets have a 50 percent chance of functional impairment. Their medical care during the first two months in the hospital exceeded $2 million. Four of the babies remained in the hospital after four months. These seven babies made their first public appearance in November 1999.[38] Many of them may need special education programs and expensive medical care throughout their life. "Money spent on octuplets," clinical bioethicist Ezekiel Emanuel warns, "is money not spent on other children with special healthcare and educational needs."[39]

IVF is sometimes preferred to artificial insemination (AI) with surrogacy because the surrogate mother is not genetically related to the child she carries. The potential legal hassles that can accompany the use of AI were poignantly illustrated by the highly publicized Whitehead case. In February 1985, William Stern entered into a surrogacy contract with Mary Beth Whitehead, who agreed to be artificially inseminated with Stern's sperm, to carry the child to term, and to relinquish her maternal rights to the Sterns after birth. In exchange, Whitehead would receive $10,000. However, shortly

TYPES OF ASSISTED REPRODUCTION

- *Artificial insemination (AI).* **Artificial insemination** involves the mechanical placement of a man's sperm in a woman's reproductive tract. AIH uses the husband's or partner's sperm; AID uses the sperm of a donor. AID is used when the husband's or partner's sperm is deficient or when he is homozygous for a genetic disorder.

- *In vitro fertilization (IVF).* In this procedure, the woman is given a series of super-ovulation, or fertility, drugs to promote multiple ovulations. Mature eggs are then removed from the ovaries through a hollow needle and mixed with sperm in a petri dish for two to three days. The healthiest fertilized eggs are transferred into the woman's uterus.

- *Gamete intrafallopian transfer (GIFT).* Eggs are harvested from the ovaries. The unfertilized eggs are mixed with sperm, loaded into a catheter, and delivered into the fallopian tube. GIFT has a slightly higher success rate than IVF. However, it requires surgery and general anesthesia, thus putting the woman at greater risk.

- *Zygote intrafallopian transfer (ZIFT).* This procedure is similar to GIFT except that the egg is fertilized outside the body and then inserted into the fallopian tube.

- *Intracytoplasmic sperm injection (ICSI).* A single sperm is injected into a mature egg. The fertilized egg is then transferred into the woman's uterus.

- *Surrogacy.* In **surrogacy** arrangements, a woman agrees to carry a child for another woman. There are several types of surrogacy, depending on whose gametes are used. With gestational surrogacy, an embryo, usually produced with gametes from one or both of the people contracting for the child, is transferred into the surrogate's uterus.

- *Cloning.* This process involves producing genetically identical individuals through asexual reproduction of a single cell.

after the birth, Whitehead changed her mind and decided she wanted to keep the child. After a long, drawn-out court battle, William Stern was awarded custody of the child.

The Use of Donor Gametes   In the United States, about 30,000 children are born each year from donor-assisted pregnancies. The use of donor gametes, as in the Whitehead case, raises several moral issues. Many people who accept reproductive technology as an extension of the normal act of procreation between a couple draw the line at the use of donor gametes. Their primary objection is that including a third party violates the exclusive procreative aspect of the marriage contract and threatens the structure of the nuclear family.

In Germany, all forms of egg, sperm, and embryo donation are illegal. In Islamic law, the use of donor gametes, especially sperm, is considered adultery. It is also regarded as adultery by some Jews.

ISLAM AND REPRODUCTIVE TECHNOLOGY

Attitudes toward adoption, surrogacy, and gamete donation in Islamic culture differ dramatically from those held by most North Americans. The official Islamic position on the use of reproductive technologies has been shaped primarily by conservative Islamic scholars and medical professionals.

Children are highly valued in Islamic cultures; however, marriage is the only acceptable avenue for reproduction. Medical or surgical treatment of infertility is regarded as a legitimate means of achieving reproduction, but, because children must be the genetic offspring of a married couple, artificial insemination is permitted only if the husband's sperm is used. The use of donor sperm or ova, donated embryos, or a surrogate uterus is forbidden because it violates the marriage contract and weakens family bonds.

Surrogacy is illegal, and contracts for surrogate pregnancy are not recognized. Surrogacy is regarded as particularly loathsome in Islamic culture because it not only denies the child a "legitimate root, . . . it is done for money, thus reducing motherhood from a 'value' to a 'price.' "[40] In addition, because the sperm or eggs of third parties cannot be involved in the marital function of reproduction, adoption is not acceptable as a solution to infertility. Like the use of donor sperm and ova, adoption is seen as violating God's will. According to the Shura:

To God belongs the dominion of the heavens and the earth. He creates what He wills (and plans). He bestows (children) male or female according to His Will (and plan). Or He bestows both males and females and he leaves barren whom He will. For He is full of knowledge and power.[41]

Islamic prohibitions on adoption, surrogacy, and the use of donor gametes have a particularly profound effect on childless women in a culture where a woman's social status and rights are dependent on motherhood. Childlessness and the failure to bear sons have had devastating economic and social consequences for Muslim women. On the other hand, unmarried professional women in the Middle East rarely have children because of the stigma attached to single motherhood. For men, polygamy and divorce are options when their wife is barren. Indeed, the fertility argument is still used to justify the continuation of polygamy.[42] However, a woman with an infertile husband has no similar option.

According to Islamic feminists, the Islamic position on reproductive technologies is grounded primarily in patriarchy rather than in concern for the well-being and rights of women and children.[43] Many Islamic feminists protest the law forbidding artificial insemination using sperm from a donor (AID) as a perpetuation of patriarchy and the idea that women and children are property. However, other Islamic healthcare ethicists argue that Islamic law promotes the common good by ensuring that fathers will take responsibility for the care of their offspring.

HONG KONG:
Report of the Committee on Scientifically Assisted
Human Reproduction (1992)

Hong Kong is one of the most densely populated places in the world, with 6 million people living in only 400 square miles. Hong Kong also boasts excellent medical facilities. Its infant mortality rate, one of the lowest in the world at 5 per 1,000, is lower than that of the United States.[44] Although Hong Kong does not enforce a one-child policy like that of mainland China, there is an effort to encourage smaller families, and most families limit themselves to a maximum of two children.

About 10 percent of married couples in Hong Kong are childless because of infertility. The Chinese reticence to discuss sexual matters is tempered by the importance placed on family. Consequently, some infertile families turn to the fertility clinics in Hong Kong, where artificial insemination using both donor sperm and the husband's sperm has been available for decades. IVG and GIFT have also been available since 1986. One of the most requested procedures is sperm separation for sex selection. This procedure appeals to many Chinese because of the strong preference for sons despite official efforts to promote gender equality.

The use of reproductive technology is met with mixed feelings in Hong Kong. As in mainland China, there is a strong Confucian emphasis on family and social responsibility. Some people find the technology both morally and religiously objectionable and an inappropriate response to childlessness. Many people are opposed to the use of donor gametes because it introduces a third party into the marriage. Most feel that reproductive technology, if it is to be legal, should be regulated by the government.

In 1987, the secretary for health and welfare appointed a committee on scientifically Assisted Human Reproduction. Its final report, issued in 1992, contained the following recommendations:

Artificial insemination: AIH should be allowed. For DI [AID], the husband's consent should be required, only banked semen should be used, the identity of the donor should be kept confidential, and the number of children sired by any one donor should be limited to three.

Access to information: Children born as a result of DI [AID] should have the right to know, upon reaching the age of majority, that the procedure was performed on their mother, without the donor's identity being revealed.

Surrogacy: Commercial surrogacy should be banned. Only genetic IVF surrogacy should be allowed and it should be restricted to infertile couples where no alternative medical treatment is possible. Only a woman who has been married and has her own children should be allowed to be a surrogate mother. Surrogacy should require the consent of both the surrogate mother and her husband.

Defenders of gamete donation point out that the use of donor gametes allows a couple to have a child who is genetically related to at least one of them. Furthermore, parenthood has long extended to adoption and stepfamilies; while a genetic relationship is important, the social aspects of parenthood are more significant.

Other moral issues raised by gamete donation pertain to the donors. Selecting a prospective parent for one's child can be as easy as logging on to the Internet and scrolling through a list of sperm or egg donors. Payment for organs is illegal, but the gamete market is fair game for profit-seeking entrepreneurs. One sample description of a sperm donor reads: "Caucasian/Irish, German, Slavic, fair skin, blond wavy hair, blue eyes, 5 ft. 11 in., 168 pounds, O positive blood."[45] Other Web sites offer colored photos and profiles of egg donors, who receive from $2,000 to $50,000 for each harvest. Eggs, in particular, have become a hot commodity on the market, with prospective parents paying premium prices for eggs from donors with "desirable" qualities. The most sought-after recruits are bright, beautiful, Caucasian college women—rekindling chilling visions of eugenic racism.

Concerns also arise about the risks to egg donors, since donation requires the use of superovulation drugs and an invasive surgical procedure to collect the eggs. Given the high cost of college education today, the financial inducement for donated eggs borders on bribery and coercion rather than voluntary consent. Because of the difficulty in obtaining eggs and the risk involved, some scientists have suggested that they be harvested from cadavers or aborted fetuses, a suggestion many people find abhorrent.

In recent cases, women have asked physicians to retrieve sperm from their dead or near-dead husband. Does a childless widow have a right to her deceased husband's sperm? Some medical ethicists argue that it helps the widow cope with the loss of her husband. The birth of their husband's child "gives them hope." Others, such as McGee, claim that it sets "a dangerous precedent to say there can be reproduction without consent." Islamic law likewise says no to this practice, since death of a spouse invalidates the marriage contract.

The emphasis on confidentiality in healthcare ethics raises questions regarding genetic knowledge when donor gametes are used. The majority of donors want their identity to remain secret. Anonymity is regarded as a mechanism for protecting both the donor and the recipient couple. Only a few states require genetic information about sperm donors, and only one requires such information in the case of eggs. Genetic information is usually not available to couples seeking the services of egg or sperm donors.

The first wave of children from donor-assisted pregnancies will be reaching maturity soon. Most will be "reproductive foundlings" who lack access to information about their genetic heritage—or at least half of it. Should donors be required to supply relevant information about their genotype to prospective parents? Do children from donor-assisted pregnancies have a right to information about their genetic heritage, or do the privacy rights of the donor take precedence? In Sweden, New Zealand, and parts of Australia, donors have a moral responsibility to their children. National registries have been set up to store and update sperm donors' medical history. In the United States and Canada, in contrast, protecting the anonymity of donors is given precedence.

Autonomy and Reproductive Technology

Women who avail themselves of the new reproductive technologies may appear to be acting autonomously. Critics of assisted reproduction, however, claim that two factors

AFRICA:
Infertility, Adoption, and Surrogate Parenthood[46]

Most Africans place a high value on having children, and life is considered incomplete without them. Because the primary purpose of marriage is to have children, infertility is considered a serious problem, and every effort is made to overcome it. If a married woman is having problems conceiving, she may "adopt" a child of a relative. Unlike adoption in the Western sense, the "adopted" child is still recognized as the child of the biological parents. However, it is believed that, by her loving and caring for this child, the spirit of the "adopted" child will attract her own natural child to her. Surrogate motherhood is also practiced in some matrilineal societies. A woman who is unable to get pregnant may arrange for her husband to impregnate another woman of her choice with the understanding that she will carry the wife's child.

Polygamy is also used as a solution to female infertility in some African cultures. If a woman has trouble getting pregnant, she may arrange for her husband to marry another woman, with the understanding that she is the mother of the new wife's first child or with the hope that the spirit of the child from this new union will attract a child to her.

may compromise women's autonomy: the technological imperative, with its pressure to have a "perfect" child, and patriarchy, which pressures women into having children that are genetically related to their husband. According to Barbara Rothman, patriarchy is implicit in assisted reproduction. If a woman has a problem with fertility, it is treated by physicians as entirely her problem.[47] However, if the husband has a problem with fertility, it is treated as a problem "of the couple." Fertility treatment is increasingly being used on fertile women whose husbands are infertile. Thus, women are being subjected to IVF treatment, with all its inherent risks, as a means of assuring the husband's genetic paternity.

Feminists have mixed reactions to assisted reproduction. The desire for children, some argue, is socially constructed. Thus, women feel socially compelled to use costly, physically and emotionally enervating reproductive technologies that demean women by turning them into "fetal containers." Commercial surrogacy, in particular, reduces women's reproductive capacities to commercial commodities. If people can make a profit from donating gametes or being a surrogate mother, a market might develop in which the financially well-off exploit the poor for their bodies. To avoid the commercialization of reproductive products and services, third parties should not be compensated beyond the medical costs incurred.

Other feminists and healthcare ethicists maintain that the new reproductive technologies increase a woman's options and autonomy. People have a right to make their own decisions about how their bodies, and the products of their bodies, will be used. Poorer women who wish to be surrogates should not be denied opportunities for economic gain and a chance to better their lives simply because of paternalistic concern over their "exploitation." They argue that women have a right to control their own bodies and to enter into contractual agreements with infertility clinics unless it can be shown that substantial harm is caused by the reproductive technologies.

The Principle of Nonmaleficence

The principle of nonmaleficence requires that we avoid harming others. Since the children born of the new reproductive technologies have not yet begun their own families, scientists are not sure of the long-term effects on future generations of technologies that involve manipulation of gametes and preembryos. However, an Australian study of 420 children found that children produced by mechanically injecting sperm into an egg cell are twice as likely as children conceived by natural means to suffer from major birth defects of the heart, genitals, and digestive tract.[48] A study of twins conceived by IVF and GIFT found that they were more likely to have low birth weights than spontaneously occurring twins.[49]

With improvement in cryogenics, women may be able to freeze healthy eggs in "egg banks" in case they should later encounter problems with fertility or decide to have a baby after the age of menopause. In addition to the risks to the woman in harvesting her eggs, there is concern that freezing may damage the eggs, which are more fragile than sperm. Any DNA damage may not become evident until several generations later.

The freezing of gametes and preembryos also raises the question of what to do with them if a couple divorce or if the donor dies. Should custody be awarded to one of the parents or a family member? Are preembryos persons with a right to life, or can they be destroyed? Should unclaimed preembryos be made available to others seeking fertility treatment?

Some healthcare ethicists fear that genetic engineering and the new reproductive technologies will reduce children to property and reduce family life to a succession of commercial transactions. According to Roman Catholic teaching, the creation of a child is the physical embodiment of the love and union of the parents. The use of assisted reproduction is rejected because it separates procreation from sexual intercourse. In his article at the end of this chapter, Leon Kass argues that moving reproduction into the laboratory erodes the meaning of marital love and destroys the natural parent/child bond.

The very nature of the infertility business, including the emphasis on confidentiality, the demand for results, and the large amounts of money involved, leaves patients vulnerable, making it easy for physicians to overstep their professional bounds. For example, in 1995, Dr. Ricardo Asch, who pioneered GIFT, was charged with prescribing an unapproved fertility drug, doing research on patients without their permission, and stealing eggs and embryos from patients to create pregnancies in others.

Infertility and the "Right to Reproduce"

Is infertility a disease or physical disability that warrants medical treatment? Infertility should be considered within its social context rather than simply as a physical state. Judged purely as a physical phenomenon, infertility is clearly not life-threatening or disabling. However, taking the social context into consideration, we find that infertility can cause great distress. Those who claim that there is a right to reproduce argue that having a genetic connection to our children is important for our well-being. For many couples, the inability to conceive a child precipitates a crisis that can lead to a serious identity crisis, depression, and strained relationships. In cultures where a woman's value is based on her ability to have children, infertility can be an even greater blow to self-esteem and bring about feelings of shame.

On the other hand, if there is a right to reproduce, should it include the right to use expensive and scarce medical resources in exercising this right? Given the global problems associated with overpopulation and lack of access to basic healthcare in many countries, including many people in the United States, is reproduction a welfare right that the state or medical insurance companies should be compelled to underwrite? Are there times when a physician should refuse patients' requests for infertility treatment? Is it the physician's business to make such judgments? If not, then who should make these decisions?

CLONING

Cloning, the process of producing genetically identical individuals through asexual reproduction, is currently the most controversial reproductive technology. Using cloning, people can produce a genetic replica of themselves, a dying child, a famous person, or a genetically enhanced individual. Couples who are infertile and have a successful IVF of an egg may choose to clone the preembryo rather than risk having no children at all. They would then have a family of cloned siblings, or time-separated twins, born at different times. Cloning may also provide a solution to genetic disease by cloning the parent who is not afflicted or, in cases where both parents are carriers, cloning a healthy, noncarrier embryo or child as a means of avoiding prenatal diagnosis and selective abortion in future pregnancies.

Methods of Cloning

There are currently two types of cloning: blastocyst (embryo) splitting, and nuclei transfer. Nuclei transfer can be subdivided into nuclei transfer using embryonic or fetal cells and nuclei transfer using adult cells.

Blastocyst (Embryo) Splitting The blastocyst, or preembryo, consists of two to eight cells. At this stage in development, cells are not yet specialized into different organ systems. Each cell is still capable of reproducing an entire organism, as occurs naturally in the case of identical twins or triplets. In October 1993, researchers at George Washington University announced that they had created the first clones of human embryos. This event touched off the first round of debates on the morality of human cloning.

Nuclei Transfer Using Embryonic and Fetal Cells In this type of cloning, the nucleus from an early embryo is transferred to an unfertilized egg from which the original nucleus has been removed. Nuclei transfer using embryonic cells has been used in cloning mice, rabbits, sheep, and cattle. The first successful cloning of vertebrate animals using nuclei transfer from tadpoles, rather than embryonic cells, occurred in 1952. In 1984, Danish embryologist Steen Willadsen succeeded in cloning the first lamb from embryonic cells. In 1997, Don Wolf at the Oregon Regional Primate Research Center announced that he had created two monkey clones using embryonic cells: Neti (an acronym for "nuclear embryo transfer infant") and Ditto.

Nuclei Transfer Using Adult Cells   Nuclei transfer using adult cells involves taking the nucleus from the cell of an adult and transferring it into a mature egg from which the nucleus has been removed. Since the new nucleus has the full complement of forty-six chromosomes, the renucleated egg and the individual who contributed the new nucleus will be virtually genetically identical, with the exception of a very small contribution of DNA material from the mitochondria of the host egg. (Mitochondria are slender microscopic filaments that provide energy to the cell.) Unlike blastocyst splitting, which is limited by the number of cells in a blastocyst, nuclei transfer from adult cells allows anyone—man or woman, adult or child—to be cloned in any quantity. Prior to Dolly, this type of cloning had never succeeded in animals.

Cloning Humans

Shortly after the birth of Dolly, an advertisement appeared on the Internet from a Bahamas-based group called Clonaid, offering to clone people for $200,000 or to save a person's cells after death for future cloning. Within the first year, Clonaid had a waiting list of more than a hundred people. In early 1998, American scientist Richard Seed announced his intention to open a human cloning clinic in the United States, hoping to produce his first human clone by 2000.[50] His goal is to produce 500 clones a year. Critics claim that Seed is a dangerous man—a "modern day Frankenstein."[51] One *New York Times* editorial compared Seed to Dr. Kevorkian: "The main difference is that Dr. Kevorkian is reckless in bringing about the end of life, whereas Dr. Seed plans to be reckless in the creation of life."[52]

In July 1998, Dr. Ryuzo Ranagimachi of the University of Hawaii announced that his team of scientists had successfully cloned mice using cumulus cells, which are found around the eggs in the ovary.[53] This method is much more efficient than the method that was used in producing Dolly. The Hawaiian scientists can create up to 200 clones a day and have even made clones of the clones. Five months later, Korean scientists Lee Bo-yon and Kim Sung-bo announced that they had cloned a human embryo from a thirty-year-old woman using the method pioneered at the University of Hawaii. However, they destroyed the clone early in its development.

In November 1998, Advanced Cell Technology, an American company, reportedly created an embryo by transferring the nucleus from the cell of an adult human into a cow egg.[54] The company plans to eventually use the technology to grow replacement tissue for humans.

Putting the Brakes on Human Cloning Research

Because biotechnology is far ahead of the debate over the morality of cloning, many countries have established temporary bans on human cloning research. Within days of the announcement of Dolly's birth, the British government, which had provided 65 percent of the funding for the Roslin Institute's cloning research, announced that it was stopping funding for cloning research.[55] In the weeks that followed, human cloning research was banned or heavily restricted in Spain, Italy, Norway, Germany, Canada, Denmark, Great Britain, and the United States. The European Commission on the Ethical Implications of Biotechnology also came out in 1997 with a statement of "condemnation of human reproductive cloning."[56]

Nearly 90 percent of Americans interviewed shortly after the announcement of Dolly's birth said they found human cloning morally repugnant.[57] The 1997 Cloning Prohibition Act in the United States outlawed the use of federal funds for research on human cloning for a period of five years. Although the act requests that the private sector refrain from human cloning research, it does not prohibit private research. A law that would permanently ban all human cloning was defeated in the U.S. Senate in 1998.

Most religious organizations are opposed to human cloning. According to the Roman Catholic Church, cloning is intrinsically wrong because it is an attempt to play God. Islamic scholar Abdulaziz Sachedina adds that cloning violates teachings about the family and the traditional role of the father in creating children. Rabbi Richard Address of the Union of American Hebrew Congregations is also against human cloning because "it violates the mystery of what it means to be human."

SELECTIONS FROM *CLONING HUMAN BEINGS*:
The Report and Recommendations of the National Bioethics Advisory Commission (NBAC), June 1997

In its deliberation, NBAC reviewed the scientific developments which preceded the Roslin announcement, as well as those likely to follow in its path . . .

In addition to concern about specific harms to children, people have frequently expressed fears that the widespread practice of . . . cloning would undermine important social values by opening the door to a form of eugenics or by tempting some to manipulate others as if they were objects instead of persons. Arrayed against these concerns are other important social values, such as protecting the widest possible sphere of personal choice, particularly in matters pertaining to procreation and child rearing, maintaining privacy and the freedom of scientific inquiry, and encouraging the possible development of new biomedical breakthroughs. . . .

Within this overall framework the Commission came to the following conclusions and recommendations:

I. The Commission concludes that at this time it is morally unacceptable for anyone in the public or private sector, whether in a research or clinical setting, to attempt to create a child using somatic cell nuclear transfer cloning. We have reached a consensus on this point because current scientific information indicates that this technique is not safe to use in humans at this time. . . .

The Commission, therefore, recommends the following for immediate action:

- A continuation of the current moratorium on the use of federal funding in support of any attempt to create a child by somatic cell nuclear transfer.

- An immediate request to all firms, clinicians, investigators, and professional societies in the private and non-federally funded sectors to comply voluntarily with the intent of the federal moratorium. . . .

Cloning and Genetic Engineering

In late 1997, the same institute that had produced Dolly announced that, by using cloning in conjunction with genetic engineering, it had created five almost identical transgenic lambs with human genes that produce factor IX, a blood-clotting substance used in treating hemophilia. Transgenic mice are also being bred to produce human antibodies. Several large drug companies are vying for the rights to breed these mice and market their antibodies.[58]

The possibility of combining genetic engineering with cloning in order to mass-produce "perfect" humans or designer humans programmed to play certain roles in society, as in Aldous Huxley's *Brave New World*, raises the ante in the cloning debate. Because genetically engineered clones are human inventions, they may be considered patentable property and denied the rights of full personhood. On the other hand, clones, because of their more desirable genomes, might become a new master race, with "natural" humans relegated to the inferior role.

Cloning and Human Dignity

According to Kantian deontology, human dignity requires that humans be treated as ends in themselves. Opponents of cloning argue that it violates human dignity in a way that natural twinning does not because it reduces people to their genetic codes. In 1772, British philosopher and scientist Robert Boyle expressed the following view of the human body: "I think the physician is to look upon the patient's body as an engine that is out of order, but yet so constituted that, by his concurrence with . . . the parts of the automaton itself, it may be brought to a better state." The idea that our bodies can be reduced to an elaborate machine with parts, which can be manipulated and analyzed, continues to dominate medicine and medical research. Reductionism removes the human body from its social and personal context and reduces it to an object to be studied and manipulated.

President Clinton, in announcing a federal ban on funding for research on human cloning, stated that "human life is unique, born of a miracle, a profound gift."[59] Cloning, opponents argue, robs the clone of his or her sense of uniqueness. The fact that twins occur naturally does not give us the right to impose sameness on other people. Clones will be burdened with genetic identities—those of their parents—that have already lived, thus inheriting a serious self-identity problem.

Supporters of human cloning for infertility treatment counter that human dignity and self-identity do not depend on genetic uniqueness. Natural twins have a sense of self-identity. Twins also frequently have a close personal relationship with each other that is the envy of many. Although genes provide the building blocks for individuals, they do not determine who we are. Genetic determinism is based on a mistaken view of human nature. Who we are is the result of the interaction between our genetic inheritance and our social and cultural environment. Clones are not drones. The idea that we could clone an army of identical Hitlers, or any group of identical people, has no scientific basis.

Redefining Parenthood and Family

Cloning, more so than reproductive technologies that require the participation of both a man and a woman, could radically redefine the meaning of parenthood and family. Clones break the connection between family and children, since a clone comes from a single parent who, unless the child's genome was genetically engineered, may also be the child's identical twin. What's more, cloning will make men reproductively superfluous. A woman who wants to clone herself would not need a man, while a man who wanted to clone himself would need a woman to provide both the egg and a womb.

On the other hand, clones could still have two social parents, and cloning may provide the only chance for some couples to have a child who is genetically related to them. The father could provide the nucleus and the mother the egg. That way, the mother would contribute at least some material—the DNA from her mitochondria—to their child. Cloning may also be the only way for a couple to avoid having a genetic disorder passed on to their children, especially if one parent carries two genes for the disorder or if the parents are morally opposed to selective abortion.

Randolfe Wicke, head of Clone Rights United Front in New York City, believes that "human cloning is a reproductive option and should be available to all."[60] Cloning, he says, is not the business of government any more than "a woman's decision to have an abortion is." Wicke says he plans to clone himself as soon as he can find a scientist who will cooperate. John Harris agrees that there is a right to procreation through cloning. We may find the idea repugnant or consider it arrogant of people such as Wicke to clone themselves or of parents to clone a dying child in order to have a replacement child or to use genetic engineering to produce the "perfect" child; however, these feelings do not, in themselves, make the practices morally wrong as long as the children's interests are protected after birth.

Consequentialist Arguments Against Cloning

Because we have little experience with human cloning, we have to rely on speculation, for the most part, in determining whether the harms outweigh the benefits. Some healthcare ethicists maintain that, because the possibility of misuse of cloning is so great, all human cloning should be banned. Cloning and genetic engineering might lead to the commodification and possibly even the mass production of children and the breakdown of parent/child relationships.

Furthermore, if human cloning is legal, what will stop people from secretly taking some of our cells to make clones of us? A piece of hair, blood, or saliva may be enough to make a clone of a former lover, a rock star, or a famous athlete. For one-stop shopping, the Armed Forces Institute of Pathology in Washington, D.C., already has a tissue bank that holds about 92 million tissue samples from civilians and military personnel around the world. Universities and biotech corporations can already buy samples from this bank for genetic research. What could you do if you discovered you were the victim of a "body bandit"? Probably not much. In the case of John Moore, in which researchers used cells from his spleen to develop a cell line for use in cancer research, the California Supreme Court ruled that Moore did not have a legal right to products developed from his body parts. This case could be used as a precedent to protect biotech entrepreneurs who clone our cells without our permission.

We do not yet know the effects of using adult cells to create clones. Dolly's DNA is already showing signs of decay typical of much older sheep. The DNA of clones like Dolly may have other defects that are not yet evident. Cloned cows are at least ten times more likely than naturally conceived cows to have health problems such as anemia.[61] Many other animals, including pigs and monkeys, are pregnant with clones in laboratories. Some of the cloned fetuses have subtle and unexpected genetic alterations that affect their development.[62] Because of these and other findings, in 1999 the Canadian government, which previously had only a voluntary moratorium on human cloning, introduced legislation that would criminalize human cloning.[63]

"We Should Not Interfere with Nature"

Some people oppose cloning on the grounds that the right to create new life belongs to God and it is wrong to infringe on God's domain. This objection is especially pertinent given the possibility that scientists may soon be able to create synthetic life. However, it needs further clarification. What do we mean by "creating" as opposed to "reproducing" life? Also, religious ethicists disagree on whether the activities of these scientists impinge on God's role as creator. According to Baylor University theologian Daniel B. McGee, "God is a presence who continues in the marvelous creative process, and we participate in that."[64]

The argument also presumes that "natural" and "good" are invariably linked, thus falling prey to the naturalistic fallacy. We are constantly interfering with nature in the name of morality. Indeed, the primary purpose of medicine is to prevent diseases by interfering with their natural course. What is meant by "unnatural"? Is it unnatural for humans to develop and use technology?

A related argument is that species have integrity as biological units and we should not disrupt the natural boundaries between species. Again, this argument assumes that "nature" and "good" are synonymous. The species-integrity argument is reminiscent of the racial-purity argument. Is the human genome sacrosanct? Why should priority be given to preserving our human genome? What is the moral value in keeping groups biologically separate? The distinction between species is not as clear as biologists once thought. Genetic exchange between species occurs in nature without human interference, not only in cloning combined with genetic engineering.

Some healthcare ethicists think the time has come to take control of our genetic destiny, including the destiny of our progeny. Our cultural evolution far outpaces our biological evolution. For example, our bodies still react to stress with a fight-or-flight response. This response may have been adaptive when the threat was a saber tooth tiger; however, it is not adaptive in the modern world. If nature is inclined to its own perfection, as some philosophers argue, perhaps our nature is now pushing us in the direction of genetic engineering. Indeed, in the face of the tremendous strain human activities are placing on the earth, maybe we should think about designing offspring who are better adapted to the modern world and have a better chance of survival. Perhaps the time has come to take charge of our evolution. The fact that genetic engineering and cloning may mark the end of human life as we know it is not in itself a moral disaster.

GENETIC TECHNOLOGY AND NONHUMAN ANIMALS

By the late 1980s, scientists were genetically altering food, taking genetic material from fish, bacteria, viruses, and insects and adding it to fruits, grains, and vegetables in order to improve the durability and quality of food. As of January 2000, about fifty genetically engineered plants had been approved for use by the U.S. government. These include plants engineered to produce their own pesticides and those engineered to survive weed-killer chemicals.[65] In the 1990s, scientists also began experimenting with mass-producing drugs by inserting human genes into bacteria. Alexion Pharmaceuticals, Inc., a Connecticut biotech company, is doing research on injecting pig embryos with human genes so they can be used as organ donors for humans. In 1998, two Holsteins, George and Charlie, were born who were cloned from genetically engineered fetal cells that included human genes so their milk would contain valuable human proteins, such as factor IX for hemophiliacs.[66]

Cloning has greatly expanded the use of genetic engineering in animals. Genetically engineered animals with human genetic material can be cloned to be used as drug factories for humans or as models for studying human diseases such as AIDS or cancer.

The Moral Standing of Genetically Engineered Animals

The Human Genome Project has made us aware of how closely related all living beings are. Living organisms have 80 percent of their DNA in common. Humans and chimpanzees differ in only 2 percent of their DNA.[67] In light of this, we need to rethink the moral wedge we currently drive between humans and nonhuman animals and the genetic exploitation of nonhuman animals to benefit humans. We need to decide at what point animals genetically engineered with human genes should receive the moral respect now reserved for humans.

The genetic manipulation of nonhuman animals and the insertion of human genes into other species may also blur the traditional line now drawn between humans and other species; indeed, it may even obliterate the concept of species. Whether this potential result is morally desirable remains to be seen.

Genetic Diversity and Species Identity

Some biologists are concerned that cloning will undermine genetic diversity and species identity. As with the human species, we ought to respect the integrity of other species. This argument, however, brings us back to the dubious equating of "natural" with "good."

We must also consider the possibility that diminished genetic diversity may lead to genetic stagnation, which will affect the ability of humans and other animals to adapt to environmental changes. There are already problems with cloned agricultural animals and plants. If genetic diversity falls below an acceptable limit, a whole herd or crop could be wiped out by a single disease. In 1970, half of the maize crop in the United States was lost to the southern corn leaf blight. The loss was attributed to lack of genetic diversity among the plants.

RESOLVING THE GENETIC ENGINEERING AND CLONING DEBATE

The ability to genetically engineer and clone humans is a milestone in history. How are we, as morally responsible citizens, going to respond to this new technology? The emphasis on patient autonomy in Western medicine has left us ill prepared to deal with biotechnologies that have far-reaching social implications. Because we share genes in common with our family and pass them on to future generations, genetics always involves others. Furthermore, germ line engineering affects future generations and the human genome itself. Autonomy, or the liberty right of parents to make their own reproductive decisions, therefore, needs to be balanced against the rights of future generations as well as against the benefits to society of eliminating genetic diseases.

We must also resist the temptation to use the temporary ban on cloning as an opportunity for sweeping the moral issues under the table or to dismiss cloning offhand as too bizarre to be morally acceptable. We should keep in mind that similar fears were voiced about IVF two decades ago. A head-in-the-sand approach may simply encourage the development of unregulated back-alley cloning clinics. Compelling and broad-based arguments are found on both sides of the cloning debate. These moral concerns are also related to the issue of abortion and the use of nonhuman animals in medical experiments. How should we balance the different moral concerns? The jury is still out regarding the acceptable limits and uses of genetic engineering and cloning.

Genealogy, Sacredness, and the Commodities Market

Aroha Te Pareake Mead, a Maori from the Ngati Awa and Ngati Porou tribes in New Zealand, is the director of the International Association of the Mataatua Declaration of Cultural and Intellectual Property of Indigenous People and a member of the Indigenous People's Bio-diversity Network. She argues that the Human Genome Project should be viewed in the context of colonial imperialism and the continuing commercial exploitation of the bodies of indigenous people and that it violates the rights and interests of indigenous people.

From the time the first European vessels reached the shores of continents long inhabited by indigenous peoples, European colonists adopted a *terra nullius** world view. "Our lands were declared vacant by papal bulls you created to justify the pillaging of our lands" (Chief Oren Lyons, Onondaga 1993). Only very recently has the world begun to concede the inaccuracy of and racism behind this view. There is an almost desperate attempt by the descendants of colonizers to consign the *terra nullius* perspective to history, but recent developments in the area of human genetic research, engineering, and human gene patents bring back haunting and painful memories to indigenous peoples of a legacy of European colonial domination.

This article addresses two specific aspects of human genetic research, the Human Genome Diversity Project and the patenting of human genetic materials. . . .

Human genetic research can be viewed in the context of colonial imperial history. It is a history which in the first wave of colonization brought about the theft of lands, extermination of indigenous peoples through military invasion and biochemical warfare. . . .

WESTERN DEVELOPMENT: A FIXATION WITH GLASS

In the early days of *terra nullius,* indigenous peoples were regarded as primitive savages. Their body parts were pickled and preserved in glass jars so scientists could study them *in vitro.* Science developed theories to rationalize gross abuses of indigenous peoples (such as using the physical size of the brain as an indicator of intelligence, an inherently male obsession)—theories which have subsequently been proven wrong.

. . . Science and technology moved away from an oral tradition based on spirituality, sacredness, and timing to one based on theories and formulae and the belief that good science can replicate anything at any time, unaffected by seasons or cultural standards. Museums, set up as display facilities, locked indigenous ancestral remains and sacred objects behind glass cases for humanity and public education. Museums are now being asked to return their collections to the rightful indigenous owners.

"Savages" were traded as slaves—as commodities—amongst settlers. People paid money for

---

**terra nullius:* A Latin legal term meaning territory belonging to no one. The general rule of the English Common Law system was that ownership could not be acquired by occupying land already occupied by another; hence, settler governments evoked *terra nullius* in the new colonies thereby refusing to acknowledge existent indigenous inhabitants. . . .

their slaves and were in turn awarded exclusive ownership property rights. The slaves were theirs to do with as they wished and no one else could interfere. Slavery wasn't considered a human rights issue at first, it was seen as a commercial transaction. It took generations of protest and resistance, and the sacrifice of thousands of lives to overturn and criminalize property rights over humans. Now property rights over human genes are being legalized.

Human genes are being treated by science in the same way that indigenous "artifacts" were gathered by museums; collected, stored, immortalized, reproduced, engineered—all for the sake of humanity and public education, or so we are asked to believe. One wonders just how far we've actually come. Is this development? Is this good science?

MY ANCESTORS ARE ALWAYS WITH ME

Central to indigenous cultures is a profound respect and understanding of sacredness. Within my own culture, Maori tribes collectively have shared values about that which is *tapu* (sacred) and that which is *noa* (common). Hair, blood, mucus, the main sources used by westerners* to collect DNA, are all *tapu*. . . . It isn't coincidental that my culture and most other indigenous cultures regard hair, blood, and mucus as being sacred. We may not have had traditional terms for DNA or genes, but we knew the importance of protecting those things which could render us vulnerable. "The taking of blood, hair and tissue samples is an affront to the religious beliefs, cultural values and sensitivities of many indigenous peoples . . ." (National Congress of American Indians, Resolution No. NV-93-118).

---

*westerners: It is understood use of the term "westerners" is not completely satisfactory as it lumps distinct groupings within western society into one amorphous category. However, the same holds true when using the term, "indigenous peoples," as it serves to marginalize strong and diverse tribal nations such as Maasai, Samburu, Ngati Awa, Mohawk, Mapuche, Yanomami, etc.

Because of our respect for our ancestors, who are in every sense *tapu*, we regard the descendants of our ancestors, all of nature, as sacred. . . . Indigenous views about the integrity of human genes, therefore, are also applicable to the integrity of all other life. "Believing in the sanctity and integrity of life even in its smallest form . . . All life forms should be treated in a way that respects their intrinsic value as living generational manifestations of creation" (Treaty for a Life forms Patent-Free Pacific, 1995). Indigenous peoples are not advocating one value for human genes and another value for all others. The call is the same— nature and living things, tangible and intangible, all are sacred. . . .

For Maori, and many others, the human gene is genealogy. A physical gene is imbued with a life spirit handed down from the ancestors, contributed to by each successive generation, and passed on to future generations. Maori have two terms to describe a human gene, both of which are interlaced with a broader reality than western scientific definitions. The first is *Ira tangata*, which is the actual word for a gene and translates as "life spirit of mortals." The second term is *whakapapa*, which means to set layer upon layer. It also means "genealogy" and is the word most commonly used by Maori to conceptualize genes and DNA.

THE SACRED AND THE PROFANE

Western science goes to great lengths to dehumanize the humanness or life-force of human genes; hence, terms such as "specimens," "materials," "properties," and "collections" are adopted as a means to ignore the essence of life contained within. For Maori, a gene has *mauri* (a life-force) as do many other things, such as rocks of special significance, sacred sites, and placenta (afterbirth). . . . It is contrary to indigenous tradition to "objectify" a gene or human organs as these are living and sacred manifestations of the ancestors; they contain a life-force that continues to exist *ex-situ*. The same perspective is carried over to issues of replication, immortalization, transgenic engineering, and cloning.

Scientists distinguish an original specimen from a synthetically reproduced "copy gene." They take the view that a copy gene no longer has a connection with the person from whom the gene was extracted because it is no longer "original." It has been "innovated" or, depending on one's values, tampered with. Accordingly, in issues such as transgenic transferal of human genes into non-human species (a practice more common than many would realize, including introduction of transgenic modified products into the food chain), ethical considerations are dismissed as "moral taint." The UK Report on the Ethics of Genetic Modification and Food Use concludes, "because a number of steps are taken 'in vitro' to purify and replicate the donor gene, for all practical purposes, the inserted material is not 'human,' in the sense that it contains DNA derived directly from a human donor. We recommend that organisms containing copy genes of human origin may be used in the food chain subject to the necessary safety assessment."

The same applies for human gene patenting. Scientists argue that because the original collected specimen is not the subject of a patent (rather, it is a reduced, innovated and synthetic copy), the copy gene is not "human" according to the reductionist objectifying ethos. This contradicts the scientific reality that in order to have a copy or a property there must first be an original—that original is genealogy, has a life spirit, and is sacred.

A gene and combinations of genes are not the sole property of individuals. They are part of the heritage of families, communities, clans, tribes, and entire indigenous nations. In saying that, there is also clarity that there is more to being human than the physical composition of our DNA. We are shaped by our cultural values, beliefs, languages, histories, spirituality, and relationship to our lands. . . .

The survival of indigenous cultures will not come about because of gene banks. . . .

THE HUMAN GENOME DIVERSITY ("VAMPIRE") PROJECT

The Human Genome Diversity Project (HGDP) promotes itself as a humanitarian project. It describes its objective, "to collect blood samples from a number of indigenous populations, essentially for studying human evolution and the history of human migrations, but also for the purposes of genetic epidemiology, and studying the predisposition of certain groups to genetic disease" (Luigi Luca Cavalli-Sforza, TIME, 7 February 1994). Cavalli-Sforza also envisions the outcomes of the research contributing to the elimination of racism: "The variation among individuals is much greater than the differences among groups. In fact the diversity among individuals is so enormous that the whole concept of race becomes meaningless at the genetic level." . . .

HGDP has shown an appalling lack of judgment, first by excluding representatives of the very peoples who were to be the objects of research from early formative meetings; secondly, by ignoring the early warning signs from indigenous peoples that they wanted dialogue with the HGDP; and more recently, they have dismissed as a "simple misunderstanding" the no-choice position left to indigenous peoples to condemn the project. Cavalli-Sforza told TIME (South Pacific) that the project "has been targeted by activists whose motives have nothing to do with science . . . [the project] is being abused by some politicians and people seeking power."

Initially, indigenous peoples simply asked for the HGDP to be halted "until its moral, ethical, socio-economic, physical and political implications have been thoroughly discussed, understood and approved by indigenous peoples" (Mataatua Declaration on the Cultural and Intellectual Property Rights of Indigenous Peoples, 1993). . . . The HGDP needs to address the substantive questions such as: Is this good science? Is this research a priority for those very peoples who are being targeted for genetic sampling? What benefits will they receive? The other side of the coin is to consider that if alleviating racism is to be an objective, then why not sample racists to find out if they have a genetic predisposition to their disabling condition? If a genetic cure for racism could be developed, it would truly be a miracle treatment!

Why do indigenous people oppose it? Far from there being a simple "misunderstanding" of the visions of the project, the HGDP is viewed by many indigenous peoples as offensive, frivolous, and disrespectful of the integrity of nature, life, the ancestors—all that is sacred. The project is based on a *terra nullius* world view that regards western models of development as rational, desirable and normal, while most indigenous peoples reject such models as irrational, destructive, and alternative. Indigenous peoples have a sacred supreme relationship with their lands and waters. They cannot be isolated or studied outside of the context of how they inter-relate with their natural heritage. That is what makes them unique. An indigenous individual is the living manifestation of his ancestors, a vessel of genealogy, knowledge, lands and waters for future generations.

The HGDP's objective to use DNA analysis to examine indigenous histories of migration is seen as *terra nullius* racism revisited. . . .

The HGDP also assumes that knowledge is, by nature, empowering to all. It isn't.

The UNESCO International Bioethics Committee suggested that there might be "confusion of social ideologies with scientific goals," but science is only of use if it improves the quality of life and society. Without that, it serves no useful purpose to humanity, only a purpose for an exclusive, minority group of western professionals. Furthermore, the very nature of the proposed research is wholly dependent on unique cultural communities, social systems, and linguistic groupings. On what basis can one justify a separation of scientific goals and social ideologies?

The project has not only failed in its protocol-setting with indigenous peoples, it lacks clarity on matters which should have been thoroughly canvassed. For instance, the extent to which governments will be involved in the project has not been clearly delineated. If the HGDP relies on government funding it almost guarantees a bias towards the stipulations of donor governments which historically are counterproductive to indigenous peoples. Most governments actively oppress indigenous peoples which is why the socio-economic statistics are as bad as they are.

The absence of a robust methodology for gaining the consent of indigenous peoples is a grave concern. The potential to cause division within communities is a tragedy destined to happen. If consent is held as an objective, then there must also be an understanding of dissent. As outsiders, who will the HGDP approach? Who will they consider to have the definitive vote? If 50 people say no, and 20 people say yes, is that informed consent? Can consent be reduced to an individual level when the very nature of genetic research implicates a wider group? What if a chief consents but members of the community oppose? That, of course, assumes that chiefs or current structures of tribal authority are equipped to deal with these matters. . . .

It needs to be stressed that indigenous peoples are not anti-science. The UNESCO Bioethics committee noted that the Mataatua Declaration on Cultural and Intellectual Property Rights of Indigenous Peoples, while calling for a halt to the HGDP, also called "for involvement in scientific research by ensuring current scientific environmental research is strengthened by increasing the knowledge of indigenous communities and of customary environmental knowledge." The 1994 Maori Congress Indigenous Peoples Roundtable meeting recommended that "indigenous research structures be established by indigenous peoples, and participation in any other national and international bodies by indigenous peoples be actively sought in order for them to monitor, approve and collect any research which affects them." The issue, therefore, is not one of anti-science. It is that most indigenous peoples do not consider the HGDP to be "good" or "sustainable" science.

A further concern is the HGDP's inability to guarantee that the collections will be protected from commercialization. The HGDP seems to be torn between western humanitarian objectives and political economic realities. . . . Will the use of patents become the distinguishing factor? The HGDP is evasive over the issue of gene patenting. Not surprisingly, one of the more recent indigenous declarations demands that the project "be asked to make an accounting of all the genetic collections they have taken from indigenous peoples and have these returned to the owners of these genes" (Beijing Declaration of Indigenous Women, 1995).

PATENTING OF HUMAN GENES: THE HAGAHAI PATENT

To understand the implications of the Hagahai patent there are at least four tiers of benefits and detriments that one must explore: (1) for the Hagahai, (2) for Papua New Guinea [PNG], (3) for all other indigenous peoples, and (4) for humanity.

The Hagahai tribe of Papua New Guinea's Madang Province number approximately 293 members whose first contact with the outside world was as recent as 1984. Their experience is similar to what many other indigenous peoples went through over 500 years ago. It is one that marvels at the wonders of European technology and recognizes the potential for development and an enhanced quality of life. Trust, hope, and awe are the operative values governing how the "outside" world and people are perceived. Guns have been replaced with needles and medical treatment. Post-contact, the Hagahai were in danger of extinction due to European diseases such as malaria and pneumonia for which they had no inbuilt immunities. Dr. Carol Jenkins, a principal researcher at the PNG Institute of Medical Research, was the European face who responded to their call for help. She provided the Hagahai with tangible and critical medical assistance and became their respected friend. This is the Hagahai reality.

On discovering genetic qualities of the Hagahai that seemed to render them immune to leukemia and degenerative neurological diseases, Jenkins and four other colleagues made a decision to take out a US patent on components of the genetic qualities of one of her Hagahai friends, and assert a worldwide patent through the World Intellectual Property Organization (WIPO) International Patent Cooperation Treaty. The Hagahai patent grants to a US government agency ownership of genetic properties of a citizen of a foreign developing country. There are many other tribes in PNG who still have not yet been "discovered." What does their future hold? "Of the estimated 3.7 million PNG population, 70% are illiterate. Only 73 of every 100 children attend primary school and only 35 complete the course" (Papua New Guinea National Report to UNCED 1992). This is the PNG reality.

"Last week Dr. Jenkins, an American citizen, was hauled off an international flight at Port Moresby's Jackson Airport by (PNG) Foreign Affairs officials who accused her of being a bio-pirate" (*Sydney Sunday Telegraph*, 31 March 1996). . . .

Patents are not a tool of humanitarian research. They are a tool of commerce and exclusive property rights that serve to give signals to others: "stay away, they're mine. I own them." . . . It is one thing to copyright research results, it is a completely different matter to patent the genetic properties of those one is researching.

The Hagahai patent and the HGDP highlight the illusiveness of informed consent, a doctrine that is as fleeting as "objectivity" and a "level playing field." What kind of discussion took place? " 'Informed Consent' is a total illusion for the indigenous peoples in PNG. The Hagahai tribe were just introduced to modern medicine, and for the first time to the sight of a white woman. Immunization of diseases unheard of in that area was quickly introduced much to the confusion of the people. Blood samples were collected much to the amusement of the locals. Sign language was the obvious mode of communication [rather] than spoken words. Obviously the work of the HGDP and the PNG [Institute of] Medical Research was much beyond the knowledge and comprehension of the locals who were subjected to this research. Would you call this 'informed consent'?" (Individual & Community Rights Advocacy Forum, Papua New Guinea, 1995).

It assumes equality amongst cultural negotiators that simply does not exist because of the difference in world view and power. The Hagahai patent is not an isolated case, and it has become a global issue because the assumptions, methodologies, and protocols that enabled it to occur have relevance to all of us. Before this, the US government attempted to patent the cell lines of a Guaymi woman. Who is next? This is the indigenous peoples' reality. . . .

WHERE IS THIS GOING?

Indigenous peoples are clear that this new field of human genetic research and gene patenting is taking science and commerce into a dimension that is uncharted in the western world, but for which there exists deeply held traditional values that tell us this is not good science or good practice.

Just where do westerners think this is going? At what point does an individual scientist, lawyer, health professional, researcher reflect on their individual activity and see where it fits into a much broader context? At this rate, immortalized genetic properties of indigenous peoples will end up on the commodities market alongside pork bellies and sausage skins. . . .

In the meantime, indigenous peoples will continue to be oppressed. More of our lands, sacred sites, and traditions will be desecrated and misappropriated. Our right to self-determination will continue to be denied. Of what benefit will the HGDP and gene patents be to us? The world is not ready to be free of racism; the greed for more land, more of nature, and more commodities has become a cancer that even geneticists cannot cure.

REFERENCES

Gale de Villa, Jill, Ed. 1992. *Environment and Development: A Pacific Island Perspective.* Philippines: South Pacific Regional Environmental Programme (SPREP) & The Asian Development Bank.

Lewontin, R. C. 1991. *The Doctrine of DNA, Biology as Ideology.* London: Penguin Books.

Mead, Aroha Te Pareake. 1994. *Global Indigenous Strategies for Self-Determination.* Report of the Maori Congress Indigenous Peoples Roundtable Meeting. Wellington: Taonga Pacific.

———. 1995. The Convention on Biological Diversity: Are Human Genes Biological Resources? In *NZ Environmental Law Reporter* 1(6), July.

———. 1995. Bicultural Issues in Human Gene Therapy and Research. In *Report on the Clinical and Research Use of Human Genes.* Auckland: NZ Health Research Council.

UNESCO International Bioethics Committee. 1995. *Report on Bioethics and Human Population Genetics Research,* Paris.

QUESTIONS FOR COMPREHENSION AND REFLECTION

1. Discuss Mead's claim that the HGDP is simply an extension of European colonial imperialism. Do you agree with her? Should the HGDP be discontinued? Support your answers.
2. Does Western science dehumanize us, as Mead claims? Compare and contrast the worldview of Western geneticists and the Maori worldview regarding the value of human life. How do you think Western geneticists involved in the HGDP should respond when their worldview conflicts with that of a culture they wish to study? Discuss how a cultural relativist and a rights ethicist might respond to this question.
3. Discuss Mead's claim that indigenous people are often not able to give true informed consent. If you were a geneticist with the HGDP, how would you resolve this problem?
4. What are some of the harms, according to Mead, of using genetic material from indigenous people for genetic research and patents? Are these harms sufficient to warrant discontinuing the practice, or do the benefits outweigh the harms? Support your answers.

ROSAMOND RHODES

Genetic Links, Family Ties, and Social Bonds: Rights and Responsibilities in the Face of Genetic Knowledge

Rosamond Rhodes is a professor at the Mount Sinai School of Medicine. In her article, she questions the presumed right to genetic ignorance based on a right to privacy. Rhodes concludes that there is no right to genetic ignorance; instead, we have a moral responsibility regarding genetic knowledge because of our family and social ties.

INTRODUCTION

An old adage tells us that blood is thicker than water. The message of the saying is that blood ties carry moral weight. A thoughtful person might wonder how to act on that advice. It had been assumed that hereditary similarities gave those of the same blood common characteristics and, hence, special responsibilities to each other. So, before modern genetics we might have considered which of our familial relations count as blood. How thick are our responsibilities to blood? And, how thin are our responsibilities to water?

Knowledge of genetics, however, complicates the message that we might previously have drawn from the saying. Since learning that all living organisms have 80% of their DNA in common, that apes differ from humans in only 2% of their DNA, and that humans differ from one another by less than .1% of their DNA, the concept of blood ties becomes much more complicated. We still need to learn which social bonds involve thick responsibilities and which ties demand less of us. As we get a clearer picture of our genetic similarities and differences, we also need to find out more about the bearing of our genetic links on our ethical obligations. . . . The point of this discussion is . . . to demonstrate the similarity that may be obscured by dazzling new technology and to point a way toward structuring our thinking about these novel circumstances in terms of traditional moral frameworks.

To approach these questions of personal decision making in the face of new genetic technology we will have to examine the presumed right to genetic ignorance and its relation to rights of privacy. We will also need an account of why the various social bonds have different strengths and why more or less demanding obligations attach to them. Certainly an analysis of these issues will have implications for the mainstream discussion of professional and institutional responsibilities with respect to genetic knowledge. I leave those extrapolations for other discussions. I offer four cases to help us focus on the issues I have identified, the cases of Tom, Dick, Harry, and Harriette.

CLINICAL CASES

Case 1—Tom

Human DNA contains 6 billion base-pairs. An average gene contains about 2,000 base-pairs. Our approximately 100,000 genes contain about 200,000,000 base-pairs of DNA. DNA is a double helix molecule of strands of just four bases, adenosine, thymine, guanine, and cytosine, referred to by their abbreviations ATCG. The genetic code is carried by triplets of these nucleotides, sequences of three bases. Only a small portion of the genetic sequences of DNA is related to our particular recognizable characteristics.

By studying families with a history of Huntington disease, however, geneticists have learned that 40 or more CAG repeats identify a person who will develop the disease. Even though the typical small number of repeats is not associated with any identifiable trait, or phenotype, an expanded number of repeats is associated with this adult onset degenerative nervous system disorder. When a parent has the disease there is a 50% chance of a child inheriting it. And when the genetic marker is inherited, if the person does not die early from some other cause, Huntington will eventually develop.

Population studies of Huntington disease have not been undertaken. Without studying the general population no one knows whether there are individuals who have long CAG repeats and no familial history of the disease. No one knows whether long CAG repeats without a family history are indications of the disease. As the technology for genetic blueprints approaches our grasp, it becomes easy to imagine that population information about the phenotypic implications of long CAG repeats could be significant to people who might have them.

Tom's family has no history of Huntington disease. If researchers were to undertake a population study to learn more about the genetics of Huntington disease should Tom volunteer to be a research subject and allow his cheek to be swabbed for collection of genetic material? Does he owe this debt to his fellows? Tom is reluctant to learn anything about himself that might give him cause to worry. Could his reluctance justify refusing to participate?

Case 2—Dick

Dick has been diagnosed with Marfan syndrome, an inherited disorder of the connective tissue. People with this syndrome are very tall and typically have heart and eye defects. Dick's cousin, Martha, is tall but it is not clear whether she too has Marfan syndrome. Martha understands that Marfan syndrome is a dominant genetic disorder, so that she would have a 50% chance of having a child with this disorder if she has the mutation causing Marfan syndrome.

She and her husband have consulted a genetic counselor because they want to have children but would want to avoid having children with this problem. The counselor explains that while the gene for Marfan syndrome has been fully mapped and cloned, each family has its own specific familial mutation. Searching for the specific mutation in the DNA of Martha's family will involve a lengthy and expensive process. A better alternative would be a linkage study to discover the pattern of this family's co-inheritance of variations in neighboring genes with the Marfan mutation. Genes that are close to one another on a chromosome tend to be inherited together. By collecting genetic samples from close relatives and comparing the patterns of linked genes, geneticists are able to identify a familial pattern and associate it with the genetic defect. Future fetuses can then be screened for the identified genetic pattern.

Martha's mother has average stature and so does her only sister. But her father, who died in a car accident, and his brother were both tall. Martha's uncle Henry has agreed to provide a blood sample for the linkage study. Martha has also asked Dick, Uncle Henry's only child, to participate in the linkage study. Does Dick have a moral responsibility to allow himself to be tested?

Case 3—Harry

After three years of deterioration and suffering, Harry's father died of Huntington disease at age 49. When his father was diagnosed all of the immediate family were invited to participate in a genetic counselling session. Harry, who was 22 years old at the time, learned that this degenerative disease of the basal ganglia is physically and mentally disabling and that he has a one in two chance of developing it. Because the number of CAG repeats tends to increase in the offspring of affected males, and because more CAG repeats indicates earlier onset of the disease, if he has inherited the genotype Harry is likely to be afflicted earlier than his father was. Although Harry's brother was tested for the genetic marker and found to be unaffected, Harry has refused the test saying that he does not want to know.

Harry and Sally have fallen in love. They want to marry and have a family. Does Harry have a moral right not to know whether he has a long CAG repeat?

Case 4—Harriette

Harriette's sister had a child who died of Tay-Sachs disease after a brief and agonizing life. Harriette's family as well as her husband's are part of a community that is known to have a significant number of Tay-Sachs disease carriers. Harriette wants to have children and she knows that Tay-Sachs is a recessive inherited disease. She knows that she and her husband could be tested and learn whether their offspring might have the disease. She and her husband have discussed the situation and decided not to be tested. Harriette says that she does not want the information to affect her choice. She has decided to take whatever she gets.

Does Harriette have the moral right to act in ignorance? Is it ethically permissible for her to take this chance for her child? If she should have one affected child, would it be her moral right to have another?

A PRESUMED RIGHT TO GENETIC IGNORANCE FROM RESPECT FOR AUTONOMY

The several societies of the genetics community and most of the authors writing on issues of genetic knowledge have embraced a policy of non-directive, value-neutral counseling. Historically, this univocal commitment can be understood as a moral stance to disassociate modern genetics from the eugenics movements of the first half of this century which directed and coerced in light of their political, economic, and social agendas. Philosophically, non-directive counseling also reflects the centrality of respect for autonomy in modern bioethics. Appropriately, the genetics community has adopted the view that value neutral, or "non-directive," counseling implies that counselors and physicians should allow their clients and patients to decide whether or not to pursue genetic testing. Less fortuitously, in their

conversations, if not explicitly in their writing, they have come to speak of their patient's right not to know. This supposed right, in turn, has become another crucial precept in the ethics of genetic counseling. Our natural psychological aversion to being coerced, the historical commitment to personal liberty in the United States, and bioethics' attachment to the principle of autonomy can all account for the genetics community's comfort with the right not to know. Yet, inclinations do not add up to an argument. This crucial moral assumption may represent an unsupported and misleading philosophical leap of faith. . . .

A RIGHT TO GENETIC IGNORANCE

When we hear the phrase, "a right not to know," it does not sound like something that we should obviously challenge. Hearing it applied in the medical context might even sound acceptable. Imagine the patient saying to his doctor, "If you find something terrible, do what you have to but I do not want to know." It is not hard to imagine the doctor justifying going along with the patient's request by maintaining that "the patient has a right not to know." However, when we begin to examine the supposed right not to know we cannot fail to notice a stark contrast to our ordinary moral thinking. This discrepancy invites us to challenge the ethical status of the right not to know.

A television commercial shows a blindfolded man test driving a car so that he can fairly assess the smoothness of its ride. That man behind the wheel might later decide that he prefers driving blindfolded. When he does not see what is in front of him he does not have to take those obstacles into account: his decision-making is simplified and he is freed from a host of troubling concerns. Even though we might sympathize with his motives, we would, nevertheless, find the prospect of his driving blindfolded totally ridiculous and morally unacceptable to such an extreme as to be not worth considering. Obviously, driving a car without being able to see where you are going puts the property and lives of others in danger. No one has the right to do that. In other words, anyone who gets behind the wheel of a car is obliged to pay careful attention to his surroundings. If he is obliged to know his situation when he is driving, he has no right to choose to be in ignorance when he drives.

This is the line of reasoning that supports negligence law. Even when people can honestly assert that they were ignorant of the hazards posed by their action or some possibly dangerous circumstance involving their property, they are still held liable for consequent harms. They are liable because they have an obligation to know: they have no right not to know.

The eighteenth-century philosopher, Immanuel Kant, is the most acknowledged source of our appreciation of the ethical significance of respect for autonomy. . . . Kant recounts the situation of someone planning a murder asking you if your friend, his intended victim, is in your house when you had previously observed your friend entering. . . . Kant argues that benevolence cannot justify lying to the murderer because you cannot know whether your lie will accomplish good or actually harm the intended victim who might have already left the house unobserved. On the other hand, you will know with certainty that your lying will undermine our general reliance on veracity and that would do "wrong to men in general." In other words, those who believe that benevolence justifies this lie are mistaken because, according to Kant's argument, concern for benevolence justifies not lying. Regardless of whether you are willing to accept Kant's conclusion in his case, the form of the argument, that benevolence cannot justify lying because benevolence is the ground for not lying, is compelling. As I see it, the argument is actually more persuasive when applied to the supposed right to genetic ignorance.

Those who have argued for a right not to know genetic information about themselves have grounded their argument on the right to have one's autonomous choices respected. Following Kant's model, I want to argue that respect for autonomy actually leads to the opposite conclusion, the obligation to pursue genetic knowledge.

Through the active history of the American bioethics movement, the principle of respect for autonomy has been a cornerstone for bioethics argument. It has supported the consensus for a strong commitment to confidentiality, sustained arguments for informed consent in research, and upheld arguments for truth-telling and patient self-determination, particularly in decisions about withholding and withdrawing treatment. Respect for autonomy entails regarding others as capable of making choices for themselves that reflect their own values and commitments. It is, in part, because we recognize that people could have good reasons for not wanting to share personal medical information with everyone that we have to respect patient confidentiality. . . . Clearly, having information has been recognized as essential for making choices. Any piece of information might change a person's choice and lead her to pursue a different course than she might have without the information or with different information. So, because it allows others to make choices according to their own lights, health care providers are ethically obligated to make available the information that may be relevant to the patient. The reason for providing information in the typical medical context is that the patient is presumed to be an autonomous agent. Without the relevant information, the patient cannot make autonomous choices. From my point of view as an individual autonomous agent (as opposed to the point of view of some professional inside or policy-maker outside of the medical context who might be inclined to limit my autonomy) when I choose to remain ignorant of relevant information, I am choosing to leave whatever happens to chance. I am following a path without autonomy. Now, if autonomy is the ground for my right to determine my own course, it cannot also be the ground for not determining my own course. If autonomy justifies my right to knowledge, it cannot also justify my refusing to be informed. I may not be aware of the moral implications of ceding autonomy by insisting on genetic ignorance, but the ramifications are there, nevertheless.

From a Kantian perspective, autonomy is the essence of what morality requires of me. The core content of my duty is self-determination. To say this in another way, I need to appreciate that my ethical obligation is to rule myself, that is, to be a just ruler over my own actions. As sovereign over myself I am obligated to make thoughtful and informed decisions without being swayed by irrational emotions, including my fear of knowing significant genetic facts about myself. When I recognize that I am ethically required to be autonomous, I must also see that, since autonomous action requires being informed of what a reasonable person would want to know under the circumstance, I am ethically required to be informed. So, if I have an obligation to learn what I can, when genetic information is likely to make a significant difference in my decisions and when the relevant information is obtainable with reasonable effort, I have no right to remain ignorant. From the recognition of my own autonomy, I have a duty to be informed. I have no right to remain ignorant. . . .

TOM, DICK, HARRY, AND HARRIETTE

. . . [W]hen we face a choice between alternative actions and when the choice turns on genetic knowledge, preserving our autonomy requires that we pursue the information. And, when we have to decide whether to assume an obligation and when the decision even in part turns on genetic knowledge, we have a moral duty to pursue that information. These strong conclusions have implications for Tom, Dick, Harry, and Harriette. None of them can claim a right to genetic ignorance. Because there is no right to genetic ignorance Tom cannot use it as a ground for refusing to participate in the population study and Dick cannot use it as a reason for not helping his cousin Martha. And as for Harry and Harriette, because they are on the brink of making important decisions that involve commitments to others, there is at least a *prima facie* reason for maintaining that they are ethically obligated to learn crucial genetic facts about themselves.

Harry is considering marriage and fatherhood but he knows that he has a 50% chance of developing Huntington disease. Because marriage and fatherhood are essentially commitments to others, he has the duty to learn whether he is likely to be able to meet these responsibilities to his future wife and children. If he worried that he might develop the disease and seriously tried to take his duties into account while still refusing genetic tests,

he would be likely to make different decisions than he would have made in the face of knowledge. For example, knowing that he was not going to develop Huntington disease might free him to take a job in Australia that would allow him better opportunities for career advancement and the development of his talents. Knowing that he was going to develop the disease might lead him to accept a less promising job that would allow him to remain geographically close to Sally's family. Taking a far-sighted view of his situation allows us to imagine that his trying to second guess what he ought to do while considering two dramatically different scenarios could lead him to do what he might otherwise have seen as wrong. His informed assessment could lead him to a different conclusion.

Harriette is considering motherhood. She knows that she may have a chance as high as one in four of having a child with Tay-Sachs disease. She and her husband have agreed to forego testing and she expresses a willingness to undertake responsibility for any children they should have. If neither she nor her husband carry the trait, or even if only one of them carries the trait, they are worrying for nothing and making choices in light of that concern that may be inappropriate for their actual situation. On the other hand, if they were to have the genetic testing and learn that they were both carriers they could consider their reproductive choices in that light.

The analysis of the presumed right to genetic ignorance has taken us some way in discerning the rights and responsibilities of genetic knowledge. Exploring the thickness of social ties may take us some steps farther in understanding more about what the individuals in our cases owe to others. . . .

CASE DISCUSSION

Because we have duties to our fellows, *Tom* has a responsibility to participate in the population study. What is being asked of him requires little effort, minuscule discomfort, and no physical risk. Yet, the information to be gained by the study could have a significant impact on the well-being and decisions of others. Because the information can be a significant good to them and because we are morally required to render service to our brethren, Tom has a duty to participate in the study.

Similarly, *Dick* is obligated to provide a blood sample for a family linkage study. His familial relationship with Martha is closer than his bond with a stranger, so it would be more terrible to ignore her need than it would be to ignore a stranger's. Compassionate concern for Martha who wants to have a child who is unaffected by Marfan syndrome should incline him to cooperate. If Dick had been particularly close lifelong friends with his cousin, or if Martha had been his sister, he might have even stronger moral reasons for trying to be of service. On the other hand, if the cousins had minimal contact in their childhood, and if they had not even spoken to one another in the past decade, his responsibility might be somewhat diminished.

Dick's case is particularly interesting because it is only his blood ties to Martha that give him an obligation to participate in the linkage study. No one else can do it for her and no one else could take his place. Dick's case makes the point that we have some of our responsibilities because of our unique ability to help, others only because of our biological ties. So morality is not entirely constructed out of socially created links. Adoption would be another relevant example. A birth mother can relinquish all of her social rights and duties to her child and the adopting parents can take them all on. But the birth mother cannot transfer her biological responsibilities. Perhaps this insight calls for collecting a blood sample from the birth mother when the child is given up for adoption so that it could provide the genetic information that her child might need from her later in life.

We have already discussed some of the issues relating to *Harry's* obligation to pursue genetic knowledge. In addition, his "fuller friendship" with Sally gives her a special claim on him. Their social relationship gives them mutual responsibilities to treat one another as partners. To use the language of feminist philosopher, Patricia Mann, they have a mutual responsibility to recognize and support one another's "social agency," which, according to Mann, is associated with "motivation, responsibil-

ity, and expectation of recognition or reward." For Harry this involves acknowledging Sally's motivation with respect to entering a marriage, the responsibilities it would entail for her, and the rewards she would anticipate and how all of that might be impacted by his developing Huntington disease. Recognizing her agency would require him to inform her of his chance of developing Huntington disease, to discuss the alternatives relating to marriage and reproduction with her as a genuine partner, and to support her agency in whatever choice she should make for herself with respect to their future.

Harry's standing with respect to his future children raises another set of concerns. What duties does he undertake when he chooses to become a father? Is there some way that he can meet his obligations to his child if [he] becomes disabled and dies before the child matures?

And as for *Harriette's* case, a lurking issue of family ties involves informing other family members about their risk for having an affected child. Was Harriette's sister obligated to inform her siblings that she had an affected child? If she were estranged from the others and lived on the other side of the country would she be bound to tell? We know that families do keep secrets. Yet, because the impact of this disease is so devastating to the affected child and the entire household, and because family relations seem to carry some moral weight, and because we should care about the projects of close friends as well as strangers, there seem to be sufficient reasons for claiming that Harriette's sister should inform her siblings regardless of their present social relationship.

The most troubling issue of family bonds related to this case, however, turns on whether there are some children who are better off not being born. A Tay-Sachs baby appears normal for the first few months. Then, between the fourth and eighth month of life, the nerves begin to be affected by a fatty substance that accumulates in the cells. The child becomes blind, deaf, unable to swallow. The muscles atrophy, response to the environment dwindles, and the relentless deterioration continues until the child is totally debilitated and develops uncontrollable seizures. Death from pneumonia or infection usually occurs between age five and eight. Are there some lives that parents have no right to create?

CONCLUSION

The cases considered in this paper have led to some troubling unanswered questions about genetic links, family ties, and social bonds. When confronting the most difficult cases, it may be useful to recall Aristotle's caution that it is difficult to decide these matters with precision. Perhaps we should sometimes be satisfied with just ruling out the worst alternatives and allowing some room for differences of opinion.

The arguments we have considered have led to some strong and perhaps surprising conclusions. The clearest conclusion is that no one has a moral right to genetic ignorance. The other noteworthy conclusion is that moral responsibility depends on a variety of factors including blood ties, social relationships, the history of an interaction, and particular features of the situation and the individuals involved.

These conclusions have obvious and forceful implications for the individuals who may have reasons for considering genetic services. They are also significant for geneticists and genetic counselors in that they present good reasons for taking a certain view on what would be right for their patients and clients to choose. However, I need to caution that my line of argument does not go so far as to over-ride the genetics community's well-modulated commitment to non-directive counseling. A vivid imagination can allow us to see that in spite of the arguments against a right to genetic ignorance, in some unusual situation a rational person could have good reasons for making another choice. Beyond that, we know that people are not ideally rational and idiosyncratic psychological facts could make a significant difference. Furthermore, the general consequences of maintaining a non-directive counseling policy could far out-weigh the alternative by encouraging people to enter the counseling setting.

The surprising conclusion of the argument against the presumed right to genetic ignorance has another significant implication. While the genetics community deserves praise for their concerted efforts to address the ethical issues raised by their new technology, they also need to be warned. Ethics draws on analogy and examples, and then requires careful argument and careful analysis that turns on careful use of technical terms. At each step it is easy to stumble and mistakes are easily compounded. It is easy to reach a wrong conclusion when you start with an inappropriate analogy, misuse a technical term, or claim to have provided ethical analysis without understanding what is involved. Misunderstandings about the nature and moral force of autonomy have led some in the genetics community to a false conclusion about genetic ignorance. That error in turn has led to extreme positions on non-directive counseling. The moral of this story is that we all have our limitations. Some are in our genes, some are not, and no one is eager to hear bad news. . . .

QUESTIONS FOR COMPREHENSION AND REFLECTION

1. Discuss whether Rhodes's position on genetic ignorance is compatible with nondirective genetic counseling. What is the obligation of a counselor if a patient wants to remain ignorant? Discuss the merits of Rhodes's analogy between a person driving blindfolded and a person who wants to remain genetically ignorant. Does her analogy effectively address the issue of autonomy and privacy in making decisions that can lead to discrimination or distress? Use Rhodes's case studies to illustrate your answers.
2. If there is no privacy right to genetic ignorance, who should control dissemination of genetic information? Discuss who—relatives, insurance companies, the government, and/or scientists—should be privy to this information and under what circumstances.

3. Discuss whether people who are at risk for genetic disorders have a moral duty to have genetic testing before reproducing. If they test positive, do they have a moral duty to refrain from having children? How might Rhodes answer these questions? Compare and contrast your answers with hers.
4. Do we have a duty of beneficence to share genetic knowledge? Apply Rhodes's argument regarding this duty to the debate over the morality of biotech companies using genetic material from indigenous people. Do indigenous people—who might carry genes that can greatly benefit humankind—have a moral obligation, based on genetic ties and social bonds between humans, to allow geneticists to make cell lines from their genetic material? Support your answers.

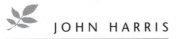

JOHN HARRIS

"Goodbye Dolly?" The Ethics of Human Cloning

John Harris is professor of bioethics and research director of the Center for Social Ethics and Policy at the University of Manchester in Great Britain, and director of the Institute of Medicine, Law and Bioethics. Harris examines some of the major official responses to cloning, including statements by the World Health Organization and President Clinton. Harris concludes that cloning is a reproductive right and is not inconsistent with human dignity.

The recent announcement of a birth in the press heralds an event probably unparalleled for two millennia and has highlighted the impact of the genetic revolution on our lives and personal choices. More importantly perhaps, it raises questions about the legitimacy of the sorts of control individuals and society purport to exercise over something, which while it must sound portentous, is nothing less than human destiny. This birth, that of "Dolly", the cloned sheep, is also illustrative of the responsibilities of science and scientists to the communities in which they live and which they serve, and of the public anxiety that sensational scientific achievements sometimes provokes. . . .

CELL MASS DIVISION

Although the technique of cloning embryos by cell mass division has for some time been used extensively in animal models, it was used as a way of multiplying human embryos for the first time in October 1993 when Jerry Hall and Robert Stillman at George Washington Medical Centre cloned human embryos by splitting early two- to eight-cell embryos into single embryo cells. . . .

INDIVIDUALS, MULTIPLES AND GENETIC VARIATION

Cloning does not produce identical copies of the same individual person. It can only produce identical copies of the same genotype. Our experience of identical twins demonstrates that each is a separate individual with his or her own character, preferences and so on. Although there is some evidence of striking similarities with respect to these factors in twins, there is no question but that each twin is a distinct individual, as independent and as free as is anyone else. . . .

The significant ethical issue here is whether it would be morally defensible, by outlawing the creation of clones by cell mass division, to deny a woman the chance to have the child she desperately seeks. If this procedure would enable a woman to create a sufficient number of embryos to give her a reasonable chance of successfully implanting one or two of them, then the objections to it would have to be weighty indeed. . . .

NUCLEAR SUBSTITUTION: THE BIRTH OF DOLLY

This technique involves (crudely described) deleting the nucleus of an egg cell and substituting the nucleus taken from the cell of another individual. This can be done using cells from an adult. The first viable offspring produced from fetal and adult mammalian cells was reported from an Edinburgh-based group in *Nature* on February 27, 1997. The event caused an international sensation and was widely reported in the world press. President Clinton of the United States called for an investigation into the ethics of such procedures and announced a moratorium on public spending on human cloning; the British Nobel Prize winner, Joseph Rotblat, described it as science out of control, creating "a means of mass destruction," and the German newspaper *Die Welt* evoked the Third Reich, commenting: "The cloning of human beings would fit precisely into Adolph Hitler's world view".

More sober commentators were similarly panicked into instant reaction. Dr Hiroshi Nakajima, Director General of the World Health Organisation said: "WHO considers the use of cloning for the replication of human individuals to be ethically unacceptable as it would violate some of the basic principles which govern medically assisted procreation. These include respect for the dignity of the human being and protection of the security of human genetic material". The World Health Organisation followed up the line taken by Nakajima with a resolution of the Fiftieth World Health Assembly which saw fit to affirm "that the use of cloning for the replication of human individuals is ethically unacceptable and contrary to human integrity and morality". . . .

HUMAN DIGNITY

Appeals to human dignity, . . . while universally attractive, are comprehensively vague and deserve separate attention. A first question to ask when the idea of human dignity is invoked is: whose dignity is attacked and how? Is it the duplication of a large part of the genome that is supposed to constitute the attack on human dignity? If so we might legitimately ask whether and how the dignity of a natural twin is threatened by the existence of her sister? The notion of human dignity is often also linked to Kantian ethics. A typical example, and one that attempts to provide some basis for objections to cloning based on human dignity, was Axel Kahn's invocation of this principle in his commentary on cloning in *Nature*.

> "The creation of human clones solely for spare cell lines would, from a philosophical point of view, be in obvious contradiction to the principle expressed by Emmanuel Kant: that of human dignity. This principle demands that an individual—and I would extend this to read human life—should never be thought of as a means, but always also as an end. Creating human life for the sole purpose of preparing therapeutic material would clearly not be for the dignity of the life created."

The Kantian principle, crudely invoked as it usually is without any qualification or gloss, is seldom helpful in medical or bio-science contexts. As formulated by Kahn, for example, it would outlaw blood transfusions. The beneficiary of blood donation, neither knowing of, nor usually caring about, the anonymous donor uses the blood (and its' donor) simply as a means to her own ends. It would also outlaw abortions to protect the life or health of the mother.

INSTRUMENTALIZATION

This idea of using individuals as a means to the purposes of others is sometimes termed "instrumentalization". Applying this idea coherently or consistently is not easy! If someone wants to have children in order to continue their genetic line do they act instrumentally? Where, as is standard practice in *in vitro* fertilisation (IVF), spare embryos are created, are these embryos created instrumentally? If not how do they differ from embryos created by embryo splitting for use in assisted reproduction?

Kahn responded in the journal *Nature* to these objections. He reminds us, rightly, that Kant's famous principle states: "respect for human dignity requires that an individual is *never* used . . . *exclusively* as a means". . . .

Kahn himself [also] rightly points out that debates concerning the moral status of the human embryo are debates about whether embryos fall within the *scope* of Kant's or indeed any other moral principles concerning persons; so the principle itself is not illuminating in this context. Applied to the creation of individuals which are, or will become autonomous, it has limited application. . . .

[Consider] the possibility of using embryo splitting to allow genetic and other screening by embryo biopsy. One embryo could be tested and then destroyed to ascertain the health and genetic status of the remaining clones. Again, an objection often voiced to this is that it would violate the Kantian principle, and that "one twin would be destroyed for the sake of another".

This is a bizarre and misleading objection both to using cell mass division to create clones for screening purposes, and to creating clones by nuclear substitution to generate spare cell lines. It is surely ethically dubious to object to one embryo being sacrificed for the sake of another, but not to object to it being sacrificed for nothing. In *in vitro* fertilisation, for example, it is, in the United Kingdom, currently regarded as good practice to store spare embryos for future use by the mother or for disposal at her direction, either to other women who require donor embryos, or for research, or simply to be destroyed. It cannot be morally worse to use an embryo to provide information about its sibling, than to use it for more abstract research or simply to destroy it. If it is permissible to use early embryos for research or to destroy them, their use in genetic and other health testing is surely also permissible. The same would surely go for their use in creating cell lines for therapeutic purposes. . . .

GENETIC VARIABILITY

So many of the fears expressed about cloning, and indeed about genetic engineering more generally, invoke the idea of the effect on the gene pool or upon genetic variability or assert the sanctity of the human genome as a common resource or heritage. It is very difficult to understand what is allegedly at stake here. The issue of genetic variation need not detain us long. The numbers of twins produced by cloning will always be so small compared to the human gene pool in totality, that the effect on the variation of the human gene pool will be vanishingly small. We can say with confidence that the human genome and the human population were not threatened at the start of the present millennium in the year AD one, and yet the world population was then perhaps one per cent of what it is today. Natural species are usually said to be endangered when the population falls to about one thousand breeding individuals; by these standards fears for humankind and its genome may be said to have been somewhat exaggerated. . . .

A RIGHT TO PARENTS

The apparently overwhelming imperative to identify some right that is violated by human cloning sometimes expresses itself in the assertion of "a right to have two parents" or as "the right to be the product of the mixture of the genes of two individuals". These are on the face of it highly artificial and problematic rights—where have they sprung from, save from a desperate attempt to conjure some rights that have been violated by cloning? However, let's take them seriously for a moment and grant that they have some force. Are they necessarily violated by the nuclear transfer technique?

If the right to have two parents is understood to be the right to have two social parents, then it is of course only violated by cloning if the family identified as the one to rear the resulting child is a one-parent family. This is not of course necessarily any more likely a result of cloning, than of the use of any of the other new reproductive technologies (or indeed of sexual reproduction). Moreover if there is such a right, it is widely violated, creating countless "victims", and there is no significant evidence of any enduring harm from the violation of this supposed right. Indeed war widows throughout the world would find its assertion highly offensive.

If, on the other hand we interpret a right to two parents as the right to be the product of the mixture of the genes of two individuals, then the supposition that this right is violated when the nucleus of the cell of one individual is inserted into the denucleated egg of another, is false in the way this claim is usually understood. There is at least one sense in which a right expressed in this form might be violated by cloning, but not in any way which has force as an objection. Firstly it is false to think that the clone is the genetic child of the nucleus donor. It is not. The clone is the twin brother or sister of the nucleus donor and the genetic offspring of the nucleus donor's own parents. Thus this type of cloned individual is, and always must be, the genetic child of two separate genotypes, of two genetically different individuals, however often it is cloned or re-cloned. . . .

WHAT GOOD IS CLONING?

One major reason for developing cloning in animals is said to be to permit the study of genetic dis-

eases and indeed genetic development more generally. Whether or not there would be major advantages in human cloning by nuclear substitution is not yet clear. Certainly it would enable some infertile people to have children genetically related to them, it offers the prospect, as we have noted, of preventing some diseases caused by mitochondrial DNA, and could help "carriers" of X-linked and autosomal recessive disorders to have their own genetic children without risk of passing on the disease. It is also possible that cloning could be used for the creation of "spare parts" by for example, growing stem cells for particular cell types from non-diseased parts of an adult.

Any attempt to use this technique in the United Kingdom, is widely thought to be illegal. . . .

The unease caused by Dolly's birth may be due to the fact that it was just such a technique that informed the plot of the film "The Boys from Brazil" in which Hitler's genotype was cloned to produce a fuehrer for the future. The prospect of limitless numbers of clones of Hitler is rightly disturbing. However, the numbers of clones that could be produced of any one genotype will, for the foreseeable future, be limited not by the number of copies that could be made of one genotype (using serial nuclear transfer techniques 470 copies of a single nuclear gene in cattle have been reported), but by the availability of host human mothers. Mass production in any democracy could therefore scarcely be envisaged. Moreover, the futility of any such attempt is obvious. Hitler's genotype might conceivably produce a "gonadically challenged" individual of limited stature, but reliability in producing an evil and vicious megalomaniac is far more problematic, for reasons already noted in our consideration of cloning by cell mass division. . . .

IMMORTALITY?

Of course some vainglorious individuals might wish to have offspring not simply with their genes but with a matching genotype. However, there is no way that they could make such an individual a duplicate of themselves. So many years later the environmental influences would be radically different, and since every choice, however insignificant, causes a life-path to branch with unpredictable consequences, the holy grail of duplication would be doomed to remain a fruitless quest. We can conclude that people who would clone themselves would probably be foolish and ill-advised, but would they be immoral and would their attempts harm society or their children significantly?

Whether we should legislate to prevent people reproducing, not 23 but all 46 chromosomes, seems more problematic for reasons we have already examined, but we might have reason to be uncomfortable about the likely standards and effects of child-rearing by those who would clone themselves. Their attempts to mould their child in their own image would be likely to be more pronounced than the average. Whether they would likely be worse than so many people's attempts to duplicate race, religion and culture, which are widely accepted as respectable in the contemporary world, might well depend on the character and constitution of the genotype donor. Where identical twins occur naturally we might think of it as "horizontal twinning", where twins are created by nuclear substitution we have a sort of "vertical twinning". Although horizontal twins would be closer to one another in every way, we do not seem much disturbed by their natural occurrence. Why we should be disturbed either by artificial horizontal twinning or by vertical twinning (where differences between the twins would be greater) is entirely unclear.

Suppose a woman's only chance of having "her own" genetic child was by cloning herself; what are the strong arguments that should compel her to accept that it would be wrong to use nuclear substitution? We must assume that this cloning technique is safe, and that initial fears that individuals produced using nuclear substitution might age more rapidly have proved groundless. We usually grant the so called "genetic imperative" as an important part of the right to found a family, of procreative autonomy. The desire of people to have "their own" genetic children is widely accepted, and if we grant the legitimacy of genetic aspirations in so many cases, and the use of so many technologies to meet these aspirations, we need

appropriately serious and weighty reasons to deny them here. . . .

We have looked at some of the objections to human cloning and found them less than plausible; we should now turn to one powerful argument that has recently been advanced in favour of a tolerant attitude to varieties of human reproduction.

PROCREATIVE AUTONOMY

We have examined the arguments for and against permitting the cloning of human individuals. At the heart of these questions is the issue of whether or not people have rights to control their reproductive destiny and, so far as they can do so without violating the rights of others or threatening society, to choose their own procreative path. We have seen that it has been claimed that cloning violates principles of human dignity. We will conclude by briefly examining an approach which suggests rather that failing to permit cloning might violate principles of dignity.

The American philosopher and legal theorist, Ronald Dworkin has outlined the arguments for a right to what he calls "procreative autonomy" and has defined this right as "a right to control their own role in procreation unless the state has a compelling reason for denying them that control". Arguably, freedom to clone one's own genes might also be defended as a dimension of procreative autonomy because so many people and agencies have been attracted by the idea of the special nature of genes and have linked the procreative imperative to the genetic imperative.

> "The right of procreative autonomy follows from any competent interpretation of the due process clause and of the Supreme Court's past decisions applying it. . . . The First Amendment prohibits government from establishing any religion, and it guarantees all citizens free exercise of their own religion. The Fourteenth Amendment, which incorporates the First Amendment, imposes the same prohibition and same responsibility on states. These provisions also guarantee the right of procreative autonomy."

The point is that the sorts of freedoms which freedom of religion guarantees, freedom to choose one's own way of life and live according to one's most deeply held beliefs are also at the heart of procreative choices. . . . Thus it may be that we should be prepared to accept both some degree of offence and some social disadvantages as a price we should be willing to pay in order to protect freedom of choice in matters of procreation and perhaps this applies to cloning as much as to more straightforward or usual procreative preferences.

. . . In so far as decisions to reproduce in particular ways or even using particular technologies constitute decisions concerning central issues of value, then arguably the freedom to make them is guaranteed by the constitution (written or not) of any democratic society, unless the state has a compelling reason for denying its citizens that control. To establish such a compelling reason the state (or indeed a federation or union of states, such as the European Union for example) would have to show that more was at stake than the fact that a majority found the ideas disturbing or even disgusting.

As yet, in the case of human cloning, such compelling reasons have not been produced. Suggestions have been made, but have not been sustained, that human dignity may be compromised by the techniques of cloning. Dworkin's arguments suggest that human dignity and indeed democratic constitutions may be compromised by attempts to limit procreative autonomy, at least where greater values cannot be shown to be thereby threatened.

In the absence of compelling arguments against human cloning, we can bid Dolly a cautious "hello". We surely have sufficient reasons to permit experiments on human embryos to proceed, provided, as with any such experiments, the embryos are destroyed at an early stage. While we wait to see whether the technique will ever be established as safe, we should consider the best ways to regulate its uptake until we are in a position to know what will emerge both by way of benefits and in terms of burdens.

QUESTIONS FOR COMPREHENSION AND REFLECTION

1. Harris claims that extensive cloning of any one genome will be limited because only a few mothers will want clones of the same child. However, is this a realistic expectation? Given the human propensity toward social conformity and the desire for popular mass-produced goods such as athletic shoes and automobiles, wouldn't it be reasonable to expect a similar public demand for the clones of widely admired people and celebrities? Support your answers.

2. Are you satisfied with the manner in which Harris addresses the question of what it means to have two parents? Explain your answer. Discuss whether Kass, author of the next reading, would be satisfied with Harris's treatment of this subject.

3. According to Confucius, rights exist only within the context of our duty to the wider community. Given the Confucian emphasis on social and familial harmony, discuss whether or not Confucius would agree with Harris that cloning is a reproductive right.

4. Do you agree with Harris that, in the absence of any compelling arguments against human cloning, we should permit research on human cloning to proceed? Support your answer.

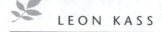

LEON KASS

The Wisdom of Repugnance: Why We Should Ban the Cloning of Humans

Leon Kass is a professor on the Committee on Social Thought at the University of Chicago. In the late 1960s and 1970s, Kass was one of the first scholars to openly express concern about the morality of human cloning. He argues that people should trust their initial feeling of repugnance toward cloning. Cloning violates some of the most important human values and turns children into commodities. The manufacture of humans by cloning, therefore, should be prohibited.

. . .

TAKING CLONING SERIOUSLY, THEN AND NOW

Cloning first came to public attention roughly thirty years ago, following the successful asexual production, in England, of a clutch of tadpole clones by the technique of nuclear transplantation. . . .

Much has happened in the intervening years. It has become harder, not easier, to discern the true meaning of human cloning. We have in some sense been softened up to the idea—through movies, cartoons, jokes and intermittent commentary in the mass media, some serious, most light-hearted. We have become accustomed to new practices in human reproduction: not just in vitro fertilization, but also embryo manipulation, embryo donation and surrogate pregnancy. Animal biotechnology has yielded transgenic animals and a burgeoning science of genetic engineering, easily and soon to be transferable to humans.

Even more important, changes in the broader culture make it now vastly more difficult to express a common and respectful understanding of sexuality, procreation, nascent life, family, and the meaning of motherhood, fatherhood and the links between the generations. . . .

Cloning turns out to be the perfect embodiment of the ruling opinions of our new age.

Thanks to the sexual revolution, we are able to deny in practice, and increasingly in thought, the inherent procreative teleology of sexuality itself. But, if sex has no intrinsic connection to generating babies, babies need have no necessary connection to sex. Thanks to feminism and the gay rights movement, we are increasingly encouraged to treat the natural heterosexual difference and its preeminence as a matter of "cultural construction." But if male and female are not normatively complementary and generatively significant, babies need not come from male and female complementarity. Thanks to the prominence and the acceptability of divorce and out-of-wedlock births, stable, monogamous marriage as the ideal home for procreation is no longer the agreed-upon cultural norm. For this new dispensation, the clone is the ideal emblem: the ultimate "single-parent child."

Thanks to our belief that all children should be *wanted* children (the more high-minded principle we use to justify contraception and abortion), sooner or later only those children who fulfill our wants will be fully acceptable. Through cloning, we can work our wants and wills on the very identity of our children, exercising control as never before. Thanks to modern notions of individualism and the rate of cultural change, we see ourselves not as linked to ancestors and defined by traditions, but as projects for our own self-creation, not only as self-made men but also man-made selves; and self-cloning is simply an extension of such rootless and narcissistic self-re-creation.

Unwilling to acknowledge our debt to the past and unwilling to embrace the uncertainties and the limitations of the future, we have a false relation to both: cloning personifies our desire fully to control the future, while being subject to no controls ourselves. Enchanted and enslaved by the glamour of technology, we have lost our awe and wonder before the deep mysteries of nature and of life. We cheerfully take our own beginnings in our hands and, like the last man, we blink.

Part of the blame for our complacency lies, sadly, with the field of bioethics itself, and its claim to expertise in these moral matters. Bioethics was founded by people who understood that the new biology touched and threatened the deepest matters of our humanity: bodily integrity, identity and individuality, lineage and kinship, freedom and self-command, eros and aspiration, and the relations and strivings of body and soul. With its capture by analytic philosophy, however, and its inevitable routinization and professionalization, the field has by and large come to content itself with analyzing moral arguments, reacting to new technological developments and taking on emerging issues of public policy, all performed with a naïve faith that the evils we fear can all be avoided by compassion, regulation and a respect for autonomy. . . .

. . . Human cloning, though it is in some respects continuous with previous reproductive technologies, also represents something radically new, in itself and in its easily foreseeable consequences. The stakes are very high indeed. I exaggerate, but in the direction of the truth, when I insist that we are faced with having to decide nothing less than whether human procreation is going to remain human, whether children are going to be made rather than begotten, whether it is a good thing, humanly speaking, to say yes in principle to the road which leads (at best) to the dehumanized rationality of *Brave New World*. This is not business as usual, to be fretted about for a while but finally to be given our seal of approval. We must rise to the occasion and make our judgments as if the future of our humanity hangs in the balance. For so it does.

THE STATE OF THE ART

. . . [F]or the tens of thousands of people already sustaining over 200 assisted-reproduction clinics in the United States and already availing themselves of in vitro fertilization, intracytoplasmic sperm injection and other techniques of assisted reproduction, cloning would be an option with virtually no added fuss (especially when the success rate improves). . . .

In anticipation of human cloning, apologists and proponents have already made clear possible uses of the perfected technology, ranging from the sentimental and compassionate to the grandiose. They include: providing a child for an infertile couple; "replacing" a beloved spouse or child who is dying or has died; avoiding the risk of genetic disease; permitting reproduction for homosexual men and lesbians who want nothing sexual to do with the opposite sex; securing a genetically identical source of organs or tissues perfectly suitable for transplantation; getting a child with a genotype of one's own choosing, not excluding oneself; replicating individuals of great genius, talent or beauty—having a child who really could "be like Mike"; and creating large sets of genetically identical humans suitable for research on, for instance, the question of nature versus nurture, or for special missions in peace and war (not excluding espionage), in which using identical humans would be an advantage. Most people who envision the cloning of human beings, of course, want none of these scenarios. That they cannot say why is not surprising. What is surprising, and welcome, is that, in our cynical age, they are saying anything at all.

THE WISDOM OF REPUGNANCE

"Offensive." "Grotesque." "Revolting." "Repugnant." "Repulsive." These are the words most commonly heard regarding the prospect of human cloning. Such reactions come both from the man or woman in the street and from the intellectuals, from believers and atheists, from humanists and scientists. Even Dolly's creator has said he "would find it offensive" to clone a human being.

People are repelled by many aspects of human cloning. They recoil from the prospect of mass production of human beings, with large clones of look-alikes, compromised in their individuality; the idea of father-son or mother-daughter twins; the bizarre prospects of a woman giving birth to and rearing a genetic copy of herself, her spouse or even her deceased father or mother; the grotesqueness of conceiving a child as an exact replacement for another who has died; the utilitarian creation of embryonic genetic duplicates of oneself, to be frozen away or created when necessary, in case of need for homologous tissues or organs for transplantation; the narcissism of those who would clone themselves and the arrogance of others who think they know who deserves to be cloned or which genotype any child-to-be should be thrilled to receive; the Frankensteinian hubris to create human life and increasingly to control its destiny; man playing God. Almost no one finds any of the suggested reasons for human cloning compelling; almost everyone anticipates its possible misuses and abuses. Moreover, many people feel oppressed by the sense that there is probably nothing we can do to prevent it from happening. This makes the prospect all the more revolting.

Revulsion is not an argument; and some of yesterday's repugnances are today calmly accepted—though, one must add, not always for the better. In crucial cases, however, repugnance is the emotional expression of deep wisdom, beyond reason's power fully to articulate it. Can anyone really give an argument fully adequate to the horror which is father-daughter incest (even with consent), or having sex with animals, or mutilating a corpse, or eating human flesh, or even just (just!) raping or murdering another human being? Would anybody's failure to give full rational justification for his or her revulsion at these practices make that revulsion ethically suspect? Not at all. On the contrary, we are suspicious of those who think that they can rationalize away our horror, say, by trying to explain the enormity of incest with arguments only about the genetic risks of inbreeding.

The repugnance at human cloning belongs in this category. We are repelled by the prospect of cloning human beings not because of the strangeness or novelty of the undertaking, but because we intuit and feel, immediately and without argument, the violation of things that we rightfully hold dear. Repugnance, here as elsewhere, revolts against the excesses of human willfulness, warning us not to transgress what is unspeakably profound. Indeed, in this age in which everything is held to be permissible so long as it is freely done, in which our given human nature no longer commands respect, in which our bodies are regarded as mere instruments of our autonomous rational wills, repugnance may be the only voice left that speaks up to defend the central core of our humanity. Shallow are the souls that have forgotten how to shudder.

Yet repugnance need not stand naked before the bar of reason. The wisdom of our horror at human cloning can be partially articulated, even if this is finally one of those instances about which the heart has its reasons that reason cannot entirely know.

THE PROFUNDITY OF SEX

To see cloning in its proper context, we must begin not . . . with laboratory technique, but with the anthropology—natural and social—of sexual reproduction.

Sexual reproduction—by which I mean the generation of new life from (exactly) two complementary elements, one female, one male, (usually) through coitus—is established (if that is the right term) not by human decision, culture or tradition, but by nature; it is the natural way of all mammalian reproduction. By nature, each child has two complementary biological progenitors. Each child thus stems from and unites exactly two lineages. In natural generation, moreover, the precise genetic constitution of the resulting offspring is determined by a combination of nature and chance, not by human design: each human child shares the common natural human species genotype, each child is genetically (equally) kin to each (both) parent(s), yet each child is also genetically unique.

These biological truths about our origins foretell deep truths about our identity and about our human condition altogether. Every one of us is at once equally human, equally enmeshed in a particular familial nexus of origin, and equally individuated in our trajectory from birth to death—and, if all goes well, equally capable (despite our mortality) of participating, with a complementary other, in the very same renewal of such human possibility through procreation. Though less momentous than our common humanity, our genetic individuality is not humanly trivial. It shows itself forth in our distinctive appearance through which we are everywhere recognized; it is revealed in our "signature" marks of fingerprints and our self-recognizing immune system; it symbolizes and foreshadows exactly the unique, never-to-be-repeated character of each human life.

Human societies virtually everywhere have structured child-rearing responsibilities and systems of identity and relationship on the bases of these deep natural facts of begetting. The mysterious yet ubiquitous "love of one's own" is everywhere culturally exploited, to make sure that children are not just produced but well cared for and to create for everyone clear ties of meaning, belonging and obligation. But it is wrong to treat such naturally rooted social practices as mere cultural constructs (like left- or right-driving, or like burying or cremating the dead) that we can alter with little human cost. What would kinship be without its clear natural grounding? And what would identity be without kinship? We must resist those who have begun to refer to sexual reproduction as the "traditional method of reproduction," who would have us regard as merely traditional, and by implication arbitrary, what is in truth not only natural but most certainly profound.

Asexual reproduction, which produces "single-parent" offspring, is a radical departure from the natural human way, confounding all normal understandings of father, mother, sibling, grandparent, etc., and all moral relations tied thereto. It becomes even more of a radical departure when the resulting offspring is a clone derived not from an embryo, but from a mature adult to whom the clone would be an identical twin; and when the process occurs not by natural accident (as in natural twinning), but by deliberate human design and manipulation; and when the child's (or children's) genetic constitution is preselected by the parent(s) (or scientists). Accordingly, as we will see, cloning is vulnerable to three kinds of concerns and objections, related to these three points: cloning threatens confusion of identity and individuality, even in small-scale cloning; cloning represents a giant step (though not the first one) toward transforming procreation into manufacture, that is, toward the increasing depersonalization of the process of generation and, increasingly, toward the "production" of human children as artifacts, products of human will and design (what others have called the problem of "commodification" of new life); and cloning—like other forms of eugenic engineering of the next generation—represents a form of despotism of the cloners over the cloned, and thus (even in benevolent cases) represents a blatant violation of the inner meaning of parent-child relations, of what it means to have a child, of what it means to say "yes" to our own demise and "replacement.". . .

. . . [I]t is impossible, I submit, for there to have been human life—or even higher forms of animal life—in the absence of sexuality and sexual reproduction. We find asexual reproduction only in the lowest forms of life: bacteria, algae, fungi, some lower invertebrates. Sexuality brings with it a new and enriched relationship to the world. Only sexual animals can seek and find complementary others with whom to pursue a goal that transcends their own existence. For a sexual being, the world is no longer an indifferent and largely homogeneous *otherness,* in part edible, in part dangerous. It also contains some very special and related and complementary beings, of the same kind but of opposite sex, toward whom one reaches out with special interest and intensity. In higher birds and mammals, the outward gaze keeps a lookout not only for food and predators, but also for prospective mates; the beholding of the many splendored world is suffused with desire for union, the animal antecedent of human eros and the germ of sociality. Not by accident is the human animal both the sexiest animal—whose females do not go into heat but are receptive throughout the estrous cycle and whose males must therefore have greater sexual appetite and energy in order to reproduce successfully—and also the most aspiring, the most social, the most open and the most intelligent animal. . . .

Through children, a good common to both husband and wife, male and female achieve some genuine unification (beyond the mere sexual "union," which fails to do so). The two become one through sharing generous (not needy) love for this third being as good. Flesh of their flesh, the child is the parents' own commingled being externalized, and given a separate and persisting existence. Unification is enhanced also by their commingled work of rearing. Providing an opening to the future beyond the grave, carrying not only our seed but also our names, our ways and our hopes that they will surpass us in goodness and happiness, children are a testament to the possibility of transcendence. Gender duality and sexual desire, which first draws our love upward and outside of ourselves, finally provide for the partial overcoming of the confinement and limitation of perishable embodiment altogether.

Human procreation, in sum, is not simply an activity of our rational wills. It is a more complete activity precisely because it engages us bodily, erotically and spiritually, as well as rationally. There is wisdom in the mystery of nature that has joined the pleasure of sex, the inarticulate longing for union, the communication of the loving embrace and the deep-seated and only partly articulate desire for children in the very activity by which we continue the chain of human existence and participate in the renewal of human possibility. Whether or not we know it, the severing of procreation from sex, love and intimacy is inherently dehumanizing, no matter how good the product.

We are now ready for the more specific objections to cloning.

THE PERVERSITIES OF CLONING

First, an important if formal objection: any attempt to clone a human being would constitute an unethical experiment upon the resulting child-to-be. As the animal experiments (frog and sheep) indicate, there are grave risks of mishaps and deformities. Moreover, because of what cloning means, one cannot presume a future cloned child's consent to be a clone, even a healthy one. Thus, ethically speaking, we cannot even get to know whether or not human cloning is feasible.

I understand, of course, the philosophical difficulty of trying to compare a life with defects against nonexistence. Several bioethicists, proud of their philosophical cleverness, use this conundrum to embarrass claims that one can injure a child in its conception, precisely because it is only thanks to that complained-of conception that the child is alive to complain. But common sense tells us that we have no reason to fear such philosophisms. For we surely know that people can harm and even maim children in the very act of conceiving them, say, by paternal transmission of the AIDS virus, maternal transmission of heroin dependence or, arguably, even by bringing them into being as bastards or with no capacity or willingness to look after them properly. And we believe that to do this intentionally, or even negligently, is inexcusable and clearly unethical.

The objection about the impossibility of presuming consent may even go beyond the obvious and sufficient point that a clonant, were he subsequently to be asked, could rightly resent having been made a clone. At issue are not just benefits and harms, but doubts about the very independence needed to give proper (even retroactive) consent, that is, not just the capacity to choose but the disposition and ability to choose freely and well. It is not at all clear to what extent a clone will truly be a moral agent. For, as we shall see, in the very fact of cloning, and of rearing him as a clone, his makers subvert the cloned child's independence, beginning with that aspect that comes from knowing that one was an unbidden surprise, a gift, to the world, rather than the designed result of someone's artful project.

Cloning creates serious issues of identity and individuality. The cloned person may experience concerns about his distinctive identity not only because he will be in genotype and appearance identical to another human being, but, in this case, because he may also be twin to the person who is his "father" or "mother"—if one can still call them that. What would be the psychic burdens of being the "child" or "parent" of your twin? The cloned individual, moreover, will be saddled with a genotype that has already lived. He will not be fully a surprise to the world. People are likely always to compare his performances in life with that of his alter ego. True, his nurture and his circumstance in life will be different; genotype is not exactly destiny. Still, one must also expect parental and other efforts to shape this new life after the original—or at least to view the child with the original version always firmly in mind. Why else did they clone from the star basketball player, mathematician and beauty queen—or even dear old dad—in the first place?

Since the birth of Dolly, there has been a fair amount of doublespeak on this matter of genetic identity. Experts have rushed in to reassure the public that the clone would in no way be the same person, or have any confusions about his or her identity: as previously noted, they are pleased to point out that the clone of Mel Gibson would not be Mel Gibson. Fair enough. But one is short-changing the truth by emphasizing the additional importance of the intrauterine environment, rearing and social setting: genotype obviously matters plenty. That, after all, is the only reason to clone, whether human beings or sheep. . . .

Curiously, this conclusion is supported, inadvertently, by the one ethical sticking point insisted on by friends of cloning: no cloning without the donor's consent. Though an orthodox liberal objection, it is in fact quite puzzling when it comes from people . . . who also insist that genotype is not identity or individuality, and who deny that a child could reasonably complain about being made a genetic copy. If the clone of Mel Gibson would not be Mel Gibson, why should Mel Gibson have grounds to object that someone had been made his clone? We already allow researchers to use blood and tissue samples for research purposes of no benefit to their sources: my falling hair, my expectorations, my urine and even my biopsied tissues are "not me" and not mine. Courts have held that the profits gained from uses to which scientists put my discarded tissues do not legally belong to me. Why, then, no cloning without consent—including, I assume, no cloning from the body of someone who just died? What harm is done the donor, if genotype is "not me"? Truth to tell, the only powerful justification for objecting is that genotype really does have something to do with identity, and everybody knows it. . . .

Human cloning would also represent a giant step toward turning begetting into making, procreation into manufacture (literally, something "handmade"), a process already begun with in vitro fertilization and genetic testing of embryos. With cloning, not only is the process in hand, but the total genetic blueprint of the cloned individual is selected and determined by the human artisans. To be sure, subsequent development will take place according to natural processes; and the resulting children will still be recognizably human. But we here would be taking a major step into making man himself simply another one of the man-made things. Human nature becomes merely the last part of nature to succumb to the technological project, which turns all of nature into raw material at human disposal, to be homogenized by our rationalized technique according to the subjective prejudices of the day.

How does begetting differ from making? In natural procreation, human beings come together, complementarily male and female, to give existence to another being who is formed, exactly as we were, *by what we are*: living, hence perishable, hence aspiringly erotic, human beings. In clonal reproduction, by contrast, and in the more advanced forms of manufacture to which it leads, we give existence to a being not by what we are but by what we intend and design. As with any product of our making, no matter how excellent, the artificer stands above it, not as an equal but as a superior, transcending it by his will and creative prowess. Scientists who clone animals make it perfectly clear that they are engaged in instrumental making; the animals are, from the start, designed as means to serve rational human purposes. In human cloning, scientists and prospective "parents" would be adopting the same technocratic mentality to human children: human children would be their artifacts.

Such an arrangement is profoundly dehumanizing, no matter how good the product. Mass-scale cloning of the same individual makes the point vividly; but the violation of human equality, freedom and dignity are present even in a single planned clone. And procreation dehumanized into manufacture is further degraded by commodification, a virtually inescapable result of allowing baby-making to proceed under the banner of commerce. Genetic and reproductive biotechnology companies are already growth industries, but they will go into commercial orbit once the Human Genome Project nears completion. . . .

Finally, and perhaps most important, the practice of human cloning by nuclear transfer—like other anticipated forms of genetic engineering of the next generation—would enshrine and aggravate a profound and mischievous misunderstanding of the meaning of having children and of the parent-child relationship. When a couple now chooses to procreate, the partners are saying yes to the emergence of new life in its novelty, saying yes not only to having a child but also, tacitly, to having whatever child this child turns out to be. In accepting our finitude and opening ourselves to our replacement, we are tacitly confessing the limits of our control. In this ubiquitous way of nature, embracing the future by procreating means precisely that we are relinquishing our grip, in the very activity of taking up our own share in what we hope will be the immortality of human life and the human species. This means that our children are not *our* children: they are not our property, not our possessions. Neither are they supposed to live our lives for us, or anyone else's life but their own. To be sure, we seek to guide them on their way, imparting to them not just life but nurturing, love, and a way of life; to be sure, they bear our hopes that they will live fine and flourishing lives, enabling us in small measure to transcend our own limitations. Still, their genetic distinctiveness and independence are the natural foreshadowing of the deep truth that they have their own and never-before enacted life to live. They are sprung from a past, but they take an uncharted course into the future.

Much harm is already done by parents who try to live vicariously through their children. Children are sometimes compelled to fulfill the broken dreams of unhappy parents; John Doe Jr. or the III is under the burden of having to live up to his fore-

bear's name. Still, if most parents have hopes for their children, cloning parents will have expectations. In cloning, such overbearing parents take at the start a decisive step which contradicts the entire meaning of the open and forward-looking nature of parent-child relations. The child is given a genotype that has already lived, with full expectation that this blueprint of a past life ought to be controlling of the life that is to come. Cloning is inherently despotic, for it seeks to make one's children (or someone else's children) after one's own image (or an image of one's choosing) and their future according to one's will. In some cases, the despotism may be mild and benevolent. In other cases, it will be mischievous and downright tyrannical. But despotism—the control of another through one's will—it inevitably will be.

MEETING SOME OBJECTIONS

The defenders of cloning, of course, are not wittingly friends of despotism. Indeed, they regard themselves mainly as friends of freedom: the freedom of individuals to reproduce, the freedom of scientists and inventors to discover and devise and to foster "progress" in genetic knowledge and technique. They want large-scale cloning only for animals, but they wish to preserve cloning as a human option for exercising our "right to reproduce"—our right to have children, and children with "desirable genes." As law professor John Robertson points out, under our "right to reproduce" we already practice early forms of unnatural, artificial and extramarital reproduction, and we already practice early forms of eugenic choice. For this reason, he argues, cloning is no big deal.

We have here a perfect example of the logic of the slippery slope, and the slippery way in which it already works in this area. Only a few years ago, slippery slope arguments were used to oppose artificial insemination and in vitro fertilization using unrelated sperm donors. Principles used to justify these practices, it was said, will be used to justify more artificial and more eugenic practices, including cloning. Not so, the defenders retorted, since we can make the necessary distinctions. And now, without even a gesture at making the necessary distinctions, the continuity of practice is held by itself to be justificatory.

The principle of reproductive freedom as currently enunciated by the proponents of cloning logically embraces the ethical acceptability of sliding down the entire rest of the slope—to producing children ectogenetically from sperm to term (should it become feasible) and to producing children whose entire genetic makeup will be the product of parental eugenic planning and choice. If reproductive freedom means the right to have a child of one's own choosing, by whatever means, it knows and accepts no limits.

But, far from being legitimated by a "right to reproduce," the emergence of techniques of assisted reproduction and genetic engineering should compel us to reconsider the meaning and limits of such a putative right. In truth, a "right to reproduce" has always been a peculiar and problematic notion. Rights generally belong to individuals, but this is a right which (before cloning) no one can exercise alone. . . .

. . . Some insist that the right to reproduce embraces . . . the right against state interference with the free use of all technological means to obtain a child. Yet such a position cannot be sustained: for reasons having to do with the means employed, any community may rightfully prohibit surrogate pregnancy, or polygamy, or the sale of babies to infertile couples, without violating anyone's basic human "right to reproduce." When the exercise of a previously innocuous freedom now involves or impinges on troublesome practices that the original freedom never was intended to reach, the general presumption of liberty needs to be reconsidered.

We do indeed already practice negative eugenic selection, through genetic screening and prenatal diagnosis. Yet our practices are governed by a norm of health. We seek to prevent the birth of children who suffer from known (serious) genetic diseases. When and if gene therapy becomes possible, such diseases could then be treated, in utero or even before implantation—I have no ethical objection in principle to such a practice (though I

have some practical worries), precisely because it serves the medical goal of healing existing individuals. But therapy, to be therapy, implies not only an existing "patient." It also implies a norm of health. In this respect, even germline gene "therapy," though practiced not on a human being but on egg and sperm, is less radical than cloning, which is in no way therapeutic. But once one blurs the distinction between health promotion and genetic enhancement, between so-called negative and positive eugenic designs. . . .

. . . [T]he principle here endorsed justifies not only cloning but, indeed, all future artificial attempts to create (manufacture) "perfect" babies.

A concrete example will show how, in practice no less than in principle, the so-called innocent case will merge with, or even turn into, the more troubling ones. In practice, the eager parents-to-be will necessarily be subject to the tyranny of expertise. Consider an infertile married couple, she lacking eggs or he lacking sperm, that wants a child of their (genetic) own, and propose to clone either husband or wife. The scientist-physician (who is also co-owner of the cloning company) points out the likely difficulties—a cloned child is not really their (genetic) child, but the child of only *one* of them; this imbalance may produce strains on the marriage; the child might suffer identity confusion; there is a risk of perpetuating the cause of sterility; and so on—and he also points out the advantages of choosing a donor nucleus. Far better than a child of their own would be a child of their own choosing. Touting his own expertise in selecting healthy and talented donors, the doctor presents the couple with his latest catalog containing the pictures, the health records and the accomplishments of his stable of cloning donors, samples of whose tissues are in his deep freeze. Why not, dearly beloved, a more perfect baby? . . .

Though I recognize certain continuities between cloning and, say, in vitro fertilization, I believe that cloning differs in essential and important ways. Yet those who disagree should be reminded that the "continuity" argument cuts both ways. Sometimes we establish bad precedents, and discover that they were bad only when we follow their inexorable logic to places we never meant to go. Can the defenders of cloning show us today how, on their principles, we will be able to see producing babies ("perfect babies") entirely in the laboratory or exercising full control over their genotypes (including so-called enhancement) as ethically different, in any essential way, from present forms of assisted reproduction? Or are they willing to admit, despite their attachment to the principle of continuity, that the complete obliteration of "mother" or "father," the complete depersonalization of procreation, the complete manufacture of human beings and the complete genetic control of one generation over the next would be ethically problematic and essentially different from current forms of assisted reproduction? If so, where and how will they draw the line, and why? I draw it at cloning, for all the reasons given.

BAN THE CLONING OF HUMANS

What, then, should we do? We should declare that human cloning is unethical in itself and dangerous in its likely consequences. In so doing, we shall have the backing of the overwhelming majority of our fellow Americans, and of the human race, and (I believe) of most practicing scientists. Next, we should do all that we can to prevent the cloning of human beings. We should do this by means of an international legal ban if possible, and by a unilateral national ban, at a minimum. . . .

QUESTIONS FOR COMPREHENSION AND REFLECTION

1. Feeling repugnance does not, in itself, signal that the object of our repugnance is immoral; repugnance can arise from cultural conditioning as well as reason. For example, people once felt deep repugnance at the thought of interracial marriages. Discuss whether Kass provides a convincing argument for his claim that our repugnance at the prospect of human cloning is based on "deep wisdom" rather than a cultural construct.
2. One of Kass's objections to cloning is that there are too many risks of mishaps and deformities. Would cloning be morally acceptable if it were perfected to the point where the chance of mishaps and deformities was significantly less than that stemming from reliance on sexual reproduction? How would Kass answer this question? How would a utilitarian philosopher respond to this question?
3. Are Kass's concerns regarding the autonomy and identity of a clone well founded? Discuss how John Harris might respond to Kass's concerns. Does Kass or Harris present the most compelling argument? Support your answer.
4. Kass argues that, while using preimplantation to create a healthy child may be morally acceptable, the use of cloning to produce a healthy child is never acceptable. Is this distinction justified? Support your answer.

GLENN McGEE

Parenting in an Era of Genetics

Glenn McGee teaches bioethics at the University of Pennsylvania. With the advance of genetic technology, parents are being offered more opportunities to enhance their children's lives. However, McGee warns that the road to genetic enhancement is paved with many sins. McGee goes on to explain the five deadly sins of parenting in the context of genetic engineering.

. . . Parenthood can feel like a laboratory in enhancement. All of us with children experience the pressure to develop the life of an infant, a young person, a young adult. Children present themselves to us as so many interwoven needs: for support, for care, for attention. The struggle to parent feels like a perilous and wonderful dance as we balance the need to transmit and inculcate values and culture with the need to give children what Joel Feinberg terms "an open future." As we make choices about our children, we pick up some cultural lessons that work not only for mundane parental decisionmaking but also for the radical possibility of making, perhaps sooner than we think, some systematic choices about the enhancement of our children through genetic technologies.

It may turn out, in this quest for some social improvement, that genes are among the least effective tools for advancing personal, familial, and social goals. Technical failings in all previously initiated trials of gene therapy suggest that our powers to induce genetic modification have perhaps been exaggerated. Is it likely that even an effective genetic therapy would revamp the human species? Not especially. Nor is it likely, conversely, that altered genes will destroy our human natures. Conventional social institutions, such as schools and churches, have a much more immediate effect on who we become, and we "conventional" parents can botch up child-making quite well without gene therapy.

There is plenty, though, to be frightened about when conversation turns to eugenics. The fear is not of genetic control but of socially prescribed blueprints of perfection, enforced by intolerant scientists-cum-bureaucrats. We have seen the results in our own century, and can at least glean from the misadventures chronicled by Daniel Kevles and others that a scientifically styled "perfect society," stratified by genes, makes little sense in a world where genetic variability turns out to be a virtue—and in which specialization and rigidity spell extinction. There are also plenty of practical examples of the danger of replacing parental responsibility with overarching social control.

How then can we put history's lessons to work in making responsible use of our social aim of improvement? First, we have to separate the dreams of eugenics from the hopes of families. The quest to improve humanity is not mere aberration, the deluded dream of social engineers. The *Newsweek* description of perfection (tall, blonde, powerful, smart children, made-to-order) is shocking, in part, because it is lifted directly from fashion magazines and television. Our culture pursues notions of "perfection," from eye color to weight to "swagger." We invest billions of dollars in the attempt to make people more intelligent and less aggressive. We call this attempt public education. As with eugenics, the goal of education is to design and inculcate skills and norms in the behaviors of offspring, from sexual mores through beliefs about history to respect for the law. Athletic activity and school lunches are designed so that children will grow up to be stronger, more capable, and smarter. Those who do not perform well in school are "failed," and miss out on college, better paying work, or social success. That families and the social order should abandon the aim at the improvement of children is unthinkable. Libraries, nutritional and environmental regulations, and the matrix of social and political institutions we have crafted testify to the necessity of this goal.

Because we make big social blunders, our programs, visionary plans, and political ambitions often do not provide the New World Order that is promised. Great plans for our children's futures can also be doomed by shortsightedness, avarice, and cowardice, or merely turn out to be unworkable or inapplicable to environmental and cultural conditions. Nonetheless, the hope for continuing improvement, "making the world better for our children," remains central to human progress and is present in the rhetoric of markets, politics, religion, and even medicine. We learn from our mistakes and work for a better future. Thus the deadly and not-so-deadly sins we need to avoid along the road to enhancement are not all related to genes, test tubes, or the Nazis. The five I explore here are instead sins we learn to avoid as parents and social stewards: Calculativeness, Overbearingness, Shortsightedness, Hasty Judgment, and Pessimism.

THE SIN OF CALCULATIVENESS

Consider, for a moment, your memories of childhood. Parents (or guardians) send children thousands of messages about appropriate behavior, communicating their hopes and fears. Some give an inordinate amount of advice and counseling. Some even set up elaborate systems of rules and procedures to instill certain habits and values. You might have been awarded two dollars for mowing the lawn, cleaning your room, and washing the dishes. You might have lost your driving or entertaining privileges for misbehaving. These thoughtful, organized systems provide a network of beliefs and structure the developmental environment. But they are not the whole experience of being a child. In fact, you may have learned much more

from the character, rules, and goals of your parents by watching what they in fact did than by obeying or disobeying the rules that they set for you. Or, the most vital and formative experiences of your childhood may not have had anything at all to do with the detailed plans that your parents agonized over. A brief, unpredictable outburst from a parent may outweigh years of regimented education. The sudden death of a grandparent or parent may change the entire family ethos. We commit the sin of calculativeness when we overemphasize the importance of planning and systematic choices in parenthood.

Like most sins, calculativeness is as much impractical as it is immoral. It is extraordinarily difficult to know what actions and words will register in the minds of our children. How will the whole package fit together: the way we treat them, the food we feed them, the genes we give them, and the rules we set for them? The most complex and sophisticated plans for a child's future can turn out to be the least effective, and we may send messages that are much more mixed than we know. . . .

Our beliefs about the "perfection" of our expected child may be much simpler or grander than we can articulate. The hopeful, infertile couple who expresses the fervent wish for any biological child, saying "all we want is a healthy baby" may not be fully conscious of the reasons why they seek not only health but also biological relation. A father who spends weeks teaching baseball to his son might actually prefer (at some deeper and more inarticulate level) that he and his son be able to have a nice conversation, or share a common goal. Because parenting is subtle, sophisticated, and enormously complicated, it is not at all surprising that we should be unaware of our own motivations—or even that we should act in ways contrary to our deeply held desires. Parenting habits are as complex as any human patterns of behavior, and can be malleable or rigid, conscientious or the thoughtless repetition of our own parents' behaviors.

Though genetic tests and therapies may not have the capacity to advance the intelligence and attractiveness of our children, faith in the efficacy of genetic technologies could lead parents to deemphasize important parts of parental responsibility. In addition, a faith in genetic modifications of offspring could encourage the emphasis by parents on narrow, artificially defined traits. Parents could have hopes of transmitting, in a simple and systematic way, all of the currently fashionable traits to their children, relying on the common images of "perfection" in the public. These images of perfection are not taken from the dreams of dictators or science-fiction novels. They are present in advertisements, polls, television programs, and movies. The perfect baby of *Cosmopolitan* or *Men's Health* might grow to be six feet tall, 185 pounds, and disease-free. His IQ is 150, with special aptitudes in biomedical science. He has blonde hair, blue eyes. He is aggressive and can play NFL football, NHL hockey, and NBA basketball, but also enjoys poetry and fine wine.

The parent who opts for such systematic control over the creation of a child puts faith in the ability of "genetic parenthood" to create a child that has particular traits. The more ordinary ways of parenting offer no such systematic options. . . . By contrast, genetic parenthood seems to offer a different kind of control. Here, parents could utterly abandon similarities, replacing them with choices that are reasoned in advance. If we thought that we could systematically impart an IQ of 150 instead of whatever mental traits we carry, we might opt to change our hereditary gift.

The "sin" of these calculated choices is not rooted in the idea that they might actually work, giving our kids 150 IQs or the appearances of gods. That much is unlikely to emerge from the polymerase chain reaction, gene-splicing, and vector technology of 1997, and may be conceptually impossible for reasons we described above. The sin is in understanding a child to be the result of systematic choices, and thus allowing genetic choices to define the child's telos. The faith that genetic enhancements can alter character (removing homosexuality or increasing thoughtfulness) lends itself to a parenthood of oppressive control. Parents that choose traits as calculative consumers might come to devalue the essential connections of relatedness and sameness in the family relationship.

. . . The sharing of similarities among members of a family could be diluted by genetic choices. A parent who is expecting a "brilliant child" could value that child only for her accomplishments, rather than for her struggles and growth. . . .

THE SIN OF BEING OVERBEARING

Hans Jonas and Joel Feinberg refer to a child's right to be open to as much freedom of identity as possible. They fear that genetic engineering, by stylizing children along the lines of rigid parental expectations, could steal this right. Children would be born into a world where their ultimate choices have been made by parents before the moment of their birth. While Jonas's fear hinges, in part, on the power of genetics to accomplish this feat, his insistence on children's continuing need for freedom is important. Genetic expectations, we noted above, could carry tremendous weight, as parents hope that children will become the sort of person whom they engineered. Already, parents who use in vitro fertilization technologies to implant the sperm of especially intelligent or athletic donors have expressed expectations of greatness from such children, insisting on endless piano lessons or daily tennis practice. . . .

We have to emphasize the responsibility that comes with new information before we spill it onto the table and write it into the chart. Parents must ask themselves of each new [prenatal diagnosis] test and procedure, "why do I want to know about X?" Honest answers may turn up more than parental curiosity. If tests for gender, intelligence, and other traits cultivate a parental mentality in which traits take center stage, it pays to consider the danger of such planning and expectations. However, as J. S. Mill, William James, and Derek Parfit have made so plain, there must be tolerance to different ways of approaching human natures. Wherever tests and procedures do not compromise the child, plural approaches to genetic modifications must be allowed. No simple, single solution will work. It makes no sense, and is generally counterproductive, to issue wholesale policy restrictions of any genetic research that is "positive" or "enhancing" in character.

Experiments in biological engineering must be tempered by respect for diversity and for each individual child. Overbearing parents can reduce the child to an instrument of their own ambitions or insecurities. This is no more appropriate when exercised through genetic technologies than when implemented by a parent who insists that a child accompany him to Klan meetings or refuse appropriate medical treatment in the name of religious beliefs a child cannot endorse. Children must be allowed to imagine and grow, and the balance to be struck is between instilling the values that parents hold and allowing the growth that could pull children away from those values. The desire for sameness can be a crippling expression of parental ego, just as the desire for a fashionably beautiful child can express self-loathing in the parent. The key is to avoid extreme measures through biological or any other means, and to temper decisions before birth with the recognition that every child has a right to make some decisions about her own identity.

THE SIN OF SHORTSIGHTEDNESS

As much as we plan for and anticipate the future, we cannot be sure what our children should or will become. We simply cannot anticipate the world of tomorrow. Within the past decade, an empire has been destroyed, Europe has formed an economic alliance, genetic testing has been developed, and computer speed has increased 10,000-fold. Economic and political prophets failed to predict a major market crash, the United States went to war with a third world country, and a U.S. physician began an assisted suicide delivery service. . . . What will the next decade, a mere ten years in the life of a child, hold in store? If you think you know, odds are you have a shortsightedness problem. Which is fine, unless it becomes the basis for designing your descendants.

One advantage of the conventional uncertainties in parenting is that just about all of our rules and practices can be changed to fit the exigencies of a changing world. For example, business schools grew to their apex during the early 1980s, then began to shrink as fewer employers recruited business majors. Savvy students quickly transferred from "entrepreneurship" into the humanities and environmental sciences. Parents with stubborn,

outmoded commitments to business school for their kids ended up with unemployed progeny or children on Prozac. Younger children are even more malleable than college students, and infants will accept the most conditioning of all. A child is receptive to language, math, rules, values, and abstract ideas. If conditions change, a child adapts. One danger of genetic engineering for positive traits, then, is the sin of shortsightedness: how can we know which traits to lock in through genetics in a world where fashions fade quickly and rigidity is a disadvantage? . . .

A parent who desires a smart child might actually be able, at some point, to increase the calculative speed of that child's brain. At present, scientists often compare the power of our minds to the power of computers. Computers are better when they are faster, so much of this research has focused on a faster brain. In ten years, though, it may turn out that calculative speed is a hindrance to thoughtfulness, imagination, and vision. A child could thus be robbed of the ability to adapt, stuck with a trait that hinders her ability to work with flexibility in the changing world. All this while expected by her parents to be brilliant.

Moreover, it is not always wise to assume that "more of a good thing is better." Genetic diversity has tremendous value because it provides the opportunity for those of many hereditary backgrounds to employ differing approaches toward maximization of the potential of a given environment. If dozens of children were created from the genes of an Einstein, would the world be a better place? Einstein was the product of a particular set of parents, experiences, and inspirations. In suburban Dallas, child of an oil baron, a cloned Einstein might as easily end up driving a truck or selling horizontal drilling rigs. He might live alone and homeless. . . .

Just as it is important for parents to allow children to develop in individual ways, there is reason for parental plans to allow for a changing world. Highly directed parental ambitions for children, such as success in a particular sport or with a particular musical instrument, can result in crushed hopes for parent and child. There are only so many slots on college and professional basketball teams, and not many will go to 5'7" men. Only one in a million musicians attends Julliard. It would be no advantage to choose male offspring, which most Americans report that they would, if suddenly 60 percent of live births were male.

Children need support—not pressure—in pursuing their own dreams within the context of family and culture. Diffuse parental hopes are more appropriate. Children need to learn courage and self-esteem, and need to be critical and functionally literate. They should have the support of their parents as they learn and grow.

THE SIN OF HASTY JUDGMENT

. . .

The perfect baby, like perfect soybeans and perfect corn, could turn out to be markedly imperfect. How difficult would it be to live an engineered life? Hans Jonas cautions of the danger of freakish accidents in genetic engineering. . . . Ironically, the more important accidents may be more likely to occur after the birth of an apparently healthy, improved baby. While medical technologies could make alterations in the physical characteristics of a newborn, we can hardly hope for the viability of those traits in our complex world. For example, wild strawberries have a much better chance of surviving against infection and parasites than engineered strawberries. The reason is that while genetic engineers controlled for particular traits, they could not control for the dozens of conditions that face a strawberry. Wild strawberries pack a variety of genetic habits. These "resistances" help them to have stable interaction with a range of circumstances. A genetically engineered strawberry, on the other hand, is a hit-or-miss proposition, with engineering emphasis placed only on particular traits.

A child who is engineered to possess positive traits might end up suffering unexpected and disastrous ills. It is extremely dangerous to move too quickly in the direction of changing human traits, lest we forget to control, or forget that we can't control, for the vast variety of human environmental conditions. Just as the gene that presumably causes sickle cell anemia codes for resistance to malaria, the gene for sonar hearing might interfere with the genetic pattern that codes for opposable thumbs or sex organs. In a strawberry, such mistakes can lead to new diseases and bad tasting fruit—in a human child, such errors become the sin of hasty judgment, and could be much more catastrophic for families.

There is also a more general point to be gleaned from our recent experience with agricultural engineering. The genetically enhanced tomato was delicious and tender when raised in lab conditions, but turned out to taste rubbery in real life. Seedless watermelons also suffer from diminished flavor. By analogy, imagine the beautiful, intelligent, even-tempered girl developed by genetic engineering. Could she survive in an imperfect world, with bad water and fatty foods? Would others hate or envy her? On paper, genetic engineering's traits look enticing. In practice, the attractiveness of other people is more random and depends on their quirks as well as assets. A perfect child would find the world of imperfection, disease, disasters, and emotions deadly or unsatisfying.

A pragmatic approach urges more cautious progress toward improving humans. Just as parents should promote malleability in their parenting, there must be room for imperfections and developmental choices. The child who is genetically crafted to 1997's models of perfection may find the world of 2014 intolerable. Instead, parents should aim to continue to update their style of parenting to match the demands of natural and social conditions. . . .

THE SIN OF PESSIMISM

In his essay, "The Moral Equivalent of War," William James argues that while war is to be avoided at all costs, humans seem to need to exercise aggression and domination during their lives. He termed the channeling of these powerful impulses into other activities, "the moral equivalent" of war. This notion of moral equivalency is useful here. Reproductive genetic enhancement may present new choices, but these choices are suffused with the "moral equivalence" of activities already present in the context of parenthood. The moral dominion of parenthood creates the context for reproductive genetic interventions. Thus while caution is intelligent, we need not treat genetics as a radically different endeavor, a slippery slope to biological castes and Frankenstein. The categorical opponents of genetic enhancement, Paul Ramsey and Jeremy Rifkin being the most notable, have utilized rigid rules to enforce the sanctity of human genetic coding. Such an ethic does little to guide our actions—it is simply naive in the light of other social pressures to apply scientific results, obtain improvements in life, and have healthy children. Ethics cannot ignore science: the problem with putting the values that are present in our culture to use in our culture is that those values can sometimes be "undermined by the conclusions of modern science."

We also would do well to consider [that] . . . the few fetal diagnoses available now are so expensive that only the wealthy use them. As a consequence, a disproportionate number of children with Downs syndrome are "almost certainly born to the less affluent." Our claim that some eugenic selection is already present in social engineering intimates another danger, then, of uncritical genetic research: it may be engineering that benefits only the powerful and wealthy. If society chooses not to concern itself with reproductive enhancement, we too have made a choice: to leave science to the scientists, and its application to political pressure and happenstance. Consider the application of genetic research in its political and economic context:

where there are therapies, there will always be pressures on a physician to offer them. The day that a gene for homosexuality is announced is too late for bioethics to put a "spin" on whether or not that gene is useful. We need to join the conversation about appropriate research before it becomes technology.

If pessimism is sinful, though, abject optimism is not its antidote. Even assuming that certain isolable ailments could be dealt with by genetic engineering, the approach to avoiding the not-so-deadly sins must be intelligent and cautious; we work toward developing protocols and therapies experimentally and gradually. This approach takes seriously the caution implicit in the "hands-off" attitude of those who would leave genetics to nature without surrendering the hope to make our condition and our nature better a little at a time. Social conversation concerning the enhancement of children is possible, and technological advancement is desirable in pediatrics. First, though, bioethicists' conversation about expensive and sophisticated genetic technologies must be connected to public conversations about parenthood. This requires us to abandon the search for an exotic ethics of enhancement, and get our hands dirty in the mundane world of the ordinary parents who will make decisions about genetic interventions and the meaning of growth and flourishing in their family and community.

QUESTIONS FOR COMPREHENSION AND REFLECTION

1. Do children, in fact, have a right to an "open future," as McGee implies? Do you agree with McGee that genetic engineering steals this right from children, especially given his concession that even cloned children may turn out to be very different from their "parents"? Is the social engineering of children, which already takes place through sending children to good schools, dance classes, churches, and other social institutions, any less problematic or calculating than genetic engineering? Do you agree with McGee that there is a morally relevant distinction between social engineering and genetic engineering? Support your answers.

2. Do parents who want the best for their children, in terms of their having a good genome, necessarily commit the sins McGee claims they do? Support your answer.

3. McGee opposes genetic engineering for "perfect" children. Is it fair, however, that some children are not born as strong, beautiful, or intelligent as other children when their parents could have made them more like everyone else? Explain.

4. McGee warns that ideas of perfection change over time and may actually work to disadvantage a child who is genetically engineered. Do you agree? Discuss your answer by contrasting your grandparents' and parents' generations' idea of the "perfect" child with your own concept of a "perfect" child.

✿ CASES FOR ANALYSIS*

1. Infertility and Androgen Insensitivity

Andrea and Carl, both age twenty-eight, come to Dr. Dakota's infertility clinic because they have been unable to conceive a child. During the initial interview, Andrea tells Dr. Dakota that she has never had a menstrual period. She also had reconstructive surgery on her vagina when she was fifteen. Genetic testing reveals that Andrea has androgen insensitivity, a rare genetic disorder in which a male fetus is unable to utilize the androgen (male hormones) necessary to stimulate the development of male characteristics. Hence, the outward development of a male with androgen insensitivity more closely resembles that of a female. Although Andrea is phenotypically a female, she is genotypically a male. When Andrea and Carl return for their follow-up, they ask Dr. Dakota about the test results. What should she tell them?

DISCUSSION QUESTIONS

1. Should Dr. Dakota tell the couple that Andrea is genotypically a male and risk devastating both of them, or should she lie and tell them that their infertility stems from another medical cause? How should she treat their infertility problem? Support your answers.
2. Discuss how Rosamond Rhodes might answer question 1. Is genetic ignorance justified in this case? Does Dr. Dakota have a right, or even a duty, to withhold genetic information from her patients in this case? Support your answers.
3. The surgeon who operated on Andrea when she was fifteen told her parents that her condition was most likely caused by fetal androgen insensitivity. However, the parents, now deceased, requested that the surgeon not inform Andrea of this but instead tell her that it stemmed from another cause. The surgeon agreed. Was the surgeon right to have acquiesced to the parents' request, or should he have informed Andrea of his diagnosis? Does the surgeon have a moral obligation to inform Andrea now of the reason for the surgery if she calls him? Support your answers.

2. Donor Eggs: "The New Solution for Aging Infertiles"

Anne Taylor Fleming and her husband had been trying for over five years to have their own child. "We had tried it all," she writes, "every high-tech and low-tech procedure then available. My body was whipped, my humor gone, my marriage frayed, our bank account depleted."[68] At forty-two and approaching menopause, she was almost ready to

---

*Names and cases are fictitious unless noted otherwise.

give up when a doctor offered her donor eggs—what Fleming calls "the new solution for us aging infertiles." For $2,500, she could buy the eggs of a high-IQ college coed. However, the price would be high for the eggs of a choice high-IQ college coed. Fleming would fill out a questionnaire about her vital statistics, such as hair color, height, hobbies, and educational achievements, and the fertility clinic would find a donor that matched these traits. The eggs would be fertilized with her husband's sperm—presto, instant baby!

"Can we meet the donor?" the Flemings asked. No, they were told, this was an anonymous donation. However, they would receive a copy of the donor's medical history.

"And best of all," the doctor pointed out, "nobody would ever have to know that this was not your real biological child. You can pass the baby off as your own, as most of my other patients who used donor sperm have been doing for years." Anne Fleming felt uncomfortable with the offer but said they would think about it.

Once she was alone, she began to have more doubts. "How can you do that?" she asked herself. "How could you bring a child into the world and not tell the truth—or outright lie—about his or her true origins?" No amount of deception would alter the fact that she was not the genetic mother and that, despite the pregnancy, this was, in effect, adoption, "if a preemptive one." What if she told the truth to the child? Would the child be traumatized? Would the child eventually go off looking for his or her genetic mother, as thousands of adoptees have done? And what about the effects on the donor? What if she later came to regret what she had done or longed to connect with her child?

On the other hand, this might be her and her husband's last chance to have the child they want so much. And at least one of them would be the genetic parent of the child. "What should we do?" she sighed.

DISCUSSION QUESTIONS

1. Discuss how an Islamic philosopher, a Kantian deontologist, and a utilitarian would respond to Anne Fleming's questions.
2. Is it right for women who are past the childbearing years to have children, especially in cases in which both parents are older? Support your answer. Discuss how a natural law ethicist might answer this question.
3. What would you do if you were in the Flemings' position? Construct an argument to support your conclusion. Break down your argument into its component parts. Which premises are descriptive statements, and which are prescriptive statements? Have you included all the relevant premises? Does the argument contain any fallacies? Do your premises support your conclusion? If not, go back and rework your argument.

3. Supermodel Gametes for Sale

In October 1999, fashion designer Ron Harris's Web site, www.ronsangels.com, caught national attention. The Web site was set up to auction off the eggs of six supermodels. The bids started at $15,000 to $150,000 for each donation, plus a 20 percent commission for Harris. In the first few days following the telling of its story on national television on October 25, 1999, the site had 5 million visits. Harris plans to expand his site, adding more supermodels—including men whose sperm will be auctioned off.

"Beauty is its own reward," states the Web page. "This is the first society to truly comprehend how important beautiful genes are to our evolution. . . .

"What is the significance of beauty? . . . Beautiful people are usually given the job of selling to, and interacting with, society. . . . The act of creating better looking, or in some organisms, more disease resistant offspring (known as Genetic Modifications), has been taking place for hundreds of years. All genetic modifications serve to improve the shape, color and traits of the organism. Every organism is trying to evolve to its most perfect state. If you could increase the chance of reproducing beautiful children, and thus giving them an advantage in society, would you?

"Any gift such as beauty, intelligence, or social skills, will help your children in their quest for happiness and success."

In addition to promoting the sale of eggs from supermodels as good evolutionary science and responsible parenting, Harris regards his Web page as a logical extension of the free-enterprise system. His philosophy is "Let the market determine the price."

Critics argue that this amounts to selling babies. It also turns beautiful children into a commodity that only the affluent can buy. The Web site, they say, sends the message that "not all eggs are created equal," thus flying in the face of this country's basic principle that "all men are created equal." Also, critics point out, there is no mention on the Web page of whether the supermodels shown in the photographs have had plastic surgery or other interventions to enhance their looks. Parents of the supermodel children may get more—or rather less—than what they bargained for.

DISCUSSION QUESTIONS

1. Discuss Harris's argument that what he is doing is simply an extension of the free-market system. Would it be an infringement of his autonomy and liberty rights to regulate or prohibit the sale of gametes on the open market, or do gametes and/or the children produced from these gametes have rights that we, as a society, ought to protect?

   Is it fair that people who have the money to buy the gametes should be able to have more beautiful children, or is being able to afford more beautiful children the same as being able to afford a more beautiful house or car? Support your answers.

2. Discuss the moral responsibilities of the supermodels whose gametes are being auctioned off. Do they have a moral obligation to disclose information about surgical alterations to enhance their beauty or to disclose genetic information that may be relevant to the health of the child? Or is the expression "Buyer beware" apropos in this situation? Do the supermodels have any moral obligations to the children that may be produced from their gametes? Support your answers.

3. Analyze Harris's statement that beautiful genes are important to our evolution. Is Harris, in fact, promoting or hindering the natural evolutionary process? Is the evolutionary effect of enterprises like his morally relevant?

4. Discuss the option to choose our children's appearance in light of philosopher John Rawls's concept of the "natural lottery" (see Chapter 1). Do parents have a moral obligation to give their child advantages such as "beauty, intelligence, or social skills?" Would or should parents of children who are not beautiful be blamed for their children's less-than-perfect appearance? Does choosing our children's appearance place a burden on them to conform to our standards, thus depriving them of an open future? Support your answers.

5. The Flemings (from case study 2) hear about Harris's Web site on national television and come to you, their genetic counselor, for advice on buying an egg from the Web site. They explain to you that, while they have used up their savings on previous infertility treatments, they can raise $60,000 by remortgaging their house. They are attracted to Harris's site because it allows them to know who the donor is. Also, neither of them is attractive, and they both have a serious weight problem. They feel that by having at least one gamete be from a supermodel their child would not have to suffer as they did. Discuss how you would advise the Flemings.

4. Jaycee: A Child Without a Parent

Jaycee was born on April 25, 1995. Shortly after the delivery, Pamela Sneel, the surrogate mother, handed the baby girl to an overjoyed Luanne Buzzanca. This was Luanne and John's fifth attempt to find a surrogate.

The month before Jaycee's birth, John filed for divorce. When Luanne sought child support, he refused on the grounds that he wasn't the baby's father. Jaycee began her life in a petri dish, the product of anonymous egg and sperm donors with no genetic ties to the Buzzancas. John also told the court that he never wanted to be a father and had only gone along with Luanne because she so desperately wanted a child. The judge ruled that not only did John have no legal obligations to Jaycee, but Luanne was not the legal mother and had to go through adoption proceedings to keep Jaycee. Luanne refused, claiming that the surrogate contract was valid. The ruling left Jaycee, the child whose conception and birth involved five different "parents," a child with no parent.

DISCUSSION QUESTIONS

1. Discuss the moral responsibilities of those involved in the creation of Jaycee. Do John Buzzanca and the gamete donors have any moral responsibilities to Jaycee? Who should be responsible for bringing up Jaycee? Should Jaycee be put up for adoption, or should the judge have granted Luanne Buzzanca legal custody? Support your answers.
2. Do physicians have a moral obligation to refrain from using reproductive technologies that might harm children? Discuss whether providers of infertility services have a moral obligation to learn about possible repercussions of different technologies and to inform patients of these possibilities. Relate your answer to the case study.
3. Discuss this case in light of both the Roman Catholic and the Islamic opposition to gamete donation and surrogacy.

5. Polly and Her Sisters: Cloning Sheep with Human Genes

In December 1997, the same scientists who brought Dolly into the limelight achieved another breakthrough with the birth of five almost identical Dorset lambs. The lambs were created by fusing a fetal lamb cell, which was altered by the addition of human genetic material, into the nucleus of a cell from a sheep's ovary. The lambs carry a gene to produce factor IX, a blood-clotting substance used in treating a rare form of hemophilia known as hemophilia B, or Christmas disease. People with hemophilia B lack factor IX, a component of blood plasma that helps it clot. The Edinburgh-based firm PPL

Therapeutics, which helped fund the research, announced that it eventually wants to establish herds of sheep carrying human genes to produce proteins and blood products for treating diseases such as hemophilia and osteoporosis.

DISCUSSION QUESTIONS

1. Is it morally acceptable to use other animals as a means only? Given that humans are a lot more like other animals than we previously believed, should moral respect be extended to other animals? Is cloning an affront to the dignity of other animals? Can cloning ever be of benefit to them? Support your answers.
2. What does it mean to be human? How many human genes must beings have before they merit the respect accorded to persons? Are these lambs part human because they carry human genes? If so, how does that affect the moral respect we should show them? Support your answers.
3. Many countries have banned the use of public money in research involving human cloning. Should this ban extend to the cloning of animals with human genetic material? Should private firms also be prohibited from cloning? Support your answers.
4. Discuss what a utilitarian might say regarding the use of specially genetically engineered and cloned lambs to produce factor IX to benefit humans with hemophilia B.

6. Born to Be Harvested: Growing Headless Humans

Many people consider the human brain to be a prerequisite for personhood. If so, then why not clone humans without brains for organ transplants and medical research? Biologists at Bath University in England have already succeeded in creating both frog and mice embryos that fail to grow heads. Says bioethicist Arthur Schafer, "Once you get over the initial revulsion—once you're past the 'yuk factor'—growing a headless human body is simply creating a sack full of organs." British biologist Jonathan Slack believes that "it is time to ponder the possibility of a headless human, cloned and grown for the express purpose of providing any needed vital organs for its anatomically complete genetic donor."[69] Dr. Slack admits that most women would shudder at the thought of having a partial embryo implanted into them. As of 2000, the technology for artificially growing such embryos was beyond our capacity.

DISCUSSION QUESTIONS

1. Many people feel extreme moral repugnance at the prospect of cloning headless humans for medical use. Is this repugnance morally justified? If so, on what grounds? Compare and contrast the cloning of headless humans for organ transplants with the current practice of harvesting organs from anencephalic infants.
2. Should women be given the option of having implants of partially cloned embryos of themselves or other family members in case organ transplants are needed in the future? Support your answer, addressing concerns of autonomy and rights ethics.
3. Is it morally permissible to pay surrogate mothers to carry headless fetuses? Would it make a difference, morally, if brainless fetuses could be grown using an artificial life-support system? Support your answers.
4. Discuss whether cloning headless human embryos is morally preferable to the current practice of using sentient nonhuman animals for organ transplants and medical

research. If so, is there a moral obligation, based on utilitarian considerations, to create headless human embryos for organ transplants and medical research? Support your answer.

7. My Father, My Son

Dianne's father was on his deathbed. Her father was an only child, and neither she nor her brother had any children. After much deliberation, Dianne decided she wanted to have her "father" as her baby. She wrote to a British geneticist asking for information on cloning. "My father," she explained in her letter, "is a remarkable man and I intend to see that he goes on in the world. . . . I am writing in the hope that you can help me find information on where human cloning may be performed now. There must be organizations that are actively pursuing cloning, and I want to contact them and see if there is a possibility of cloning my father. I have little time left to pursue this venture, and I would greatly appreciate your assistance." Dianne also offered to be the host mother for the clone of her father.

Derek, who read Dianne's correspondence on the Internet, was horrified at her request. "The desire to clone a passed-on loved one," he responded, "seems to me to be grotesque. It brings to mind the Stephen King book *Pet Sematary*. The clone would be a disappointment to the donor's relatives, in that the original personality could never be completely duplicated. Additionally, the clone would not be able to live its own life; it would be forced to live in a predefined, unattainable role."

DISCUSSION QUESTIONS

1. Are Derek's misgivings valid? Does the fact that the donor's relatives might be disappointed or the concern that the clone may be deprived of an open future override Dianne's reproductive autonomy? If so, should these criteria be considered any time a woman wants to have a child, through sexual procreation, in order to carry on the inheritance of herself and the father of the child? Support your answers. Discuss how a libertarian might respond to these questions.
2. Applying utilitarian theory, discuss whether the clone of Dianne's father would be harmed by being a clone and, if so, whether the harms outweigh the benefits.
3. Would it make a difference morally if Dianne's father consented to being cloned? What if he was unable to give his informed consent to being cloned or was opposed to the cloning? Support your answers.
4. Research suggests that clones from adult cells might inherit aging DNA that may cause premature aging and increase the risk of cancer. If this is found to be true, should it preclude human cloning from adult cells, especially those of older adults like Dianne's father? On the other hand, parents have children through sexual reproduction knowing that the children may inherit genes that lead to premature death. Should the risk factors associated with cloning be treated like any other "genetic disorder" that leads to premature death? Support your answers.

8. Germ Line Therapy and Huntington's Disease

As a teenager, Benjamin Cooper, who is now thirty-two, saw both of his parents slowly degenerate and eventually die of Huntington's disease, an insidious inherited neurological disease that does not usually manifest itself until people are middle-aged or older. Benjamin's father lost his job when he was forty-eight due to symptoms associated with the then undiagnosed disease. After the disease was diagnosed, his father was denied medical insurance by his next employer. Benjamin and his wife, Shamir, desperately want to have children of their own; however, they are aware that their children will probably inherit the disease. Benjamin also knows that he will eventually manifest symptoms of Huntington's disease and wants to have a family soon so he can enjoy his children as long as possible. They have considered using donor sperm, but, being a Muslim, Shamir is opposed to the use of donor sperm. Benjamin would also prefer to have a child that is genetically related to him.

Shamir Cooper, who is a physician at a teaching hospital, hears about a research study on germ line therapy using retroviral probes to replace the deleterious Huntington gene with a healthy gene. After she and her husband discuss the study, they volunteer to be subjects. Less than two years later, they give birth to a pair of twin boys. Neither baby carries the gene for Huntington's disease.

DISCUSSION QUESTIONS

1. Was germ line therapy morally justified in this case? Is it morally relevant that germ line therapy was still in an experimental stage? Support your answers, using good arguments.
2. Discuss what a utilitarian, a rights ethicist, and an Islamic ethicist would think about the morality of the Coopers' decision.
3. Should medical insurance companies be allowed to refuse coverage for people with genetic disorders such as Huntington's disease? If not, how should insurance companies raise the money to cover the medical expenses of people suffering from genetic disorders? Who should bear the burden of covering these costs? Do employers have a moral right to refuse to hire or provide medical coverage for people with costly and disabling genetic disorders? Support your answers.
4. Following the birth of the twins, the Coopers' neighbors, Bert and Brenda Calvin, decide they also want germ line therapy for their next child. Both of the Calvins are short, and they feel this has hindered them in their careers as well as in their social life. Their only child, Zachery, has been taunted by bullies at school because of his short stature. They also want to have a probe carried out for the "gay gene"—a gene purportedly associated with homosexual tendencies—because of the social ostracism suffered by Brenda Calvin's Uncle Bob, who eventually committed suicide. Compare and contrast this case with that of the Coopers. Would the Calvins be morally justified in using germ line therapy for their next child? Is germ line therapy or enhancement justified to spare a child from social discrimination and ostracism? What if the Calvins also asked the physician to add genes for enhanced intelligence and beauty? Support your answers.

9. Cloning the Woolly Mammoth[70]

Japanese biologist Kazufumi Goto has a dream. He wants to resurrect the long-extinct woolly mammoth. Goto and his team of scientists have been combing the permafrost of Siberia, the old stomping grounds of the woolly mammoth, in hopes of coming across frozen viable tissue and cells. His partner in the project, genetic engineer Akira Iritani of Kinki University in Japan, has a successful Frozen Zoo project that preserves the sperm of endangered species. If the team is able to find mammoth sperm, they can use it to fertilize a living elephant egg. Then the egg of the offspring of the mammoth-elephant hybrid would be fertilized with mammoth sperm, creating a hybrid three-quarters mammoth. However, because the gestation period of elephants is 600 days and because it takes up to fifteen years for a female elephant to reach maturity, this procedure is not as practical as cloning. "I'm fifteen years older than Goto," says Iritani. "I can't wait thirty years to see a mammoth."[71]

Instead, Goto and Iritani hope to find somatic cells in a specimen of frozen mammoth that are capable of being cloned. Goto has already scouted out a site near Yakutia, the capital city of the Siberian province, for a mammoth park along the lines of the fictional Jurassic Park for dinosaurs, where the resurrected woolly mammoths could live as they did over 11,000 years ago.

DISCUSSION QUESTIONS

1. Is it morally acceptable to clone long-extinct species such as the woolly mammoth? Make a list of premises. Go over the premises and eliminate those that contain fallacies. Which premises support the conclusion that such cloning is morally acceptable? Which premises support the opposite or a different conclusion? Based on this analysis, what advice would you give Goto and Iritani regarding their project?
2. Would it be morally permissible to clone extinct humanoid species, such as Neanderthal man, if scientists could find a way to overcome the problems associated with cloning older DNA? Support your answer.
3. If scientists succeed in cloning extinct species of animals, including humanoid species, should they be able to get a patent on the genome of these species? Support your answer.
4. Scientists in the next few years may be able to create synthetic life. Discuss the moral issues involved in synthesizing more complex life, such as mammoths or human beings. Would synthetic humans have the same moral value and dignity as humans created from sexual reproduction? Would it make a difference if the synthetic humans were a more intelligent species than *Homo sapiens*? Support your answers.

C H A P T E R   6

Human and Animal Experimentation

In 1932, the U.S. Public Health Service initiated the Tuskegee syphilis study to learn more about the progression of untreated syphilis. The study, which included 412 men with syphilis, has been called "the most notorious case of prolonged and knowing violation of subjects' rights."[1] The subjects were recruited from among poor, illiterate black men living in the Macon County, Alabama, area. The men were led to believe that they were receiving medical treatment for their condition. Despite the discovery in the late 1940s that penicillin could cure syphilis, treatment was withheld from the nearly 300 surviving participants in the study. The survivors were given a $50 bonus to be used to help pay their funeral expenses in exchange for permission to have their bodies autopsied.

In 1972, Peter Buxtum, a public health official working for the Public Health Service, expressed concern to a reporter about the morality of the ongoing study. When the story of the study hit the newsstands, there was immediate public outrage. The study, which was discontinued as a result of the publicity, opened the way for public discussion of several social and ethical issues in medical experimentation, including informed consent, exploitation of vulnerable subjects, and the need for standards of professional ethics.

RESEARCH, EXPERIMENTATION, AND THERAPEUTIC TREATMENT

Modern medicine depends on scientific research. **Research** involves the orderly investigation or scientific study of a phenomenon in order to gain new knowledge. Research can be conducted through observation, a study of the literature on the topic, or experimentation.

Experimentation Using Live Subjects

An **experiment** is "a scientific procedure used to test the validity of a hypothesis, to gain further evidence or knowledge, or to test the usefulness of a drug or type of therapy that has not been tried previously."[2] This chapter focuses on experimentation using live subjects. The term *subject* includes human and nonhuman animals who are directly subjected to a procedure or action by an experimenter. We will use the term *animal experimentation* to refer only to experimentation using nonhuman animals, in accordance with the common use of this term.

Therapeutic and Nontherapeutic Experiments

In biomedical research, a distinction is generally made between therapeutic and nontherapeutic experiments. The primary purpose of therapeutic experiments is to benefit the subject by relieving suffering and restoring health. Therapeutic experiments may involve the use of experimental therapy or drugs, such as a new type of heart surgery or vaccination, on patients who stand to benefit from the procedure. The concept of experimental treatment implies that there is some ambiguity as to the effectiveness and/or safety of a particular treatment.

Nontherapeutic experiments, in contrast, generally are not directly related to any illness or susceptibility the subjects may have. Their primary purpose is not to benefit the individual subjects but to contribute to the development of knowledge and the greater good of society. An example of a nontherapeutic experiment is an experiment on healthy women to determine the effect of a new estrogen drug on bone density. Many experiments using human subjects, as well as the vast majority of medical experiments using nonhuman animals, are nontherapeutic.

In practice, there is no clear distinction between therapeutic and nontherapeutic experiments. In addition, therapeutic experiments are never carried out for the sole purpose of benefiting the patient. A drug intended to benefit a patient-subject in a therapeutic experiment may have unanticipated toxic side effects. The extra procedures involved in therapeutic research, such as drawing blood or taking tissue samples, also involve some risk. While therapeutic experimentation may inadvertently cause subjects more harm than benefit, nontherapeutic experimentation may indirectly benefit subjects. For example, the women in the estrogen experiment may benefit by lowering their risk of osteoporosis. Both therapeutic and nontherapeutic experiments may also benefit subjects by providing them with needed medical care that they could not afford otherwise or by requiring subjects to engage in healthier life-styles.

The researchers' intent is one criterion distinguishing the two types of experiments. However, researchers may claim—and even convince themselves—that their primary intent is to benefit the patient-subject when, in fact, it is not. Researchers may rationalize risky experiments as being therapeutic in order to secure funding or institutional approval. In an experiment at New York's Willowbrook Institute for retarded children, researchers gave children live hepatitis B viruses in order to study the disease and develop a vaccine. The parents gave consent on behalf of their children without being informed of the considerable health hazards associated with hepatitis. Researchers justified the experiment as therapeutic, claiming that the children would likely have contracted hepatitis in the institutional setting anyway. By artificially inducing the disease in an experimental setting, they argued, they actually benefited the children because they received better monitoring and medical care and possibly gained increased resistance to more virulent strains of the virus. Critics, in turn, maintained that better monitoring for hepatitis and improvements in medical care could have been achieved without artificially inducing the disease in the children. The moral justification of this experiment is still being debated among healthcare ethicists.

Experimental Design

The most widely used experimental design in medical research is the **randomized clinical trial (RCT),** in which subjects are randomly assigned to either an experimental group or a control group. The experimental group receives the experimental treatment, and the control group receives either the standard treatment, no treatment, or a placebo. A **placebo** is an inactive substance or treatment. The RCT allows experimenters to assess the effect of a particular treatment or drug while balancing other unknown variables. Double-blind RCTs, in which researchers are kept ignorant of which subjects are receiving the treatment and which are receiving the placebo, were not widely used until the 1950s. The purpose of this experimental design is to minimize researchers' influence on the outcome of the experiment.

Despite its success as a research tool, the RCT has its critics. Hans Jonas, for example, in his article at the end of this chapter, questions the morality of using placebos because it involves deception. Advocates of RCTs counter that no deception is involved because subjects give their informed consent to the research design and are aware that they may be given a placebo. On the other hand, because physicians are unaware of which group their patient is in, double-blind RCTs risk undermining the doctor/patient relationship, which depends on the physician's acting in the best interests of his or her patient.

RCTs also raise the question of the fairness of denying the control group the benefits of the experimental treatment, especially in studies of drug treatments for potentially fatal diseases such as AIDS and cancer. In 1994, the U.S. National Institute of Allergies and Infectious Diseases interrupted a study on the effects of the drug zidovudine on the transmission of AIDS from pregnant women to their children after preliminary data revealed a statistical difference in the rates of transmission of women receiving zidovudine and of those receiving the placebo. In their article at the end of this chapter, George Annas and Michael Grodin question the RCT research design used in the AIDS studies on pregnant women in Africa, Asia, and the Caribbean because of the availability of drug regimens that are effective in reducing HIV transmission.

Some healthcare ethicists favor an alternative to the traditional RCT, which uses a placebo treatment for the control group. They suggest that when there is already an effective treatment the control group should receive the conventional treatment and the other group the experimental treatment. While they acknowledge that this alternative may not be as informative or precise as the traditional RCT, they counter that it is more humane.

THE HISTORY OF MEDICAL EXPERIMENTATION[3]

Human experimentation did not have a significant impact on the course of Western medicine until the twentieth century. Prior to this time it was carried out by individual physicians on only a few subjects. Although the use of humans in medical research is mentioned in ancient Greek, Roman, and Arab medical treatises, it was probably relatively rare. The most frequent type of experimentation mentioned was the testing of toxic substances on condemned criminals.

The Rise of Modern Medical Experimentation

In the late eighteenth century, English country physician Edward Jenner (1749–1823) observed that farmers and milkmaids who had contracted smallpox from their pigs or cattle acquired some degree of immunity to more virulent forms of smallpox. Using material from the pustules of smallpox victims, Jenner inoculated his one-year-old son with an experimental vaccine. When his experiment failed, Jenner modified the inoculation and tried it again, on a neighborhood boy. This time the inoculation was a success.

Almost a century later, French microbiologist Louis Pasteur (1822–1895) conducted his famous experiments involving a rabies antidote using dogs as subjects. Although the antidote was successful, Pasteur was reluctant to try it on humans. Several months later, a distraught mother whose nine-year-old son had been mauled by a rabid dog came to him for help. After consulting with his colleagues, and with the boy near death, Pasteur finally agreed to administer a series of inoculations to the boy. The boy recovered. The findings of these two early experiments have saved countless human lives.

Nonhuman Animal Subjects and the Antivivisection Movement

Some early medical experiments used nonhuman animals as subjects. Louis Pasteur was one of the first scientists to systematically use nonhuman animal subjects as a prelude to performing the same experiments on human subjects.

The use of animals in medical experiments in the United States began in earnest in 1871 when Harvard professor Henry Bowditch established one of the first animal vivisection labs in the country in order to bring Harvard "into conformity with continental European standards." **Vivisection** involves cutting or operating on a live animal for the sake of scientific research. Not all animal research involves vivisection.

The New England Anti-Vivisection Society (NEAVS) was founded in 1895 "to expose and oppose secret or painful experiments upon living animals, lunatics, paupers, or criminals."[4] However, their early legislative efforts to restrict vivisection failed because of the strenuous opposition of the well-organized medical establishment. "I should not feel like putting any limit to the service [vivisection] of animals if it means saving the life of one child," President Eliot of Harvard testified.[5]

The British antivivisection movement was more successful. In 1876, the British Cruelty to Animals Act was amended to include vivisection. While not outlawing vivisection, it regulated the use of anesthetic on live animals in painful scientific experiments and the euthanasia of animals who suffered as a result of experimentation.

Many early vivisectionists accepted the Cartesian view that nonhuman animals were simply machines incapable of feeling pain. The growing evidence that animals do feel pain and are capable of suffering has contributed in recent years to more humane practices, as well as to attempts to find replacements for animal experimentation.

Human Experimentation Between 1900 and 1940

Nonhuman animals were not the only unwilling experimental subjects sacrificed in great numbers in the name of medical progress. The use of nonconsenting human subjects also became commonplace in the first half of the twentieth century. The discovery in the 1890s of the role of germs in causing disease and the increasing professionalization of medicine led to an increase in both human and animal experimentation. In 1900, U.S. Army pathologist and bacteriologist Walter Reed (1851–1902) recruited American servicemen and Spanish workers to participate in a study on the role of mosquitoes as transmitters of yellow fever. Subjects were given $100 in gold for participation and an extra $100 if they contracted yellow fever. If the subjects died of yellow fever, the money went to their heirs. Although Reed's experiment would be considered immoral today, it was significant in the history of human experimentation because it included both formal contracts with subjects and rewards for participating in hazardous experimentation.

For the most part, however, experimenters had little concern with obtaining the consent of subjects used in human experimentation. Children in orphanages, inmates of mental institutions, and patients in public hospitals were all used in medical experiments. One of the most popular sources of human subjects was prisons. Because of their restricted and regimented life-style, prisoners, like lab rats kept in cages, made ideal human subjects. In 1906, Dr. Richard P. Strong performed a series of experiments with cholera, using condemned prisoners in Bilibid Prison in Manila in the Philippines. Thirteen subjects died as a result of the experiments. Those who survived were compensated with cigars and cigarettes. Strong received a professorship of tropical medicine at Harvard University for his work.

Between 1918 and 1922, hundreds of prisoners at San Quentin Prison in California were given injections or implants of testicular substances from animals. Others received testicle transplants from executed prisoners. In an experiment in Colorado, 800 prisoners served as guinea pigs for a tuberculosis vaccine.

One of the few experiments in the United States in which the morality of the research was actively challenged was a study conducted by Hideyo Noguchi (1876–1928) to determine whether lutein could be used to diagnose syphilis. With the cooperation of fifteen New York physicians, Noguchi rounded up 400 subjects, most of whom were inmates of orphanages and mental hospitals or patients in public hospitals. Although Noguchi and some of the other physicians first tested lutein on themselves, with no ill effects, they did not inform the subjects about the nature of the experiment or obtain their permission. Despite considerable public criticism, Noguchi was never prosecuted for his exploitation of the subjects, and no formal ethics codes evolved as a result of this case.

World War II

During World War II, physicians in Nazi Germany conducted medical experiments using concentration camp inmates. The horror and magnitude of these medical experiments, some of which are described by Arthur Caplan in his article at the end of this chapter, shook the world to its core. While Nazi medicine is often portrayed as an aberration or the work of madmen, Caplan reminds us that it stemmed from the same

GERMAN GUIDELINES ON HUMAN EXPERIMENTATION (1931)

Guidelines on human experimentation were first published as a circular of the Reich Minister of the Interior in 1931 and remained in force until 1945. These guidelines were reputed to be the first of their kind. Although the guidelines tended to emphasize scientific progress and medical authority over patient rights and autonomy when it came to therapeutic experiments, the requirements for informed consent in nontherapeutic experimentation were relatively stringent. It is interesting to note the incongruity between the guidelines and Nazi practice. These guidelines are testimony to the inadequacy of ethical guidelines that are not supported by wider cultural values. The following are excerpts from the guidelines:

1. In order that medical science may continue to advance, the initiation in appropriate cases of therapy involving new and as yet insufficiently tested means and procedures cannot be avoided. Similarly, scientific experimentation involving human subjects cannot be completely excluded as such, as this would hinder or even prevent progress in the diagnosis, treatment, and prevention of disease.

The freedom to be granted to the physician accordingly shall be weighed against his special duty to remain aware at all times of his major responsibility for the life and health of any person on whom he undertakes innovative therapy or performs an experiment. . . .

5. Innovative therapy may be carried out only after the subject or his legal representative has unambiguously consented to the procedure in the light of relevant information provided in advance.

Where consent is refused, innovative therapy may be initiated only if it constitutes an urgent procedure to preserve life or prevent serious damage to health and prior consent could not be obtained under the circumstances. . . .

12. . . . The following additional requirements shall apply to scientific [nontherapeutic] experimentation.

(a) experimentation shall be prohibited in all cases where consent has not been given;

(b) experimentation involving human subjects shall be avoided if it can be replaced by animal studies . . . ;

(c) experimentation involving children or young persons under 18 years of age shall be prohibited if it in any way endangers the child or young person;

(d) experimentation involving dying subjects is incompatible with the principles of medical ethics and shall therefore be prohibited.

13. While physicians and, more particularly, those in charge of hospital establishments may thus be expected to be guided by a strong sense of responsibility toward their patients, they should at the same time not be denied the satisfying responsibility (*Verantwortungsfreudigkeit*) of seeking new ways to protect or treat patients or alleviate or remedy their suffering where they are convinced, in the light of their medical experience, that known methods are likely to fail.

academic and scientific roots as the medical culture in the United States and other Western countries.[6] Indeed, Germany is the birthplace of scientific medicine, and Germany's 1931 Guidelines on Human Experimentation are thought to be the first of their kind. The same German medical schools that graduated the Nazi physicians served as a model for medical schools in many other countries, including the United States and Japan. Indeed, when Dr. Gerhard Rose, head of tropical medicine at Germany's distinguished Robert Koch Institute, was sentenced by the Nuremberg Tribunal following World War II for "murders, tortures, and other atrocities committed in the name of medical science,"[7] he argued in his defense that American physicians had been complicit in similar medical experiments.

World War II was a turning point in human experimentation. In the United States, individual experiments were replaced by well-organized, extensive, federally funded projects. Concerns about informed consent and the rights of subjects were eclipsed by the overriding social goal of winning the war. There was also a temporary decline in animal experimentation as the antivivisection movement gained momentum and animal researchers were put to work saving human lives. A 1949 poll showed that 40 percent of Americans opposed vivisection. However, human subjects were not so lucky, nor did the often appalling experiments performed on nonconsenting humans during World War II—not just in the United States, but also in Japan, Britain, Australia, and other countries involved in the war—receive much publicity.

The use of prisoners as subjects in biomedical research became increasingly common in the United States during World War II. American prisoners were used in experiments involving sleeping sickness, malaria, gonorrhea, and induced gas gangrene. The benefits of using prisoners for research were so great that no one opposed it. In the laissez-faire climate that characterized the "gilded age of research," laws were loose and institutional review boards nonexistent. In addition, the money allocated for research grants increased many times over during the years following the war.

In 1941, President Franklin Roosevelt created the Office for Scientific Research and Development (OSRD). In addition to carrying out weapons research, the OSRD was mandated to find solutions to health problems that afflicted combat soldiers. Subjects for the patriotic research were gleaned from orphanages, institutions for the feeble-minded, mental institutions, and prisons. At Joliet Prison in Illinois, the University of Chicago, with the permission of the warden, took over one whole floor for the purpose of carrying out malaria research on 500 prisoners who agreed to be in the study. Four hundred prisoners at Stateville Prison in Illinois were used in a study of malaria that eventually led to a cure. Both the researchers and the prisoner-subjects in these studies were publicly praised for their contribution to the war effort. When the war ended, prisoners continued to be used as subjects.

While for all practical purposes it is now illegal for those receiving federal money to use prisoners in clinical research on experimental drugs, it is still legal under some state laws, and research on HIV drugs is being conducted by pharmaceutical companies in prisons in some states, including Florida and Texas.[8] This research has reopened the question of the moral permissibility of using prisoners as subjects, especially prisoners who volunteer to take part in medical experiments. Cathy Potler of the New York City Board of Corrections writes, "While we must never forget the historical abuse of prisoners as subjects in drug experimentation, we should not take a protectionist or paternalistic posture that could result in a different kind of abuse—denying prisoners the

CULTURAL WINDOWS

JAPANESE EXPERIMENTS IN BIOLOGICAL WARFARE

While the atrocities committed by Nazi physicians have been heavily publicized, Germany was not alone in using war as an excuse for ignoring moral protocol in medical experimentation. How did Japanese physicians justify such experiments?

Prior to the 1860s, Japanese medical tradition was dominated by the Confucian ideals of jin (benevolence) and respect for order and authority. In fact, the term for medicine in Japan is *jinjyutsu* (the art of jin). Respect for authority was further reinforced by the traditional Japanese belief in the inviolable authority of the state and the emperor. In medicine, respect for authority expressed itself in a paternalistic and authoritarian relationship between physicians and their patients, as well as in physicians' uncritical acceptance of prevailing cultural norms. Physicians thought of themselves as members of a group rather than as individuals. To question tradition or express an individual opinion was considered a sign of arrogance.

During the late nineteenth century, Japan became more open to ideas from the West. The government hired foreign advisers to provide information on modernization in areas such as industry and medicine. The Japanese government was drawn to the German medical model because of Germany's success in science and technology. The German model was also highly authoritarian. Combined with Japanese physicians' emphasis on paternalism and respect for authority and social order, the German model contributed to the neglect of the development of any concept of patient rights. "Research," writes medical historian Rihito Kimura, "became the supreme interest at many university hospitals, and patients who presented interesting cases were treated as research material."[9] The good of society was elevated above the rights and autonomy of the individual patient.

opportunity to benefit from clinical trials."[10] While extra precautions are needed in obtaining informed consent because prisons "jeopardize the ability of a prisoner to make a fully and uncoerced decision to join a clinical trial,"[11] this difficulty has to be weighed against the proportional benefits to the prisoners of participation in research, especially in cases where the experimental treatment is the only potential treatment for the disease under study. There may also be wider social benefits in addition to potential benefits for the prisoners. Because of the prevalence of HIV and AIDS among prisoners, they may be the best population for studying the effects of new treatments, thus expediting the release of effective treatments into society at large.

On the other hand, allowing the use of prisoners as subjects in clinical trials for HIV drugs is a foot in the door for others to use prisoners as subjects in clinical trials that might not be as potentially beneficial. Given the poor level of healthcare in most prisons and the desperation of many prisoners to receive adequate healthcare, as well as the lack of privacy and freedom in prisons, we need to ask whether we want to open that door—at least at this time. In addition, up to 54 percent of patients who take anti-

The official ethics of the medical profession in Japan at this time did not extend to human experimentation, which was subject to no review boards or government regulations. The medical profession came under the control of the militaristic state, which exploited the physicians' respect for order and authority for its own ends. In 1938, the Japanese government established the Ministry of Health and Welfare. One of the primary goals of this agency was to strengthen the health of the nation in order to win the war against China.

Between 1930 and 1945, Japan conducted experiments on the use of anthrax, cholera, typhoid, and typhus for biological warfare. The main testing site was a Chinese prison, where more than three thousand people died in biomedical experiments.[12] The Japanese also used special planes for dropping germ-bombs. At least eleven Chinese cities were targets of germ-warfare attacks. In one experiment, fleas carrying bubonic plague were dropped on a city, causing more than a hundred deaths.[13] Eight American bomber pilots, captured in Tokyo and sentenced to death, were used in vivisection experiments. As in Nazi Germany, many of the physicians who designed and participated in these experiments were professors and scientists at prestigious research institutes.

Following the war, there was a radical shift in Japanese medical education away from the German authoritarian model. In 1951, the Japan Medical Association issued an ethics statement that ushered in a return to the earlier Confucian value of jin and the importance of physicians' and medical researchers' putting the welfare of patients first. The Japanese medical profession is also beginning to question authority. During the 1960s, medical students in many universities took a stand against what they regarded as authoritarian medical faculties. The American influence on postwar Japan has also contributed to dialogue on patient autonomy and patient rights. It is no longer acceptable in Japan to compromise human dignity by undertaking medical experimentation for the sake of the state.

HIV drug combinations develop a resistance to these drugs and may not be good candidates for future, more effective drug combinations.[14]

CODES OF CONDUCT

Following World War II, several efforts were made to establish codes of conduct that required researchers to follow certain research protocols rather than rely on their conscience. One of the first and most important of these codes was the Nuremberg Code.

The Nuremberg Code

The Nuremberg Code was drawn up in 1947 in Nuremberg, Germany, by a panel of American physicians and judges sitting in judgment over twenty-three German

THE NUREMBERG CODE (1947)

1. The voluntary consent of the human subject is absolutely essential. This means that the person involved should have legal capacity to give consent; should be so situated as to be able to exercise free power of choice, without the intervention of any element of force, fraud, deceit, duress, overreaching, or other ulterior form of constraint or coercion; and should have sufficient knowledge and comprehension of the elements of the subject matter involved as to enable him to make an understanding and enlightened decision. . . .

2. The experiment should be such as to yield fruitful results for the good of society, unprocurable by other methods or means of study, and not random and unnecessary in nature.

3. The experiment should be so designed and based on the results of animal experimentation and a knowledge of the natural history of the disease or other problem under study that the anticipated results will justify the performance of the experiment.

4. The experiment should be so conducted as to avoid all unnecessary physical and mental suffering and injury.

5. No experiment should be conducted where there is an a priori reason to believe that death or disabling injury will occur; except, perhaps, in those experiments where the experimental physicians also serve as subjects.

6. The degree of risk to be taken should never exceed that determined by the humanitarian importance of the problem to be solved by the experiment.

7. Proper preparations should be made and adequate facilities provided to protect the experimental subject against even remote possibilities of injury, disability, or death.

8. The experiment should be conducted only by scientifically qualified persons. . . .

9. During the course of the experiment the human subject should be at liberty to bring the experiment to an end. . . .

10. During the course of the experiment the scientist in charge must be prepared to terminate the experiment at any stage, if he has probable cause to believe . . . that a continuation of the experiment is likely to result in injury, disability, or death to the experimental subject.

physicians and scientists accused of committing medical crimes in the Nazi concentration camps. The creators of the Nuremberg Code felt that the Hippocratic Oath, with its focus on the therapeutic nature of the individual physician/patient relationship, was not sufficient to protect the autonomy and rights of human subjects in medical research.

EGYPT AND THE MIDDLE EAST:
Medical Research

Learning about the perspective of another culture can help medical professionals move beyond cultural norms and be more sensitive to the goals valued in other cultures. For example, a public health program officer who administers Ford Foundation research grants for the Middle East was dismayed when she learned that one of the research projects at a prestigious Egyptian medical school entailed giving children medical treatment that was not standard and might be life-threatening. When she met with the practitioners, she was surprised to find that, rather than being insensitive, they were well intentioned, sincere, and enthusiastic about the care of their patients.[15] The problem, she later realized, was not that the doctors were insensitive but that they placed a higher value on the pursuit of scientific knowledge and medical technology than on the welfare of their individual patients.

The lack of regulation of medical research and the social inequality reflected in a two-tier healthcare system have led to a situation in which human research subjects are gleaned from the poorest segments of the population—people obtaining medical care from government rather than private hospitals. The use of human subjects does not reflect fundamentally different moral values, but rather different priorities. In this case, calling attention to the importance of patient autonomy over that of the nonmoral value of medical progress encouraged Egyptian researchers to rethink their priorities and give more attention to patient autonomy.

The Nuremberg Code replaced the physician-centered, paternalistic approach of the Hippocratic Oath with a subject-centered, human rights approach. The first principle in the code states that "the voluntary consent of the human subject is absolutely essential." Under the Nuremberg Code, prisoners, children, and patients in mental institutions were no longer eligible to be used as subjects in experiments. Despite its moral impact, the legal authority of the Nuremberg Code was limited to the trial of the Nazi war criminals.

Change was slow in other parts of Europe and North America, in part because of the prevailing belief that the Nuremberg Code was relevant only to the Nazi experience.[16] Because the Nazi experiments had been conducted during wartime, the Nuremberg Code seemed irrelevant to peacetime research. The fact that those who carried out the crimes were physicians was downplayed; instead, the evildoers were portrayed as Hitler's henchmen.[17] Following the Nuremberg trials, the majority of physicians continued to be guided by the Hippocratic Oath. Some researchers interpreted the Hippocratic Oath as permitting experiments to be conducted without the informed consent of subjects, relying on the belief that the physician could be trusted to make the best decisions for the patient-subjects. As late as 1987, the U.S. Supreme Court refused to endorse the Nuremberg Code as binding on all research.

THE DECLARATION OF HELSINKI, WORLD MEDICAL ASSOCIATION (1964; REVISED 1989)

Introduction

It is the mission of the physician to safeguard the health of the people. His or her knowledge and conscience are dedicated to the fulfillment of this mission. . . .

Medical progress is based on research which ultimately must rest in part on experimentation involving human subjects. . . .

Because it is essential that the results of laboratory experiments be applied to human beings to further scientific knowledge and to help suffering humanity, the World Medical Association has prepared the following recommendations as a guide to every physician in biomedical research involving human subjects. . . . The standards as drafted are only a guide to physicians all over the world. Physicians are not relieved from criminal, civil and ethical responsibilities under the laws of their own countries.

I. Basic Principles

1. Biomedical research involving human subjects must conform to generally accepted scientific principles and should be based on adequately performed laboratory and animal experimentation and a thorough knowledge of the scientific literature. . . .

5. Every biomedical research project involving human subjects should be preceded by careful assessment of predictable risks in comparison with foreseeable benefits to the subject or to others. Concern for the interests of the subject must always prevail over the interests of science and society.

6. The right of the research subject to safeguard his or her integrity must always be respected. Every precaution should be taken to respect the privacy of the subject and to minimize the impact of the study on the subject's physical and mental integrity and on the personality of the subject. . . .

9. In any research on human beings, each potential subject must be adequately informed of the aims, meth-

The Declaration of Helsinki

The World Medical Association (WMA), established during World War II, considered the Nuremberg Code to be too stringent. Adoption of the Nuremberg Code, it argued, would seriously hamper medical research, particularly pediatric and psychiatric research, because of its restrictive policy on informed consent and subject selection. The requirement that patient-subjects sign consent forms was viewed as an intrusion on the privacy of the patient/physician relationship. Prisoner-subjects were also considered too valuable to eliminate from consideration as experimental subjects. Research involving prisoners continued in the United States into the 1970s, when political pressures forced the government to stop such research on the grounds that prisoners could not give true informed consent because of their inherently coercive environment.

ods, anticipated benefits and potential hazards of the study and the discomfort it may entail. He or she should be informed that he or she is at liberty to abstain from participation in the study and that he or she is free to withdraw his or her consent to participation at any time. The physician should then obtain the subject's freely-given informed consent, preferably in writing. . . .

11. In case of legal incompetence, informed consent should be obtained from the legal guardian in accordance with national legislation. . . . When the subject is a minor, permission from the responsible relative replaces that of the subject in accordance with national legislation. . . .

II. Medical Research Combined with Professional Care (Clinical Research)

1. In the treatment of the sick person, the physician must be free to use a new diagnostic and therapeutic measure, if in his or her judgment it offers hope of saving life, reestablishing health or alleviating suffering.

2. The potential benefits, hazards and discomfort for a new method should be weighed against the advantages of the best current diagnostic and therapeutic methods. . . .

6. The physician can combine medical research with professional care, the objective being the acquisition of new medical knowledge, to the extent that medical research is justified by its potential diagnostic or therapeutic value for the patient.

III. Non-Therapeutic Biomedical Research Involving Human Subjects

1. In the purely scientific application of medical research carried out on a human being, it is the duty of the physician to remain the protector of the life and health of that person on whom biomedical research is being carried out.

2. The subjects should be volunteers— either healthy persons or patients for whom the experimental design is not related to the patient's illness. . . .

4. In research on man, the interest of science and society should never take precedence over considerations relative to the well-being of the subject.

In 1964, the WMA issued the Declaration of Helsinki, subtitled "Recommendations Guiding Physicians in Biomedical Research Involving Humans." It was an attempt to provide a compromise between the rigorous demands of the Nuremberg Code regarding informed consent and the demand for human subjects. The declaration affirms the paternalism inherent in the Hippocratic Oath by permitting physicians to invoke therapeutic privilege, which allows them to withhold information from patients and override the need for informed consent for therapeutic research on patients unable to give their consent. This exception was justified by the expectation that researchers searching for cures for diseases could be trusted not to use unethical means in achieving their goal. While this may be true in the majority of cases, noble intentions can be sidetracked by other goals. The Tuskegee Study, which started out with the praiseworthy intent of providing poor black men with medical care, soon shifted its focus to increasing scientific knowledge.

The Declaration of Helsinki has been amended several times since 1964. In 1999, the WMA met in Santiago, Chile, to provide guidance on emerging research issues such as the increasing trend toward international studies and the different standards of research ethics for rich communities and poor communities. The WMA also plans to address the use of placebos in studies involving diseases for which an effective treatment is already available when it revises the declaration, possibly as early as fall 2000.[18]

Henry Beecher's Exposé of Unethical Research in the United States

In 1966, Henry Beecher, of the Harvard Medical School, published a landmark article, "Ethics and Clinical Research," that contained descriptions of twenty-two experiments in the United States in which subjects were not informed of the considerable risks involved. Among them were the Tuskegee syphilis study, the Willowbrook hepatitis study, and an experiment in which live cancer cells were injected into unsuspecting patients at the Brooklyn Jewish Chronic Disease Hospital. While these experiments were certainly not of the magnitude of those conducted in Nazi Germany, Beecher's exposé demonstrated that unethical research can take place anywhere. His article brought home the need to regulate the power of medical researchers rather than rely solely on their good will and discretion.

Institutional Review Boards (IRBs)

In 1966, the U.S. Surgeon General announced that institutions receiving Public Health Service grants must create institutional review boards (IRBs) to protect human subjects and balance the interests of subjects with the interests of society and medical science. IRBs generally consist of about fifteen people from different walks of life, including physicians, hospital administrators, ethicists, clergy, and lawyers.

Although IRBs have gone a long way toward protecting the rights of human subjects, many people feel they do not go far enough. Because it takes a long time to put IRBs together and most meet only a few times a year, there is tension between the need to protect the rights of subjects and the need to handle research reviews in a timely fashion.

The U.S. Department of Health and Human Services believes that the current system, which relies on IRBs to approve experimental protocols and to monitor adherence to the codes of ethical conduct, is inadequate to deal with the changes that took place in research and medicine during the 1990s.[19] Experiments involving gene therapy and genetic engineering, for example, involve complex moral issues that many IRBs are unable to handle not only because they may lack members with expertise in the field, but also because of the unknown consequences of these procedures on individuals and society.

In 1999, the Department of Health and Human Services cited nearly 150 institutions for ignoring federally mandated rules designed to protect human subjects.[20] In a crackdown of several prestigious research institutions, the research privileges of Duke University were suspended for five days because of failure to obtain full, informed consent from subjects in some of its studies. The inadequacies of the institutional review boards in many of these institutions were cited as part of the problem. Infractions included approving research projects without having sufficient information, failing to monitor serious side effects in trials, using informed-consent documents that required

THE ISLAMIC CODE OF MEDICAL ETHICS, ISLAMIC ORGANIZATION OF MEDICAL SCIENCES (1981)

In Islamic countries, research is guided by the requirements of Islam, which prohibits exploitation of humans.[21] Despite this, it is not uncommon for researchers to put scientific knowledge above the welfare and rights of subjects. This problem is aggravated by the scarcity of IRBs and similar committees to review research protocols.

The problem of unethical research was addressed in the 1981 Islamic Code of Medical Ethics, which was endorsed at the First International Conference on Islamic Medicine, held in Kuwait in 1981. It states:

There is in Islam no censorship of scientific research, be it academic to reveal the signs of God in His creation, or applied for the solution of a particular problem.

Within this freedom of research, however, there shall be no subjugation of man, no harming, withholding of treatment, deceiving or otherwise exploiting him. Neither shall there be any cruelty to animals experimented upon.[22]

patients to waive their legal rights, and involving researchers in a conflict of interest by naming them as members of the IRB.

Whereas most human experimentation in the past was federally funded and was conducted at one site by one researcher, human experiments, some funded by private corporations, now may involve thousands of subjects at many sites across the country and across the world. The recent emergence of for-profit IRBs also creates the potential for conflicts of interest. What is needed, some healthcare ethicists argue, is a clearly stated code of ethics to guide IRBs.

The Belmont Report and the Four Principles

The exposure of the Tuskegee syphilis study in 1972 by the public media shocked the nation into demanding more stringent guidelines for human experimentation. In 1974, Congress established the National Commission for the Protection of Human Subjects of Biomedical and Behavioral Research. The Belmont Report, issued by the commission in 1979, states that four basic principles should be observed in research using human subjects: beneficence, nonmaleficence, respect for autonomy, and justice.[23] These four principles, discussed in depth in Chapter 1, have since become the foundation of American healthcare ethics. The Belmont Report also states that parents or legal surrogates can make choices on behalf of children. As a result of this effort and similar efforts in other countries, most of the problems and abuses that plagued early human research have been sharply reduced.

Physicians as Researchers

The Hippocratic Oath symbolizes the relationship of trust between the physician and the patient. It requires physicians to help the sick and to do no harm, even if doing so would bring about greater social utility. In therapeutic research, as Jonas points out in his article, the physician plays the role of a "double agent" in which the physician's role as caretaker can conflict with the quest for scientific results.

Codes of conduct for researchers such as the Declaration of Helsinki and the Belmont Report have tried to provide a workable compromise between the Hippocratic Oath and the goals of medical research. Provision 2.07(2) of a 1989 American Medical Association statement on research proclaims, "In conducting clinical investigation, the investigator should demonstrate the same concern and caution for the welfare, safety, and comfort of the person involved as required of a physician who is furnishing medical care to a patient independent of any clinical investigation."

Is this a realistic goal? Should practicing physicians be permitted, as they are as of 2000, to conduct medical research on their patients or to recruit subjects from among their own patients for other researchers, or should the roles of physician and researcher be kept separate? Some healthcare ethicists maintain that the participation of physicians in research contributes to an erosion of trust in the medical profession. In the Hippocratic tradition, patients must ultimately trust that their physician will provide the best possible treatment. Medical experimentation, some critics argue, substitutes subject for patient. Its purpose is to test a scientific hypothesis rather than to act in the patient-subject's best interests. Patients participating in therapeutic experiments may feel betrayed when they learn that they have been treated as subjects rather than patients, thus weakening trust. Furthermore, if patient-subjects are led to believe that an experiment is therapeutic, as in the Tuskegee Study, they may forgo other treatment options.

Many healthcare ethicists maintain that the patient-physician relationship allows physicians to use an experimental treatment only if they believe it is more likely than the traditional treatment to benefit their patients. Indeed, when the only treatment available is an experimental treatment, it may be in the patients' best interests to enlist them as subjects.

THE STATE AND BIOMEDICAL RESEARCH

The Nazi era, in which physicians became the tools for achieving political goals, illustrated all too painfully the vulnerability of medical professionals to political pressures, for better or worse. Following World War II, the U.S. government became increasingly influential in determining the course of biomedical research, primarily through control of funding. In the final year of the war, the National Institutes of Health (NIH) received about $700,000. In 1955, this figure was $139 million; by 1965, it had escalated to $1.2 billion.[24] The greater availability of funds for research led to a dramatic increase in both nontherapeutic experimentation and the demand for nonhuman animals as subjects.

Research and National Security

In 1977, former CIA director Stanfield Turner disclosed that his agency had conducted covert brainwashing experiments on prisoners and patients who were mentally ill. CIA agents had also slipped LSD and other psychotropic drugs into patrons' drinks at bars in New York and San Francisco. The purpose of this long-term, $25 million experiment was to study the usefulness of these drugs for brainwashing. The study was fueled by the fear that communists might use LSD to brainwash converts. The CIA also financed studies on hypnosis, electroshock, lobotomy, and sensory deprivation.

Because of the power of the state and the importance it attaches to national security, government research is perhaps most vulnerable to the lure of unethical conduct. Easy access to information about citizens, unlimited funding, secrecy, the power to implement a research program, and the difficulty of suing the federal government all grant state-sponsored research an immunity from accountability that private research institutes don't have.

The Atomic Energy Commission (AEC) Radiation Experiments

During World War II and the Cold War between the United States and the Soviet Union that followed, the Atomic Energy Commission (AEC) was given unprecedented power, including complete immunity from liability for gross negligence and harm. The AEC "became a world unto itself, a quasi-government and private corporation in one. It preempted local and state laws, and it could ignore any federal law but the Atomic Energy law. As an economic enterprise the AEC quickly became larger than most countries."[25] One of the AEC's projects was a series of experiments on the effects of radiation on humans.

In the 1980s, the Freedom of Information Act was expanded, and many of the radiation experiments previously shielded from the public eye under the cover of "national security" were made public. In 1986, Senator Edward Markey's office issued a report titled "American Nuclear Guinea Pigs: Three Decades of Radiation Experiments on U.S. Citizens." The public was stunned. Several thousand American citizens, including pregnant women, people with mental disabilities, soldiers, hospital patients, prison inmates, federal workers, and people who happened to live downwind from testing sites, had been unwitting subjects in massive experiments on the effects of radiation. Between 1948 and 1953, for example, the Defense Department deliberately released radioactive material into the air in order to gather data on the feasibility of using radiation weapons to kill or debilitate enemy soldiers. The scientists who conducted the experiments were aware of the dangers of radiation, including a possible increase in birth defects; however, they believed that the benefits in terms of national security and improvements in the U.S. nuclear arsenal outweighed the risks to the "experimental subjects."

Perhaps even more disconcerting was the complicity of some of America's most prestigious institutions of higher learning in the radiation research. At Vanderbilt University in Nashville, Tennessee, for example, more than eight hundred pregnant women, most of whom were recruited from poor and remote Appalachian towns, were fed radioactive iron without their knowledge or consent.

Until 1994, when Energy Secretary Hazel O'Leary declared that the victims of the U.S. nuclear experiments should receive compensation, the U.S. government steadfastly denied pleas for recognition from people who had been exposed to radiation from the experiments. In 1997, President Bill Clinton announced that all human research conducted in the name of national security would have to conform to the rules for informed consent and that participating scientists would have to notify subjects of the names of sponsoring government agencies.

The United States was not the only country to carry out nuclear weapons experiments without regard for the consent or safety of the people involved. British nuclear tests in Australia exposed aborigines living in the test areas to harm from radiation. No attempt was made to warn the aborigines of the impending tests.

Conflicts of Interest

The involvement of government in biomedical experimentation creates conflict between the achievement of political goals and the protection of human subjects. The power of the state magnifies the already unequal balance of power between experimenters and subjects.

The interests of researchers in the pursuit of scientific knowledge may also conflict with the objectives of the funding government agency. The openness required by academic freedom and scientific inquiry can be severely compromised when universities and medical schools participate in classified government research. In addition, the trust citizens have in the ability of the state to protect them can be seriously damaged when they discover that the government has involved them in dangerous experiments.

Federal Drug Testing Laws

In many countries, including the United States, federal laws require that new drugs and medical treatments be tested first on nonhuman animals and then, if there are no or only minimal adverse effects, on human subjects. In order to meet these requirements, researchers often look to sources such as public hospitals and prisons for subjects. Much animal experimentation is carried out to satisfy legal requirements. According to animal rights advocates, most of this research is unnecessary.

The drug testing laws raise the cost of new drugs and medical procedures because of the tremendous investment of time and money they require companies to put into research and development. AIDS activists in particular have challenged the long, drawn-out process involved in moving a drug from experimental to treatment status. They argue that it is unethical and paternalistic to keep off the market drugs that have shown promise in preliminary trials, such as the antiviral drug DDI.[26] They argue further that patients have a right to make their own informed decisions regarding the use of experimental drugs.

Most physicians and pharmaceutical companies disagree. In part because of fear of malpractice and other lawsuits and in part because of concern for the well-being of their patients, they want to ensure that a treatment has been thoroughly tested and meets legal requirements before they use it. Patients who are seriously ill, they point out, tend to be unrealistically optimistic about the curative effects of experimental drugs and treatments, making them vulnerable to exploitation. Medical insurance companies also want to know that a particular treatment is cost-effective before they pay for it.

INFORMED CONSENT

In 1970, a double-blind experiment was conducted to determine whether the side effects of the contraceptive pill were physical or psychological. The subjects were mostly poor, Mexican-American women who had come to a San Antonio clinic for contraception.[27] Seventy-six of the women received a placebo, while another group was given the Pill. Although the women consented to being part of an experiment, they were not informed that they might be given a placebo. However, they were all told to use a vaginal contraceptive cream because the Pill might not be "completely effective." As a result of the experiment, ten of the women receiving the placebo became pregnant.

Several years passed before the informed-consent requirement of the Nuremberg Code was incorporated into biomedical research. Informed consent protects the rights and dignity of persons and gives them precedence over the scientific goals of the researcher. Although informed consent is also required in therapeutic treatment, it is particularly important in experimentation because of the greater risks to subjects. Informed consent has three aspects:

1. The subject must be properly informed.
2. The subject must be competent.
3. The consent must be freely given.

Informing Prospective Subjects

Prospective subjects should be adequately informed of the nature and risks of the experiment as well as alternatives in the case of therapeutic experimentation so they can make an autonomous decision about whether or not to participate. This requirement rules out the deliberate withholding of pertinent information about the nature of the experiment, such as that in the San Antonio contraceptive study and the Tuskegee syphilis study. Subjects should also be informed that they can withdraw from the experiment at any time.

According to some healthcare ethicists, informed consent is incompatible with the use of placebos. Even though subjects may be informed that they are participating in a randomized clinical trial, they cannot make informed decisions about withdrawing from the experiment and seeking an alternative treatment for their condition if they do not know whether or not they are already receiving an experimental treatment.

Others protest that the "informed" part of informed consent is unrealistic in many cases. Utilitarian considerations may militate against revealing all information to subjects. Therapeutic privilege, which the AMA allows under exceptional circumstances, has been invoked to justify the withholding of certain information as being in the best interests of the patient-subject. It is also argued that the great social benefits of withholding pertinent information may, in some experiments, outweigh any harm to the individual subjects. In the San Antonio study, for instance, the researchers claimed that the benefits of thousands of women who were previously concerned about the harmful side effects of switching to the Pill outweighed the harms to the subjects of the experiment.[28]

Opponents of informed consent as a requirement for participation in medical experiments also claim that most subjects are unable to understand the relevant scientific information about the research and thus are unable to make a genuinely informed decision. They argue that researchers are in the best position to decide what is in the best interests of prospective subjects.

The view that informed consent should not be required because laypeople are incapable of understanding scientific information is unacceptable to most healthcare ethicists. The fact that the information may be difficult to understand does not mean it is impossible to understand. Researchers should present the relevant information in a way that prospective subjects can understand—preferably in writing, since this gives prospective subjects an opportunity to review the information on their own and ensures that all pertinent information is covered. A person who cannot understand the relevant information about the study, they argue, should not be used as a subject in the research.

Consent and Competency

In order for informed consent to be freely given, subjects should be capable of acting autonomously; that is, they must be competent moral agents. **Competency** involves the ability to understand the consequences of one's choices and actions and to make thoughtful and autonomous decisions based on that understanding. There are no clear-cut guidelines for determining competency. At what age do people become competent? Are people with mental disabilities always incompetent? If so, is it justifiable for a third party, such as a parent or a guardian, to consent on their behalf? Should experimentation using incompetent subjects be ruled out?

Great Britain, along with some states in the United States, prohibits nontherapeutic experimentation that poses more than minimal risks to children and incompetent adults. Some researchers object to this restriction, arguing that it has had a major detrimental effect on research into the causes and cures of mental illness, including Alzheimer's disease and dementia. They suggest that patients in the early stages of Alzheimer's disease and patients with mental illness be permitted to sign an "advance waiver" during periods of lucidity agreeing to their participation in future research into their condition. However, whether such a waiver constitutes informed consent is questionable.

Surrogate Consent

The U.S. Department of Health and Human Services permits surrogates to give consent to therapeutic psychiatric research using incompetent patients. In 1999, the New York Department of Health expanded this permission to include "slightly risky" experimentation on mentally ill or disabled adults who are unable to give informed consent, arguing that this type of research promises "great benefits to others in the future."[29] These regulations have been challenged by mental health advocates who fear that they permit psychiatric patients to be "used as human guinea pigs."[30] On the other hand, a prohibition on the use of mentally ill patients as subjects would preclude schizophrenic and Alzheimer's patients who do not respond to conventional treatments from receiving an experimental treatment that might benefit them.

Some scientists claim that we may be underestimating the competency and ability to make autonomous choices of people with mental illness. In a 1998 study, schizophrenic patients participating in randomized clinical trials of different antipsychotic medications were first given informed-consent forms to read and sign. The study found that the patients were able to understand the material in the forms. Even one week later, the patients were able to answer most of the questions asked about "the study's procedures and goals, patients' available choices as participants, their physicians' responsibilities to the investigation, and potential ill effects of antipsychotic drugs that were to be given in the trial."[31] The study concluded that many people with severe psy-

**THE AMERICAN MEDICAL ASSOCIATION POSITION
ON SURROGATE CONSENT (1984)**

2.07(4), Minors or mentally incompetent persons may be used as subjects only if:

i. The nature of the investigation is such that mentally competent adults would not be suitable subjects.

ii. Consent, in writing, is given by a legally authorized representative for the subject under circumstances in which an informed and prudent adult would reasonably be expected to volunteer himself or his child as a subject.

chiatric conditions are capable of giving informed consent if researchers are willing to develop strategies to use with potential subjects to "boost their capacity to consent."

Coercion, Enticement, and Consent

The circumstances under which experiments are carried out can affect a subject's ability to consent. Residents of institutions such as prisons, nursing homes, and mental hospitals, because of the very nature of the highly structured institutional setting, are generally under pressure to behave in certain ways. This pressure, in turn, may compromise their ability to freely consent to participate in an experiment. Even patients in ordinary hospitals, because of the duress of their illness and the desire to please their physicians, may go along with any suggestion made by their physician.

The use of rewards and enticements, such as in Walter Reed's study on yellow fever, may also be a form of coercion, especially in cases in which potential subjects need the money. In the United States, the widespread use of people who lack medical insurance and who volunteer to be in experiments in order to receive medical care and/or financial compensation might be considered a form of coercion. In the absence of universal medical care, should people without access to healthcare be restricted from participating in medical experiments, or would excluding them be paternalistic and infringe on their autonomy?

Is Informed Consent Enough?

The institutionalization of medical experimentation and the emphasis on scientific knowledge as an end in itself can relegate the rights and welfare of living subjects to the back seat. Thus, it is important that informed consent be obtained and the welfare of subjects protected. However, informed consent alone is not sufficient. Researchers first have to determine whether the experimental procedure in question is at the stage at which it is appropriate to test it on human, or even nonhuman, subjects. This is especially important in relatively new fields such as gene therapy, in which knowledge of the procedure is limited even among the well-educated public and hopes that a cure will follow may be unrealistically high.

Obviously, absolute informed consent is impossible. There will always be more information that a prospective subject can be told regarding a particular experiment, and there will always be factors that limit our freedom to give genuinely autonomous consent. However, informed consent should still be the ideal. Just how close we should come to the ideal before involving people as subjects in an experiment remains subject to debate.

THE SELECTION OF SUBJECTS

In 1996, Janssen Pharmaceutical paid physicians $3,600 for each patient they enrolled in a study of a migraine drug. That same year, Wyeth-Ayerst paid $4,581 for each patient enrolled in a study of a drug for hormone replacement in women.[32] In the past, most of the recruitment of human subjects for medical research was carried out by universities or hospitals under the watchful eye of their institutional review boards. However, with the rise of cost-conscious HMOs and their adverse effect on many physicians' earnings, some physicians are looking for new sources of income. The drug companies have stepped in to meet the demand. Since 1990, the recruitment of patients as research subjects by their personal physicians has become a multibillion-dollar business, with top recruiters earning up to a million dollars a year from drug companies. In 1997, more than two-thirds of drug trials were being carried out by private doctors rather than at research facilities in universities and hospitals, a reversal of the 1989 figure.[33]

Pharmaceutical companies from Europe and North America also use people in the developing world who are HIV positive to test anti-AIDS drugs. Between 1990 and 1997, the number of HIV-positive people worldwide tripled and was expected to reach 40 million by 2000. Ninety-five percent of infected people live in undeveloped countries, most in sub-Saharan Africa, where in 1999 an estimated 23 million people were HIV positive.[34]

Ninety-five percent of people with AIDS living in the developing world receive no treatment because of the prohibitive costs of anti-AIDS drugs. Anti-AIDS cocktails can cost up to $40,000 a year; consequently, the new drugs developed from this research will be used primarily in the West. The researchers for some of the drug companies target poor people—particularly pregnant women who are HIV positive—who cannot afford treatment and welcome any help they can get. Before people can take part in experiments, however, they must first consent to being taken off the drugs when the experiment is completed. Many subjects are unable to read or understand the consent forms and sign them mainly out of desperation. Enrolling in medical experiments may be the only chance they have to receive treatment, even though it may be limited.

The Principle of Descending Order

What criteria should be used in selecting subjects for biomedical experimentation? Jonas suggests using the "principle of descending order" in selecting subjects. This principle requires researchers to select the least vulnerable people as subjects, a reversal of the normal procedure of gleaning subjects from the most vulnerable populations, such as prisoners, the sick and disabled, and the impoverished. According to Jonas, physicians and researchers should be the first to act as subjects in medical experiments, since they are best qualified to understand the risks and benefits. Although the sick are most available, they should not be used as subjects even in therapeutic experiments.

Besides imposing additional burdens and risks on people who are already suffering, Jonas argues, using patients as subjects undermines the physician/patient trust. This issue is becoming more important with the recent trend of using subjects recruited by their private physicians.

Arthur Caplan takes a somewhat different approach. According to him, research is based on voluntary cooperation between the researcher and subjects. If competent patients want to participate in therapeutic experiments, they should be able to do so. However, like Jonas, Caplan opposes the practice of seeking out subjects from groups that are more vulnerable and will not directly benefit from the research.

Vulnerable Groups

The experiments in the Nazi concentration camps, as well as the Willowbrook hepatitis study and the Tuskegee syphilis study, raised public awareness about the need to protect vulnerable people, especially in nontherapeutic experiments. Two main groups are considered vulnerable subjects for research. The first includes those who lack the capacity to give informed consent, such as children and adults with mental or intellectual impairment. Membership in this group depends, to some extent, on one's definition of personhood. For example, if fetuses are persons, they should not be exposed to experimentation that may harm them. Animal rights activists also include nonhuman animals in this group.

The second group includes people who are vulnerable to manipulation or coercion because of fear, ignorance, poverty, or pressure to participate. Prisoners, residents of institutions, economically disadvantaged people who lack access to adequate healthcare, and those unfamiliar with the nuances of the research fall into this second group. Because of the financial incentives for physicians, patients of physicians who are paid to recruit subjects for drug studies may also be subjected to subtle pressure to enroll in a study, especially if they lack adequate health insurance to pay for prescription drugs. Some healthcare ethicists, including George Annas and Michael Grodin in their article on international AIDS experimentation, oppose recruiting subjects by offering financial incentives or health services they would otherwise be unable to afford. Others argue that, while poverty may render some people more vulnerable to being harmed by experiments, they still have the right to decide what risks to take, especially if participation in an experiment is the only way to receive quality medical treatment.

According to some ethicists, college students attending institutes conducting research also fall into this second group. Because there is an unequal power relationship between faculty and students, students are vulnerable to pressure from faculty. Faculty members may even offer extra credit to students to be subjects in experiments. Some medical schools prohibit the use of students in research that poses more than minimal risk or that interferes with their studies. While some people protest this policy as paternalistic, others claim that it is elitist in that medical students are given greater protection than other people from being exploited in biomedical experiments. Some researchers justify the use of students in experiments as being educational for the students. In addition, most experiments using college students as subjects are relatively innocuous and do not harm the students or compromise their integrity.

Pregnant and nursing women are also considered vulnerable by the U.S. Department of Health because of risks to fetuses and nursing infants, who are unable to give their consent. This policy is controversial, since it restricts the autonomy of these women and prevents them from participating in therapeutic experiments that might benefit them. Most libertarians argue that when there is a conflict between the well-being of a pregnant woman and that of her fetus, the woman, not the government or the medical profession, has the moral right to resolve it. Those who believe that the fetus is a person maintain that, while it is morally acceptable for people to put themselves in harm's way, they do not have the right to expose another person—in this case, the fetus—to harm.

Racism, Sexism, and the Use of Marginalized Groups as Subjects

Subject selection in research often reflects the prejudices of society. The use of marginalized groups in risky nontherapeutic experiments reflects the tacit belief that certain groups of people don't count as much or even are dispensable. Experiments in the United States that researchers would never have considered carrying out on economically advantaged white subjects have been carried out on black and Hispanic subjects. Scientific justification is often given for this bias. The scientists who oversaw the Tuskegee Study, for example, regarded it as a "natural experiment" because "such people" were all infected and would not seek treatment for their syphilis. This racist and mistaken assumption was used to justify withholding treatment from the men even after the discovery of penicillin as a cure.

People with mental disabilities are also viewed by some well-educated research physicians as less than human. In a 1971 Department of Defense study, subjects were specifically selected because of their "low-educational level . . . low-functioning quotient."[35] "Mentally enfeebled" patients, most of whom were also poor and black, were irradiated in order to determine the effects of radiation on soldiers on an atomic battlefield. The research continued even after it came to the attention of the institutional review board at the University of Cincinnati, where it was being conducted.

At the other extreme, the almost exclusive use of white males in past therapeutic research reflects the belief that the white male is the archetypal human. Because women and minorities have been excluded from or underrepresented in most medical research, they have not benefited from the results to the same extent as men. Women, for example, have been underrepresented in studies on cardiovascular disease, even though it is the leading cause of death in women. Also, despite the fact that women use over 90 percent of diet pills, nearly all of the testing has been done on men.[36]

The barriers to women's participation in medical research are being challenged as a violation of the principle of justice, since women are denied the benefits not only of experimental treatments but also of informed treatment when a new drug is released on the market. Because most new drugs have not been tested on women, the effect of the drugs on women and fetuses is unknown, even though they may be routinely prescribed to women—including pregnant women. Another issue is the practice in medical research (and society) of defining women but not men primarily by their reproductive role. Studies show that sperm can be damaged by exposure to certain chemicals and drugs.[37] Should women who are sexually active or pregnant have the same right as men to make an informed decision about participating in medical research?

Between 1990 and 1994, major policy changes were made regarding the inclusion of women in research. The NIH now requires that grant recipients include appropriate numbers of women and minorities unless inclusion can be shown to be unsuitable for health reasons or other circumstances. In 1997, the U.S. Food and Drug Administration proposed a rule that ensured that women who had a life-threatening disease would not be excluded from drug trials because they are of childbearing age.[38]

International Research, Human Rights, and Cultural Relativism

Concern for human rights in medical experiments has become more urgent with the globalization of medical experimentation. Some countries have no official ethical guidelines for human experimentation, thus allowing governments in economically developed nations and multinational corporations to conduct morally questionable experiments. Instead of simply paying lip service to the concept of universal moral principles, Annas and Grodin maintain, researchers should make an active commitment to universal human rights. Multinational researchers also need to understand the social customs of their host country and how these customs influence the carrying out of universal moral principles.

Africa, in particular, has been targeted by many AIDS researchers because of the high prevalence of HIV infection and untreated AIDS in many African nations. Some healthcare ethicists are concerned that the maternal/fetal HIV transmission experiments in Africa are exploiting the impoverished in order to gain knowledge that will benefit developed countries. Impoverished people suffering from AIDS will accept any medical assistance, even experimental, as "better than nothing." It is also unlikely that these people would volunteer to be in an experiment that will have no long-term benefit for their community—or, in most cases, for themselves—if poverty were not a factor.

Subject Selection and Justice

Justice requires that subjects be able to share in the benefits of the research, especially in therapeutic experimentation. A primary criticism of the AIDS research in Africa is that the participants do not share in the fruits of the experiments. The withdrawal of effective treatment from subjects after the experiments have ended has upset healthcare providers in some countries. Dr. Peter Cleaton-Jones, a member of the ethical committee at the University of Witwatersrand, South Africa, which cooperated with the project, had second thoughts about the experiments. "Companies from abroad," he says, "come to this country to circumvent ethics."[39] South Africa is currently engaged in negotiations with the German company carrying out the experiments to continue to supply the drugs to people used as subjects.

How should the burdens and benefits of medical experimentation be distributed? Some healthcare ethicists argue that it is unfair that certain people, such as people in wealthy nations, reap the benefits of biomedical research without making a reciprocal contribution by volunteering to be subjects. Others, including Jonas, maintain that people have no duty to contribute to biomedical research and medical progress because it is inherently wrong to sacrifice an individual for the social good. Medical progress, because it is not essential to the well-being or survival of the human species, is an optional goal. People who volunteer to be subjects in nontherapeutic experiments are performing acts of altruism and heroism. While we owe these heroes a duty of gratitude, we do not have a duty to society based on reciprocity and justice.

INTERNATIONAL ETHICAL GUIDELINES FOR BIOMEDICAL RESEARCH INVOLVING HUMAN SUBJECTS, THE WORLD HEALTH ORGANIZATION (WHO) AND THE COUNCIL FOR INTERNATIONAL ORGANIZATIONS OF MEDICAL SCIENCES (CIOMS) (1993)

Because of the bias of many researchers against other cultures, WHO and CIOMS have developed a set of guidelines for international research. The intent of the guidelines is to help countries—especially developing countries—form national policies on biomedical research, to assist researchers in applying universal moral standards at the local level, and to define mechanisms for protecting human subjects used in medical research. Following are excerpts from the guidelines.

General Ethical Principles

All research involving human subjects should be conducted in accordance with three basic ethical principles, namely respect for persons, beneficence and justice. It is generally agreed that these principles, which in the abstract have equal moral force, guide the conscientious preparation of proposals for scientific studies. In varying circumstances they may be expressed differently and given different moral weight, and their application may lead to different decisions or courses of action. The present guidelines are directed at the application of these principles to research involving human subjects. . . .

The Guidelines

Informed Consent of Subjects
Guideline 8: Research involving subjects in underdeveloped communities

Before undertaking research involving subjects in underdeveloped com-

EXPERIMENTATION ON CHILDREN AND FETUSES

Baby Fae was born in 1984 with a malformed heart that left her with only half of a functioning heart. She was taken to the Loma Linda University Medical Center in California, where twelve days after her birth a surgical team headed by Dr. Leonard Bailey performed a heart transplant on her using the heart of a baboon. Baby Fae lived only twenty days with the new heart. She was the fourth person to receive a **xenograft,** a transplanted organ from another species. The other three people all died shortly after their transplants.

Following Baby Fae's ill-fated heart transplant, questions were raised about the ethics of the experimental surgery, especially since no attempt had been made to find a human heart. Objections were also raised by animal rights advocates regarding the sacrifice of a healthy animal for an experiment that had dubious benefits. Although Bailey admitted that it was "an oversight on our part not to search for a human donor from the start," he defended his action on the grounds that human hearts suitable for transplant were scarce. He also pointed out that he had performed more than 150 organ transplants on nonhuman animals and believed that the procedure might work on Baby Fae.

Experimentation on Children

Children are vulnerable to exploitation in biomedical experimentation because of their dependence on adults to make decisions for them. While many ethicists oppose

munities, whether in developed or developing countries, the investigator must ensure that:

—persons in underdeveloped communities ordinarily will not be involved in research that could be carried out reasonably well in developed communities;

—the research is responsive to the health needs and the priorities of the community in which it is carried out.

—every effort will be made to secure the ethical imperative that the consent of individual subjects be informed; and

—the proposals for the research have been reviewed and approved by an ethical review committee that has among its members or consultants persons who are thoroughly familiar with the customs and traditions of the community. . . .

Selection of Research Subjects
Guideline 10: Equitable distribution of burdens and benefits

Individuals or communities to be invited to be subjects of research should be selected in such a way that the burdens and benefits of the research will be equitably distributed. Special justification is required for inviting vulnerable individuals and, if they are selected, the means of protecting their rights and welfare must be particularly strictly applied. . . .

Externally Sponsored Research
Guideline 15: Obligations of the sponsoring and host countries

Externally sponsored research entails two ethical obligations:

—An external sponsoring agency should submit the research protocol to ethical and scientific review according to the standards of the country of the sponsoring agency, and the ethical standards applied should be no less exacting than they would be in the case of research carried out in that country.

—After scientific and ethical approval in the country of the sponsoring agency, the appropriate authorities of the host country, including a national or local ethical review committee or its equivalent, should satisfy themselves that the proposed research meets their own ethical requirements.

the use of children as subjects in nontherapeutic experiments, most sanction their use in therapeutic experiments if the risk is minimal. Prohibiting therapeutic experimentation on children, it has been argued, discriminates against children much as the exclusive use of white males as subjects in low-risk therapeutic experiments discriminates against women and minorities. Furthermore, therapeutic experimentation on children is essential if we are to improve medical treatment for childhood diseases.

As with any biomedical experimentation, it is tempting to justify as therapeutic any experiment that holds out any hope of benefit to the subject-patient. But was Baby Fae's heart transplant a therapeutic experiment? Given that she was critically ill and in all likelihood would have died without intervention, did even the very low probability of success outweigh the suffering she endured as a result of the experimental surgery? Would Baby Fae have consented to the transplant had she been able?

Parents and Surrogate Consent

The inability of children to give informed consent is a primary issue in pediatric research. Although surrogate consent is prohibited by the Nuremberg Code, several other national and international codes of ethics—including the Declaration of

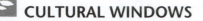

CULTURAL WINDOWS

MULTINATIONAL RESEARCH IN SOUTHEAST ASIA

Some Western researchers are turning to Southeast Asia, where there is little government regulation of medical experimentation. Much of the research violates international agreements. Extensive drug and contraceptive testing, as well as genetic and psychosurgical research, is being carried out on poor subjects without their informed consent.[40] Thailand, for example, is one of the primary sites for multinational AIDS research.

Some governments and medical communities in Southeast Asia are responding by formulating guidelines to prevent exploitation of the poor by Western researchers. In 1985, the Thailand National Research Council developed guidelines for human experimentation. Two years later, the Philippine Council for Health Research and Development published its National Guidelines for Biomedical Research Involving Human Subjects. The Philippine guidelines were modeled on the World Medical Association's Helsinki Code.

Unfortunately, there is little compliance with these guidelines among physicians and researchers in Thailand and the Philippines. Indeed, Southeast Asian researchers often willingly assist Western researchers in carrying out experiments that would be condemned in the West.

In response, Southeast Asian health-care ethicists are looking to their traditional ethics as well as to Western bio-ethics. Southeast Asian ethics is influenced by Hinduism, Buddhism, Islam, and Christianity. The Hindu and Buddhist principle of ahimsa (no harm), for example, clearly conflicts with some of the research being conducted in Southeast Asia. In addition, one of the five precepts of Buddhism prohibits deception, which raises questions about the morality of using placebos in double-blind trials in medical research.

Christianity, with its emphasis on compassion and respect for human dignity, has also contributed to the development of bioethics in Southeast Asia. In 1983, the Center for Biomedical Ethics Development was established in Indonesia to promote bioethics and Christian values in medicine. The Southeast Asian Center of Bioethics was established in the Philippines in 1987 by a group of Catholic physicians and priests to encourage ethical reflection and dialogue on ethical issues.

Several medical schools now offer courses in medical ethics. In addition, efforts are being made in many Southeast Asian countries to establish institutional review committees to evaluate the ethical and scientific value of research proposals.

Helsinki—permit parents to consent to nontherapeutic research on behalf of their children. The American Medical Association also permits surrogate consent if the surrogate would reasonably agree to be a subject in the experiment.

Between 1946 and 1956, physicians gave radioactive calcium and iron to retarded children at a state school in Massachusetts in order to study the long-term effects of exposure to radiation. When the study was made public, the physicians claimed that they were following accepted scientific procedures, although they did apologize for not first obtaining the consent of the parents. But what if the parents had given consent? Do parents have the right to give consent for their children to be used in medical experiments? Can parents always be trusted to act in their children's best interest? After all, the parents in the Willowbrook study had consented to their children being used in the hepatitis experiment.

Parents are often disadvantaged when it comes to giving informed surrogate consent, even in therapeutic experiments. Unlike the child who is experiencing the disease, parents, at least in most cases, have only secondhand knowledge of the disease. The process by which parental consent is obtained can be problematic. In the Willowbrook case, parental consent was sought at a public meeting at which parents were informed about the prospective experiment. The solicitation of surrogate consent in group forums can lead to "group thinking" rather than autonomous decision making.

In the case of seriously ill newborns, the technical complexities involved in intensive neonatal therapy leave most parents dependent on the physician's judgment. The distress of seeing their child desperately ill leaves many parents willing to agree to any treatment, experimental or otherwise, that holds out any hope of cure. In the case of Baby Fae, for example, questions were raised about whether the parents understood or had been properly informed about the procedure and its bleak prognosis.

Research on Embryos and Fetuses

Biomedical experimentation on embryos and fetuses is almost exclusively nontherapeutic. Although the U.S. Congress in 1965 banned the use of federal money for research in which a human embryo is "subjected to risk of injury or death," this ban does not apply to privately funded research, nor does it prohibit the use of aborted fetuses.

The two primary reasons for fetal and embryo research are to find cures for debilitating disease and to learn more about human development. In 1998, Dr. Curt Freed of the University of Colorado transplanted cells from forty-five- to fifty-five-day-old aborted fetuses into twenty patients with Parkinson's disease. Preliminary experiments indicated that after receiving fetal implants patients experienced significant improvement in their motor skills. Scientists also use brain cells from aborted fetuses in an effort to find cures for neurological disorders such as Huntington's disease and spinal-cord injuries.

Most cadavers of fetuses used in fetal research are acquired from abortion clinics. Human embryos are also used in genetic and biomedical research. In the past, embryo research was conducted primarily on surplus embryos obtained from infertility clinics. However, since spare embryos are generally of lower quality than those used for implants, several biotech firms have turned to anonymous gamete donors for sperm and eggs. These companies then fertilize the eggs, thus creating a ready supply of human embryos for experimental use.[41] While embryo farming is illegal in some countries, for example, Australia, it is legal in the United States. Should embryo farming and embryo research be permitted? What about nontherapeutic experimentation on living fetuses who are going to be aborted? Is using nonsentient human fetuses and embryos preferable to using sentient nonhuman animals?

EXPERIMENTATION USING NONHUMAN ANIMALS

In the early hours of the morning on May 18, 1984, five men and women broke into the University of Pennsylvania's Head Trauma Research Center, where neurosurgery professor Thomas Gennarelli conducted head-injury experiments on baboons. The group stole videotapes of the experiments and ransacked the lab. The videotapes showed gruesome scenes of terrified baboons being held in vises as their heads were smashed by pistons while researchers joked around, as well as operations being performed on primates without regard for their pain or for standard research procedures. As they left the lab, the five intruders wrote the initials ALF on the wall. ALF (the Animal Liberation Front) is a radical animal rights organization founded in England in the mid-1970s.

The release of the stolen videotapes to the media sparked a worldwide debate on the ethics of using nonhuman animals in medical experiments. Gennarelli defended his research, claiming the animals had been properly treated, and accused the ALF of setting back medical research. Both the University of Pennsylvania and the National Institutes of Health, which awarded the lab a new grant to repair the damages, supported Dr. Gennarelli. In 1985, however, the secretary of health and human services stopped federal funding for the head-injury program. Congress also passed more stringent laws regulating the use of nonhuman animals in biomedical research.[42]

The Legal and Moral Status of Nonhuman Animals

Do humans have obligations to other animals? Do other animals have rights that we ought to respect, as the ALF claims? An estimated 20–120 million nonhuman animals are killed annually in the United States in experiments designed to benefit humans.[43] While the trend worldwide is toward using fewer nonhuman animals in experiments, there was an increase during the 1990s in their use in biotechnology and genetics.[44] Scientists are genetically engineering "designer" animals for specific research purposes. Human genes are being inserted into other animals so they can be used as "drug factories" or harvested for organ transplants. Mice are being genetically altered for use in research on diabetes, cancer, Alzheimer's disease, and epilepsy.[45]

Animal experimentation enjoys more support in the United States than in most Western countries. Both the NIH and the AMA strongly support it. In Britain, Canada, and many other European countries, on the other hand, the number of nonhuman animals used in experiments has dropped by over half since the 1970s.[46]

In 1968, Canada became the first country to create animal care committees in all research facilities using nonhuman animals in research. In Canada, mammals have been largely replaced by fish in experiments. Britain passed the Animals (Scientific Procedures) Act in 1986. This act, which is probably the strictest of its kind in the world, extended the protection offered by the 1876 Cruelty to Animals Act. In 1992, the European Commission established the European Center for the Validation of Alternative Methods. In 1996, the Netherlands passed a law stating that animals have "intrinsic value" and, as sentient beings, are entitled to the moral concern shown toward human subjects in research.

Scientists and physicians, like the general public, have mixed feelings about animal experimentation. Women, younger people, and recent PhDs in science are the most likely to oppose animal experimentation; farmers, hunters, and clergy are the most

✿ EXPERIMENTS USING NONHUMAN ANIMALS[47]

Toxicity tests: Animals are force-fed or forced to inhale varying quantities of a substance in order to determine potential adverse side effects or the lethal dose (LD) at which a given percent of animals die over a preestablished time period. Following the experiment the animals are killed and their tissues examined.

Psychology research: Animals are used in experiments that include electric shock, "punishment," induced fighting and killing, brain damage, mutilation, drug addiction, maternal deprivation, and overcrowding.

Weapons tests: Animals are used to study the effects of atomic blasts, radiation, chemical and biological warfare, and laser weapons on the body.

Biotechnology: Animals are genetically engineered, and sometimes cloned, for use in medical experiments, to produce drugs for human use, and for organ transplants.

Genetics: Animals are used in the development of gene therapy and in experiments to learn more about genetic inheritance and genetic disease in humans.

✿ CULTURAL WINDOWS

THE ISLAMIC VIEW ON ANIMAL EXPERIMENTATION

Muslims, like Judeo-Christian ethicists, believe that humans are superior to other animals. However, Muslims also believe that other animals possess a psyche and are conscious. All species have moral standing and form one community. Animal experimentation, therefore, is strictly regulated in Islamic countries.

According to Muslim scholar Al-Hafiz B. A. Masri, humans have a moral responsibility to be active protectors of the welfare of other animals as well as to avoid cruelty. The Hadith of the Holy Prophet Muhammad lists cruelty to animals as the third of four sins: "The grievous things are: Polytheism; disobedience to parents; the killing of breathing things. . . ." The use of animals in biomedical experimentation is permitted only if the same moral codes that apply to human subjects are applied to animal subjects. Painful and disfiguring experimentation on nonhuman animals, such as that in the head-trauma experiments, is prohibited.

---

likely to favor it.[48] Among philosophers, Aristotle believed that only humans had souls or minds and that other animals were inferior beings whom nature made "for the sake of man." His worldview was Christianized by Thomas Aquinas, who wrote, "By divine providence they [dumb animals] are intended for man's use in the natural order. Hence it is not wrong for man to make use of them, either by killing or in any other way whatever."[49] Aquinas backed up his views with biblical scripture, which says that

CULTURAL WINDOWS

INDIAN MORAL PHILOSOPHY AND ANIMAL EXPERIMENTATION

Attitudes toward animal experimentation in India have been shaped by several schools of thought, including Hinduism, Buddhism, and Jainism.

Hindus, like traditional Western philosophers, believe that nonhuman animals do not have rights. However, unlike Western philosophers, who regard humans as fundamentally different from other animals, Hindus believe in the unity of all life. Humans with bad karma may be reincarnated into nonhuman animals. Nevertheless, a lower form of life cannot demand a duty from a higher form of life. This does not mean that we can use nonhuman animals in biomedical experimentation. Salvation requires observation of the principle of ahimsa. Doctrinal Hinduism, therefore, does not permit the use of nonhuman animals in biomedical research. Practical modern Hinduism, however, permits medical uses of animals but "*if and only if (1) the benefits humans receive far outweigh the pain animals endure, and (2) the use of animals is necessary* (that is, the benefits are not otherwise attainable)."[50]

Unlike Hinduism, which sees compassion toward other animals primarily as a means of achieving salvation, Buddhist and Jainist traditions regard nonhuman animals as sentient beings with at least some degree of free will. Therefore, they tend to take a stronger stand against animal experimentation than do Hindus. The principle of ahimsa, which is central in both Buddhist and Jainist philosophies, requires that we do no harm. This entails avoiding biomedical experiments that cause suffering to nonhuman animals as well as to humans. Indian law, however, requires that medicines first be tested on nonhuman animals. Pharmaceutical companies owned by Jainists, in addition to treating the animal subjects with compassion during the experiments, rehabilitate and then release them when the experiment is over. Both Jainists and Buddhists also strongly encourage the development of alternatives to animal experimentation.

humans were created in God's image and were given dominion over other creatures (Genesis 1:26). Of course, not all Christians interpret this passage as condoning unrestricted research on nonhuman animals.

The belief that humans are separate from and morally superior to other animals was embraced by René Descartes (1596–1650), the "father of modern philosophy." According to him, nonhuman animals are merely organic machines, much like clocks, without souls, free will, or consciousness. Francis Bacon (1561–1626), one of the founders of the scientific method, also accepted the prevailing view and enthusiastically endorsed vivisection for the pure joy of learning. Because of the tremendous success of science in generating results and new technologies, few people bothered to question the morality of sacrificing nonhuman animals to achieve some of this success.

Challenges to traditional anthropocentrism came from several fronts. These challenges are summarized in the article at the end of this chapter by Judith A. Boss and

Alyssa V. Boss. In his book *The Descent of Man* (1871), Charles Darwin argued that other animals are clearly capable of reasoning and deliberating. Rather than humans being special creations, there is no fundamental difference between humans and the higher animals in their mental faculties. The utilitarians were among the first advocates of the welfare of nonhuman animals. According to Jeremy Bentham (1748–1832), nonhuman animals deserve our moral consideration even if they are not capable of reasoning, since it is not reason but the capacity to suffer that is morally relevant.[51] Australian utilitarian Peter Singer continues this tradition.

Eastern philosophy, particularly that of Gandhi, also had an enormous influence on the animal rights movement. Gandhi once said, "The greatness of a nation can be judged by the way its animals are treated. . . . Vivisection is the blackest of all the black crimes that man is at present committing against God and His fair creation." In most of Asia, the use of nonhuman animals in biomedical research is limited by three things: (1) the principle of ahimsa, or noninjury to living beings, (2) the belief in the unity or interconnectedness of all being, and (3) the concepts of karma and reincarnation. In order to overcome the negative effects of karma, one must practice ahimsa, or compassion toward other animals.

Utilitarian Arguments

Utilitarians adopt a cost/benefit approach to animal experimentation in which the benefits to humans are weighed against the pain and suffering of the animals. Although many, if not most, animal researchers are concerned with reducing the suffering of their subjects, they also claim that animal experimentation has been vital to past success in medicine and is necessary for continued progress. The development of vaccines for infectious diseases including diphtheria, rabies, whooping cough, and poliomyelitis has relied heavily on animal experimentation. Animal experimentation has also led to the development of new antibiotics and other drugs that have saved thousands of human lives, as well as to advances in open-heart surgery and organ transplants.

Not all utilitarians support animal experimentation. Peter Singer, whose 1975 book *Animal Liberation* launched the current animal rights movement, argues that the benefits to humans in most cases do not outweigh the tremendous suffering of animal subjects. Utilitarians also question the use of the term *necessary suffering* in the context of animal experimentation, since the suffering of animals is often regarded as "unnecessary" only when it does not facilitate human ends or human well-being. Thus, talk of "necessary suffering" may mask a degraded view of other animals as things. The suffering caused to a hundred dogs or mice may be deemed "necessary," while the same experiment performed on one severely retarded human is condemned as a moral outrage. This discriminatory practice is not justified by utilitarian theory. Even if we rate human cognitive pleasures higher than those of other animals, as does John Stuart Mill, the pain of other animals is still a concern.

The conviction that it is wrong to perform experiments on mentally impaired or marginalized humans has fueled the conviction that it is similarly wrong and contrary to the principle of justice to perform experiments on other animals. The claim that humans are a superior form of life does not entitle humans to exploit other animals any more than superior humans are entitled to exploit their inferiors. According to Singer, we are engaging in what he calls speciesism if we do not grant equal consideration to other animals cognitive ability equal to that of humans, such as infants or mentally impaired people, whom we would not use in nontherapeutic experiments. Singer defines *speciesism* as "a prejudice or attitude of bias in favor of the interests of members of one's own species and against those of members of another species."[52] His rule of thumb for avoiding speciesism is that "we should give the same respect to the lives of animals as we give to the lives of those humans at a similar mental level." Animal experimentation can be justified only if it is also morally permissible to use humans with low cognitive functioning as subjects. Indeed, if our concern is to benefit humans, using brain-damaged humans may be preferable to using nonhuman animals, because the experimental results would be more accurate.

Some opponents of animal experimentation take another tack, arguing that it is misleading to extrapolate results from experiments on other species to effects on humans. Of the 209 new drugs marketed in the United States between 1976 and 1985, for example, 52 percent had "serious postapproval risks" not predicted by animal experimentation. Important medical advances have also been held back because of misleading results. Under the standards set by the National Cancer Institute, of the nineteen chemicals known to cause cancer in humans when ingested, only seven cause cancer in mice and rats. In addition, in the 1960s scientists concluded, based on numerous animal experiments, that inhaled tobacco smoke does not cause lung cancer. For many years, the tobacco industry used these studies to prevent the government from putting warning labels on cigarette packs and to discourage physicians from advising their patients to give up smoking. Research on birth defects also relies heavily on animal research, yet most has not been helpful. In fact, the incidence of birth defects in humans is on the rise, as is that of cancer and heart disease.

Animal experimentation opponents point out that 90 percent of human disease, including 80 percent of cancer cases, is primarily the result of unhealthy life-styles and is avoidable. Instead of focusing on cures for these diseases, they argue, we should focus on preventative measures. The NIH in 1991 granted more money in research dollars for animal research than for research on humans.[53] The millions of dollars spent every year on animal experimentation would be better spent on epidemiological studies and on preventative measures that could save human lives. The fact that medical science relied on animal experimentation in the past to solve medical problems rather than developing alternatives does not mean that it was necessary or that we should continue to do so in the future.

Advocates of animal experimentation, while acknowledging that most health problems can be avoided through life-style changes, respond that some health concerns, such as the development of vaccines and cures for infectious diseases, can be addressed only through the use of animal experimentation. They also claim that nonhuman animals in fact make good models for studies of human diseases and that the great majority of experiments provide results that can be applied to humans. One researcher writes:

> In truth, there are no basic differences between the physiology of laboratory animals and humans. Both control their internal biochemistry by releasing endocrine hormones that are all essentially the same; both humans and laboratory animals send out similar chemical transmitters from nerve cells and the central and peripheral nervous systems, and both react in the same way to infection or tissue injury.[54]

However, if there is so little physiological difference between humans and laboratory animals, can we realistically continue to deny these animals moral standing?

Rights, Duties, and Nonhuman Animals

The animal rights movement is an outgrowth of the animal welfare movement. Most animal rights activists believe that all nontherapeutic animal experimentation is immoral. While they may not deny that animal experimentation has benefited humans, they claim that some things, no matter how beneficial the consequences may be, are simply wrong. Rights, in other words, trump utilitarian considerations.

According to Tom Regan, there is a fundamental right not to be harmed simply to benefit others. Any being that has interests and desires to satisfy those interests can be harmed. Benefits to oneself and others are morally acceptable only if no one else's rights are violated in achieving those benefits. Instead of using human cognitive ability as the gold standard of moral standing, as does Singer, Regan argues that there is no morally significant cognitive difference between humans and other adult mammals. The interests of humans or more cognitively developed beings, therefore, do not ipso facto override the interests of other animals. While nonhuman animals, like children and incompetent humans, may lack the cognitive ability to be moral agents, they can still be moral patients with rights and interests that we ought to respect. Fairness entails that the strong not misuse their power by frustrating the interests of the weak.

Carl Cohen, in contrast, in his article at the end of this chapter, argues that other animals have no rights that humans are bound to respect. Moral rights and duties, according to him, arise from an implicit social contract among members of the community. Since only rational, autonomous agents can enter into a contract and exercise claims against one another, humans have no moral duties toward other animals who, presumably, lack the capacity to make moral choices. Our only duty regarding nonhuman animals is to protect them from severe, unnecessary pain.

One drawback of this model of rights is that is eliminates noncompetent humans as holders of rights. Some critics of Cohen, including Singer, argue that using nonhuman animals in experiments gives researchers the green light to go ahead and use humans at the same cognitive level as nonhuman animals. Cohen disagrees. He argues that noncompetent humans have rights, even though they are incapable of claiming these rights, simply because they are members of a group whose members normally have rights. This is a questionable jump. As a member of a university community, I have certain rights; however, these rights don't automatically extend to anyone who is related to me. Why draw the community boundary around species membership? Why not draw it around all sentient beings, as Singer does? In addition, even if we restrict the community to members of the human species, the fact that rights may arise from our having membership in a social contract does not mean that this membership is the only source of rights. Rights may also arise from interests, as Regan argues.

The Future of Animal Research

Both abolitionists and animal welfare advocates encourage the use of alternatives to animals as subjects in biomedical research. In 1959, British scientists William Russell and Rex Burch published *The Principles of Humane Experimental Technique*, in which they set out three goals for researchers: replacement, reduction, and refinement. Nonhuman animal subjects can be replaced in many cases by tissue or cell cultures, one-cell organisms, in vitro tests, observation of patients, epidemiological and clinical studies, cadavers, computer simulation, and mechanical models. For example, researchers at a Dutch pharmaceutical company in 1999 created a latex rat, known as a PVC-Rat, that can be used instead of real rats in research on microsurgical procedures.[55] The number of nonhuman animal subjects used can be reduced by using statistical means and by reviewing the mounds of past data for information on the effects of certain chemicals rather than retesting these chemicals on animals. Finally, laboratories and the design of experiments can be refined to cause less suffering to animals. Boss and Boss discuss the concept of alternatives to animal research in more depth in their article. In 1993, the U.S. Congress directed the NIH to develop a plan for implementing the three R's.

Even if we reject the claim that other animals have inherent moral worth, we should stop and consider how our life-styles may cause suffering to other animals. To maintain that the value of other animals is less than that of humans does not excuse the exploitation of animals in experiments that provide little benefit to humans or that are conducted to further research on diseases preventable by life-style changes. Virtue and the duty of nonmaleficence require that we at least stop depending on the suffering of other animals for cures to diseases that we cause by engaging in unhealthy life-styles.

Seventeen out of the top twenty drug companies test new drugs on electronic human models, using computer-assisted virtual testing to determine whether proceeding to human testing is justified.[56] While virtual testing and alternatives such as tissue cultures will probably never completely replace human or animal experimentation, they will eliminate some of the riskier experiments.

USING THE RESULTS OF UNETHICAL EXPERIMENTS

In 1899, Bayer, a German dyestuff company, realized that it could make vast profits in the new pharmaceutical industry. It has since become one of the largest pharmaceutical companies in the world, with Aspirin, a registered Bayer trademark, the standard remedy for a wide array of illnesses. Part of Bayer's success was due to its research and development program. The ready availability of captive human subjects in Nazi Germany provided a unique opportunity for pharmaceutical companies such as Bayer to test their new drugs, as well as the effectiveness of existing drugs, under a wide variety of conditions. Bayer, which at the time of World War II was part of the I. G. Farben industrial empire that supplied Zyklon-B gas to the Nazi concentration camps, was one of the companies that enlisted the cooperation of the notorious Dr. Josef Mengele to test its products on twins at Auschwitz. According to Eva Mozes Kor, who filed a class-action suit against the company, representatives from Bayer "monitored and supervised those experiments, and used them as a form of research and development for its corporate benefit."[57] Healthy inmates in the camps were first given various infections delivered through pills, powders, injections, and enemas. Various medications were then administered to determine their effectiveness in combating the different infections.

As another example, Caplan describes in his article a hypothermia experiment that used an estimated 300 inmates, about 80 to 90 of whom died. The results of these experiments may have saved hundreds of lives.[58] Nazi physicians and scientists who carried out research on human subjects in the concentration camps believed that they were morally justified in sacrificing the interests of the few to benefit the many. While we may condemn the research, the results of these experiments yielded useful scientific information. Should data acquired by immoral means be used?

"Bad Ethics, Therefore Bad Science"

The "bad ethics, therefore bad science" argument is often used to dismiss debate over the use of results from unethical research. The first version of this argument states that experiments that are grossly immoral and violate the rights of the subjects, such as the Nazi experiments, cannot possibly generate any valid scientific results. Likewise, some animal rights activists argue that animal experimentation cannot generate valid results for human medicine. This argument, however, is based on the fallacy of false cause. Although in a perfect and just world we might wish it were so, in actual fact no logical causal connection exists between the morality of the research design and the scientific validity of the research findings.

The second version of this argument is more compelling. It states that even if the results of immoral research are scientifically valid they should be excluded from the body of scientific knowledge. Added to the insult to those who may be subjects in such experiments is the fear that legitimating the results will encourage other scientists to become complacent about the rights and welfare of their subjects and tempt less scrupulous researchers to resort to morally questionable experimentation in order to gain notoriety in their field. It was this self-serving and arrogant disregard for the rights of human subjects in research that led to the establishment of IRBs in the 1970s.

Utilitarianism and Beneficiaries of Unethical Experimentation

Because utilitarians consider only future consequences, the past, although it may be regrettable, is not morally relevant except to the extent that using data from immoral experiments might encourage similar experiments in the future. If the data can be used to save lives, they should probably be used. In the case of the hypothermia experiments, for example, we need to ask whether the long-term benefits of the experiments outweigh the pain and suffering of the 300 people used in the study. The findings of the German study have been used to design hypothermia-protective devices that protect the neck and head and may already have saved many lives.

Is it fair for people who played no role in these experiments to be denied cures that may save their lives? On one hand, we don't refuse a dying person an organ transplant because the donor was killed by a drunk driver. Also, using the organs of victims of drunk driving does not cause or encourage drunk driving. Instead, we deal with the drunk-driving issue independently of any good that might come out of accidents. Similarly, we might argue, steps for dealing with unethical experimentation should not include suppressing the results from past experiments. Furthermore, how should we purge scientific findings that have become commonplace in medicine? What about freedom of speech?

On the other hand, many ethicists believe that, even if utility justifies using data from research such as the hypothermia experiments, we should still make a commitment never to use data from past experiments that violated human rights and dignity.

Eva Mozes Kor, who survived Dr. Mengele's experiments, appealed to all scientists and doctors to pledge to promote a universal ideal that states: "Treat the subjects of your experiments in the manner that you would want to be treated if you were in their place."[59]

In a results-oriented system in which promotion and fame are based on producing research results, the temptation to engage in unethical research is powerful. As the Nazi experience poignantly illustrates, ethical codes and committees are not a sufficient guarantee that the rights and welfare of subjects used in research will be protected—the medical ethics codes in Germany in the 1940s were among the most sophisticated in the world. Nor can we count on ethics committees to always put human rights and animal welfare before medical progress. More than any other force, the public has been the most effective watchdog. As citizens and as members of institutions where medical research is conducted, we have a moral duty to be vigilant and to call researchers to task when they stray outside the limits of moral decency.

HANS JONAS

Philosophical Reflections on Experimenting with Human Subjects

Philosopher Hans Jonas is one of the pioneers in healthcare ethics. According to Jonas, it is inherently wrong for medical researchers to sacrifice the individual for the good of society or for medical progress, and informed consent is not sufficient to justify the use of human subjects. Subjects should be recruited from those who are most knowledgeable about the research and most capable of understanding its implications.

Experimenting with human subjects is going on in many fields of scientific and technological progress. It is designed to replace the over-all instruction by natural, occasional experience with the selective information from artificial, systematic experiment which physical science has found so effective in dealing with inanimate nature. Of the new experimentation with man, medical is surely the most legitimate; psychological, the most dubious; biological (still to come), the most dangerous. I have chosen here to deal with the first only, where the case *for* it is strongest and the task of adjudicating conflicting claims hardest. . . .

THE PECULIARITY OF HUMAN EXPERIMENTATION

Experimentation was originally sanctioned by natural science. There it is performed on inanimate objects, and this raises no moral problems. But as soon as animate, feeling beings become the subjects of experiment, as they do in the life sciences and especially in medical research, this innocence of the search for knowledge is lost and questions of conscience arise. The depth to which moral and religious sensibilities can become aroused over these questions is shown by the vivisection issue. Human experimentation must sharpen the issue as it involves ultimate questions of personal dignity and sacrosanctity. . . .

. . . The question is inherently philosophical as it concerns not merely pragmatic difficulties and their arbitration, but a genuine conflict of values involving principles of a high order. May I put the conflict in these terms. On principle, it is felt, human beings *ought not* to be dealt with in that way (the "guinea pig" protest); on the other hand, such dealings are increasingly urged on us by considerations, in turn appealing to principle, that claim to override those objections. Such a claim must be carefully assessed, especially when it is swept along by a mighty tide. Putting the matter thus, we have already made one important assumption rooted in our "Western" cultural tradition: The prohibitive rule is, to that way of thinking, the primary and axiomatic one; the permissive counter-rule, as qualifying the first, is secondary and stands in need of justification. We must justify the infringement of a primary inviolability, which needs no justification itself; and the justification of its infringement must be by values and needs of a dignity commensurate with those to be sacrificed. . . .

"INDIVIDUAL VERSUS SOCIETY" AS THE CONCEPTUAL FRAMEWORK

The setting for the conflict most consistently invoked in the literature is the polarity of individual versus society—the possible tension between the individual good and the common good, between private and public welfare. . . . We concede, as a matter of course, to the common good some pragmatically determined measure of precedence over the individual good. In terms of rights, we let some of the basic rights of the individual be overruled by the acknowledged rights of society—as a matter of right and moral justness and not of mere force or dire necessity (much as such necessity may be adduced in defense of that right). But in making that concession, we require a careful clarification of what the needs, interests, and rights of society are, for society—as distinct from any plurality of individuals—is an abstract and, as such, is subject to our definition, while the individual is the primary concrete, prior to all definition, and his basic good is more or less known. Thus the unknown in our problem is the so-called common or public good and its potentially superior claims, to which the individual good must or might sometimes be sacrificed, in circumstances that in turn must also be counted among the unknowns of our question. Note that in putting the matter in this way—that is, in asking about the right of society to individual sacrifice—the consent of the sacrificial subject is no necessary part of the *basic* question.

"Consent," however, is the other most consistently emphasized and examined concept in discussions of this issue. This attention betrays a feeling that the "social" angle is not fully satisfactory. If society has a right, its exercise is not contingent on volunteering. On the other hand, if volunteering is fully genuine, no public right to the volunteered act need be construed. There is a difference between the moral or emotional appeal of a cause that elicits volunteering and a right that demands compliance. . . .

. . . "No one has the right to choose martyrs for science" was a statement repeatedly quoted in the November, 1967, *Daedalus* conference. But no scientist can be prevented from making himself a martyr for his science. At all times, dedicated explorers, thinkers, and artists have immolated themselves on the altar of their vocation, and creative genius most often pays the price of happiness, health, and life for its own consummation. But no one, not even society, has the shred of a right to

expect and ask these things in the normal course of events. They come to the rest of us as a *gratia gratis data.* . . .

WHAT SOCIETY CAN AFFORD

"Can Society afford . . . ?" Afford what? To let people die intact, thereby withholding something from other people who desperately need it, who in consequence will have to die too? . . . The specific question seems to be whether society can afford to let some people die whose death might be deferred by particular means if these were authorized by society. Again, if it is merely a question of what society can or cannot afford, rather than of what it ought or ought not to do, the answer must be: Of course, it can. If cancer, heart disease, and other organic, noncontagious ills, especially those tending to strike the old more than the young, continue to exact their toll at the normal rate of incidence (including the toll of private anguish and misery), society can go on flourishing in every way.

Here, by contrast, are some examples of what, in sober truth, society cannot afford. It cannot afford to let an epidemic rage unchecked; a persistent excess of deaths over births, but neither—we must add—too great an excess of births over deaths; too low an average life expectancy even if demographically balanced by fertility, but neither too great a longevity with the necessitated correlative dearth of youth in the social body; a debilitating state of general health; and things of this kind. These are plain cases where the whole condition of society is critically affected, and the public interest can make its imperative claims. The Black Death of the Middle Ages was a *public* calamity of the acute kind; the life-sapping ravages of endemic malaria or sleeping sickness in certain areas are a public calamity of the chronic kind. Such situations a society as a whole can truly not "afford," and they may call for extraordinary remedies, including, perhaps, the invasion of private sacrosanctities. . . .

For what objectives connected with the medico-biological sphere should this reserve be drawn upon—for example, in the form of accepting, soliciting, perhaps even imposing the submission of human subjects to experimentation? We postulate that this must be not just a worthy cause, as any promotion of the health of anybody doubtlessly is, but a cause qualifying for transcendent social sanction. Here one thinks first of those cases critically affecting the whole condition, present and future, of the community we have illustrated. Something equivalent to what in the political sphere is called "clear and present danger" may be invoked and a state of emergency proclaimed, thereby suspending certain otherwise inviolable prohibitions and taboos. We may observe that averting a disaster always carries greater weight than promoting a good. Extraordinary danger excuses extraordinary means. This covers human experimentation, which we would like to count, as far as possible, among the extraordinary rather than the ordinary means of serving the common good under public auspices. Naturally, since foresight and responsibility for the future are of the essence of institutional society, averting disaster extends into long-term prevention, although the lesser urgency will warrant less sweeping licenses.

SOCIETY AND THE CAUSE OF PROGRESS

Much weaker is the case where it is a matter not of saving but of improving society. Much of medical research falls into this category. As stated before, a permanent death rate from heart failure or cancer does not threaten society. So long as certain statistical ratios are maintained, the incidence of disease and of disease-induced mortality is not (in the strict sense) a "social" misfortune. I hasten to add that it is not therefore less of a human misfortune, and the call for relief issuing with silent eloquence from each victim and all potential victims is of no lesser dignity. But it is misleading to equate the fundamentally human response to it with what is owed to society: it is owed by man to man—and it is thereby owed by society to the individuals as soon as the adequate ministering to these concerns outgrows (as it progressively does) the scope

of private spontaneity and is made a public mandate. It is thus that society assumes responsibility for medical care, research, old age, and innumerable other things not originally of the public realm (in the original "social contract"), and they become duties toward "society" (rather than directly toward one's fellow man) by the fact that they are socially operated.

Indeed, we expect from organized society no longer mere protection against harm and the securing of the conditions of our preservation, but active and constant improvement in all the domains of life: the waging of the battle against nature, the enhancement of the human estate—in short, the promotion of progress. This is an expansive goal, one far surpassing the disaster norm of our previous reflections. It lacks the urgency of the latter, but has the nobility of the free, forward thrust. It surely is worth sacrifices. It is not at all a question of what society can afford, but of what it is committed to, beyond all necessity, by our mandate. Its trusteeship has become an established, ongoing, institutionalized business of the body politic. As eager beneficiaries of its gains, we now owe to "society," as its chief agent, our individual contributions toward its *continued pursuit*. I emphasize "continued pursuit." Maintaining the existing level requires no more than the orthodox means of taxation and enforcement of professional standards that raise no problems. The more optional goal of pushing forward is also more exacting. We have this syndrome: Progress is by our choosing an acknowledged interest of society, in which we have a stake in various degrees; science is a necessary instrument of progress; research is a necessary instrument of science; and in medical science experimentation on human subjects is a necessary instrument of research. Therefore, human experimentation has come to be a societal interest.

The destination of research is essentially melioristic. It does not serve the preservation of the existing good from which I profit myself and to which I am obligated. Unless the present state is intolerable, the melioristic goal is in a sense gratuitous, and this not only from the vantage point of the present. Our descendants have a right to be left an unplundered planet; they do not have a right to new miracle cures. We have sinned against them, if by our doing we have destroyed their inheritance—which we are doing at full blast; we have not sinned against them, if by the time they come around arthritis has not yet been conquered. . . .

THE MELIORISTIC GOAL, MEDICAL RESEARCH, AND INDIVIDUAL DUTY

Nowhere is the melioristic goal more inherent than in medicine. To the physician, it is not gratuitous. He is committed to curing and thus to improving the power to cure. Gratuitous we called it (outside disaster conditions) as a *social* goal, but noble at the same time. Both the nobility and the gratuitousness must influence the manner in which self-sacrifice for it is elicited, and even its free offer accepted. Freedom is certainly the first condition to be observed here. The surrender of one's body to medical experimentation is entirely outside the enforceable "social contract."

Or can it be construed to fall within its terms—namely, as repayment for benefits from past experimentation that I have enjoyed myself? But I am indebted for these benefits not to society, but to the past "martyrs," to whom society is indebted itself, and society has no right to call in my personal debt by way of adding new to its own. Moreover, gratitude is not an enforceable social obligation; it anyway does not mean that I must emulate the deed. . . .

THE "CONSCRIPTION" OF CONSENT

But here we must realize that the mere issuing of the appeal, the calling for volunteers, with the moral and social pressures it inevitably generates, amounts even under the most meticulous rules of consent to a sort of *conscripting*. And some soliciting is necessarily involved. . . . [I]n this area sin and guilt can perhaps not be wholly avoided. And this is why "consent," surely a non-negotiable minimum requirement, is not the full answer to the problem. Granting then that soliciting and therefore some degree of conscripting are part of the situation, who may conscript and who may be conscripted? Or less harshly expressed: Who should issue appeals and to whom?

The naturally qualified issuer of the appeal is the research scientist himself, collectively the main carrier of the impulse and the only one with the technical competence to judge. But his being very much an interested party (with vested interests, indeed, not purely in the public good, but in the scientific enterprise as such, in "his" project, and even in his career) makes him also suspect. The ineradicable dialectic of this situation—a delicate incompatibility problem—calls for particular controls by the research community and by public authority that we need not discuss. They can mitigate, but not eliminate the problem. We have to live with the ambiguity, the treacherous impurity of everything human.

SELF-RECRUITMENT OF THE COMMUNITY

To whom should the appeal be addressed? The natural issuer of the call is also the first natural addressee: the physician-researcher himself and the scientific confraternity at large. With such a coincidence—indeed, the noble tradition with which the whole business of human experimentation started—almost all of the associated legal, ethical, and metaphysical problems vanish. If it is full, autonomous identification of the subject with the purpose that is required for the dignifying of his serving as a subject—here it is; if strongest motivation—here it is; if fullest understanding—here it is; if freest decision—here it is; if greatest integration with the person's total, chosen pursuit—here it is. With the fact of self-solicitation the issue of consent in all its insoluble equivocality is bypassed *per se*. Not even the condition that the particular purpose be truly important and the project reasonably promising, which must hold in any solicitation of others, need be satisfied here. By himself, the scientist is free to obey his obsession, to play his hunch, to wager on chance, to follow the lure of ambition. . . .

It would be the ideal, but is not a real solution, to keep the issue of human experimentation within the research community itself. Neither in numbers nor in variety of material would its potential suffice for the many-pronged, systematic, continual attack on disease into which the lonely ex-ploits of the early investigators have grown. Statistical requirements alone make their voracious demands. . . . How then can our mandatory faith be honored when the recruitment for experimentation goes outside the scientific community, as it must in honoring another commitment of no mean dignity? We simply repeat the former question: To whom should the call be addressed?

The Fundamental Privilege of the Sick

In the course of treatment, the physician is obligated to the patient and to no one else. He is not the agent of society, nor of the interests of medical science, nor of the patient's family, nor of his co-sufferers, or future sufferers from the same disease. The patient alone counts when he is under the physician's care. By the simple law of bilateral contract (analogous, for example, to the relation of lawyer to client and its "conflict of interest" rule), the physician is bound not to let any other interest interfere with that of the patient in being cured. But manifestly more sublime norms than contractual ones are involved. We may speak of a sacred trust; strictly by its terms, the doctor is, as it were, alone with his patient and God.

There is one normal exception to this—that is, to the doctor's not being the agent of society vis-à-vis the patient, but the trustee of his interests alone: the quarantining of the contagious sick. This is plainly not for the patient's interest, but for that of others threatened by him. (In vaccination, we have a combination of both: protection of the individual and others.) But preventing the patient from causing harm to others is not the same as exploiting him for the advantage of others. . . .

The Principle of "Identification" Applied to Patients

On the whole, the same principles would seem to hold here as are found to hold with "normal subjects": motivation, identification, understanding on the part of the subject. But it is clear that these conditions are peculiarly difficult to satisfy with regard to a patient. His physical state, psychic preoccupation, dependent relation to the doctor, the submissive attitude induced by treatment—every-thing connected with his condition and situation makes the sick person inherently less of a sovereign person than the healthy one. Spontaneity of self-offering has almost to be ruled out; consent is marred by lower resistance or captive circumstance, and so on. In fact, all the factors that make the patient, as a category, particularly accessible and welcome for experimentation at the same time compromise the quality of the responding affirmation that must morally redeem the making use of them. This, in addition to the primacy of the physician's duty, puts a heightened onus on the physician-researcher to limit his undue power to the most important and defensible research objectives and, of course, to keep persuasion at a minimum.

Still, with all the disabilities noted, there is scope among patients for observing the rule of the "descending order of permissibility" that we have laid down for normal subjects, in vexing inversion of the utility order of quantitative abundance and qualitative "expendability." By the principle of this order, those patients who most identify with and are cognizant of the cause of research—members of the medical profession (who after all are sometimes patients themselves)—come first; the highly motivated and educated, also least dependent, among the lay patients come next; and so on down the line. An added consideration here is seriousness of condition, which again operates in inverse proportion. Here the profession must fight the tempting sophistry that the hopeless case is expendable (because in prospect already expended) and therefore especially usable; and generally the attitude that the poorer the chances of the patient the more justifiable his recruitment for experimentation (other than for his own benefit). The opposite is true.

Nondisclosure as a Borderline Case

Then there is the case where ignorance of the subject, sometimes even of the experimenter, is of the essence of the experiment (the "double blind"–control group–placebo syndrome). It is said to be a necessary element of the scientific process. Whatever may be said about its ethics in regard to normal subjects, especially volunteers, it is an outright betrayal of trust in regard to the patient who believes that he is receiving treatment. Only supreme importance of the objective can exonerate it, without making it less of a transgression. The patient is definitely wronged even when not harmed. And ethics apart, the practice of such deception holds the danger of undermining the faith in the *bona fides* of treatment, the beneficial intent of the physician—the very basis of the doctor-patient relationship. In every respect, it follows that concealed experiment on patients—that is, experiment under the guise of treatment—should be the rarest exception, at best, if it cannot be wholly avoided.

This has still the merit of a borderline problem. The same is not true of the other case of necessary ignorance of the subject—that of the unconscious patient. Drafting him for nontherapeutic experiments is simply and unqualifiedly impermissible; progress or not, he must never be used, on the inflexible principle that utter helplessness demands utter protection. . . .

"IDENTIFICATION" AS THE PRINCIPLE OF RECRUITMENT IN GENERAL

If the properties we adduced as the particular qualifications of the members of the scientific fraternity itself are taken as general criteria of selection, then one should look for additional subjects where a maximum of identification, understanding, and spontaneity can be expected—that is, among the most highly motivated, the most highly educated, and the least "captive" members of the community. From this naturally scarce resource, a descending order of permissibility leads to greater abundance and ease of supply, whose use should become proportionately more hesitant as the exculpating criteria are relaxed. An inversion of normal "market" behavior is demanded here—namely, to accept the lowest quotation last (and excused only by the greatest pressure of need); to pay the highest price first.

The ruling principle in our considerations is that the "wrong" of reification can only be made "right" by such authentic identification with the cause that it is the subject's as well as the re-

searcher's cause—whereby his role in its service is not just permitted by him, but *willed*. That sovereign will of his which embraces the end as his own restores his personhood to the otherwise depersonalizing context. To be valid it must be autonomous and informed. The latter condition can, outside the research community, only be fulfilled by degrees; but the higher the degree of the understanding regarding the purpose and the technique, the more valid becomes the endorsement of the will. . . .

THE RULE OF THE "DESCENDING ORDER" AND ITS COUNTER-UTILITY SENSE

We have laid down what must seem to be a forbidding rule to the number-hungry research industry. Having faith in the transcendent potential of man, I do not fear that the "source" will ever fail a society that does not destroy it—and only such a one is worthy of the blessings of progress. But "elitistic" the rule is (as is the enterprise of progress itself), and elites are by nature small. The combined attribute of motivation and information, plus the absence of external pressures, tends to be socially so circumscribed that strict adherence to the rule might numerically starve the research process. This is why I spoke of a descending order of permissibility, which is itself permissive, but where the realization that it is a *descending* order is not without pragmatic import. . . . The poorer in knowledge, motivation, and freedom of decision (and that, alas, means the more readily available in terms of numbers and possible manipulation), the more sparingly and indeed reluctantly should the reservoir be used, and the more compelling must therefore become the countervailing justification.

Let us note that this is the opposite of a social utility standard, the reverse of the order by "availability and expendability": The most valuable and scarcest, the least expendable elements of the social organism, are to be the first candidates for risk and sacrifice. . . . It is also the opposite of what the day-to-day interests of research clamor for, and for the scientific community to honor it will mean that it will have to fight a strong temptation to go by routine to the readiest sources of supply—the suggestible, the ignorant, the dependent, the "captive" in various senses. . . . This price—a possibly slower rate of progress—may have to be paid for the preservation of the most precious capital of higher communal life.

NO EXPERIMENTS ON PATIENTS UNRELATED TO THEIR OWN DISEASE

Although my ponderings have, on the whole, yielded points of view rather than definite prescriptions, premises rather than conclusions, they have led me to a few unequivocal yeses and noes. The first is the emphatic rule that patients should be experimented upon, if at all, *only* with reference to *their disease*. Never should there be added to the gratuitousness of the experiment as such the gratuitousness of service to an unrelated cause. . . .

. . . Experiment as part of therapy—that is, directed toward helping the subject himself—is a different matter altogether and raises its own problems, but hardly philosophical ones. As long as a doctor can say, even if only in his own thought: "There is no known cure for your condition (or: You have responded to none); but there is promise in a new treatment still under investigation, not quite tested yet as to effectiveness and safety; you will be taking a chance, but all things considered, I judge it in your best interest to let me try it on you"—as long as he can speak thus, he speaks as the patient's physician and may err, but does not transform the patient into a subject of experimentation. Introduction of an untried therapy into the treatment where the tried ones have failed is not "experimentation on the patient."

Generally, and almost needless to say, with all the rules of the book, there is something "experimental" (because tentative) about every individual treatment, beginning with the diagnosis itself; and he would be a poor doctor who would not learn from every case for the benefit of future cases, and a poor member of the profession who would not make any new insights gained from his treatments available to the profession at large. Thus, knowledge may be advanced in the treatment of any patient, and the interest of the medical art and all

sufferers from the same affliction as well as the patient himself may be served if something happens to be learned from his case. But this gain to knowledge and future therapy is incidental to the *bona fide* service to the present patient. He has the right to expect that the doctor does nothing to him just in order to learn.

In that case, the doctor's imaginary speech would run, for instance, like this: "There is nothing more I can do for you. But you can do something for me. Speaking no longer as your physician but on behalf of medical science, we could learn a great deal about future cases of this kind if you would permit me to perform certain experiments on you. It is understood that you yourself would not benefit from any knowledge we might gain; but future patients would." This statement would express the purely experimental situation, assumedly here with the subject's concurrence and with all cards on the table. In Alexander Bickel's words: "It is a different situation when the doctor is no longer trying to make [the patient] well, but is trying to find out how to make others well in the future."

But even in the second case, that of the nontherapeutic experiment where the patient does not benefit, at least the patient's own disease is enlisted in the cause of fighting that disease, even if only in others. It is yet another thing to say or think: "Since you are here—in the hospital with its facilities—anyway, under our care and observation anyway, away from your job (or, perhaps, doomed) anyway, we wish to profit from your being available for some other research of great interest we are presently engaged in." From the standpoint of merely medical ethics, which has only to consider risk, consent, and the worth of the objective, there may be no cardinal difference between this case and the last one. I hope that the medical reader will not think I am making too fine a point when I say that from the standpoint of the subject and his dignity there is a cardinal difference that crosses the line between the permissible and the impermissible, and this by the same principle of "identification" I have been invoking all along. Whatever the rights and wrongs of any experimentation on any patient—in the one case, at least that residue of identification is left him that it is his own affliction by which he can contribute to the conquest of that affliction, his own kind of suffering which he helps to alleviate in others; and so in a sense it is his own cause. It is totally indefensible to rob the unfortunate of this intimacy with the purpose and make his misfortune a convenience for the furtherance of alien concerns. The observance of this rule is essential, I think, to at least attenuate the wrong that nontherapeutic experimenting on patients commits in any case. . . .

CONCLUSION

There would now have to be said something about nonmedical experiments on human subjects, notably psychological and genetic, of which I have not lost sight. But I must leave this for another occasion. I wish only to say in conclusion that if some of the practical implications of my reasonings are felt to work out toward a slower rate of progress, this should not cause too great dismay. Let us not forget that progress is an optional goal, not an unconditional commitment, and that its tempo in particular, compulsive as it may become, has nothing sacred about it. Let us also remember that a slower progress in the conquest of disease would not threaten society, grievous as it is to those who have to deplore that their particular disease be not yet conquered, but that society would indeed be threatened by the erosion of those moral values whose loss, possibly caused by too ruthless a pursuit of scientific progress, would make its most dazzling triumphs not worth having. Let us finally remember that it cannot be the aim of progress to abolish the lot of mortality. Of some ill or other, each of us will die. Our mortal condition is upon us with its harshness but also its wisdom—because without it there would not be the eternally renewed promise of the freshness, immediacy, and eagerness of youth; nor would there be for any of us the incentive to number our days and make them count. With all our striving to wrest from our mortality what we can, we should bear its burden with patience and dignity.

QUESTIONS FOR COMPREHENSION AND REFLECTION

1. What is the "rule of descending order"? What does Jonas mean when he says that this rule runs contrary to social utility? Who—Jonas or the utilitarians—presents the stronger argument regarding criteria for subject selection? Support your answers.
2. What is the difference between volunteering and complying? How can we know if a subject is truly volunteering? Is it ever permissible to use a subject without his or her informed consent? Support your answers.
3. What is the "principle of identification"? Discuss how this principle applies in borderline cases. Use specific case studies to illustrate your answer.
4. What would Jonas most likely think about the practice of professors using their students as subjects in low-risk, nontherapeutic experiments? Would you agree with Jonas? Would it make a difference if students were paid or given credit for their participation? Support your answers.

ARTHUR L. CAPLAN

How Did Medicine Go So Wrong?

Arthur Caplan is director of the Center for Bioethics at the University of Pennsylvania School of Medicine in Philadelphia. After examining the role physicians played in the medical experiments conducted in Nazi concentration camps, Caplan asks if there are parallels to the Nazi experience in other countries or if it was unique in medical history. He also discusses the morality of using the results derived from the Nazi experiments.

IS MORAL INQUIRY INTO NAZI MEDICAL CRIMES IMMORAL?

. . .

The myriad crimes carried out under medical supervision in Germany prior to and during World War II were so heartless, cruel, and inhumane that it is not at all evident why it is necessary to subject them to moral analysis. Is there any reason to conduct an ethical analysis of Nazi medical crimes? The conduct of German biomedicine during the Nazi era was *prima facie* abhorrent and indisputably immoral. There is no need for an argument to prove that what happened was evil.

Despite the obvious immorality of biomedicine's role in the Holocaust, there is, nevertheless, a need for moral inquiry; it is necessary to understand how those who committed horrific crimes on a massive scale were able to persuade themselves that what they were doing was ethically correct. As difficult as it is to accept, some physicians, public health officials, nurses, and government agencies killed, maimed, tortured, or did not protest these activities because they believed it was morally correct to perform them. . . .

WHY DOES BIOETHICS HAVE SO LITTLE TO SAY ABOUT THE HOLOCAUST?

. . .

There has been almost no discussion of the roles played by medicine and science during the Nazi era in bioethics literature. Rather than see Nazi biomedicine as morally bad, the field of bioethics has generally accepted the myths that Nazi biomedicine was either inept, mad, or coerced. By subscribing to these myths, bioethics has been able to avoid a painful confrontation with the fact that many who committed the crimes of the Holocaust were competent physicians and health care professionals acting from their moral convictions. Not one of the doctors or public health officials on trial at Nuremberg pleaded for mercy on the grounds of insanity. A few claimed they were merely following legitimate orders, but no one alleged coercion.

The bitter reality is that the ranks of physicians, scientists, and public health officials who committed terrible acts against innocent persons included competent health professionals and scientists, some of international renown. Mainstream German medicine supported the rise of the Nazi party to power. Some of its leaders helped create the scientific foundation for the euthanasia program that was instituted to eliminate the disabled, demented, deformed, and, eventually, Jews and Gypsies. Others helped design the death camps. Most were neither mad nor coerced into cooperation with the Nazi regime. They believed what they were doing was right. . . .

It is often presumed, if only tacitly, by those who teach bioethics that those who know what is ethical will not behave in immoral ways. What is the point of doing bioethics, of teaching courses on ethics to medical, nursing, and public health students, if the vilest and most horrendous of deeds and policies can be justified by moral reasons? Bioethics has been speechless in the face of the crimes of Nazi doctors and biomedical scientists precisely because so many of these doctors and scientists believed they were doing what was morally right to do. . . .

EXPERIMENTATION IN THE CAMPS

Although the role of mainstream medicine and science in the Holocaust has been underplayed, there has been at least an acknowledgment that medicine and science perpetrated heinous crimes in the name of experimentation in the concentration camps. Yet, the scope of experimentation conducted in the camps is not widely understood.

There were at least 26 different types of experiments conducted for the explicit purpose of research in concentration camps or using concentration camp inmates in Germany, Poland, and France during the Nazi era. Among the studies in which human beings were used in research were the analysis of high-altitude decompression on the human body; attempts to make sea water drinkable; the efficacy of sulfanilamide for treating gunshot wounds; the feasibility of bone, muscle, and joint transplants; the ability to treat burns caused by incendiary bombs; the efficacy of polygal for treating trauma-related bleeding; the efficacy of high-dose radiation in causing sterility; the efficacy of phenol (gasoline) injections as a euthanasia agent; the efficacy of electroshock therapy; the symptoms and course of noma (starvation-caused skin gangrene); the postmortem examination of skeletons and brains to assess the effects of starvation; the efficacy of surgical techniques for sterilizing women; and the impact of stress and starvation on ovulation, menstruation, and cancerous growths in the reproductive organs of women. A variety of other studies were carried out on twins, dwarves, and those with congenital defects. Some camp inmates were used as subjects to train medical students in surgery. Jewish physicians in one camp surreptitiously recorded observations about the impact of starvation on the body.

The question of whether any of these activities carried out in the name of medical or scientific research upon unconsenting, coerced human beings deserves the label of *research* or *experimentation* is controversial. When the description of research is broadened further to include the intentional killing of human beings in order to establish what methods are most efficient, references to "research" and "experimentation" begin to seem completely strained. Injecting a half-starved, young girl with phenol to see how quickly she will die or trying out various forms of phosgene gas on camp inmates in the hope of finding cheap, clean, and efficient modes of killing so the state can effectively prosecute genocide is not the sort of activity associated with the term *research*. But murder and genocide are not the same as intentionally causing someone to suffer and die to fulfill a scientific goal. Killing for scientific purposes, while certainly as evil as murder in the service of racial hygiene, is, nonetheless, morally different. The torture and killing that were at the core of Nazi medical experiments involve not only torture and murder but also the exploitation of human beings to serve the goals of science. To describe what happened in language other than that of human experimentation blurs the nature of the wrong-doing. The evil inherent in Nazi medical experimentation was not simply that people suffered and died but that they were exploited for science and medicine as they died.

Isolating these crimes from the realm of biomedical experimentation is to draw a line that inappropriately weakens mainstream medicine and science's connection with dastardly acts. Doctors and scientists, many holding university and medical school appointments, did make men, women, and children suffer and die in the name of advancing knowledge in science and medicine.

The ethical issues raised by experimentation in the camps was forcefully brought to my attention by a physiologist, Robert Pozos, who was then in the department of physiology at the University of Minnesota in Duluth. . . .

Pozos, an expert in the field of hypothermia, had been wrestling with this issue, as had others in the field of physiology, for many years. When he raised the question with me about the ethics of using information from heinous experiments, I assumed that the data had not been cited previously in scientific literature. This assumption was false. The findings had been cited by dozens of scientists from many countries in numerous peer-reviewed publications. As I subsequently discovered, Pozos himself had previously cited the data. Nevertheless, it took courage for him to raise the question of the ethics of using this data. Many of Pozos' scientific peers and predecessors had simply ignored the moral issues involved and had cited the Nazi experiments on camp residents without comment or discussion. Pozos told me that the Nazi hypothermia research was widely known among experts in the physiology of exposure to cold temperatures in the US, Canada, Britain, Japan, and the Soviet Union. He also said there might be further information on the experiments stored in archives in Germany or elsewhere. Should these documents be found, would it be right for him or anyone else to examine them and publish their findings?

The experiments done in the concentration camps on hypothermia were undertaken to solve a problem of special importance to the German armed forces. In the first months of the war, German aviation and naval leaders were very concerned about the loss of pilots and seamen from exposure to cold. . . .

The military had turned to the medical branch of the Luftwaffe for answers. The military physicians felt that the best way to learn about the limits of human endurance to cold and techniques for revival was to conduct a series of experiments in which men would be exposed to cold temperatures under controlled conditions. At first, their discussions presumed the use of German military volunteers, but eventually it was decided that the fastest way to proceed was to use inmates in concentration camps. By exposing human beings to potentially lethal cold temperatures answers might be more readily available. However, the shift to exposures to lethal temperatures led the military to turn away from the use of volunteers in carefully controlled trials to the use of camp inmates who would be experimented upon under primitive and crude circumstances.

Two sets of experiments involving hypothermia were actually performed. The first set involved inmates at the Dachau concentration camp. German military physicians from the physiology department at the University of Kiel came to the camp to supervise the experiments. They were concerned that the results be generalizable to Aryan men so they tried to select political prisoners and dissidents who were not Jews or Gypsies as their subjects.

The university physiologists worked under the supervision of SS physician Sigmund Rascher, who administered Dachau. He was a personal favorite of Heinrich Himmler, chief of the SS. Subjects were selected from among camp inmates with an eye toward their race, health, and age and then were fed an improved diet to make them more suitable subjects. After a few weeks, the men were brought to a special unit in the camp where a vat had been built containing ice and freezing water. The men were immersed until they became unconscious. Vital signs of those thus exposed were monitored and recorded. The suffering endured by the subjects was enormous. Various techniques were used to try and revive those who did not die. Those who did die were autopsied on the spot. . . .

Both sets of experiments were cruel, inhumane, and immoral. Those involved suffered a great deal. About one-quarter of the subjects died. Their suffering was so great that some of those who assisted in the experiments tried to take action to help the subjects, thereby casting doubt over the reliability of the findings that were reported. Nonetheless, the researchers believed that the information they obtained, at least in the first series of experiments, was accurate and valid. The findings were presented at a meeting of military physicians in Berlin. The German armed forces apparently used the findings in the design of survival suits for soldiers and in developing resuscitation policies for those exposed to cold temperatures.

Pozos believed and continues to believe that the findings produced by the hypothermia studies are of scientific value. Other experts in hypothermia agree. Pozos and some other physiologists believe that these studies are the only source of information concerning both the response of the body to prolonged extremes of cold temperature under conditions of total immersion and of the efficacy and reliability of certain resuscitation techniques. . . .

One line of response to the issue of citing Nazi data is to shed doubt on their validity. And there are many reasons to doubt that the findings of the hypothermia studies . . . are either valid or the only source of life-saving information. But in another sense, haggling over the merits of the methodology of Nazi science misses a more important point. Some experts not only believe the data in the hypothermia . . . studies are valid; they have long been referenced in biomedical literature. . . .

A summary report prepared for the American military about the hypothermia experiments has been cited in the peer-reviewed literature of medicine more than two dozen times since the end of World War II, most recently in a physiology textbook published in 1989. Not only were the data examined and referenced, but they were applied. British air–sea rescue experts used the Nazi data to modify rescue techniques for those exposed to cold water. The force of the question "Should the data be used?" is diminished not only because there are reasons to doubt the reliability and exclusivity of the data but also because the question has already been answered: Nazi data have been used by many scientists from many nations.

There is another moral issue that does not hinge on the answer to the question of whether the research was well-designed or whether the findings are of enduring scientific value. How did physicians and scientists convince themselves that murderous experimentation was morally justified?

No one understood the need for justification more clearly than the doctors and scientists put on trial for their crimes after the conclusion of the war. The defendants admitted that dangerous and even lethal experiments had been conducted on unconsenting persons in prisons and other institutions. Some protested attempts by the prosecution, in its effort to highlight the barbarity of what they had done, to demean or disparage the caliber of their research. No one apologized for their role in various experiments conducted in the camps. Instead, those put on trial attempted to explain and justify what they had done, often couching their defense in explicitly moral terms.

THE ETHICS OF EVIL

Probably the most succinct precis of the moral arguments brought forward by physicians, public health officials, and scientists in defense of their participation both in experimentation in the concentration camps and in the "final solution" can be found in the transcripts of the Nuremberg trials. The first group of individuals to be put on trial by the Allies were physicians and public health officials. The role they had played in conducting or tolerating cruel and often lethal experiments in the camps dominated the trials. As it happens, the same arguments that were brought forward in defense of the camp experiments were also used to justify participation in mass murder and attempts at the forced sterilization of camp inmates. . . .

One of the most common moral rationales given at the trials was that no wrong had been done because those who were subjects had volunteered. Prisoners might be freed, some defendants argued, if they survived the experiments. The prospects of release and pardon were mentioned very frequently during the trial since they were the basis for the claim that people participated voluntarily in the experiments. On this line of thinking, experimentation was justified because it might actually benefit the subjects.

The major flaw with this moral rationale is simply that it was false. In 1989, the British newspaper, the *London Sunday Observer*, found a man who had survived the hypothermia experiments, which involved prolonged submersion in tanks of freezing water. The man now lives in Belgium. He had been sent to Dachau because of his political beliefs. He said that the researchers told him that if he survived the hypothermia experiments and then the decompression experiments, he might be freed. He was not. He said no prisoners were. However, he was given a medal by the Reich on the recommendation of the experimenters. The medal was given in recognition of the contributions he had made to medical science!

Granted, Nazi researchers did not keep their promises. But what if they had? Would arduous, even potentially lethal experimentation be justified by the promise of freedom if the subject survived the research? The answer to this position clearly seems to be no. It seems extremely coercive to tell a condemned prisoner that his only chance at freedom or even survival is to survive an arduous experiment. Consent means nothing where such an offer is concerned. Moreover, it seems immoral to even accept the offer of participation in painful, disabling, and potentially lethal experimentation as legitimate.

Another of the key rationales on the part of those put on trial was that only people who were doomed to die were used for biomedical purposes. Time and again the doctors who froze screaming subjects to death or watched their brains explode as a result of rapid decompression stated that only prisoners condemned to death were used. It seemed morally defensible to physicians and scientists to learn from what they saw as the inevitable deaths of camp inmates.

This line of argument does not lack contemporary advocates. Jack Kevorkian, who rocketed to fame as the man who assisted Janet Adkins in committing suicide in the back of his Volkswagen van in a suburban Detroit campground, has long advocated dispatching prisoners condemned to die in such a way that we can . . . use them for research. . . .

But putting aside the immoral grounds for condemning Jews, Gypsies, POWs, and others to death, are those who are condemned to die fair game for biomedical experimentation? The answer would seem to be no if only because even the condemned are not to be treated as mere instruments. Indeed, the very justification of the morality of capital punishment depends on the treatment of those who are doomed to die as more than things or objects.

A third ethical rationale for performing brutal experiments upon innocent subjects was that participation in lethal research offered expiation to the subjects. By being injected, frozen, or transplanted subjects could cleanse themselves of their crimes. Suffering prior to death as a way to atone for sin seemed to be a morally acceptable rationale for causing suffering to those who were guilty of crimes.

The problem with this ethical defense is that those who were experimented on or made to suffer by German physicians and scientists were never guilty of any crime other than that of belonging to a despised ethnic or racial minority or for holding unacceptable political views. Even if those who were experimented upon or killed had been guilty of some serious crime, would it have been moral to use medical experimentation or the risk of death as a form of punishment or expiation? It is hard to see how these goals square with the goals of medicine or health care. It is impossible to see how such a position is persuasive with respect to incompetent persons and minor children.

A fourth moral rationale, one that is especially astounding even by the standards of self-delusion in evidence throughout the trial proceedings, was that scientists and physicians had to act in a value-neutral manner. To use a philosophical description, some of those who had tortured, maimed, and killed pled logical positivism in their defense. Although they did not actually use these words, they maintained that scientists and doctors are not responsible for and have no expertise about values and thus could not be held accountable for their actions.

> . . . if the experiment is ordered by the state, this moral responsibility of experimenter toward the experimental subject relates to the way in which the experiment is performed, not the experiment itself.

Some researchers only felt themselves responsible for the proper design and conduct of their research. They felt no moral responsibility for what had occurred in the camps because they did not have any expertise concerning moral matters. They claimed to have left decisions about these matters to others.

The view that scientists must leave moral matters to others has some resonance in contemporary debates about medicine and science. But there are few who would argue that physicians or scientists have immunity for the consequences of their actions simply because they are not experts in values. Most people are not professors of religion, law, or philosophy, and yet, we hold each other accountable for our actions.

The fifth moral justification for what happened presented by many of the defendants was that they had done what they did for the defense and security of their country. All actions were done to preserve the Reich during "total" war. . . .

Total war, in which the survival of the nation hangs in the balance, justifies exceptions to ordinary morality, the defendants maintained. Those who had run the camps, made the selections on the ramps, and had conducted war-related research had done so at the legitimate request of state authorities. They had followed legitimate orders from legitimate authorities in order to preserve their nation. Allied prosecutors had much to ponder in thinking about this defense in light of the fire-bombing of Dresden and Tokyo and the dropping of nuclear bombs on Hiroshima and Nagasaki.

Arguments about what total war permits in terms of morality raised tough issues for the Allied prosecutors and continue to raise hard questions for us now. Those who build or might fire nuclear weapons must confront the issue on a daily basis. However, none of the issues in contemporary bioethics that so often elicit analogies to Nazism—genetic engineering, fetal tissue research, abortion, or euthanasia—have a plausible connection to rationales concerning the rights of the state to compel behavior in times of war. Whatever the motives and moral thinking are of those who perform abortions or terminate medical care, the requirements of total war play no role and thus have no analogy to this aspect of Nazi conduct.

The last rationale is the one that appears to carry the most weight among all the moral defenses offered. Many who conducted lethal experiments or actively engaged in genocide argued that it was reasonable to sacrifice the interests of the few in order to benefit the majority.

The most distinguished of the scientists who was put on trial, Gerhard Rose, the head of the Koch Institute of Tropical Medicine in Berlin, said that he initially opposed performing potentially lethal experiments to create a vaccine for typhus on camp inmates. But he came to believe that it made no sense not to risk the lives of 100 or 200 men in pursuit of a vaccine when 1000 men a day were dying of typhus on the Eastern front. What, he asked, were the deaths of 100 men compared to the possible benefit of getting a prophylactic vaccine capable of saving tens of thousands? Rose, because he admitted that he had anguished about his own moral duty when asked by the Wehrmacht to perform the typhus experiments in a concentration camp, raises the most difficult and most plausible moral argument in defense of lethal experimentation.

The prosecution encountered some difficulty with Rose's argument. The defense team for Rose noted that the Allies themselves justified the compulsory drafting of men for military service throughout the war, knowing many would certainly die, on the grounds that the sacrifice of the few to save the many was morally just. Moreover, they also pointed out that throughout history medical researchers in Western countries used versions of utilitarianism to justify dangerous experiments on prisoners and institutionalized persons.

Justifying the sacrifice of the few to benefit the majority is a position that must be taken seriously as a moral argument. However, in the context of the Nazi regime, it is fair to point out that sacrifice was not born equally by all as is true of a compulsory draft that allows no exceptions. It is also true that many would argue that no degree of benefit should permit intrusions into certain fundamental rights.

Crude utilitarianism is a position that sometimes rears its head in contemporary bioethical debate. Some argue that we ought not spend scarce social resources on certain groups within our society such as the elderly so that other groups, such as children, may have greater benefits. Those who want to invoke the Nazi analogy may be able to show that this form of crude utilitarian thinking does motivate some of the policies or actions taken by contemporary biomedical scientists and health care professionals.

In closely reviewing the statements that accompany the six major moral rationales for murder, torture, and mutilation conducted in the camps—freedom was a possible benefit, only the condemned were used, expiation was a possible benefit, a lack of moral expertise, the need to preserve the state in conditions of total war, and the morality of sacrificing a few to benefit many—it becomes clear that the conduct of those who worked in the concentration camps was sometimes guided by moral rationales. These positions need to be understood and critically assessed if we are to clearly understand the values that allowed biomedical scientists and health care professionals to participate in inhumane experimentation and genocide. . . .

QUESTIONS FOR COMPREHENSION AND REFLECTION

1. According to Caplan, why are bioethicists reluctant to engage in moral inquiry about the Nazi medical war crimes? What are some of the myths that have allowed modern physicians and healthcare ethicists to minimize the role physicians played in the experiments in Nazi concentration camps? To what extent do, or did, you accept these myths?

2. Compare and contrast some of the experiments performed by Nazi physicians with those performed by American physicians, such as the Tuskegee syphilis study and the Atomic Energy Commission radiation studies.

3. Discuss the moral issues involved in using the results of immoral medical experiments. How morally questionable must an experiment be before it becomes morally unacceptable to use the results? Illustrate your answer using the Nazi hypothermia and typhus vaccine experiments, as well as the Atomic Energy Commission radiation studies, the Willowbrook hepatitis study in the United States, or the AIDS studies in Africa (see the reading by Annas and Grodin).

GEORGE J. ANNAS AND MICHAEL A. GRODIN

Human Rights and Maternal-Fetal HIV Transmission Prevention Trials in Africa

George Annas and Michael Grodin are professors at the Health Law Department of Boston University School of Public Health and cofounders of Global Lawyers and Physicians. Annas and Grodin maintain that the AIDS trials in Africa do not take the rights and welfare of the subjects seriously. The only way for wealthy nations to avoid exploitation when conducting experiments in impoverished, developing countries is to insist on informed consent and ensure that, if the experimental treatment proves beneficial, the impoverished population receives the treatment.

INTRODUCTION

Since the adoption of the Universal Declaration of Human Rights by the United Nations General Assembly in 1948, the countries of the world have agreed that all humans have dignity and rights. In 1998, the 50th anniversary of the Universal Declaration of Human Rights, the Declaration's aspirations have yet to be realized, and poverty, racism, and sexism continue to conspire to frustrate the worldwide human rights movement. The human rights and public health issues of maternal-fetal human immunodeficiency virus (HIV) transmission prevention trials in Africa, Asia, and the Caribbean are not unique to acquired immunodeficiency syndrome (AIDS) or to those countries. Open discussion of these issues provides an opportunity to move the real human rights agenda forward. This is why Global Lawyers and Physicians (GLP), a transnational organization dedicated to promoting and protecting the health-related provisions of the Universal Declaration of Human Rights, joined with Ralph Nader's Public Citizen organization to challenge the conduct of a series of AIDS clinical trials in these developing countries.[1]

THE CLINICAL TRIALS

In 1994, the first effective intervention to reduce the perinatal transmission of HIV was developed in the United States in AIDS Clinical Trials Group (ACTG) Study 076. In that trial, use of zidovudine administered orally to HIV-positive pregnant women as early as the second trimester of pregnancy, intravenously during labor, and orally to their newborns for 6 weeks reduced the incidence of HIV infection by two thirds (from about 25% to about 8%).[2] Six months after stopping the study, the US Public Health Service recommended the ACTG 076 regimen as the standard of care in the United States. In June 1994, the World Health Organization (WHO) convened a meeting in Geneva at which it was concluded (in an unpublished report) that the 076 regime was not feasible in the developing world. At least 16 randomized clinical trials (15 using placebos as controls) were subsequently approved for conduct in developing countries, primarily in Africa. These trials involve more than 17,000 pregnant women. Nine of the studies, most of them comparing shorter courses of zidovudine, vitamin A, or HIV immunoglobulin with placebo, are funded by the Centers for Disease Control and Prevention (CDC) or the National Institutes of Health (NIH).

Most of the public discussion about these trials has centered on the use of placebos.[1] The question of placebo use is a central one in determining how a study should be conducted. But we believe the more important issue these trials raise is the question of whether they should be done at all. Specifically, when is medical research ethically justified in developing countries that do not have adequate health services (or on US populations that have no access to basic health care)? This question is especially pertinent since February 1998 when, on the basis of a Thailand study that demonstrated that a short course of zidovudine reduced HIV transmission by 50%, CDC, NIH, and the United Nations Program on AIDS (UNAIDS) officials announced that they would recommend that the use of placebo be halted in all mother-to-fetus transmission studies.

RESEARCH ON IMPOVERISHED POPULATIONS

The central issue involved in doing research with impoverished populations is exploitation. Harold Varmus, speaking for NIH, and David Satcher, speaking for CDC, both seem to realize this. They wrote in the *New England Journal of Medicine* last year that "trials that make use of impoverished populations to test drugs for use solely in developed countries violate our most basic understanding of ethical behavior."[3] However, instead of trying to demonstrate how the study interventions, such as a shorter course of zidovudine (AZT), could actually be delivered to the populations of the countries in the studies, they assert that the studies can be justified because they will provide information that the host country can use to "make a sound judgment about the appropriateness and financial feasibility of providing the intervention."[3] However, what these countries require is not good intentions, but a real plan to deliver the intervention, should it be proven beneficial.

Unless the interventions being tested will actually be made available to the impoverished populations that are being used as research subjects, developed countries are simply exploiting them in order to quickly use the knowledge gained from the clinical trials for the developed countries' own benefit. If the research reveals regimens of equal efficacy at less cost, these regimens will surely be implemented in the developed world. If the research reveals the regimens to be less efficacious, these results will be added to the scientific literature, and the developed world will not conduct those studies. Ethics and basic human rights principles require not a thin promise, but a real plan as to how the intervention will actually be delivered. Actual delivery is also, of course, required to support even the utilitarian justification for the trials, which is to find a simple, inexpensive, and feasible intervention in as short a time frame as possible because so many people are dying of AIDS. No justification is supportable unless the intervention is actually made widely available to the relevant populations.

Neither NIH nor CDC (nor the host countries) has a plan that would make the interventions they are studying available in Africa, where more than two thirds of the people in the world reside who are infected with HIV. As an example, Varmus and Satcher point out that the wholesale cost of zidovudine in the 076 protocol is estimated to be in excess of $800 per mother and infant and that this amount is far greater than what most developing countries can pay for standard care. The CDC estimates the cost of the "short course" zidovudine regimens being investigated to be roughly $50 per person. The cost of merely screening for HIV disease, a precondition for any course of therapy, is approximately $10, and all pregnant women must be screened to find the cases to treat. These costs must be compared with the total per capita health care expenditures of the countries where this research is being conducted. Given this fact, African countries involved in the clinical trials (or some other funder) must make realistic assurances that if a research regimen proves effective in reducing mother-to-fetus transmission of HIV, resources will be made available so that the HIV-positive pregnant women in their countries will receive this regimen.

However, the mere assertion that the interventions will be feasible for use in the developing countries is simply not good enough, given our experience and knowledge of what happens in Africa now. For example, we already know that effectively treating sexually transmitted diseases such as syphilis, gonorrhea, and chancroid with the simple and effective treatments that are now available can drastically lower the incidence of HIV infection. Yet, these inexpensive and effective treatments are not delivered to poor Africans. For example, a recent study showed that improving the treatment of sexually transmitted diseases in rural Tanzania could reduce HIV infections by 40%.[4] Nonetheless, this relatively inexpensive and effective intervention is not delivered. Vaccines against devastating diseases have also been developed with sub-Saharan African populations as test subjects.[5] Nonetheless, even though vaccines such as the group A meningococcal meningitis vaccine are inexpensive and effective, they are not adequately delivered to the relevant sub-Saharan African populations.[5]

CULTURAL RELATIVISM OR UNIVERSAL HUMAN RIGHTS?

In their article in the *New England Journal of Medicine*, Varmus and Satcher sought to bolster their ethical position by quoting the chair of the AIDS Research Committee of the Uganda Cancer Institute, who wrote in a letter to Dr. Varmus:

> These are Ugandan studies conducted by Ugandan investigators on Ugandans. . . . It is not NIH conducting the studies in Uganda, but Ugandans conducting their study on their people for the good of their people.[3]

Two points are especially striking about Varmus' and Satcher's using this justification. First, their justification is simply not accurate. If NIH and CDC were not involved in these studies, these agencies would not have to justify them; indeed, the studies would not have been undertaken. These US agencies *are* involved—these trials are not just Ugandans doing research on other Ugandans. Second, and more importantly, the use of this quotation implies support for an outdated and dangerous view of cultural relativism.

Even if it were true that the studies in question were done by Ugandans on Ugandans, this would not mean that the United States or the international community could conclude that they should not be criticized. (This rationale did not inhibit criticism of apartheid in South Africa, genocide in Rwanda, or torture and murder in the Congo.) Human Rights Watch, referring to repression in Central Africa, said in its December 1997 review of the year on the issue of human rights that the slogan "African solutions to African problems" is now used as a "thin cover" for abusing citizens.[6] That observation can be applicable to experimentation on citizens as well.

The other major justification both NIH and CDC use for the trials is the consensus reached at the June 1994 meeting of researchers at WHO. Of the many analogies that have been drawn between the HIV transmission prevention trials and the US Public Health Service's Tuskegee syphilis study, perhaps most striking is their reliance on professional consensus instead of ethical principle to justify research on poor, black populations. As historian James Jones wrote in his book *Bad Blood,* which was written about the Tuskegee experiment: "The consensus was that the experiment was worth doing, and in a profession whose members did not have a well-developed system of normative ethics, consensus formed the functional equivalent of moral sanction."[7]

Neither researcher consensus nor host country agreement is ethically sufficient justification for choosing a research population. As the National Research Council's Committee on Human Genome Diversity properly put it, in the context of international research on human subjects, "[s]ensitivity to the specific practices and beliefs of a community cannot be used as a justification for violating universal human rights."[8] Justice and equity questions are also important to the ability of individual research subjects to give informed consent.

INFORMED CONSENT

Research subjects should not be drawn from populations who are especially vulnerable (e.g., the poor, children, or mentally impaired persons) unless the population is the only group in which the research can be conducted and the group itself will derive benefits from the research. Even when these conditions are met, informed consent must also be obtained. In most settings in Africa, voluntary, informed consent will be problematic and difficult, and it may even preclude ethical research. This is because, in the absence of health care, virtually any offer of medical assistance (even in the guise of research) will be accepted as "better than nothing" and research will almost inevitably be confused with treatment, making informed consent difficult.

Interviews with women subjects of the placebo-controlled trial in the Ivory Coast support this conclusion. For example, one subject, Cecile Guede, a 23-year-old HIV-infected mother participating in a US-financed trial, told the *New York Times,* "They gave me a bunch of pills to take, and told me how to take them. Some were for malaria, some were for fevers, and some were supposed to be for the virus. I knew that there were different kinds, but I figured that if one of them didn't work against AIDS, then one of the others would."[9] The *Times* reporter who wrote the front-page story, Howard W. French, said, "For Ms Guede, the reason to enroll in the study last year was clear: it offered her and her infant free health care and a hope to shield her baby from deadly infection. . . . [T]he prospect of help as she brought her baby into the world made taking part in the experiment all but irresistible."[9]

Persons can make a gift of themselves by volunteering for research. However, it is extremely unlikely that poor African women would knowingly volunteer to participate in research that offered no benefit to their communities (because the intervention would not be made available) and that would only serve to enrich the multinational drug companies and the developed world.[8] Thus, a good ethical working rule is that researchers should presume that valid consent cannot be obtained from impoverished populations in the absence of a realistic plan to deliver the intervention to the population. Informed consent, by itself, can protect many subjects of research in developed countries, but its protective power is much more compromised in impoverished populations who are being offered what looks like medical care that is otherwise unavailable to them.

THE INTERNATIONAL COMMUNITY AND THE AIDS PANDEMIC

If the goal of the clinical trials is to reduce the spread of HIV infection in developing countries, what strategy should public health adopt to achieve this end? It is not obvious that the answer is to conduct clinical trials of short-term zidovudine treatment. In the developed world, for example, HIV-infected women are advised not to breast-feed their infants because 8% to 18% of them will be infected with HIV from breast milk.[10] However, in much of the developing world, including in most African countries, WHO continues to recommend breast-feeding because the lack of clean water still makes formula-feeding more dangerous. As long as this recommendation stays in effect, and is followed, even universal use of the ACTG 076 regimen, which would lower the overall newborn infection rate by about 16%, would only likely serve to reduce the incidence of HIV infection in infants by about the same amount that it is increased by breast-feeding (8% to 18%). A more effective public health intervention to improve the health of women and their children may be to put more efforts into providing clean water and sanitation. This will help not only to deal with HIV, but also to alleviate many other problems, including diarrheal diseases.

President Jacques Chirac of France was on target in his December 1997 speech to the 10th International Conference on Sexually Transmitted Disease and AIDS in Africa, which was held in the Ivory Coast. President Chirac proposed creating an international "therapy support fund" that is primarily funded by European countries (the former colonial powers in Africa).[11] Although he put emphasis on the new drugs available for AIDS treatments, it would be more useful to consider the public health priorities of the countries themselves, for example, prevention, especially in areas such as sanitation, water supply, nutrition, education, and the delivery of simple and effective vaccines and medical treatments for sexually transmitted diseases.

CONCLUSION

Actual delivery of health care requires more than just paying lip service to the principles of the Universal Declaration of Human Rights; it requires a real commitment to human rights and a willingness on the part of the developed countries to take economic, social, and cultural rights as seriously as political and civil rights.

REFERENCES

1. Lurie P, Wolfe SM. Unethical trials of interventions to reduce perinatal transmission of human immunodeficiency virus in developing countries. *N Engl J Med.* 1997;337:853–856.
2. Connor EM, Sperling RS, Gelber R, et al. Reduction of maternal-infant transmission of human immunodeficiency virus type 1 with zidovudine treatment. *N Engl J Med.* 1994;331:1173–1180.
3. Varmus H., Satcher D. Ethical complexities of conducting research in developing countries. *N Engl J Med.* 1997;337:1003–1005.
4. Grosskurth H, Mosha F, Todd J, Mwijarubi E, et al. Impact of improved treatment of sexually transmitted diseases on HIV infection in rural Tanzania: randomized controlled trial. *Lancet.* 1995;346:530–536.
5. Robbins JB, Towne DW, Gotschlich EC, Schneerson R. 'Love's labours lost': failure to implement mass vaccination against group A meningococcal meningitis in sub-Saharan Africa. *Lancet.* 1997;350:880–882.
6. Clines FX. Rights group assails US on land mines and ties with China. *New York Times.* December 5, 1997:A13.
7. Jones JH. *Bad Blood: The Tuskegee Syphilis Experiment.* New York, NY: Free Press, 1981.
8. Committee on Human Genome Diversity. Evaluating Human Genetic Diversity. Washington, DC: National Academy Press; 1997:65.
9. French HW. AIDS research in Africa: juggling risks and hopes. *New York Times.* October 9, 1997:A1.
10. Van de Perre P. Postnatal transmission of human immunodeficiency virus type 1: the breast-feeding dilemma. *Am J Ob Gyn.* 1995;173:483–487.
11. Bunce M. Chirac seeks worldwide relief for AIDS in Africa. *Boston Globe.* December 8, 1997:A2.

1. Does the prospect of finding a cheaper alternative to the ACTG 076 treatment, which might benefit people in poor countries, justify the use of placebos in experiments in these countries? Does the fact that subjects might temporarily benefit from the experiments, even though the benefits stop once the experiment is terminated, morally justify using them in the experiment? Support your answers. Discuss how both Caplan and a utilitarian might answer these questions.

2. The AIDS studies in Africa have been compared to the Tuskegee syphilis study in the United States. Is this comparison valid? Support your answer.

3. Discuss the use of placebos in biomedical experiments. Is the use of placebos in randomized clinical trials inconsistent with genuine informed consent? Is the use of placebos justified in the AIDS studies in Africa? Under what circumstances, if any, is the use of placebos in medical experiments morally justified? Support your answers.

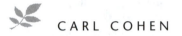

CARL COHEN

Do Animals Have Rights?

Carl Cohen is a philosophy professor at the University of Michigan. Cohen defends the traditional Kantian view of moral agency and rights. According to him, rights are based on self-assertion rather than interests. Since only moral agents can assert moral claims, only moral agents have rights. Thus, we do not violate the rights of nonhuman animals by doing research on them. Cohen also argues that we have a moral obligation to increase the use of nonhuman animals in research because doing so benefits humans.

Whether animals have rights is a question of great importance because if they do, those rights must be respected, even at the cost of great burdens for human beings. A right (unlike an interest) is a valid claim, or potential claim, made by a moral agent, under principles that govern both the claimant and the target of the claim. Rights are precious; they are dispositive; they count.

You have a right to the return of money you lent me; we both understand that. It may be very convenient for me to keep the money, and you may have no need of it whatever; but my convenience and your needs are not to the point. You have a *right* to it, and we have courts of law partly to ensure that such rights will be respected.

If you make me a promise, I have a moral right to its fulfillment—even though there may be no law to enforce my right. It may be very much in your interest to break that promise, but your great interests and the silence of the law cut no mustard when your solemn promise—which we both well understood—had been given. Likewise, those holding power may have a great and benevolent interest in denying my rights to travel or to speak freely—but their interests are overridden by my rights.

A great deal was learned about hypothermia by some Nazi doctors who advanced their learning by soaking Jews in cold water and putting them in refrigerators to learn how hypothermia proceeds.

We have no difficulty in seeing that they may not advance medicine in that way; the subjects of those atrocious experiments had rights that demanded respect. For those who ignored their rights we have nothing but moral loathing.

Some persons believe that animals have rights as surely as those Jews had rights, and they therefore look on the uses of animals in medical investigations just as we look at the Nazi use of the Jews, with moral loathing. They are consistent in doing so. If animals have rights they certainly have the right not to be killed, even to advance our important interests.

Some may say, "Well, they have rights, but we have rights too, and our rights override theirs." That may be true in some cases, but it will not solve the problem because, although we may have a weighty *interest* in learning, say, how to vaccinate against polio or other diseases, we do not have a *right* to learn such things. Nor could we honestly claim that we kill research animals in self-defense; they did not attack us. If animals have rights, they certainly have the right not to be killed to advance the interests of others, whatever rights those others may have.

In 1952 there were about 58,000 cases of polio reported in the United States, and 3,000 polio deaths; my parents, parents everywhere, trembled in fear for their children at camp or away from home. Polio vaccination became routine in 1955, and cases dropped to about a dozen a year; today polio has been eradicated completely from the Western Hemisphere. The vaccine that achieved this, partly developed and tested only blocks from where I live in Ann Arbor, could have been developed *only* with the substantial use of animals. Polio vaccines had been tried many times earlier, but from those earlier vaccines children had contracted the disease; investigators had become, understandably, exceedingly cautious.

The killer disease for which a vaccine now is needed most desperately is malaria, which kills about 2 million people each year, most of them children. Many vaccines have been tried—not on children, thank God—and have failed. But very recently, after decades of effort, we learned how to make a vaccine that does, with complete success, inoculate mice against malaria. A safe vaccine for

humans we do not yet have—but soon we will have it, thanks to the use of those mice, many of whom will have died in the process. To test that vaccine first on children would be an outrage, as it would have been an outrage to do so with the Salk and Sabin polio vaccines years ago. We use mice or monkeys *because there is no other way*. And there never will be another way because untested vaccines are very dangerous; their first use on a living organism is inescapably experimental; there is and will be no way to determine the reliability and safety of new vaccines without repeated tests on live organisms. Therefore, because we certainly may not use human children to test them, we will use mice (or as we develop an AIDS vaccine, primates) *or we will never have such vaccines*.

But if those animals we use in such tests have rights as human children do, what we did and are doing to them is as profoundly wrong as what the Nazis did to those Jews not long ago. Defenders of animal rights need not hold that medical scientists are vicious; they simply believe that what medical investigators are doing with animals is morally wrong. Most biomedical investigations involving animal subjects use rodents: mice and rats. The rat is the animal appropriately considered (and used by the critic) as the exemplar whose moral stature is in dispute here. Tom Regan is a leading defender of the view that rats do have such rights, and may not be used in biomedical investigations. He is an honest man. He sees the consequences of his view and accepts them forthrightly. In *The Case for Animal Rights* (Regan, 1983) he wrote,

> The harms others might face as a result of the dissolution of [some] practice or institution is no defense of allowing it to continue. . . . No one has a right to be protected against being harmed if the protection in question involves violating the rights of others. . . . No one has a right to be protected by the continuation of an unjust practice, one that violates the rights of others. . . . Justice *must* be done, though the . . . heavens fall. (pp. 346–347)

That last line echoes Kant, who borrowed it from an older tradition. Believing that rats have rights as humans do, Regan (1983) was convinced that killing them in medical research was morally intolerable. He wrote,

On the rights view, [he means, of course, the Regan rights view] we cannot justify harming a single rat *merely* by aggregating "the many human and humane benefits" that flow from doing it. . . . Not even a single rat is to be treated as if that animal's value were reducible to his *possible utility* relative to the interests of others. (p. 384)

If there are some things that we cannot learn because animals have rights, well, as Regan (1983) put it, so be it.

This is the conclusion to which one certainly is driven if one holds that animals have rights. If Regan is correct about the moral standing of rats, we humans can have no right, ever, to kill them—unless perchance a rat attacks a person or a human baby, as rats sometimes do; then our right of self-defense may enter, I suppose. But medical investigations cannot honestly be described as self-defense, and medical investigations commonly require that many mice and rats be killed. Therefore, all medical investigations relying on them, or any other animal subjects—which includes most studies and all the most important studies of certain kinds—will have to stop. Bear in mind that the replacement of animal subjects by computer simulations, or tissue samples, and so on, is in most research a phantasm, a fantasy. Biomedical investigations using animal subjects (and of course all uses of animals as food) will have to stop.

This extraordinary consequence has no argumentative force for Regan and his followers; they are not consequentialists. For Regan the *interests* of humans, their desire to be freed of disease or relieved of pain, simply cannot outweigh the *rights* of a single rat. For him the issue is one of justice, and the use of animals in medical experiments (he believes) is simply not just. But the consequences of his view will give most of us, I submit, good reason to weigh very carefully the arguments he offers to support such far-reaching claims. Do you believe that the work of Drs. Salk and Sabin was morally right? Would you support it now, or support work just like it saving tens of thousands of human children from diphtheria, hepatitis, measles, rabies, rubella, and tetanus (all of which relied essentially on animal subjects)—as well as,

now, AIDS, Lyme disease, and malaria? I surely do. If you would join me in this support we must conclude that the defense of animal rights is a gigantic mistake. I next aim to explain why animals *cannot* possess rights.

WHY ANIMALS DO NOT HAVE RIGHTS

Many obligations are owed by humans to animals; few will deny that. But it certainly does not follow from this that animals have rights because it is certainly not true that every obligation of ours arises from the rights of another. Not at all. We need to be clear and careful here. Rights entail obligations. If you have a right to the return of the money I borrowed, I have an obligation to repay it. No issue. If we have the right to speak freely on public policy matters, the community has the obligation to respect our right to do so. But the proposition *all rights entail obligations* does not convert simply, as the logicians say. From the true proposition that all trees are plants, it does not follow that all plants are trees. Similarly, not all obligations are entailed by rights. Some obligations, like mine to repay the money I borrowed from you, do arise out of rights. But many obligations are owed to persons or other beings who have no rights whatever in the matter.

Obligations may arise from commitments freely made: As a college professor I accept the obligation to comment at length on the papers my students submit, and I do so; but they have not the right to *demand* that I do so. Civil servants and elected officials surely ought to be courteous to members of the public, but that obligation certainly is not grounded in citizens' rights.

Special relations often give rise to obligations: Hosts have the obligation to be cordial to their guests, but the guest has not the right to demand cordiality. Shepherds have obligations to their dogs, and cowboys to their horses, which do not flow from the rights of those dogs or horses. My son, now 5, may someday wish to study veterinary medicine as my father did; I will then have the obligation to help him as I can, and with pride I shall—but he has not the authority to demand such help as a matter of right. My dog has no right to daily exercise and veterinary care, but I do have the obligation to provide those things for her.

One may be obliged to another for a special act of kindness done; one may be obliged to put an animal out of its misery in view of its condition—but neither the beneficiary of that kindness nor that dying animal may have had a claim of right.

Beauchamp and Childress (1994) addressed what they called the "correlativity of rights and obligations" and wrote that they would defend an "untidy" (pp. 73–75) variety of that principle. It would be very untidy indeed. Some of our most important obligations—to members of our family, to the needy, to neighbors, and to sentient creatures of every sort—have no foundation in rights at all. Correlativity appears critical from the perspective of one who holds a right; your right correlates with my obligation to respect it. But the claim that rights and obligations are *reciprocals,* that *every* obligation flows from another's right, is false, plainly inconsistent with our general understanding of the differences between what we think we *ought* to do, and what others can justly *demand* that we do.

I emphasize this because, although animals have no rights, it surely does not follow from this that one is free to treat them with callous disregard. Animals are not stones; they feel. A rat may suffer; surely we have the obligation not to torture it gratuitously, even though it be true that the concept of a right could not possibly apply to it. We humans are obliged to act humanely, that is, being aware of their sentience, to apply to animals the moral principles that govern us regarding the gratuitous imposition of pain and suffering; which is not, of course, to treat animals as the possessors of rights.

Animals cannot be the bearers of rights, because the concept of rights is essentially *human;* it is rooted in, and has force within, a human moral world. Humans must deal with rats—all too frequently in some parts of the world—and must be moral in their dealing with them; but a rat can no more be said to have rights than a table can be said to have ambition. To say of a rat that it has rights is to confuse categories, to apply to its world a moral category that has content only in the human moral world.

Try this thought experiment. Imagine, on the Serengeti Plain in East Africa, a lioness hunting for her cubs. A baby zebra, momentarily left unattended by its mother, is the prey; the lioness snatches it, rips open its throat, tears out chunks of its flesh, and departs. The mother zebra is driven nearly out of her wits when she cannot locate her baby; finding its carcass she will not even leave the remains for days. The scene may be thought unpleasant, but it is entirely natural, of course, and extremely common. If the zebra has a right to live, if the prey is just but the predator unjust, we ought to intervene, if we can, on behalf of right. But we do not intervene, of course—as we surely would intervene if we saw the lioness about to attack an unprotected human baby or you. What accounts for the moral difference? We justify different responses to humans and to zebras on the ground (implicit or explicit) that their moral stature is very different. The human has a right not to be eaten alive; it is, after all, a human being. Do you believe the baby zebra has the *right* not to be slaughtered by that lioness? That the lioness has the *right* to kill that baby zebra for her cubs? If you are inclined to say, confronted by such natural rapacity—duplicated with untold variety millions of times each day on planet earth—that neither is right or wrong, that neither has a *right* against the other, I am on your side. Rights are of the highest moral consequence, yes; but zebras and lions and rats are totally amoral; there is no morality for them; they do no wrong, ever. In their world there are no rights.

A contemporary philosopher who has thought a good deal about animals, referring to them as "moral patients," put it this way:

> A moral patient lacks the ability to formulate, let alone bring to bear, moral principles in deliberating about which one among a number of possible acts it would be right or proper to perform. Moral patients, in a word, cannot do what is right, nor can they do what is wrong. . . . Even when a moral patient causes significant harm to another, the moral patient has not done what is wrong. Only moral agents can do what is wrong. (Regan, 1983, pp. 152–153)

Just so. The concepts of wrong and right are totally foreign to animals, not conceivably within their ken or applicable to them, as the author of that passage clearly understands.

When using animals in our research, therefore, we ought indeed be humane—but we can never violate the rights of those animals because, to be blunt, they have none. Rights do not *apply* to them.

But humans do have rights. Where do our rights come from? Why are we not crudely natural creatures like rats and zebras? This question philosophers have struggled to answer from earliest times. A definitive account of the human moral condition I cannot here present, of course. But reflect for a moment on the kinds of answers that have been widely given:

- Some think our moral understanding, with its attendant duties, to be a divine gift. So St. Thomas said: The moral law is binding, and humans have the power, given by God, to grasp its binding character, and must therefore respect the rights that other humans possess. God makes us (Saint Augustine said before him) in his own image, and therefore with a will that is free, and gives us the power to recognize that, and therefore, unlike other creatures, we must choose between good and evil, between right and wrong.

- Many philosophers, distrusting theological justifications of rights and duties, sought the ground of human morality in the membership, by all humans, in a moral community. The English idealist, Bradley, called it an organic moral community; the German idealist, Hegel, called it an objective ethical order. These and like accounts commonly center on human interrelations, on a moral *fabric* within which human agents always act, and within which animals never act and never can possibly act.

- The highly abstract reasoning from which such views emerge has dissatisfied many; you may find more nearly true the convictions of ethical intuitionists and realists who said, as H. A. Prichard, Sir David Ross, and my friend and teacher C. D. Broad, of happy memory, used to say, that there is a direct, underivative, intuitive cognition of rights as possessed by other humans, but not by animals.

- Or perhaps in the end we will return to Kant, and say with him that critical reason reveals at the core of human action a uniquely moral will, and the unique ability to grasp and to lay down moral laws for oneself and for others—an ability that is not conceivably within the capacity of any nonhuman animal whatever.

To be a moral agent (on this view) is to be able to grasp the generality of moral restrictions on our will. Humans understand that some things, which may be in our interest, *must not be willed;* we lay down moral laws for ourselves, and thus exhibit, as no other animal can exhibit, moral autonomy. My dog knows that there are certain things she must not do—but she knows this only as the outcome of her learning about her interests, the pains she may suffer if she does what had been taught forbidden. She does not know, cannot know (as Regan agrees) that any conduct is wrong. The proposition *It would be highly advantageous to act in such-and-such a way, but I may not because it would be wrong* is one that no dog or mouse or rabbit, however sweet and endearing, however loyal or attentive to its young, can ever entertain, or intend, or begin to grasp. Right is not in their world. But right and wrong are the very stuff of human moral life, the ever-present awareness of human beings who can do wrong, and who by seeking (often) to avoid wrong conduct prove themselves members of a moral community in which rights may be exercised and must be respected.

Some respond by saying, "This can't be correct, for human infants (and the comatose and senile, etc.) surely have rights, but they make no moral claims or judgments and can make none—and any view entailing that children can have no rights must be absurd." Objections of this kind miss the point badly. It is not individual persons who qualify (or are disqualified) for the possession of rights because of the presence or absence in them of some special capacity, thus resulting in the award of rights to some but not to others. Rights are universally human; they arise in a *human moral world,* in a moral *sphere.* In the human world moral judgments are pervasive; it is the fact that all humans including infants and the senile are members of that moral community—not the fact that as individuals they have or do not have certain special capacities, or merits—that makes humans bearers of rights. Therefore, it is beside the point to insist that animals have remarkable capacities, that they really have a consciousness of self, or of the future, or make plans, and so on. And the tired response that because infants plainly cannot make moral claims they must have no rights at all, or rats must have them too, we ought forever put aside. Responses like these arise out of a misconception of right itself. They mistakenly suppose that rights are tied to some identifiable individual abilities or sensibilities, and they fail to see that rights arise only in a community of moral beings, and that therefore there are spheres in which rights do apply and spheres in which they do not.

Rationality is not at issue; the capacity to communicate is not at issue. My dog can reason, if rather weakly, and she certainly can communicate. Cognitive criteria for the possession of rights, Beauchamp said, are morally perilous. Indeed they are. Nor is the capacity to suffer here at issue. And, if *autonomy* be understood only as the capacity to choose this course rather than that, autonomy is not to the point either. But *moral autonomy*—that is, *moral self-legislation*—is to the point, because moral autonomy is uniquely human and is for animals out of the question, as we have seen, and as Regan and I agree. In talking about autonomy, therefore, we must be careful and precise.

Because humans do have rights, and these rights can be violated by other humans, we say that some humans commit *crimes*. But whether a crime has been committed depends utterly on the moral state of mind of the actor. If I take your coat, or your book, honestly thinking it was mine, I do not steal it. The *actus reus* (the guilty deed) must be accompanied, in a genuine crime, by a guilty mind, a *mens rea*. That recognition, not just of possible punishment for an act, but of moral duties that govern us, no rat or cow ever can possess. In primitive times humans did sometimes bring cows and horses to the bar of human justice. We chuckle at that practice now, realizing that accusing cows of crimes marks the primitive moral view as inane. Animals never can be criminals because they have no moral state of mind.

Mistakes parallel to this in other spheres may be helpful to think about. In the Third Part of *The Critique of Pure Reason*, Immanuel Kant explained with care the metaphysical blunders into which we are led when we misapply concepts of great human import. In our human experience, for example, the concepts of time and space, the relations of cause and effect, of subject and attribute, and others, are essential, fundamental. But, forgetting that these are concepts arising only within the world of our human experience, we sometimes are misled into asking: Was the world caused, or is it uncaused? Did the world have a beginning in time, or did it not? Kant explained—in one of the most brilliant long passages in all philosophical literature—why *it makes no sense to ask such questions*. Cause applies to phenomena we humans encounter *in* the world, it is a category of our experience and cannot apply to the world as a whole. Time is the condition of our experience, not an absolute container in which the world could have begun. The antinomies of pure reason, and after those the paralogisms of pure reason, Kant patiently exhibited as confusions arising from the misapplication of the categories of experience. His lesson is powerful and deep. The misapplication of concepts leads to error and, sometimes, to nonsense. So it is with rights also. To say that rats have rights is to apply to the world of rats a concept that makes good sense when applied to humans, but which makes no sense at all when applied to rats.

WHY ANIMALS ARE MISTAKENLY BELIEVED TO HAVE RIGHTS

From the foregoing discussion it follows that, if some philosophers believe that they have proved that animals have rights, they must have erred in the alleged proof. Regan is a leader among those who claim to *argue* in defense of the rights of rats; he contends that the best arguments are on his side. I aim next to show how he and others with like views go astray. Bear in mind that Regan's book is long, its argument tortuous and at times convoluted. In what follows I must compress the report of his views, obviously; but I promise to be fair and to hold Regan responsible for nothing that he does not clearly say. We know—if we are agreed that rats are not the holders of rights—that Regan must have got off the track. Examining *The Case for Animal Rights,* let us see if we can find the faulty switch.

Much of Regan's (1983) book is devoted to a general treatment of the nature of ethical thinking and theory, to discussions of animal consciousness and animal awareness, and to detailed critiques of the views of others whom he thinks in error. Regan sought to show, patiently and laboriously, that the common belief that we do have obligations to animals, although they have no rights, has not been defended satisfactorily. That belief cannot be justified, he contended, by direct duty views of which he finds two categories: those depending on the obligation to be kind or not to be cruel, and those depending on any kind of utilitarian calculation.

None of this counterargument could possibly establish his conclusion that animals do have rights, unless Regan had proved that his listing of all alternative conflicting views was exhaustive, which it was not, and unless he had proved conclusively that every such candidate is untenable, which he did not do. . . .

The case is built entirely on the principle that allegedly *carries over* almost everything earlier claimed about human rights to rats and other animals. What principle is that? It is the principle, put in italics but given no name, that equates moral agents with moral patients:

> *The validity of the claim to respectful treatment, and thus the case for the recognition of the right to such treatment, cannot be any stronger or weaker in the case of moral patients than it is in the case of moral agents.* (Regan, p. 279)

But hold on. Why in the world should anyone think this principle to be true? Back [W]here Regan first recounted his view of moral patients, he allowed that some of them are, although capable of experiencing pleasure and pain, lacking in other capacities. But he is interested, he told us there, in those moral patients—those animals— that are like humans in having *inherent value.* This is the key to the argument for animal rights, the possession of inherent value. How that concept functions in the argument becomes absolutely crit-ical. I will say first briefly what will be shown more carefully later: *Inherent value* is an expression used by Regan (and many like him) with two very different senses—in one of which it is reasonable to conclude that those who have inherent value have rights, and in another sense in which that inference is wholly unwarranted. But the phrase, *inherent value* has some plausibility in both contexts, and thus by sliding from one sense of inherent value to the other Regan appears to succeed . . . in making the case for animal rights.

The concept of inherent value first entered the discussion in the seventh chapter of Regan's (1983) book, at which point his principal object is to fault and defeat utilitarian arguments. It is not (he argued there) the pleasures or pains that go "into the cup" of humanity that give value, but the "cups" themselves; humans are equal in value because they are humans, having inherent value. So we are, all of us, equal—equal in being moral agents who have this inherent value. This approach to the moral stature of humans is likely to be found quite plausible. Regan called it the "postulate of inherent value"; all humans, "The lonely, forsaken, unwanted, and unloved are no more nor less inherently valuable than those who enjoy a more hospitable relationship with others" (p. 237). And Regan went on to argue for the proposition that all moral agents are "equal in inherent value." Holding some such views we are likely to say, with Kant, that all humans are beyond price. Their inherent value gives them moral dignity, a unique role in the moral world, as agents having the capacity to act morally and make moral judgments. This is inherent value in Sense 1.

The expression *inherent value* has another sense, however, also common and also plausible. My dog has inherent value, and so does every wild animal, every lion and zebra, which is why the senseless killing of animals is so repugnant. Each animal is unique, not replaceable in itself by another animal or by any rocks or clay. Animals, like humans, are not just things; they live, and as unique living creatures they have inherent value. This is an important point, and again likely to be thought plausible; but here, in Sense 2, the phrase *inherent value* means something quite distinct from what was meant in its earlier uses.

Inherent value in Sense 1, possessed by all humans but not by all animals, which warrants the claim of human rights, is very different from inherent value in Sense 2, which warrants no such claim. The uniqueness of animals, their intrinsic worthiness as individual living things, does not ground the possession of rights, has nothing to do with the moral condition in which rights arise. Regan's argument reached its critical objective with almost magical speed because, having argued that beings with inherent value (Sense 1) have rights that must be respected, he quickly asserted (putting it in italics lest the reader be inclined to express doubt) that rats and rabbits also have rights because they, too, have inherent value (Sense 2).

This is an egregious example of the fallacy of equivocation: the informal fallacy in which two or more meanings of the same word or phrase have been confused in the several premises of an argument (Cohen & Copi, 1994, pp. 143–144). Why is this slippage not seen at once? Partly because we know the phrase *inherent value* often is used loosely, so the reader is not prone to quibble about its introduction; partly because the two uses of the phrase relied on are both common, so neither signals danger; partly because inherent value in Sense 2 is indeed shared by those who have it in Sense 1; and partly because the phrase *inherent value* is woven into accounts of what Regan (1983) elsewhere called the *subject-of-a-life criterion,* a phrase of his own devising for which he can stipulate any meaning he pleases, of course, and which also slides back and forth between the sphere of genuine moral agency and the sphere of animal experience. But perhaps the chief reason the equivocation between these two uses of the phrase *inherent value* is obscured (from the author, I believe, as well as from the reader) is the fact that the assertion that animals have rights appears only indirectly, as the outcome of the application of the principle that moral patients are entitled to the same respect as moral agents—a principle introduced at a point in the book long after the important moral differences between moral patients and moral agents have been recognized, with a good deal of tangled philosophical argument having been injected in between.

I invite readers to trace out this equivocation in detail; my limited space here precludes more extended quotation. But this assurance I will give: there is no argument or set of arguments in *The Case for Animal Rights* that successfully makes the case for animal rights. Indeed, there *could* not be, any more than any book, however long and convoluted, could make the case for the emotions of oak trees, or the criminality of snakes.

Animals do not have rights. Right does not apply in their world. We do have many obligations to animals, of course, and I honor Regan's appreciation of their sensitivities. I also honor his seriousness of purpose, and his always civil and always rational spirit. But he is, I submit, profoundly mistaken. I conclude with the observation that, had his mistaken views about the rights of animals long been accepted, most successful medical therapies recently devised—antibiotics, vaccines, prosthetic devices, and other compounds and instruments on which we now rely for saving and improving human lives and for the protection of our children—could not have been developed; and were his views to become general now (an outcome that is unlikely but possible) the consequences for medical science and for human well-being in the years ahead would be nothing less than catastrophic.

Advances in medicine absolutely require experiments, many of which are dangerous. Dangerous experiments absolutely require living organisms as subjects. Those living organisms (we now agree) certainly may not be human beings. Therefore, most advances in medicine will continue to rely on the use of nonhuman animals, or they will stop. Regan is free to say in response, as he does, "so be it." The rest of us must ask if the argument he presents is so compelling as to force us to accept that dreadful result.

REFERENCES

Beauchamp, T. L., & Childress, J. F. (1994). *Principles of biomedical ethics* (4th ed.). New York: Oxford University Press.

Cohen, C., & Copi, I. M. (1994). *Introduction to logic* (9th ed.). New York: Macmillan.

Regan, T. (1983). *The case for animal rights.* Berkeley: University of California Press.

1. Cohen acknowledges that inhumane treatment of nonhuman animals is wrong when we can achieve the same results using alternative methods. Discuss whether his claim that researchers have a moral obligation to treat nonhuman animals humanely is consistent with his claim that animals have no rights.

2. Cohen argues that nonhuman animals feel pain and that researchers should not subject them to unnecessary suffering. What does he mean by unnecessary suffering? To what extent does this criterion limit the type of experimentation that is morally permissible? Compare and contrast Cohen's position on the significance of suffering in the moral justification of experiments using nonhuman animals with that of a utilitarian such as Peter Singer. Which presents the more compelling argument? Support your answers.

3. Does Cohen do an effective job of discrediting the argument that nonhuman animals have rights? Support your answer. Discuss how a rights ethicist such as Regan might respond to Cohen's criticism of his position.

4. Do you agree with Cohen's claim regarding the qualitative gap between humans and other animals? Discuss how Cohen would respond to the argument that scientists who justify using nonhuman animals in experiments on the grounds that they are not like humans find themselves in a moral dilemma, since there would be no point in using nonhuman animals in psychology and learning experiments if they were not like us.

JUDITH A. BOSS AND ALYSSA V. BOSS

Paradigm Shifts, Scientific Revolutions and the Moral Justification of Experimentation on Nonhuman Animals

Judith Boss is assistant director of curriculum affairs at Brown University Medical School and a visiting scholar with the Center for the Study of Human Development at Brown University. Alyssa Boss is a Providence lawyer. Both are former college ethics teachers. Boss and Boss argue that the biological sciences are currently undergoing a paradigm shift in which people are questioning the use of nonhuman animals in experimentation. After presenting the arguments for and against animal experimentation, including those of Cohen, Singer, and Regan, Boss and Boss conclude that the present level of animal experimentation cannot be morally justified.

An estimated 70 to 120 million nonhuman animals are killed every year in scientific experiments.[1] The justifications for the use of nonhuman animals in scientific experiments to benefit humans are based on two conflicting paradigms or models regarding the nature of human and nonhuman animals. . . .

. . . A paradigm shift, we will argue, is presently taking place in the biological sciences. The effect of this shift is currently being experienced in the conflict and uncertainty over what policies to adopt regarding the use of nonhuman animals in scientific experiments.

THE TRADITIONAL PARADIGM UNDERLYING "ANIMAL" EXPERIMENTATION

The traditional paradigm is based on a pseudo-scientific, anthropocentric, religious worldview which fails to stand up under philosophical and scientific scrutiny. It is based on the premise that there is a distinct line separating humans and other animals. Because of this, it is perfectly acceptable and even, according to some, morally required to use other animals in experiments to benefit humans or increase our knowledge.

The traditional paradigm forms the basis of the current approach to biological science, or what [Thomas] Kuhn calls "normal science." The term "normal science" refers to "research firmly based upon one or more past scientific achievements, achievements that some particular scientific community acknowledges for a time as supplying the foundation for its further practice."[2] The purpose of education and textbooks is not to question or even explicate the basic paradigm, but to explain the accepted theories of normal science and to illustrate the successful application of these theories. In this way, the traditional paradigm is passed on to future generations of scientists. Only those who are willing to work within the accepted paradigm are welcome to participate in the community of scientists. Those who question the paradigm of "normal science" or refuse to accept it must either work in isolation or join a fringe group.

The traditional paradigm regarding "animal" experimentation was heavily influenced by the Greek philosophers, such as Aristotle, who argued that reason is an activity of the soul. Only the soul, which is non-material and hence not restricted by the laws of nature, can act freely. Humans have a soul; nonhuman animals don't. This paradigm, which was Christianized by Thomas Aquinas, forms the basis of what is referred to as "traditional morality"—the notion that only humans have intrinsic moral value. This philosophical tradition has been one of the most deeply rooted obstacles to serious consideration of the rights of nonhuman animals. . . .

CHALLENGES TO THE TRADITIONAL PARADIGM

Challenges to the traditional paradigm have come from several fronts including Galileo's discovery that the earth is not the center of the universe, Darwinian evolutionary theory, Piaget's finding that logical thought can occur without language, concern for the rights of human subjects following the holocaust of World War II, the civil rights movement, and the environmental movement. The increasing evidence of irrational human brutality, and the alarming acceleration in the past few decades of environmental destruction because of human activities including the extinction of thousands of species of plants and animals every year, has caused many people to rethink the traditional paradigm and to realize that humans are not separate from nature but a part of nature. It is becoming apparent, as we stand on the brink of ecological disaster, that it is the human animal, more than any other, that needs to be restrained and have order imposed on it. . . .

Many nonhuman animals are . . . clearly capable of reasoning and remembering. If they were not, it would be pointless to use them as subjects in learning experiments. Nonhuman animals obviously have concepts of food and danger, and they show evidence of having expectations of future events, such as rewards and punishments. A recent article in *Scientific American* states that "computers have mastered intellectual tasks such as chess and integral logic, but they have yet to attain the skills of a lobster in dealing with the real world."[3]

Behavioral evidence also supports the claim that other animals, like young humans, have memory without language. And memory depends on concept formation. Because we don't know how other animals do this without a system of conventional symbols does not mean that they don't do it. To use an analogy, if we adopted an ornithocentric or bird-centered worldview, we might claim that flying stands at the summit of all other achievements. Because all birds need feathers in order to fly, we might conclude that feathers are essential for flying. However, this is clearly false, since bats and butterflies and airplanes are also capable of flying. Of course, we are readily able to admit that non-birds are capable of flying, since our perception is not shaped by an ornithocentric worldview. However, if it were, we would probably devise all other sorts of other theories that are compatible with our paradigm to "explain" what these other beings are doing in the air without actually flying.

The claim that only humans are self-conscious or have a concept of self is also hard, if not impossible, to substantiate scientifically. The same criteria that we use in concluding that other humans are self-conscious—the formation and use of concepts, the realization that a particular experience is happening to them, the ability to learn from their experience, the efforts to protect themselves from harm—all point to the presence of self-consciousness in other animals. However, when scientists do try to apply the same criteria to humans and nonhuman animals, their observations are discounted amid accusations of anthropomorphism—one of the cardinal sins of normal science. In this way, traditional science avoids having to confront its anthropocentric assumptions by engaging in circular reasoning.

If nonhuman animals are incapable of making decisions or choices based on reason, they would be useless in learning experiments. "If we refuse to impute mental processes to other animals," notes philosopher and animal liberation advocate Peter Singer, "the logical consequence of this view of 'scientific methods' is that experiments on animals cannot teach us anything about human beings. As amazing as it may seem, some psychologists have been so concerned to avoid anthropomorphism that they have accepted this conclusion."[4]

Thus, applying the traditional paradigm of "normal science" to scientific experimentation on nonhuman animals involves accepting contradictory premises: that other animals are fundamentally different from humans and that other animals are enough like humans that we can use them in research to make relatively accurate generalizations about human physiology and learning. This flaw in the old paradigm is becoming increasingly apparent with the rapid growth of the animal liberation and animal welfare movements in the past few decades. . . .

Another challenge to the traditional paradigm came through changes in our attitudes regarding the use of non-consenting humans in nontherapeutic experiments. Prior to World War II, there were very few regulations. . . .

As a result of . . . growing public awareness, strict regulations regarding human experimentation have been put in place to prevent the use in scientific experiments of humans lacking the cognitive or political power to assert their rights. The conviction that it is wrong to perform experiments on mentally defective, imprisoned or similarly marginalized humans has fueled the similar conviction that it is wrong and contrary to the principle of justice to do the same to other animals.

The impassioned battle for equal rights for all groups of humans during the various civil rights movements also fueled a demand for respect for the rights of other animals as well. The principle of equality among humans is not based on an empirical description of actual equality of humans but upon a moral ideal of equal concern for the well-being of others. An implication of this concern is that equal respect should apply to all beings regardless of their particular abilities, their intelligence or social standing. Indeed, many people who were engaged in the movements for equal rights for humans, such as Mahatma Gandhi, Mary Wollstonecraft, Lord Shaftesbury, Susan B. Anthony, Elizabeth Cady Stanton, and Horace Greeley, to name only a few, were also involved in the animals rights movement.[5] These people in turn, and in particular Gandhi who was adamantly opposed to the exploitation of nonhuman animals, had a large impact on the American Civil Rights movement of the 1960's. Gandhi's basic philosophy centered on the interconnectedness of all life and the importance of extending moral respect to all living beings if we are to ever have a peaceful world.

MAKING THE SHIFT

Because of the heavy investment of traditional scientists in a particular paradigm, scientific revolutions rarely occur overnight or even in a single generation. This is especially true in areas of science which are insulated from the general public and whose publications are primarily in journals geared only toward others in the field or related fields. In the early stages of the development of a new paradigm, attention tends to be focused on the development of new alternatives.[6]

The emergence of a new paradigm from competing alternatives, according to Kuhn, is generally "preceded or accompanied by fundamental philosophical analysis of the contemporary research tradition."[7] In light of this observation, it should come as no surprise that many of the leaders of the animal rights movement are social reformers, philosophers and ethicists who came from outside of normal science.

Paradigm shifts generally occur when a new paradigm eventually gains enough adherents to make their voice heard. Since 1980, the membership of animal protection groups, while still representing a minority of the population, has increased five to tenfold.[8] Supporters of a new paradigm are generally members of the laity or restricted to a narrow subdivision, generally newcomers, of the scientific community who are not committed to the traditional rules of normal science. . . .

Paradigm shifts are more likely to occur during a time of crisis, when normal science is unable to solve a particular problem. The threat of global ecological disaster, while still denied by many scientists, may be such a crisis. As such it requires that humans, as a species, reassess their relationship to the earth as well as to their technology. New paradigms require that people see the world, including other species of animals, in a radically new way. This means a complete re-evaluation of the traditional anthropocentric morality which allows us to exploit other animals and the environment. Because the use of "animal" research in the scientific and medical research community is so thoroughly entrenched, there is tremendous resistance to doing so.

When a paradigm shift occurs, there is inevitably conflict and heated debate as the two competing views openly clash. When a paradigm shift occurs, some of the old problems that were considered trivial or non-existent, such as the morally significant difference between humans and other animals and the rights and welfare of nonhuman animals and the environment, become the "very archetypes of significant scientific advancement."[9]

According to Kuhn, "normal science—that put forth in traditional textbooks—often suppresses fundamental novelties because they are necessarily subversive of its basic commitments."[10] One of the present commitments is to the use of nonhuman animals in scientific research. "Once a pattern of animal experimentation becomes the accepted mode of research in a particular field," Singer notes, "The process is self-reinforcing and difficult to break."[11] A whole system of rewards, including tenure, the award of research grants, publication and scientific achievement, is invested in acceptance of the traditional paradigm. For this reason, arguments in support of animal research based on the benefits derived from it are essentially unresolvable. Even if valuable discoveries have been made using nonhuman animals, we cannot say how successful medical and scientific research would have been if it had been compelled, from the beginning, to develop alternative methods of investigation or if it had addressed itself to a different set of medical problems, such as preventive medicine or world health or environmentally-related issues. . . .

Kuhn points out that when scientists and other people who are heavily invested in a particular paradigm are confronted with an anomaly, they will "devise numerous articulation and ad hoc modifications of their theory in order to eliminate any apparent conflict."[12] For example, religious organizations, who have traditionally been guardians of the anthropocentric morality that underlies the traditional paradigm, have become increasingly involved in the environmental movement. This, however, places churches in the uncomfortable position of being accused of being one of the primary causes of the current crisis by condoning exploitation of the earth's resources for human advancement, while at the same time trying to promote themselves as the beneficent caretakers of the earth. . . .

[A] more radical alternative paradigm has been put forth by feminist theologians, such as Sallie McFague, author of *The Body of God: An Ecological Theology* (1993). Using the Big Bang theory as support for the unity and common source of all being, the universe is envisioned in this paradigm as the incarnated body of God, rather than as being separate from and the creation of a transcendent, disembodied God. While the implications of this paradigm have yet to be worked out by its proponents, it would seem to require us to acknowledge the divinity and intrinsic moral worth of all beings, including laboratory animals, rather than just humans.

The strategy of making ad hoc modifications in theories in order to avoid conflict or having to give up the traditional paradigm also occurs among scientists. For example, R. G. Frey and W. Paton, defenders of the use of nonhuman animals in scientific experiments, admit that equality in terms of life and interests of some humans and some nonhuman animals is a problem that needs to be taken more seriously when designing experiments. According to the principle of justice. "When individuals are treated differently, we need to point to a difference between them that justifies the differences in treatment."[13] Mere difference in species is not enough to justify differences in treatment by scientists any more than is mere difference in group membership sufficient to justify paying a woman or an African-American less or denying them a job. To discriminate solely on the bases of gender or race constitutes sexism or racism. To discriminate solely on the basis of species consti-

tutes what Singer terms "speciesism." Singer's rule of thumb for avoiding speciesism is that "we should give the same respect to the lives of animals as we give to the lives of those humans at a similar mental level."[14]

Applying this rule to animal experimentation, Frey and Paton observe that:

> We do not do to defective humans all that we presently do in our laboratories to quite healthy animals. My interest is in why we do not. If the justification is that we think human life of greater value than animals' life, then we must be prepared to face the facts, at least on the grounds I suggested, that (i) not all human life is of the same value and (ii) some human life has a value so low as to be exceeded by some animal life.[15]

However, rather than relinquish the traditional paradigm, Frey and Paton conclude that, in accordance with the principle of justice as explicated by Singer and Rachels, experimentation on healthy sentient mammals also justifies similar experimentation on humans with similar or lower capacities.

One of the weaknesses of the alternative based on this version of the principle of justice is that it is still basically anthropocentric in that it respects nonhuman life only to the extent that it resembles sentient human life. Indeed, Singer limits his opposition to scientific experimentation using nonhuman animals primarily to those done on mammals.

Another alternative paradigm is that based on rights ethics rather than the principle of justice. Traditional morality supports a model of rights based on self-assertion. The model of rights adopted by most civil rights and animals rights activists, on the other hand, is based on interests. According to the self-assertion model, a right "is a claim, or potential claim, that one party may exercise against another. Rights arise, and can be intelligibly defended, only among beings who actually do, or can, make moral claims against one another."[16] This model, which is steeped in traditional dualistic ethics, assumes that only humans have rights, since "nonhuman animals lack this capacity for moral choice."[17]

However, this description of human and non-human animals is inaccurate. Many nonhuman animals, as well as small children, respond with indignation, which is anger at an injustice, when their interests or needs are ignored or thwarted. They certainly seem to be recognizing and responding to moral claims. Another problem with this concept of rights is that we do recognize and protect, though not to the same extent that we protect the rights of adults,[18] the rights of small children and humans with severe brain damage despite the fact that they are not generally recognized as being capable of free moral judgment, and in some cases have no potential for rationality.

Under the self-assertion model of rights, being able to claim one's rights boils down to having the power, generally political power, to successfully assert oneself. Basing rights on one's power to assert oneself, or the presence of an effective agent who will act on one's behalf, allows us to disregard not only the rights of nonhuman animals but also the rights of disempowered groups of humans who lack the political power or force of law to exercise their moral claims.

Philosophical concepts and the paradigms they support do not exist in a vacuum but have real-life consequences. This model of rights has contributed to the belief that humans in positions of power, such as scientists and medical doctors, have the right to assert their power over and exploit other species of animals in the name of science with little concern for their welfare, and in ways that would be considered as cruel and immoral if done by someone in a lesser position of power. Indeed, as was pointed out earlier, this model of rights was used at one time to justify the use in scientific experiments, without their informed consent, of groups of people who lacked political power.

The second model of rights, which is part of a newly emerging non-anthropocentric paradigm, is based on the principle of equal consideration of interests. The existence of interests is based on the capacity for suffering and for enjoyment. Humans are seen as members of a wider animal community, or a web of life, rather than as being a special and unique creation. All sentient animals, including humans, have an interest in doing that which brings pleasure as well as an interest in avoiding harm and suffering. Beings, however, have a right to pursue only their legitimate interests—that is, those interests that do not prevent others from pursuing their similar interests. Under this model of rights, benefits to oneself and others are morally acceptable only if no one else's rights have been violated in achieving these benefits. For example, we can't sacrifice the life of one child in a medical experiment to save the lives of fifty others.

Not all animals have the same interests. There are distinctly human rights, such as the right to religious freedom and the right to a formal education, that other animals lack since they have no interest in organized religion or formal schooling. On the other hand, all sentient animals, including humans, cats and mice, have an interest in not being tortured, not because they are capable of rational thought, but because they have the capacity to feel pain. In recognition of this, the Animal Welfare Act prohibits experiments that cause nonhuman animals unnecessary pain.

The need for one's space also does not ground a distinctive human right but one belonging to all territorial animals. Property or territorial rights belong to more than just humans since squirrels and mice and many other animals also need property or territory for collecting food and raising their young. This right is recognized and minimally respected in the Animal Welfare Act and its amendments regulating minimum space requirements for different "laboratory animals," so called. The Animal Welfare Act also expects experimenters to respect animals' interests in health care, proper nutrition and a clean living space. However, it does not recognize their liberty rights or right to life. Rachels notes in this regard that

> While it is generally acknowledged by philosophers that liberty and freedom from coercion are essential if we humans are to develop and lead the types of lives where we can exercise our powers as rational agents, it is also true that liberty is necessary for many nonhuman animals if they are to live the sorts of lives, and thrive, in ways that are natural to them.[19]

In justifying the conscription of nonhuman animals for scientific experiments, the argument that humans can only be used if they give their informed consent, but other animals can be used because they are incapable of giving informed consent, is simply illogical and a good candidate for doublethink. Because other animals have an interest in liberty, field experiments are morally preferable to ones where animals are held captive in laboratories or where there is insufficient space for them to pursue their interests.

Despite the claims of those who adhere to the traditional paradigm, which assigns moral value based on the possession of autonomy and rationality, the moral relevance of sentience, rather than intelligence, is recognized in the prohibition against the use of severely mentally retarded humans in painful non-therapeutic medical research. However, if a higher degree of intelligence does not justify one human using another merely sentient human in scientific research, without their consent, then how can it entitle humans to exploit sentient nonhuman animals for the same purpose?

The clash between competing paradigms can result in deep chasms and misunderstandings between the factions because of the difference in basic assumptions and the different use of key terms. . . . In the great majority of cases, scientists using nonhuman animals in their research have motives which are noble and aimed at benefiting humans.

At the same time, we can all improve. Martin Luther King, Jr. once said that the "Universe bends toward justice." There are times in all our lives when, upon reflection, we realize that the end does not always justify the means and that we can do better in making this a more compassionate and just world.

SEEKING VIABLE ALTERNATIVES

The claim that putting an end to all or most research using nonhuman animals would bring scientific progress to a halt is surely an exaggeration, as well as an indication of how some scientists are unable to see beyond the old paradigm. In fact, it was not too long ago that some scientists felt that the use of human subjects, without their consent, was necessary for scientific progress. Similarly, "those scientists who have convinced themselves that there can't be viable scientific alternatives to the use of animals in research," Tom Regan contends, "are captives of mental habits that science abhors."[20] Rather than stopping all research, scientists are now being called by the newly emerging paradigm and the new ethics to redirect their practice from using nonhuman animals toward using more just alternative methods of scientific research.

The current paradigm shift is marked by a growing interest in the topic of alternatives to research using nonhuman animals. The concept of alternatives was developed by two British scientists, W. M. Russell and L. R. Burch, in 1959 and involves the principle of the "Three R's": Replacement, Reduction and Refinement.

The first "R," replacement, refers to situations where techniques, such as mathematical and computer models and tissue cultures, can be substituted for those using nonhuman animals. Also, in some cases, informed, consenting human subjects could be used in place of nonhuman subjects. For example, there is no shortage of people with AIDS who would like to volunteer to be subjects in experiments designed to find a cure for AIDS.[21] The fact that it might be less convenient to carry out research on humans instead of captive animals does not in itself justify using nonhuman animals. When alternative, morally acceptable techniques are available, they ought to be used.

Reduction refers to cutting back, whenever possible, on the number of nonhuman animals used in experiments. This involves the elimination of experiments that test trivial hypotheses or hypotheses whose truth or falsity is already sufficiently established, poorly designed experiments, and the use of nonhuman animals in experiments for duplication of drugs by competing firms. When nonhuman animals are used, the minimum number necessary for results should be used. For example, the National Cancer Institute in the course of only a few years has reduced the number of rodents used in cancer research by 80–90%. The Institute is switching to the use of cell culture screening systems which are turning out to work better than the standard nonhuman animal model systems.[22]

The third "R," refinement, refers to the modification of techniques to reduce the pain and distress suffered by laboratory animals. In line with this, animal welfare legislation now requires that principal investigators minimize animal pain and distress in their research projects.

We would also like to add a fourth "R": Respect. The experimental design should be compatible with respect, not only for nonhuman animal subjects, but also, if you are a user, for yourself as a researcher. Do you feel you are compromising your own moral dignity or that of those who work with you by participating in this experiment? Using captive animals places the experimenter in a position of superiority. When we hold a position of power over others—humans or nonhuman animals—this often turns into contempt for those we have power over, as well as a numbing toward their suffering. In experimentation using nonhuman animals, this contempt might be exhibited not only in a debased attitude toward "laboratory animals" but toward nonhuman animals in general.

A last question to ask is whether the experimental design can pass the test of publicity. The test of publicity states that we should do only those actions which a reasonable person or persons would deem morally acceptable. How do others, especially those new to the field or outside the field, respond to the experiment? Young children, especially, have not yet been socialized in the traditional paradigm which teaches them to regard other animals as "things." Consequently, they often develop close relationships with members of other species such as a cat or dog. Would you feel good about using one of your childhood animal companions in your experiment? If not, why not?

Philosopher David Hume believed that although reason may inform our moral decisions, it is sentiment or feeling that actually moves us to act on these decisions.[23] In deciding whether it is morally acceptable to use nonhuman animals in your particular experiment, you should listen to others—especially young people and others who are not so heavily invested in the old traditional paradigm; then listen to your own heart.

CONCLUSION

It is only by reference to religious myths and paradigms that we can justify a strict moral separation of humans and other animals. Science does not provide the criteria for such a division. As Mary Midgley points out: "Animals are not just one of the things with which people amuse themselves, like chewing-gum and water skis, *they are the group to which people belong*. We are not just rather like animals; we *are* animals."[24] . . .

The anthropocentric religious worldview began breaking up long before Darwin, with the knowledge that the earth is not the center of the universe but just another celestial body. The job was, in theory at least, completed by Darwin with the finding that human beings are not the center or apex of creation but, rather, members of a widely diverse animal community. However, knowledge alone does not mean abandonment of an entrenched worldview. Sometimes this process takes centuries.

While the moral ideal under the new ethics and the emerging post-modern paradigm would be to cease all non-therapeutic or coercive research on captive nonhuman animals, the four "R's" at least point us in this direction. . . .

As the "universe bends toward justice," if in fact this is happening, one can only hope that our concept of moral community will grow and become more inclusive. This new worldview is also going to force people to reexamine their attitudes toward other animals as sources of food, clothing, amusement and tethered companionship as well. Albert Schweitzer once said that we are not truly civilized if we concern ourselves only with the relation of humans to other humans. What is important is the relation of humans to all life.[25] Perhaps someday the new paradigm that will eventually replace the traditional paradigm will be similar to that espoused by Albert Schweitzer and Mahatma Gandhi and be based on respect for all living beings regardless of their resemblance to humans.

Until that time, the growing concern for the welfare and rights of nonhuman animals manifested in laws such as the Animal Welfare Act and in policy statements of such groups as the National Institutes of Health (1985), the Council for International Organizations of Medical Science (1985), and other professional groups are surely steps in the right direction and, as such, are to be applauded.

NOTES

1. Peter Singer, *Animal Liberation* (New York: Random House, 1990), p. 37.
2. Thomas Kuhn, *The Structure of Scientific Revolutions* (Chicago: University of Chicago Press, 1970), p. 10.
3. John Searle, Paul M. Churchland, and Patricia Smith Churchland, "Artificial Intelligence: A Debate," *Scientific American* 262 (1990), p. 25.
4. Peter Singer, *op. cit.*, p. 52.
5. *Ibid.*, pp. 221–222.
6. Kuhn, *op. cit.*, p. 76.
7. *Ibid.*, p. 70.
8. Andrew N. Rowan, "The Alternatives Concept," *Animal Welfare Information Newsletter* 2 (1991), p. 8.
9. Kuhn, *op. cit.*, p. 103.
10. *Ibid.*, p. 5.
11. Singer, *op. cit.*, pp. 90–91.
12. Kuhn, *op. cit.*, p. 78.
13. James Rachels, "Why Animals Have a Right to Liberty," in Tom Regan and Peter Singer (eds.), *Animals Rights and Human Obligations,* second edition (Englewood Cliffs, NJ: Prentice-Hall, 1989), p. 98.
14. Singer, *op. cit.*, p. 21.
15. Raymond G. Frey and William Paton, "Vivisection, Morals, and Medicine: An Exchange," *Journal of Medical Ethics* 9 (1983), p. 95.
16. Carl Cohen, "The Case for the Use of Animals in Biomedical Research," *New England Journal of Medicine* 315 (1986), p. 865.
17. *Ibid.*, p. 866.
18. Damme, "Infanticide: The Worth of an Infant under Law," *Medical History* 22 (1978), p. 1.
19. James Rachels, "Why Animals Have a Right to Liberty," from Tom Regan and Peter Singer, *Animal Rights and Human Obligations, op. cit.*, p. 120.
20. Tom Regan, *The Case for Animal Rights* (Berkeley, CA: The University of California Press, 1983), p. 455.
21. Rowan, *op. cit.*, pp. 1–2.
22. *Ibid.*, p. 2.
23. David Hume, *Enquiry Concerning the Principles of Morals,* Reprinted from the Edition of 1777 (LaSalle, IL: Open Court, 1946).
24. Mary Midgley, "The Concept of Beastliness: Philosophy, Ethics and Animals' Behavior," *Philosophy* 48 (1973), p. 114.
25. Albert Schweitzer, *The Philosophy of Civilization* (New York: Macmillan Co., 1949).

QUESTIONS FOR COMPREHENSION AND REFLECTION

1. According to Boss and Boss, what is the "traditional paradigm" and how does it support animal experimentation? Do you agree with Boss and Boss that this paradigm cannot be scientifically justified? Support your answers.
2. Do you agree with Boss and Boss that a paradigm shift away from animal experimentation is taking place in the biological sciences? Illustrate your answer with specific examples, particularly ones since 1994, when their article was published. If such a shift is occurring, is it morally desirable? Discuss how Cohen would most likely answer these questions.
3. Using the arguments presented in the article, discuss whether you think all nontherapeutic animal experimentation should be abolished or strictly limited. If so, discuss policies that might be implemented to stop or limit animal experimentation. If not, discuss what policies, if any, should be implemented to regulate animal experimentation.

1. Placebo Surgery and Parkinson's Disease

Researchers at the University of Colorado are studying the effects of using cells from embryos to replace brain cells destroyed by Parkinson's disease. When fifty-five-year-old George Doeschner's physician told him about the experimental surgery, Doeschner, who first developed symptoms of Parkinson's disease twelve years ago, applied to be part of the experiment. In Denver, Doeschner was prepped for surgery and sedated. A hole was drilled through his skull. The hole was then sewn up without any embryonic cells being inserted.

Doeschner was part of a double-blind placebo trial, in which half of the subjects received placebo surgery rather than the real thing. Doeschner was well aware that he might be part of the control group. He was also told that a fake operation could leave him a "vegetable." However, he believed that the benefits outweighed the risks. "I wanted to do something that would help everybody who has Parkinson's."[60]

DISCUSSION QUESTIONS

1. The National Institutes of Health agree with Doeschner. In fact, they even require placebo surgeries in certain types of research. Critics of placebo surgery, on the other hand, point out that no surgery, even fake surgery, is risk-free. Analyze the two positions. What are some premises that could be used in support of each position? Which argument is most compelling, and why?
2. Some ethicists object to using severely ill patients in experiments, arguing that these patients are unable to give genuine informed consent. Bioethicist Arthur Caplan, for example, maintains that the experiment in which Doeschner participated was not morally justified. "Consent is irrelevant," according to Caplan. "When you're dealing with desperate illness, people will consent to anything."[61] Discuss Caplan's position.
3. Imagine that you are Doeschner. Your wife and children are very opposed to your being part of the experiment because of the risks involved. They plead with you to wait until the experimental surgery has been approved by the FDA and then to have it. To what extent, if any, should their opposition to your participation in the experiment be taken into consideration in making your decision? Support your answer.
4. Discuss the moral issues involved in using cells from human embryos or fetuses to treat patients with Parkinson's disease.

2. Recruiting Patients as Research Subjects[62]

When the drug company SmithKline Beecham P.L.X. offered Dr. Arcan $1,610 for each patient he could recruit for a study on a new drug to shrink the prostate gland, he willingly agreed. During the routine checkup of one of his patients, sixty-four-year-old Thomas Parham, Dr. Arcan suggested that he join the drug study. When Parham asked why, since he had never had a problem with his prostate, Dr. Arcan replied that the experimental drug might prevent future problems. Trusting his advice, Parham agreed to be a subject in the experiment.

It turned out that Parham should not have been in the experiment because he had been hospitalized the previous year for a heart condition that disqualified him from the study. However, because Dr. Arcan had stated in the paperwork that the heart condition was not serious, the drug company granted an exemption.

Shortly after joining the study, Parham began complaining of fatigue, a symptom of a slowed heart rate. Dr. Arcan dismissed the complaint as emotional. A few weeks later, Parham asked to be dropped from the study. Days later, he was taken to the hospital and given a pacemaker. Parham was unable to prove that the experimental drug had aggravated his heart condition.

DISCUSSION QUESTIONS

1. Discuss the moral issues involved in physicians' recruiting their own patients as subjects for research. Under what conditions, if any, is this practice morally justified? Was it justified in this case study? Is the fact that the drug company paid Dr. Arcan to recruit subjects morally relevant? Would your answer be different if Dr. Arcan had told Parham he was getting paid to recruit Parham and had offered to share the money with him? Support your answers.
2. Referring to the Nuremberg Code and the Helsinki Declaration, discuss whether Parham's rights were violated. Did Parham give his informed consent to be in the study? Discuss what would constitute informed consent in this case and what legal or institutional controls should be put in place to ensure that patients' rights are protected in cases where physicians recruit their patients as subjects.
3. Approval of a new drug by the FDA requires that it first be tested on human subjects. Given this requirement, discuss how drug companies should recruit human subjects for their research.
4. Do physician-recruiters have a moral duty to enroll as subjects themselves in medical research? Discuss your answer in light of Jonas's rule of descending order.

3. Prisoners as Subjects in AIDS Research

A disproportionate number of prison inmates are HIV positive. In 1990, more than 20 percent of men admitted to the New York State prison system were HIV positive. Others become infected while in prison, mainly as a result of intravenous drug use.[63] In 1999, recently released prisoners accounted for one-sixth of AIDS cases in the United States.[64] Because of the difficulty in recruiting enough human subjects to receive FDA approval for new drugs, the University Center for AIDS Research, in collaboration with the Apollo Pharmaceutical Company, approaches the State Department of Corrections with a research proposal.

Dr. Kim, leader of the research team, opens the meeting by describing the experimental design. "Half of the group—500 inmates—will receive the new experimental drug," she explains. "The others will receive AZT, an existing treatment."

Dr. Silva, the chief medical officer of the Department of Corrections, nods. "There's no doubt that our prison medical facilities are overburdened. Allowing the research to be carried out here would provide a level of quality of medical care that we are currently unable to give to our prisoners who are HIV positive."

"That may be," responds Ms. Digby, assistant director of the State Department of Corrections. "But I think the solution is to improve the existing medical facilities by lobbying for more state support for our prisons, not to take advantage of prisoners as research subjects just so they can get proper medical care."

Dr. Kim interjects. "Except, as it is now, there are many benefits for prisoners in the study—better healthcare and living quarters. It may even save their lives."

"But it is these very incentives," Ms. Digby replies, "that diminish a prisoner's ability to give informed consent, since researchers are taking advantage of the conditions of deprivation in prison. How can a prisoner make a truly informed choice if it is his only option for getting proper medical care or escaping the boredom of prison life?"

"On the other hand," Dr. Kim counters, "is it fair to deny prisoners who are HIV positive the benefits of enrolling in studies on experimental treatments just because we may have to take additional precautions in obtaining their informed consent?"

"I agree with Dr. Kim," Mr. Potter from the ACLU adds. "It's a denial of a basic right to equal treatment to refuse prisoners access to experimental treatments because of their confinement or living conditions. To do so would be to add to their punishment in a way that is undeserved. It's true that prison life does restrict inmates. But it's even more paternalistic to deny prisoners the right to give their consent to take part in research."

"But prison is different than life outside," Ms. Digby replies. "Nothing is private here; there is no 'right to confidentiality' here. And there is a strong stigma attached to being HIV positive. Infected inmates are often shunned and even brutally attacked by other prisoners. Being in the study will be tantamount to wearing a neon sign flashing 'I'm HIV positive.' I'm not saying that we shouldn't approve the research; but, if we grant permission, we need some way to protect the prisoners who are subjects from discrimination and violence."

Mr. Potter shakes his head. "Risk or even death is a way of life in prison. The only place in prison where people don't die is in the research units. What is it that you are protecting them from?"[65]

"These men will probably also suffer from discrimination from the parole boards, who will be more reluctant to grant parole to someone who is HIV positive simply out of concern for public safety," says Ms. Digby in response. "Even if they do win parole, there is the problem of discrimination in employment, housing, and insurance because of their HIV status."

"Using prisoners in AIDS research could also increase discrimination against prisoners in general, since it sends a message to the public that prisoners are much more likely than the general population to be infected," Dr. Silva adds. "This could have repercussions for ex-prisoners who are not infected."

"It is true that there is a tradeoff here," Mr. Potter adds, "but to forbid prisoners to participate has even worse repercussions. Despite their limited options, it should be the prisoners themselves who make the final decision."

DISCUSSION QUESTIONS

1. Using a utilitarian cost/benefit analysis, discuss whether the use of prisoners in AIDS research is morally justified. What other moral considerations are relevant? Taking these considerations into account, create an argument regarding the moral permissibility of using prisoners as subjects in this case study.

2. If it is determined that using prisoners as subjects is morally permissible, who should be doing the research? Should private pharmaceutical companies be involved in research? Is it morally acceptable for prisons to benefit financially from research or to participate in medical research as a means of upgrading their healthcare systems?

Should prisoners receive compensation for their participation in clinical trials? Support your answers.

3. The prison officials decide to put together an eight-member institutional review board (IRB) to review this proposal and any future research proposals. Discuss who should be a member of the IRB and why.

4. Create a policy statement for the IRB regarding the use of prisoners in medical experiments and obtaining their informed consent. Compare and contrast your policy to those currently existing in law and in ethics codes on human research.

4. Excluding Women from Research

Twenty-six-year-old Lydia Nez, a graduate student in applied mathematics, has sickle cell disease. Although she is usually in good health and avoids, as best she can, situations that might precipitate a sickle cell crisis, the periodic attacks have left her feeling concerned about her future, including job prospects and obtaining private health insurance after she graduates. Her younger brother, Miguel, frequently needs blood transfusions because of the same condition. Several weeks ago, Miguel Nez enrolled in a study on an experimental drug for controlling sickle cell disease. Since this time, he has had no symptoms of the disease.

Encouraged by her brother's experience, Lydia Nez inquires about enrolling in the study, which is still in the process of recruiting new subjects. The experimental drug, she believes, may be her only hope for controlling her condition.

"I am sorry," the recruiter replies to her inquiry, "but we are only accepting men for this study."

"Why?" asks Nez. "Both my brother and I have sickle cell disease, and you accepted him for the study. What does my being a woman have to do with being accepted or rejected?"

"Women can become pregnant," the recruiter smiles.

"But I'm not pregnant," Lydia protests. "In fact, I'm not even sexually active, and I'm quite willing to keep things that way for the duration of the study. Miguel, on the other hand, has recently married, and he and his wife are trying to get pregnant. And I recently read a study that found that toxic substances can cause genetic abnormalities in sperm."

"Well, I don't know about that," the recruiter replies. "Anyway, it's different with men—as I said, they can't get pregnant. We can't take chances with women of child-bearing age. After all, you may change your mind or who knows what. And we do, as you can surely understand, have a duty to protect fetal life. Besides, we'll get more accurate data from the study if we use only men and don't have to deal with the effect of gender. That means that the drugs may be available soon. If the drug is approved, which hopefully will happen in the next five years, you can get it from your physician," the recruiter reassures her. "So everyone ends up benefiting and no one is put at undue risk."

"But if this new drug has never been tested on women, how will I know that it is safe for me?" Lydia asks in frustration. "And what if I am married then and even pregnant when the drug is finally available?"

The recruiter stands up and walks toward the door. "Look, rules are rules. They are for your protection." He opens the door and gestures for her to leave. "Thank you for stopping by."

DISCUSSION QUESTIONS

1. Analyze the arguments put forth by both the recruiter and Lydia Nez. Which person makes the stronger argument? What premises, if any, might you add to each argument? Would it make a difference if Nez were pregnant or sexually active? Support your answers.

2. Discuss the moral issues involved in the practice, in recruiting subjects for biomedical research, of defining women but not men primarily by their reproductive role. Should women who are fertile have the same right as men to make an informed decision regarding the risks and benefits of participating in medical research? What if a woman is pregnant or not using contraception? Support your answers. Discuss how a utilitarian and a rights ethicist might respond to these questions.

3. Do researchers have a moral duty to open studies to both men and women that offer potential benefits not available in ordinary treatment to all adults? Discuss the moral obligations of the researchers in this case study.

5. The Unwilling War Veteran

You are a physician in a veterans' hospital. In the past two months, twenty-seven patients have been admitted with a mysterious and fatal disease. All of them were stationed on the same military base in the Middle East, and you suspect that biological weapons may be to blame. Six of the patients have already died, and all but one of the remaining are in critical condition. Some of the veterans' family members have also begun to develop symptoms, leading you to fear that the disease may be contagious.

Dr. Kwame, another physician in the hospital, is a well-known researcher on Gulf War diseases. So far, her experiments have not yielded any leads for a cure. Her one hope is that your patient who is recovering from the disease carries an antibody. With your permission, she approaches him and asks if she can take blood and tissue samples for experimentation, as well as try out some experimental procedures on him. The patient answers, "No, I've already been through enough, and I just want to put this behind me."

DISCUSSION QUESTIONS

1. Would it be morally permissible in this case to pressure the patient to participate in the experiment? Who should try to convince the patient—the patient's physician or Dr. Kwame? What arguments might you use to try to get the patient's cooperation?

2. What are the moral rights and duties of the patient in this case? Does he have a duty to society to participate in this experiment? Discuss how Hans Jonas and Arthur Caplan might answer this question.

3. Unable to get the patient's permission, Dr. Kwame asks you if you will take extra blood and urine samples, as well as sneak in an experimental treatment with his regular medication. Reluctantly, you agree. She then develops a potential vaccine based on the stolen blood samples. Would it be morally permissible to test the vaccine on the dying patients even though they are no longer able to give their consent for the experiment? If the vaccine is a success, would it be morally permissible to market the vaccine if it was developed using ethically questionable means? Support your answers.

6. Whooping Cough and Children as Subjects

In March 1994, the U.S. Department of Health sponsored a randomized clinical trial involving a new vaccine against pertussis (whooping cough). The study was carried out in Sweden and Italy, because, unlike in the United States, most of the children in these countries had not been vaccinated. Consent for the children to participate in the study was first obtained from their parents.

The study came under sharp criticism from a leading Italian epidemiologist, since the current vaccine against pertussis is effective. Rather than being used as subjects in a study on a new vaccine, he argued, all the children should have been vaccinated against this potentially fatal disease with the existing vaccine. Defenders of the study responded that in Italy and Sweden withholding the vaccine from the children in the control group did not put them at extra risk because they would not normally have been vaccinated. Thus, the chances of the children in the control group catching whooping cough were the same as they had been before the children were enlisted as subjects in the experiment.

DISCUSSION QUESTIONS

1. Does justice require that the existing vaccine, even though it may not be as effective as the new vaccine, be used with children in Italy and Sweden, as it is with children in the United States? How do the benefits and risks to the children in the experiment weigh against the benefits to future children who might have access to the new vaccine?
2. Was the use of children as subjects in this experiment morally justified? Did withholding the existing vaccine exploit the children's circumstances? Support your answers. Discuss how Jonas might respond to these questions.
3. Discuss whether the parents had the right to give surrogate consent for their children to be used in this study. Discuss how you would have responded had you been approached regarding the participation of your child in this study.
4. Compare and contrast the moral issues involved in this study with those involved in the AIDS studies in Africa.

7. Of Mice and Men

About 10 million mice and rats are used annually in medical research. In the 1980s, scientists at Yale successfully transplanted foreign genes into mice. Mice, who share about 85 percent of their genes with humans, have since become the most popular nonhuman animals used in medical research. At the Induced Mutant Resource Lab, part of the Jackson Laboratory in Bar Harbor, Maine, mutant mice models are studied to determine their usefulness for scientific research. When the lab first opened in 1993, it distributed about one hundred mutant mice. By 1998, it was shipping 80,000 mutant mice to research labs at a cost of approximately $10 to $70 per mouse.[66]

Transgenic mice are used for research on diabetes, epilepsy, cancer, heart disease, drug addiction, obesity, and HIV. These mice, who are genetically bred to get sick, may be born without an immune system or may suffer from gross obesity, seizures, or other medical problems. On the other hand, the use of transgenic mice has contributed to a 50 percent reduction in the use of other animals in research, since more accurate research results can be achieved with transgenic mice.

DISCUSSION QUESTIONS

1. Some healthcare ethicists, including zoologist John McArdle of the Alternative Research & Development Foundation, oppose the widespread use of mice in medical research. "They're not pieces of lab equipment," says McArdle. "They certainly suffer during research."[67] Discuss under what conditions, if any, it is morally permissible to use mice as research subjects. For example, is the use of transgenic mice justified in medical experiments that save human lives? In medical experiments for conditions that are not fatal to humans? In medical experiments for health problems related to human life-style choices, such as smoking or drug use? Support your answers.

2. Many transgenic mice carry human genes. Does this fact alter their moral value as research subjects? Should there be different moral standards regarding the use of animals who are genetically more closely related to humans? If so, why? Support your answers.

3. Does the decrease in the use of other animals in medical research justify the creation and use of genetically altered mice if it contributes to a significant overall decrease in the number of nonhuman animals being used in lab experiments? Discuss how a utilitarian, a Muslim healthcare ethicist, an animal welfare advocate, and an animal rights advocate might answer this question. Which presents the strongest argument? Support your answer.

4. In April 1999, Animal Liberation Front (ALF) activists broke into labs at the University of Minnesota, smashed laboratory equipment, destroyed research information, and stole forty-eight transgenic mice. Was their action morally justified, or are they simply terrorists? Role-play a discussion between one of the members of the ALF and one of the research scientists on the ethics of this action. Analyze the merits and weaknesses of each argument.

8. The Alien Abduction[68]

What was previously passed off as imagination and science fiction turns out to be true! At 3:07 A.M., a strange-looking craft was found floating off the coast of Florida. Upon investigation, it was found to be an elaborate laboratory. The survivors told of their grisly experiences as subjects in laboratory experiments run by an alien species. Apparently, the aliens had been using human subjects in research for at least sixty years. Human fetuses were removed from abducted pregnant women and used as subjects in experiments on ectogenesis and in research on genetic engineering and organ transplants. The human subjects were housed in small pens, which were kept clean and well supplied with food and water. The aliens also used an anesthetic or amnesiac when they performed operations. Most of the subjects were painlessly euthanized when they were no longer needed. Others were returned to their homes on the surface until they were needed for further tests. Several human subjects, especially those bred in the laboratory, refused to leave, protesting vociferously when rescuers tried to remove them from their pens.

Because of the availability of human subjects, the alien species has been able to make tremendous strides in improving the quality of their lives on earth. They apparently are a highly advanced, intelligent life-form that communicates entirely by telepathy. They are unable to understand human language, which sounds to them like babbling. They regard humans as a much lower form of life and see no moral problem in using humans to benefit their own species. Indeed, they believe the use of human subjects in their research is a moral duty, since it has done so much to benefit their own species.

DISCUSSION QUESTIONS

1. If you could communicate with the aliens, what arguments might you use to try to convince them that they should not be using human subjects in their research? Do you agree with them that higher species have a moral right, and perhaps even a moral duty, to use lower species as a means of advancing themselves? Support your answers. Apply your answers to the issue of human experimentation on sentient nonhuman animals.

2. What criteria should be met for the experiments to be ethical? Is the fact that many of these humans were bred solely for the purpose of experimentation morally relevant? What if they had been genetically engineered with alien genes? If the research was unethical, would the rescuers be justified in using research results left behind in the lab related to cures for lethal diseases such as AIDS and cancer? Support your answers.

3. According to the Helsinki Declaration, incompetent subjects, as the humans were considered by the aliens, may be used in medical experiments if the experiments have therapeutic value for the subjects. The Nuremberg Code, in contrast, prohibits experimentation on nonconsenting subjects. Discuss the merits of the two codes in light of this case study.

4. Most of the humans who were bred in the alien laboratories refused to be "rescued." Does their refusal constitute consent to be included in the alien experiments? Is forcefully rescuing these human subjects morally justified if an alien ship is waiting nearby to retrieve them and the humans express a desire to return to the aliens? Support your answers.

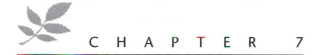

Organ Transplantation

Dr. Christiaan Barnard's first meeting with Louis Washkansky to discuss the possibility of performing a heart transplant was uneventful. The dying, fifty-five-year-old Washkansky appeared to show little interest in finding out more about this radically new operation. According to Barnard's account of their meeting, Washkansky's immediate response was "That's fine with me—I'm ready and waiting for it." After Barnard spoke further about giving him a new heart, Washkansky replied, "So I'm ready to go ahead." And nothing more was said. As Barnard turned to leave the room, he noticed Washkansky simply return to his book, a Western. Barnard reflected:

> How . . . could he return to pulp fiction after being suddenly cast into the greatest drama of his life? . . . No man in the history of the world had ever met the surgeon who was going to cut out his heart and replace it with a new human one—at least, not until this moment, which was now being lost somewhere in a Western novel.[1]

This incident is indeed revealing. Barnard pondered about Washkansky's lack of enthusiasm given the historic and medical magnitude of the operation. Nevertheless, Barnard himself made no further effort to engage his patient in conversation. He could have explored the patient's expectations and fears, but he did not. He let his patient escape into pulp fiction.

Washkansky was the first human to receive a heart transplant. He received his "new" heart on December 3, 1967, and lived with it for eighteen days before dying of lobar pneumonia on December 21. Washkansky's death was a crushing blow to Barnard. In his own words, Barnard "crash-landed." But he was not about to give up. At Washkansky's autopsy, Barnard realized the importance of continuing.

> I had not failed. I had succeeded. The first attempt, with all its pain and sorrow, had been made for the second. To now turn back would be to deny the first—*to turn away from Louis Washkansky's dream.*[2]

Note that, in what appears to be an unexamined projection, Barnard describes *his* goal as being Washkansky's.

In any case, Barnard approached fifty-eight-year-old retired dentist Philip Blaiberg as a candidate for the second heart transplant. The following accounts give two renditions of the encounter. First is the condensed account given by Blaiberg:

Professor Barnard spoke in low tones. "I feel like a pilot who has just crashed. . . . Now I want you, Dr. Blaiberg, to help me by taking up another plane as soon as possible to get back my confidence." . . .

"Professor Barnard," I said at once, "I want to go through with it now more than ever—*not only for my sake but for you and your team who has put so much into your effort to save Louis Washkansky.*"[3] (italics added)

What is particularly revealing is Blaiberg's identification with what he perceived as Barnard's, and his team's, mission to successfully perform the transplant. If this account is accurate, it would have been incumbent on Barnard to discuss Blaiberg's expectations with him further in order to ensure more genuinely informed consent to the procedure, but no record of any such conversation exists.

In contrast, Barnard's account of his meeting with Blaiberg depicts a patient who seems less than willing to discuss the details of the operation or his own fears and expectations. When Barnard raised the prospect of a heart transplant, Blaiberg's response, according to this second account, was "The sooner, the better . . . I'll co-op . . . cooperate in every way." And that was it.

This account is also revealing. Whether Blaiberg's or Barnard's account is more accurate, one thing seems certain: Barnard did not make the necessary effort to engage his patient further in conversation. Further discussion would have been essential not only to clarify the realistic aims of the procedure, but also to explore and clear up any unrealistic expectations and unavoidable fears.

This episode is instructive with regard to communication and its effect on informed consent. First, there is a critical need for physicians to separate self-interest from the interests of the patient. Otherwise, distortions may be created by patients and sustained by physicians. Second, if the surgeon demonstrates an inability or unwillingness to engage in open, honest discussion about the procedure, including its risks and benefits and the patient's expectations regarding the operation and its outcome, meaningful consent is in effect annulled.

A SKETCH OF THE ETHICAL ISSUES

We cannot help but feel a profound sense of awe when we contemplate the intricacies of organ transplantation. The passage of one organ into another body is complex. The donor's organ must be excised at precisely the right time in order for the organ to remain properly oxygenated, and exact criteria for determining brain death must be established to ensure proper timing for removal of the organ from a dead body. In addition, the recipient must be properly prepared. Surgical methods for excising the donor organ have become more precise, enabling surgeons to more successfully implant the organ into its new "home" and to seamlessly join the organ and its blood vessels. Also, more effective immunosuppressant agents allow the recipient's body to accept the new organ. While cyclosporine was a big advance over previous agents, the new immunosuppressant FK-506 is claimed to be even better. All these improvements have brought about a boom in the transplant business, and typical survival rates continue to improve. For example, 70 percent of renal, heart, and liver transplant patients survive up to five years. Sight has been restored in nearly 85 percent of corneal transplants for cases of blindness.[4]

A fair share of moral problems, however, accompany this monumental success. In fact, organ transplantation is a clear example of technical progress outpacing moral sensitivity and responsibility. Despite its ability to save lives and offer a better quality of life to numerous patients, organ transplantation elicits several moral concerns.

Typical Objections to Transplantation

Those opposed to organ transplantation argue that transplantation research illustrates modern medicine's ethos of the technological imperative; that is, because the technical means—in this case, transplantation technologies—to alleviate a problem exist, we feel compelled to use those means. Furthermore, it is argued, organ transplantation using cadaver organs violates respect for the deceased. The bodies of the deceased in many cultures are viewed as symbols deserving of respect. However, it can be argued that symbols should not assume more importance than the reality they are meant to represent. Even if we agree that the newly dead should be treated with reverence, we can argue that different obligations exist toward the newly dead and toward those who still live.

A related argument against organ transplants is that maintaining bodily integrity is crucial. In the case of a kidney transplant, for example, transplantation from a living donor disrupts bodily integrity. According to the religious idea of **stewardship,** while alive we are stewards over our bodies, which are gifts given to us in trust by God. Yet this stewardship position assumes a certain set of religious premises. Our pluralist society, with its various religious beliefs, enjoys no religious consensus regarding the justifiability of organ transplantation. Many major religions do accept organ transplantation, while others find it questionable. Therefore, arguments against transplantation based on premises other than religious claims carry more weight.

Some opponents of organ transplantation maintain that it leads to a view of the body as a commodity with interchangeable parts and that the use of these body parts is unnatural and could lead to a diminished respect for persons' individual rights. Because of the severe shortage of donor organs, it is feared that certain categories of patients—such as patients who are near brain death, those in persistent vegetative states, or infants who are anencephalic—may be viewed more as potential organ donors than as patients who can still be treated. Also, certain contexts of transplantation, for example, interracial transplants, could lead to exploitation. Minorities and other vulnerable groups could be unfairly targeted as potential organ donors. For example, Dr. Barnard's first heart transplant involved a white recipient and a black donor. This fear of exploitation could be alleviated by constructing rigorous procedural rules and protocols. For instance, it is a rule that members of the healthcare team who care for the patients must not be involved in any way with the transplantation.

There are also questions about what constitutes "medical success" for a transplant recipient. Does the mere fact of survival signal success? A certain length of survival? Quality of life? Whose quality of life are we talking about? Can we make fair decisions about retransplants when there is less likelihood that a retransplant will extend the recipient's life?

Another concern involves autonomy and consent. Genuine informed consent has many ramifications. Were the donor and the recipient sufficiently informed? Was the consent voluntary? Were the donor and the recipient competent in consenting? What role should the families of donors have? Practically speaking, families appear to

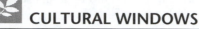

CULTURAL WINDOWS

BODILY INTEGRITY:
Japanese and Jewish Views

Emiko Namihira, a Japanese anthropologist, tells of a terrible airline crash a number of years ago in Japan. The entire crew and all the passengers of a Japan Air Lines flight perished. At the crash sight, officials cordoned off a large area to search for bodies. While they conducted their official search for remains, family members were permitted to go on-site to help in the effort to collect body parts! They were allowed the opportunity to help in restoring some bodily integrity to their deceased family members. In Japan, bodily integrity is critically important. Although it was virtually impossible to collect all body parts for all the victims, the individual families of the victims formed their own community in a collective effort to restore at least a semblance of wholeness to the dead bodies.

This emphasis in Japan on maintaining bodily integrity has its source in numerous philosophical and religious traditions in Japan. To begin with, traditional Japanese philosophy has never considered a dualistic relationship between the mind and the body. For Japanese, mind and body are not two separate entities but instead work together in a mutually defining and interactive way. Mind, or mental activity, cannot be understood apart from body, or bodily activity. Together they form the self. Upon bodily death, selfhood is affected, so there is a long-established taboo against violating the corpse through autopsy.

A Buddhist expression of this position was put forth by Kukai (774–835), the founder of Shingon Buddhism, who emphasized the notion of being a buddha in and through our bodies. This same idea is expressed in Shinto, the indigenous religion of Japan. For example, Motoori Norinaga (1730–1801) pointed out that the body–mind unity can be bodily expressed through

exercise the final say over the donation of a family member's organs. Should they have veto power over an individual's prior consent?

On a broader level, how many resources should we allocate to transplantation research when other areas of need exist, including cancer prevention, maternity care, nursing home care, and chronic pain programs? On a narrower level, how do we choose equitably among the various transplant candidates? Given the severe shortage of available organs, is it fair for single individuals to receive multiple organs when these organs can be distributed among more people?

Who Is Adrian Kantrowitz?

In addition to the objections already mentioned, organ transplantation gives rise to a host of other ethical concerns. Some were highlighted during the first heart transplant, performed by Christiaan Barnard at Cape Town, South Africa. Philosopher Gregory Pence provides an insightful analysis of these issues.[5] The principal ethical issues originally centered around the tremendous pressure surgeons and institutions

poetic speech. In both Buddhist and Shinto teachings, the body is a living expression of the self. Thus, every effort must be made to sustain bodily wholeness.

Jewish instructions regarding issues in medical ethics stem primarily from the Old Testament, or Hebrew Scripture, and the Talmud, which forged the legal framework for scriptural teachings. These teachings and interpretations became systematized through legal codes such as that of Moses Maimonides in the twelfth century and the *Shulhan Arukh* (the Prepared Table) in the sixteenth century. These works contain special instructions regarding the human body and how it ought to be treated. There is a strong belief in the notion of "stewardship," the belief that our bodies are given to us by God in temporary trust and only God has full ownership.

According to Jewish tradition, the body is purified right after death by being ritually washed. Every effort is made to keep the body whole. Jewish teachings emphasize that this enables the body to be resurrected when the Messiah arrives. This belief in the holiness of the body and the need to maintain bodily integrity explains why incisions and cremation are generally prohibited and why Jewish families often insist on burying parts of the body that may have been amputated along with the body of the deceased. Furthermore, dissecting a corpse for anatomical research is permitted only under certain strict circumstances: if required by law; if the deceased has given prior consent; if necessary in order to save another person's life, for example, as by detecting possible hereditary factors that may lead to death. Even in these cases, final approval must be given by both the family and their rabbi. These stipulations were reinforced in 1953 by Israel's parliament, the Knesset, when it passed the Anatomy and Pathology Law. Despite these restrictions, Orthodox Jews staged protests in the 1960s alleging that the sanctions were being abused and autopsies were taking place without familial and rabbinical approval. Nevertheless, the 1953 ruling has persisted.

faced, and continue to face, to be the first to successfully perform certain procedures. This pressure to be pioneers in their specialties often provokes degrees of professional territorialism among physicians. For instance, some American surgeons were highly critical of the fact that Barnard was the first surgeon to perform a transplant. Not only was Barnard trained in America, but it was felt that Norman Shumway of Stanford, California, who had been preparing for the procedure for some time, should have been the pioneer. Critics argued further that at the time of Barnard's operation immunosuppressant agents were inadequately developed, so the survival of a heart recipient was likely to be of short duration. They questioned whether Barnard's operation was truly in his patient's best interest or whether his motive was actually to achieve prestige and fame.

Who is Adrian Kantrowitz? He was the first surgeon to perform a heart transplant on a newborn infant, using the heart of an anencephalic baby. The infant who received the heart lived only for a few hours. The point we are making is this: Had Kantrowitz performed this delicate operation before Barnard's transplant, he, not Barnard, would have made the headlines.[6]

ISLAMIC VIEWS ON BODILY INTEGRITY

Muslims maintain a strict belief in the so-called stewardship we have over our bodies. We do not totally own our bodies; our bodies and lives are given to us as gifts from Allah. Muslims generally resist autopsies because of their prevailing belief in the resurrection of the body after death. A passage in the Quran states:

(O man) follow not that whereof thou hast no knowledge. Lo! the hearing and the sight and the heart—of each of these it will be asked.

This passage is interpreted as referring to the moment of resurrection after death; that is, when the body is resurrected, the heart, hearing, and sight need to be present, since they will be cross-examined.[7] Nevertheless, Muslims believe that while we are alive we are the temporary guardians of our bodies, so despite a widespread reluctance to donate organs, a transplant that may save another's life is encouraged.

A review of Muslim teachings reveals various opinions and interpretations of fundamental precepts. For example, all Muslims believe that it is crucial to maintain bodily integrity. At the same time, there are times when this may not be possible. According to one interpretation, what matters is how we use our body while still alive and whether its use is for a just cause. A jihad (holy war) constitutes a just cause, so in this case Muslims are called to sacrifice self for others. In another interpretation, saving another's life by using the organs of someone who has died has priority over maintaining the bodily integrity of the deceased.

What about donating body parts while still alive? The matter then becomes more complex. For instance, some Muslim commentators hold that the donation of a sole existing organ, such as the heart or the liver, while one is still alive is wrong because it is an instance of suicide. In Islamic law, suicide is forbidden, since one's body is given in temporary trust from Allah and is not one's property. On the other hand, the donation of one of a pair of organs, such as a kidney or a lung, is permitted under certain conditions. First, the donor must freely consent without any degree of coercion; this means that there must not be any economic exploitation, such as offering monies to a donor in poverty. Second, the donation itself must not seriously threaten the donor's health. Third, although Muslims can receive organs from non-Muslims, Muslims are commonly forbidden to donate organs to non-Muslims. Muslim teachings point to the value of sustaining Muslim lives if at all possible.[8] Islamic law further prohibits the use of organs from those who are classified as "terminally ill" and thus not yet brain dead. The meaning of "terminally ill" is, in itself, vague; since Islamic law accepts the brain death standard, removal of organs from someone not yet dead generally constitutes murder unless some prior consent was obtained from the patient and authorization given by the family.

The first heart transplant is instructive in demonstrating that celebrity status is bestowed on those who are medical pioneers. In the highly visible field of organ transplantation, this status brings with it huge amounts of financial support in the form of research endowments. Not only does the individual surgeon cull the honors, but the institution profits as well. For example, the University of Pittsburgh Medical Center's Presbyterian Hospital continues to be one of the most prestigious transplant centers in the world, to a great extent due to the pioneering efforts of transplant surgeon Thomas Starzl, who performed both the first human liver transplant, in 1963, and the first baboon-to-human liver transplant, in 1992.

This situation raises a related issue—the role of the media. In their effort to report the facts, journalists often engage in a style of reporting that tends to sensationalize an event. This usually involves taking events out of context and sometimes misrepresenting and even distorting facts. Media accounts are powerfully influential in that they bias the public's expectations of medicine and new medical treatments. Media inaccuracy needs to be taken into account whenever "medical miracles" are touted.

While on the surface public recognition of breakthrough medical procedures may appear to be justified, it opens up some hard-hitting ethical questions. One question involves the relationship between federal funding for research and the institutions that receive this funding. Does the acquisition of sizable research funding compromise the mission of universities and their programs? Shouldn't universities maintain a critical distance between societal values and governmental and political priorities?

Another question pertains to broader concerns regarding overall allocation of funds. For example, research funding for transplant programs at Pittsburgh–Presbyterian is quite sizable, yet many other programs affect more people. Should programs dealing with heart-disease prevention and treatment, cancer, chronic pain, and pediatrics lose funding to transplantation research? Shifting funds from these programs means they will inevitably be diminished or dropped.

Determining Death

Another ethical concern is determining the clinical and legal criteria of death. In the case of liver, pancreas, and heart transplants, the donor must be dead before the removal of the organ. Otherwise, removal of the organ would constitute murder. Because advances in medical technology, such as the ventilator, enable the heart and lungs to continue to function while the patient is kept alive, exact criteria for determining the death of a patient are necessary.

In 1969, the Harvard Ad Hoc Committee on Brain Death set forth specific criteria to determine **brain death,** which is defined as the irreversible dysfunction of both the cortical region of the brain and the brain stem. The Harvard criteria, described in Chapter 8, revolve around the absence of spontaneous reflexes associated with the brain stem. This absence must be attested to by two physicians, twenty-four hours apart. Furthermore, these physicians must have no role in any potential organ transplantation.

Since brain death is accepted as a legal definition of death in many countries, brain dead donors are not being killed for their organs, but the brain death standard raises other questions. For example, what about harvesting organs from patients who either are in a persistent vegetative state or are anencephalic? A persistent vegetative state occurs when the higher brain function is lost due to a temporary lack of oxygen.

CULTURAL WINDOWS

BRAIN DEATH IN JAPAN

The Diet, Japan's legislative body, has not accepted total brain death as the legal definition of death. Japan shares this resistance against brain death with Israel. In fact, the two countries are the only developed nations that do not officially recognize brain death. Many Japanese physicians remain wary of setting forth exact empirical criteria for determining death. This attitude may be supported by Buddhist teachings, particularly those based on the Abhidharma texts, which address issues of personal identity and existence. These teachings provide little basis for citing the brain as the determinative feature of human identity, which is not associated with simply a single physical organ. Since Buddhist teachings do not assign any special status to the brain, the dysfunction of the brain does not necessarily mean death. Buddhist teachings allude to the metaphor of Indra's Net, a net that holds a bril-liant jewel at every knot. Human identity is compared to a jewel in the net. Just as each jewel is reflected in all the others, each individual identity is reflected in the whole of all other beings. This image is a powerful one in Buddhism.

According to traditional Shinto teachings, which form the cornerstone of many Japanese beliefs, life in some sense is still present in the body as long as the body remains warm. This is one reason why the Japanese are reluctant to perform autopsies on newly "dead" bodies. Moreover, Shinto customs reflect the belief that a waiting period is required before actually proclaiming a person dead, since it is possible that the soul may reenter the body. Survivors pray that the soul will return to the body. Thus, using a brain death criterion may declare a person to be dead prematurely. Shinto holds that death occurs when the soul departs the body,

In anencephaly, the cerebral hemispheres of the brain are absent. In both conditions, higher brain performance is dysfunctional or lacking altogether, yet since the brain stem remains intact there is no brain death. Therefore, harvesting organs in these two situations is unjustifiable, at least in American culture, in which legal death entails both biological death (irreversible cessation of brain stem activity) and the permanent loss of consciousness (irreversible loss of the neocortex).

PROCURING ORGANS

In 1996, more than 55,000 patients were on organ transplant waiting lists throughout the United States. In that same year, nearly 20,000 organ transplants were performed, and of those who remained on waiting lists an estimated 4,000 patients died. This means that over 60 percent of the nation's organ donation potential was not achieved.[9]

but when this occurs is not known with certainty.[10]

For the Japanese, if any one organ is central, it is the heart, not the brain. Japanese have traditionally placed more importance on the heart than on the brain as being critical to personal identity. The Japanese word for heart, *kokoro*, does not mean "anatomical heart" as much as "self." In contrast, American culture assigns more importance to the brain as the primary organ in determining personal identity.[11]

Despite Japan's ongoing resistance to the concept of brain death, on June 17, 1997, the Diet approved a bill stipulating that a brain dead person can be defined as dead if that same person has given prior consent both for organ transplantation and for being diagnosed as brain dead. Brain death is therefore allowed only in strict utilitarian circumstances—to enable heart transplants. This ruling in effect allows for heart transplants, which have been officially prohibited in Japan for nearly three decades. However, since the ruling took effect, many Japanese have still been hesitant to donate their hearts upon their death. A study released by the Japanese government showed that only 2.6 percent of Japanese had signed donor cards, and a number of Japanese have died waiting for hearts, even after passage of the bill.[12]

The 1997 bill, however, did lead to Japan's first legal heart transplant, which took place on February 28, 1999. The donor was a man in his forties who had consented to donate his heart, liver, and kidneys if he was determined to be brain dead. In a coma after suffering a stroke and a brain hemorrhage, he was pronounced brain dead, and his organs were removed. This case was only the second heart transplant in Japanese history. The first occurred in 1968; since then, heart transplantation had been officially banned until the 1997 ruling. However, despite the new ruling and Japan's first legal heart transplant, many Japanese physicians are still reluctant to think of brain death as real death, partly due to the uncertainty in applying medical criteria in order to determine brain death.

Procuring Organs from Cadavers

How do we form a fair method and policy for obtaining organs? The need for organs far exceeds what is available. While many Americans seem to favor the idea of receiving an organ if it means keeping them alive, many are apparently reluctant to commit themselves to be official organ donors.

The majority of organs used for transplantation come from cadavers. In the United States, a high value is placed on the principle of altruism, consistent with the autonomy model, in which altruism is an exercise of self-determination that goes beyond the call of duty. Unless there is some indication to the contrary, most Americans feel that it is unjustifiable to use another's organs. Thus, organ donation offers an opportunity to act altruistically. Since individual autonomy is valued, it is up to the individual to decide whether to donate organs on his or her death. One problem, however, is that, even though we cherish individual autonomy in principle, in actual practice the family often has the final say. Thus, even if individuals have signed their donor cards or indicated on their driver's license their willingness to donate organs, the family's veto of the request contributes to the wholesale shortage of available organs.

Some states legally require healthcare professionals to request consent from the family to use the organs of deceased family members in the hope that this **required request** will encourage consent. Yet obtaining consent in this way has not met with success. One reason is that hospital staff naturally find it difficult to approach family members, who are already going through their own personal grief. Furthermore, sudden deaths in which an organ becomes immediately available may occur near institutions that do not perform transplants, and the hospital staff may be less aware of transplantation issues and benefits.

Another suggested way to procure organs is to adopt the system of **presumed consent,** used in countries such as France and Singapore. In contrast to the U.S. presumption of refusal to donate organs unless stipulated otherwise, presumed consent assumes that individuals are willing to donate their organs unless they have given a clear indication of refusal. Family members still have the final say.

Another possible approach is a policy of reciprocity, whereby a person's chances of obtaining an organ are greater if he or she has previously indicated a willingness to donate. For instance, in Singapore, those who register as eventual donors acquire priority for receiving kidneys if they ever need them.

Even though most organs for transplantation come from cadavers, it is inaccurate to refer to them as "donor" organs unless the deceased previously requested that they be used for transplant. Moreover, cadaver organs are becoming scarcer, leading to an increased reliance on live donors, particularly donors who are related to the recipient.

Procuring Organs from Living Donors

In the United States, there are four legal conditions regarding the procuring of organs from living donors. First, the donor must give genuine consent. This means that the donor must be sufficiently informed as to potential risks and benefits, the consent must be voluntary and free of coercion, and the donor must be competent to make the request. Second, the donor must be in a sound state of health, both physically and mentally. Third, the intended transplantation must have a good chance of success. This condition is problematic, since what constitutes a "good chance of success" is not quite clear. For instance, is a 50 percent chance of survival considered "good"? Fourth, the living donor and the recipient must either be related to each other or be spouses. This is another problematic requirement. Why limit organ donation to family members when what really matters is correct tissue match and positive medical outcome? This last requirement implies some suspicion regarding the motives of strangers who donate organs.

These conditions raise additional questions. Is donation of organs by children precluded? Suppose a child offers to donate his or her bone marrow or kidney to a sibling. At what age does such an offer become sufficiently autonomous? In Canada, it is illegal in nine provinces to use minors and mentally disabled adults as donor organs. Furthermore, if we restrict organ donation to family members could emotional pulls become so strong that they compromise an autonomous decision? We can easily imagine family members so pulled by their attachment to the patient that their reasoning becomes impaired. What about emotional blackmail, which occurs when a family member feels pressured into donating an organ without really desiring to do so? From a medical

MUSLIMS AND LIVE ORGAN DONORS

Whom do Muslims look to as potential live donors? First, they consider those whom they regard as "outcasts," including enemies, prisoners, felons, and others who are deemed harmful to Islamic society. Then they consider those who voluntarily donate their organs. However, these volunteers must meet certain conditions:

- The voluntary donation must not be made under any sort of pressure. Muslims strictly forbid the selling and buying of organs. The marketing of organs is viewed as an "inhuman act" for a variety of reasons. First, since the body is in total trust to Allah, it is not completely owned by us. There can be no legal sale transactions regarding that which is in temporary trust. Second, the removal of organs with its accompanying injuries to the body and health cannot be justified on the basis of one's economic situation. Third, sanctioning the trade in organs would result in the blatant exploitation by the affluent of vulnerable classes such as the destitute, children, and the mentally disabled, as has been documented in Egypt. Fourth, on a broader scale, the richer countries would most likely exploit developing countries. At the same time, this prohibition does not preclude voluntarily offering a gift to an organ donor.

- The organ donation must not endanger the donor's health.

- Muslims are forbidden to donate to non-Muslims; however, non-Muslims can donate to Muslims.

Muslims can make voluntary consent as well as a signed will that takes effect when the donor is deceased. Even without this prior consent, in certain cases the final decision can be made by the Office of the Attorney General. Furthermore, proxy consent can be made for minors and the mentally disabled.

Muslim culture draws a strict line of separation between those who are deceased with relatives and those who are deceased without relatives. For example, autopsies and the removal of the eyes for eye banks can be performed on those deceased without relatives, whereas these practices are generally prohibited on those deceased with relatives. Despite this, however, Islamic law provides more protection for the rights of the deceased than do other countries. For example, in India, it is permitted to remove the cornea from anyone who is deceased, and France holds to the notion of presumed consent.

In determining how organs are to be distributed, Muslim physicians themselves decide who the recipients will be, using one of two possible strategies. First, they can draw lots, relying on the will of Allah. This method might be used if there are several potential recipients, all of whom are histocompatible. Drawing lots is based on the example of Muhammad, whose wives drew lots to determine who would accompany him during his travels. Second, they can decide on the grounds of seeking the maximal benefit for the respective recipients. This entails ensuring the best possible match between donor and recipient. Physicians also need to ascertain that there is a strong likelihood the organ recipient will recover following the procedure.[13]

perspective, we can also ask what medical benefit the donor receives. There seems to be no real medical benefit, while there are certainly medical risks, depending on the procedure. For instance, kidney donation involves risks that are not minor, and these risks are accompanied by soreness and inconvenience. Even if the donor understands the risks and still chooses to donate a kidney, should medical professionals think twice about going ahead with the procedure, since the donor receives no real medical gain? On the other hand, as a general rule, physicians accept research subjects who do not stand to gain medically from the experimental procedure.

Procuring Fetal Tissue

The prospect of transplanting cells from aborted fetuses has generated a unique set of moral issues. Researchers believe that fetal tissue can be used to help patients suffering from serious degenerative diseases such as Parkinson's disease, Alzheimer's disease, acquired immune deficiency syndrome (AIDS), and Huntington's disease. Some patients suffering from these conditions have already received brain tissue from aborted fetuses. They seem to be showing signs that fetal tissue, which is less likely to be rejected, offers a better chance of effective therapy for these conditions. Scientists also believe that fetal tissue transplants can aid patients suffering from diabetes, skin diseases, and certain types of blindness.

There is already a long history of research on fetal tissue, particularly in studies related to cancer and infectious diseases. However, the road to fetal tissue transplant research has been rocky. In the late 1980s, the National Institutes of Health (NIH) established an advisory group, the Human Fetal Tissue Transplantation Research Panel, to look into the transplantation of fetal tissue and to come up with sound guidelines. The members on the panel agreed that the guidelines must prohibit both paying for fetal tissue and specifying certain individuals to receive the tissue, such as family members of the donor. The panel seemed opposed to giving women any unfair incentive to procure an abortion.

However, in the face of opposition by various groups because fetal transplant research would involve tissue from induced abortions, the Bush administration in 1988 banned further federal funding of such research. Much of the opposition came from anti-abortionists, who argued that permitting fetal research on aborted fetuses would lead to further widespread legitimization of abortion. They also held that such research would induce persons to deliberately have abortions in order to alleviate certain conditions, such as Alzheimer's disease. Congress tried to overturn the ban by inserting a clause in the NIH Reauthorization Act, but the bill was vetoed by President Bush.

The ban did not halt fetal tissue research, however, and laboratory studies continued. Nor did the ban prohibit private funding of transplant research. Nevertheless, the impetus was slowed over the five years the moratorium remained in existence. On January 22, 1993, President Clinton removed the ban on federal funding. Since then, scores of grant proposals regarding fetal tissue research have been submitted for government funding. Fetal tissue research on transplantation is still in its experimental phase, yet studies give increasing evidence that transplanting fetal cells can be useful for treating a number of serious conditions. However, the ethical issues persist. The most critical ethical issue concerns fetal tissue transplantation's link with induced abortions. In his article at the end of this chapter, Kevin O'Rourke presents an ethical analysis of the issue.

WHO GETS AN ORGAN?

In 1995, when thirty-four-year-old Sandra Jensen requested a heart-lung transplant, she was turned down by both the Stanford University and the University of California at San Diego medical centers. She was not even allowed to be on the waiting list of candidates. Why? She suffered from Down syndrome, and physicians unfairly lumped her in the category of those who lacked the mental capacity to understand and cooperate with the posttransplant regimen.

Little did they know that Jensen was, in fact, quite competent enough to challenge the decision. In fact, she had always been an active spokesperson for the rights of the mentally disabled. When George Bush signed the Americans with Disabilities Act in 1990, she was present at the signing. She defied the decision not to place her on the waiting list for a transplant and eventually won her plea. In 1996, at Stanford, she was given a new heart and lungs. She died sixteen months later from problems associated with the transplant.

This case poignantly demonstrates one of the most bitter pills regarding the distribution of organs for transplantation. Aside from the questions of who gets an organ and on what grounds, there is a preliminary question: Who becomes eligible as a transplant candidate to begin with?

Who Gets on the Waiting List?

Some perplexing questions arise regarding whether a person should be admitted to an organ transplantation waiting list. What standards would be fair? Jensen was initially overlooked as a candidate because of a mental competency standard based on ability to follow through with a rather complicated posttransplant regimen. Unfortunately, she was unfairly stereotyped. (Stereotyping was also an issue in the Baby Doe case, which we will discuss in Chapter 8.) Is this competency standard a fair gauge for determining candidacy status? The following criteria have been either used or proposed for consideration. Whether they are ethically defensible is the subject of debate.

"The Green Screen"   The term *green screen,* coined by Dr. Clive Callender, the head of Howard University's transplant center, refers to whether or not a patient has an insurance carrier. Transplants are expensive procedures. Liver transplants, for example, can cost up to $250,000. If insurance coverage is used as a criterion for admittance to the waiting list for transplants, access to organs would be denied for at least 37 million uninsured Americans, most of whom are members of racial minorities.

The Sickest   According to some, patients who are most ill or suffer from the most complications should have priority on the waiting list, yet due to their condition these same patients are less likely to succeed with a new organ. Nevertheless, the Department of Health and Human Services (DHHS) is now urging that priority be assigned to the sickest patients.

Support System   Many centers deem it necessary that any candidate have a system of social and familial support. Given the complicated follow-up regimen after the transplant operation, the medical outcome is adversely affected by the absence of such support.

Age   Some commentators suggest that lines regarding eligibility for organs should be drawn at certain ages. For example, at the Stanford University Medical Center, the line is drawn at age sixty for receiving lungs. In the United Kingdom, those past the age of sixty are no longer eligible for kidney transplants. Should chronological age be the standard, or should physiological age—the state of health relative to each individual—be considered instead?

Unrehabilitated and/or Self-destructive Behavior   A controversial criterion for exclusion involves those who exhibit so-called unrehabilitated behavior. Much of this debate concerns alcoholics who need liver transplants. Should unrehabilitated alcoholics be placed on the list? Alcoholism is recognized as a disease as well as a form of indirectly self-destructive behavior. Chronic smoking can also be viewed as indirectly self-destructive behavior. Should smokers be permitted on waiting lists for lung transplants? Are prisoners entitled to be placed on waiting lists for organs? What about the eligibility of those who engage in more direct acts of self-destruction, such as those who have attempted suicide? For example, overdosing on Tylenol surely damages the liver, and the person who survives such an overdose may need a liver transplant. The underlying issue is the degree of personal responsibility for the particular behavior and whether this should be a factor in determining candidacy for an organ.

A Closer Look at the DHHS Proposal

In a major move to allocate organs according to uniform criteria, the National Organ Transplant Act was enacted in 1984. Five years later, the DHHS charged the United Network in Organ Sharing (UNOS) with the task of overseeing fair allocation of organs. However, in 1994, the DHHS expressed an interest in managing the distribution process. As of 1999, the UNOS directs the policy.

In order to assess the recent proposal by the DHHS to distribute organs, we need to review the current policy. The UNOS allocates organs according to criteria that first consider regional proximity. There are sixty-three regions throughout the United States. When an organ becomes available, local candidates in the region where that organ is available are the first ones considered. Then the center considers candidates in the wider regional area. If no regional candidates are found for that specific organ, then a search for a likely candidate is opened up nationally.

This regionally based approach has some problems. First, there are discrepancies in waiting time for those on waiting lists. For example, in Michigan and Ohio, the typical waiting period for a liver is about 370 days, whereas the waiting period is about 96 days in Louisiana and Mississippi.[14] This means that, depending on the region, sicker patients who are waiting for organs may die while those who are less sick receive transplants. Ninety-five percent of organ recipients in South Carolina were well enough to be able to live at home.[15] Meanwhile, many sicker patients in neighboring states were unable to receive organs.

A second problem involves liver transplant candidates who do not have the options available to other candidates, such as those waiting for kidneys. Patients on waiting lists for kidneys have the alternative treatment of kidney dialysis. According to an American Medical Association account:

> In 1996, for instance, more than 60% of liver transplants were done in the same area where the organs were procured, and more than 50% went to patients who were not

sick enough to be hospitalized. At the same time, however, nearly 400 would-be recipients died in hospitals in other areas. The total number of waiting-list deaths [for liver transplant candidates] in 1996 was 953.[16]

Due to these problems, as well as the wholesale shortage of available organs, the DHHS has proposed to overhaul the regionally based system and make it more national in scope. According to Secretary Donna Shalala, the DHHS hopes to reorganize the allocation system so that those most in medical need of an organ can be more easily identified and targeted as the most appropriate recipients.

This proposal, however, has its own share of problems. The DHHS move has stirred up quite a bit of controversy. First, smaller centers feel threatened. Since larger centers tend to care for sicker patients, smaller centers may be put out of business, while larger metropolitan centers stand to gain. Second, this proposal opens up a turf battle between the DHHS and the UNOS regarding management and control over the whole process of procurement. Many critics claim that the new proposal shifts management to government. Walter Graham, executive director for the UNOS, fears it would "politicize the allocation policy."[17] From a medical perspective, the most serious argument against the proposal is that it targets the sickest patients, whose prospect for longer-term survival is probably lowest, as the first line of organ recipients. This constitutes, in effect, a waste of good organs.

Responsibility and Social Worth

Should we adopt standards other than "sickest patients first"? Clearly, the criterion of medical outcome makes good sense, but what about other standards, such as social worth? For example, many critics point out that Pennsylvania's Governor Casey made it to the top of the waiting list for a heart due to his political influence. These same critics reasonably argue that criteria of social worth are suspect for many reasons, the most important being that they are certainly discriminatory in nature. Allocating organs according to race, nationality, religion, and social class seems unfair, and using occupation and social contribution as factors is a clear violation of Kant's second formation of the categorical imperative, in which he exhorts us to treat others as persons as ends in themselves.

On the other hand, our allocation should be socially responsible. For instance, if there is a choice between two recipients, a serial murderer and a judge, is it responsible to randomly select the organ recipient? What if the serial murderer wins? Would that be a conscientious choice?

Psychosocial Issues Regarding the "Gift Exchange"

Many tales of transplantation focus on the donor. When the donor happens to be a stranger, we tend to suspect motives, as in the following account of the "fishing buddy." This suspicion leads us to ask what motivates people to donate their organs.

> Rick Wilson fished alongside Frank Rembert for three days—the two had not known each other previously—then offered him a kidney. Rembert, who had experienced kidney failure a year earlier, had been on dialysis and waiting lists for kidneys. Now, thanks to Wilson's donation, he had a transplant and was recovering. Wilson, the donor, was also still recovering two months after surgery, with pain along his incision and unable to return to work for another month or so. . . .

. . . Indeed, Wilson's offer of a kidney was suspect to many. Wilson and Rembert were themselves aware that the donation would be questioned: "[They] fibbed a bit. To avoid arousing suspicion, they told doctors that they had known each other for several years. . . . 'They most often drilled me on how long I've known Frank and where we fished together. . . . So we had to collaborate stories. . . . We got pretty good stories going.'"[18]

The gift exchange of organ donation is exceedingly complex. According to French anthropologist Marcel Mauss, in his 1954 essay *The Gift,* a gift exchange essentially has three parts: giving, accepting, and repaying. Using the insights of Mauss, medical sociologist Mary Ann Lamanna points out the irony behind the expression "gift exchange." The term *gift* denotes something freely given without conditions, whereas *exchange* conveys some sort of trade. In any case, there are certain issues pertaining to accepting the gift. Recipients may have problems with accepting gifts, depending on how such acceptance affects the recipient's self-esteem, self-empowerment, and level of dependency. This is what Renee Fox and Judith Swazey refer to as the "tyranny of the gift."[19] The situation is all the more compounded if the gift is from a stranger, as in the case of the fishing buddy.

Note that media campaigns have a way of assigning priorities when it comes to organ transplants. The media create their own viewing "community," so showing the face of a child in need of a transplant situates that child in a sort of communal relationship with viewers. This inclusion in a "community" creates an unfair advantage over those on the waiting list who are not shown to the public, suggesting the significance of the bonding process that takes place within a communal relationship. Strangers are not included in that bonding process; therefore, we tend to be more suspicious of strangers' motives.

Multiple Listing

Beyond any measure of doubt, the demand for transplantable organs far exceeds the available supply. In view of this situation, what would be the most ethically sound way to allocate organs that become available? Among those who are on waiting lists, how do we fairly choose who receives what? In her article at the end of this chapter, Tracy Miller gives an insightful overview of the development of policies for bringing about the equitable distribution of organs. She also cites the unique example of New York State, which in July 1990 became the first state to officially ban multiple listing for potential organ recipients.

This brings us to another problematic area: patients currently on a waiting list who also choose to be placed on other waiting lists at other transplant centers, thus increasing their chance of being selected sooner for an organ. It also gives them an advantage over those who do not list with other centers. Patients who do not list with other centers primarily do not know enough about the process and/or are not able to afford it.

Is it justifiable to allow patients to place themselves on multiple waiting lists? Following are some typical arguments in support of multiple listing:

- Multiple listing allows patients to exercise their personal autonomy and freedom to increase their chances of treatment.
- Patients gain wider access to available organs.

- Multiple listing is particularly advantageous for transient patients who live in different regions during the year.

- Multiple listing is advantageous for smaller centers. Prohibiting multiple listing would mean that most patients would prefer to list at larger, more prestigious centers, jeopardizing the existence of smaller centers.

The most common arguments that oppose multiple listing follow:

- Although multiple listing benefits the more affluent patient, it provides an unfair advantage over patients who cannot afford to be on multiple lists.

- Under the End Stage Renal Dialysis Program, the federal government incurs the costs of all treatment and tests having to do with end-stage kidney disease. When patients place themselves on multiple lists, evaluative tests are repeated at the various centers at which patients choose to be listed. This duplication becomes quite costly, and the government and taxpayers pick up the tab. This is fiscally unfair.

- There is the likelihood of less continuity of care for patients who multiple-list.

The UNOS first allowed multiple listing in August 1987 and then reversed its decision in January 1988. However, because of a strong backlash and protestations by patient advocate groups who upheld persons' rights to have control over their access to healthcare, the UNOS again changed its position in May 1988, granting patients the right to multiple-list. Two years later, New York became the first state to officially ban multiple listing, deciding that the umbrella of individual rights does not override the unfair gain that multiple-listed patients have over those who cannot afford to multiple-list.

LIVER TRANSPLANTS AND SELF-DESTRUCTIVE BEHAVIOR

"Julie Smith" is thirty-one years old. In an attempt to end her life, she took a heavy overdose of extra-strength Tylenol capsules. The amount of acetaminophen she ingested was enough to cause severe liver damage, and she developed fulminant hepatic, or intense liver, failure. Her liver damage was so severe that it eventually impaired her brain function. She was desperately in need of a healthy liver. Within days, she entered into a coma. At this point, receiving a liver would mean nearly a 100 percent chance of survival. If she had to wait any longer, however, Smith's condition would worsen and make her a less viable candidate. The time for a new liver was now.

However, Smith's personal history raised some questions. She came from a rather dysfunctional family. Her parents, now divorced, were alcoholics. Her mother remarried, and her stepfather grew marijuana that he pressured Smith into selling. Smith herself was married and had a six-year-old daughter from a previous marriage. She was in an abusive relationship, and she and her husband were undergoing therapy. At the same time, her husband had initiated divorce proceedings.

Smith had been an administrator at a psychiatric hospital's outreach center; she was fired from the hospital after being arrested for selling her stepfather's marijuana. Within the past six months, she had been drinking heavily and had occasionally taken cocaine. According to the psychiatrist's report, she is an alcoholic and multiple-drug abuser and is under severe marital strain. Should Smith be activated on the waiting list for a liver?[20]

At least 60,000 Americans die every year of some type of liver disease. Of those who are on waiting lists for a liver, 10 percent die before one becomes available. Despite the acute shortage of livers, the demand continues to grow. Smith is in need of a liver. She has developed rapid and intense liver failure, and the longer she remains in this condition, the lower the chances of a successful transplant. She is now at the point at which a transplant would be highly successful, and timing is urgent. Given her suicide attempt, as well as her family situation, is she a feasible candidate for a transplant? The consensus among the staff caring for Smith is that she should not be placed on the waiting list, for a number of reasons. She has an extensive history and pattern of drug abuse and dependency. Furthermore, she lives in a dysfunctional family system, so there would be little family support.

The staff compares Smith's situation to that of an alcoholic. Whether alcoholics should be placed on waiting lists remains one of the most volatile issues related to the fair distribution of organs. According to the transplant policies in a number of hospitals, alcoholics can be considered as feasible candidates for a transplant only if they meet certain conditions:

- They must have abstained from alcohol for at least the past six months.
- There cannot be any injury beyond the liver, or extrahepatic damage.
- There must not be a psychiatric condition associated with the alcoholism.
- The patient must have some measure of socioeconomic security.
- The patient must have a reasonably sound family support system.[21]

The Responsibility Factor

Many critics argue that, especially in view of the severe shortage of organs, alcoholics are not entitled to be activated on the waiting list for liver transplants. Their arguments center around the idea of personal accountability. They contend that, even if alcoholism is viewed as a disease, alcoholics could have sought treatment at some earlier point. If they did not, then they are irresponsible and do not deserve to receive such a scarce resource. Critics consider personal accountability a fair factor in assessing the situation of alcoholics. They contend that, because alcohol-related end-stage liver disease could have been averted, individuals who deliberately and knowingly engage in this form of self-destructive and addictive behavior should not acquire priority on the waiting list for transplants. Individuals who are not personally responsible for having developed end-stage liver disease should have priority over the irresponsible alcoholic. Moss and Seigler, in their article at the end of this chapter, argue along these lines.

Others, however, disagree. They argue that using personal responsibility as a criterion for allocating organs leads to dangerous and arbitrary moral evaluations of others and that this is indefensible. Medical treatments should not rest on the medical team's moral judgments of their patients. Furthermore, linking alcoholism to moral weakness brings up all sorts of problems. Alcoholism is not simply a matter of individual responsibility. For instance, women are more prone to liver damage when they drink alcohol, and Asians are less prone to developing liver disease. In addition, at what point can the behavior of alcoholics be said to be truly voluntary? Cohen and Benjamin's article reflects this counterargument. Indeed, many variables besides personal responsibility appear to be involved. As one writer puts it:

> . . . in our assessment of drinkers we need to verify that they drank at all, determine the amount they drank, determine whether they were aware the amount was excessive, determine definitively whether the drink was from habit or addiction, determine the genetic disposition to addiction, and determine whether the histologic diagnosis was informed by the drinking history in the assignment of etiology.[22]

Personal responsibility involves awareness and education, and persons who take risks are often unaware of the extent to which the risk is dangerous. In this regard, we need to learn more about the role of personal responsibility in cases of addiction. Surely, there is some deliberate choice that leads to a habit and then to the addiction, but how voluntary is that choice? What if studies indicate a genetic factor that leads to a predisposition to alcohol? Furthermore, if we use personal responsibility as a criterion, why would we not apply it across the board to all medical situations? In point of fact, we don't as a rule apply personal responsibility to general medical practice. Why make an exception in the case of liver transplants?

The Likelihood-of-Success Factor

In the case described above, how compliant would Smith be with her postoperative therapy? Compliance is critical to the success of a transplant, and hospital policies often establish the need for a supportive family network. Yet is this assumption well founded? The existence of a family network does not necessarily ensure postoperative compliance. Why would a person without family necessarily be less compliant, especially if other support systems are available? Physician Colin Atterbury asserts that this policy is actually a social criterion disguised in a quasi-medical form.[23]

It is clear that success is measured not only in terms of the operation itself but in its long-range outcome. Will Smith be able to return to a somewhat useful life? If so, for how long? Smith's long past history of drug abuse seems to stack the cards against her. Therefore, it is important to establish whether it is likely that she will continue to show a pattern of drug dependency. Her drug abuse, as well as her weak familial support system, led the staff to question Smith's appropriateness as a candidate for a liver transplant.

The issue becomes further complicated when we consider that certain conditions make an individual more predisposed to liver disease from alcohol use. For example, in the presence of a viral liver infection, only a slight intake of alcohol may produce thoroughly damaging effects. Should persons who suffer from such conditions be held subject to the same standards as persons who have alcoholic dependency?

Mark Aulisio and Robert Arnold argue that Smith's case is not merely analogous to that of an alcoholic. Though the focus of others is on her suicide attempt, her condition does involve alcoholism. In this respect, she clearly does not meet certain requirements and should not be activated on the list for a liver. They state further that the combination of her alcoholism, drug abuse, and suicide attempt make her cooperation in a posttransplant regimen highly unlikely. Despite the fact that predicting the outcome with absolute certitude is impossible, we still need to make responsible decisions based on reasonable probabilities.

MARKETING ORGANS

Arguments Opposing the Sale of Organs

Despite the radical shortage of organs and the increasing demand for transplantation, there is a rather strong reaction against the idea of commercializing the procurement and distribution of organs. The idea has evoked such intense disapproval that we will first consider this opposition. In order to address the subject reasonably, we need to examine the issue from all perspectives—those of the seller, the buyer, and the context in which such transactions occur. From a libertarian perspective, a commercial exchange may be a justified expression of individual liberties. But against the backdrop of poverty in which such transactions occur, can they genuinely be said to involve free trade and consent? Following are the leading arguments against selling and buying organs.

Coercion   Are donor-sellers truly autonomous? Since most are poor and live in impoverished circumstances that lead to social exploitation, are they in fact coerced by virtue of their condition? On the other hand, the mere fact of poverty and monetary incentive does not necessarily preclude making an autonomous decision. The issue is to what degree we are sufficiently autonomous. Material conditions by themselves may not so much jeopardize autonomy, but rather create a context whereby the reasoning process is compromised. When this occurs, coercive elements become a greater factor.

We can argue that all persons have a right to engage in behavior that incurs some level of risk to themselves, in this case, the donation of organs. Would prohibiting the selling of organs violate this right? In response, we need to consider three components: donors, physicians, and the role of medicine. To start with, is the donor sufficiently informed? As we described earlier in our discussion of informed consent, in order to give informed consent to surgery, the patient needs to understand the risks and benefits involved. Will poor donors be less informed of the risks? By virtue of their circumstances, they are subject to exploitation by others. For an impoverished donor, the incentive of a monetary payment may well inflate the benefits over the risks in a benefit/risk calculation. However, if we do not allow poor people to donate their organs, are we acting paternalistically? From the physicians' point of view, surgery should be performed only for medical reasons, not for monetary ones. The sale of organs shuffles this motivation around. As for the role of medicine, commercializing organs would impose a market ideology that eventually would override all other concerns, with profit becoming the driving force in medicine. This is already a major fear in the face of the current corporatization of American healthcare.

The Canadian government has recently become more sensitive to the dangers in marketing organs. Many Canadians have traveled abroad to shop for organs, with quite a few going to China and India. There is also evidence that some Americans have acted as brokers for Canadians seeking to buy organs. Canada is moving to legislate against any activity that involves the selling and buying of organs. The marketing of organs as described above would become a criminal offense.

Social Harm and the Threat to Altruism   Commercializing the "gift exchange" would diminish the significance we place on altruism. The sale of organs conflicts with our notion of the organ as a gift by viewing organs within a market-driven context in which organs are treated merely as another commodity. Western countries, in prohibiting the

CHINA AND CONDEMNED PRISONERS

The first heart transplant in China occurred rather recently, in 1992, at a Beijing hospital. China first started performing organ transplants in the early 1980s, after cyclosporine had been proven to be a more effective immunosuppressive agent in organ transplantation. The circumstances for the first heart transplant are revealing. The transplanted heart, grafted onto a fifteen-year-old girl, was harvested from a condemned prisoner who was given a lethal injection. The girl lived for another six months.

There is mounting evidence that more prisoners are being executed by lethal injection.[24] Lethal injection enables the organs to remain oxygenated during the complex process of removing and transplanting the prisoners' organs. As in the past, some prisoners in China continue to be executed by being shot in the back of the head, a style of execution that still allows for the retrieval of organs such as the heart.

In 1984, China established Temporary Rules Concerning the Utilization of Corpses or Organs from the Corpses of Executed Criminals. The rules stipulated that executed prisoners' organs could be used for transplantation under certain conditions: if the prisoner gives his or her prior consent; if the prisoner's family provides consent; if no one claims the prisoner's corpse.[25] Since enactment of the rules, the use of prisoners' organs for transplantation has become big business in China. In fact, according to various reports, the primary source of organs, particularly kidneys, is executed prisoners.

Citizens from other countries, such as Taiwan (which previously had marketed organs but banned the practice officially in 1994) and countries in the Pacific Rim and even Canada, continue to "shop" in China, where they can obtain organs almost immediately. For example, Thais in need of kidney transplants often go to China, where for a sizable sum of money they can buy kidneys from executed prisoners. According to the report of one case, payment was made up-front, before the buyer-patients boarded their flights. Furthermore, some of the monies were given to the prisoners' family after they were executed.[26] Another report stated that some Canadians traveled to China to purchase organs, operating through U.S. brokers for a substantial fee.[27] In 1998, two men were arrested in New York City for arranging the purchase of organs from executed Chinese prisoners. One was a former procurator who oversaw executions in the Chinese province of Hainan.[28]

This situation has raised hard questions for many Chinese as well as for the international community. First, can a condemned prisoner offer genuine consent to donate his or her organs? Second, to what extent can medical professionals be involved in state-sanctioned executions without violating their professional medical ethics? Third, could viewing condemned prisoners as potential sources for organs lead to abuses, including commercial exploitation? Critics point out that the practice of transplanting organs from

continued on page 430

continued from page 429 *executed prisoners will inevitably lead to an increase in capital punishment, given the increasing societal demand for organs. According to a recent Amnesty International report, China handed down over 6,000 death sentences in 1996, twice as many as in the previous two years combined.*[29]

The sale of organs remains officially illegal in China, violating official policy statements such as the 1984 rules and a 1994 policy statement of the Transplant Society. Despite this formal ban, however, the sale of organs has become a lucrative trade involving prison officials, local politicians, and medical professionals.

trade in organs, share the view of the World Health Organization (WHO), which has strictly forbidden physicians to take part in any transplantation they believe involves the commercialization of organs.

On another note, many fear that if we had the choice to either give or sell an organ, many of us would likely choose to sell. Donors themselves would not really benefit from the sale. Even though they would be paid for their organs, they would stand the chance of not being paid enough to compensate for their donation. Also, there are more medical risks to donors than most donors realize. From an egalitarian point of view, the trade in organs would widen the gap between the affluent and the poor, as well as the gap between richer and poorer countries. Furthermore, since most donors would be poor and thus more likely to suffer from insufficient healthcare, there would be an increased likelihood of unhealthier organs being used.

Arguments Supporting the Sale of Organs

Some support the idea of providing financial incentives to organ donors. Supporters argue that allowing financial incentives would be advantageous for two primary reasons: (1) It upholds our respect for individual autonomy; (2) it helps abate the current organ shortage. James Blumstein, a spokesperson for this position, challenges what he terms one of our culture's "sacred cows"—the value we place on altruism as opposed to monetary motives. Any talk about commercializing the sale of organs and providing financial incentives is immediately met with sharp antagonism. A cultural mind-set favors the notion of altruism and disfavors financial incentives. Such altruism is a "moral imperative" among Americans.

Given this mind-set, we still need to face hard-hitting reality. With 30,000 Americans on organ transplant waiting lists and 200 added each month, the supply of available organs continues to diminish. Furthermore, in just about every other facet of medicine, financial incentives exist that have an impact on decision making in healthcare. Blumstein states:

> Principles of competition and incentives have influenced the rest of the health policy arena in the past decade. Those principles are strikingly at odds with the strongly held, fundamental principles of altruism and communitarianism that are so widespread in the organ transplantation arena.[30]

Blumstein proposes that the burden of proof in criticisms of the market approach lie with those who feel that the market approach should remain illegal. He questions the arguments typically raised against marketing organs. We address these arguments—and the counterarguments—below.

Are Donor-Sellers Coerced? Blumstein proposes that the commercialization of organs should first start with cadavers by a system of "forward contracting." Even if we associate risk factors with possible coercion, do we not regularly make other risk choices without necessarily being coerced? He feels that safeguards can be set up in order to prevent coercion.

What impact would a cadaver market have on the donor's family? For instance, if a family member "forward contracts," that is, stipulates that his or her viable organs be transplanted upon death and compensation be given to the donor's family, it may be an expression of personal autonomy, but doesn't it also take away the feeling of grieving family members that they themselves have chosen to give the gift of life to another? Blumstein responds that, though the family's emotional gratification is important, it should never override an individual's own expression of autonomy in executing a forward contract.

Will the Sale of Organs Lead to a Reduction in Altruism? No available data in the United States support this concern. The sale of organs was officially banned in the United States in 1984. Data from other countries, including India and Egypt, indicate that the organ trade has brought about an increase in the number of available organs. Blumstein suggests that we conduct an experiment in the United States, allowing financial incentives for organ donation in order to obtain adequate data.

This experiment should start with the sale of cadaver organs. Marketing does not preclude altruistic acts of donation. On the contrary, marketing and altruism can coexist. Moreover, quite a few other life-saving treatments involve marketing, including transplantation alternatives such as dialysis and the allocation of artificial body parts and organs. Perhaps, according to Blumstein, we are so opposed to legalizing the sale of organs because people would in fact choose to engage in it. Blumstein states:

> Indeed, when one carefully examines the argument for preserving altruism by outlawing market transactions, one wonders whether the real fear is that legalization of market transactions will in fact work; that is, given a choice, people would choose to participate in a market and would abandon altruism. Unpacked, the argument to outlaw market exchanges to preserve altruism is in reality *an argument to coerce altruism.*[31] (italics added)

Is It Unfair That the Rich Stand a Better Chance of Obtaining Organs? Fairness seems to dictate that organs should be distributed according to medical needs, not financial status. This is certainly a problem, considering the rampant inequities in wealth. On the other hand, isn't wealth already a factor in organ transplantation in the United States? For example, a number of wealthy organ recipients from other countries have obtained organs in Pittsburgh. Blumstein proposes that we establish some type of public subsidy for those who are financially stressed, comparable to the government funding available for all patients, regardless of income, suffering from end-stage renal disease.

From another perspective, why prohibit the more affluent from choosing to obtain an organ? For instance, AZT is very expensive and, unfortunately, may be acquired only by those who can afford it. Why treat organ transplants differently? All

CULTURAL WINDOWS

INDIA AND THE ORGAN TRADE

India is a land of contrasts. A small pocket of enormous wealth resides within its immense population, while most of the country remains impoverished. Evidence of this inequity can be seen in the abject poverty in the major cities of Calcutta and Bombay. At the same time, India is becoming increasingly sophisticated in technology while still holding on to its rich and ancient religious heritage, especially as manifested in the majority Hindu tradition. India's other religious traditions are Jainism, Islam, Christianity, and a remnant of Buddhism.

India is a country where the practice of buying and selling kidneys is becoming more widespread. Indeed, many Indians desperately in need of kidneys seem to have little in the way of alternatives. India's medical system does not have an established dialysis program to provide maintenance for those suffering from renal disease, nor does it have any policy for utilizing cadaver kidneys for transplanta-

tion. In India, cadaveric transplantation and ICU sustenance of organs for those who are brain dead are not common. Furthermore, India lacks a welfare safety net. For those suffering from renal failure and in dire need of a kidney, the options are limited: They can either obtain a kidney from a living donor, related or unrelated, or receive no kidney at all. Thus, the purchase of kidneys from living donors is often practiced, raising all sorts of issues.

The purchase of kidneys, and, for that matter, any other organ, is certainly not universally accepted in India, and there are strong arguments against the practice. Some of the most vocal arguments stem from religious perspectives that contend that our bodies are given to us as gifts, and we therefore have no right to treat them as simple objects. This is the stewardship argument, which is especially prominent in Christian teachings. Hindu, Jain, and Muslim teachings also underscore the

other dimensions of transplantation involve money, so why shouldn't the organ itself? Blumstein points out what he regards as a fundamental inconsistency in the arguments against marketing organs: Organ transplantation is regarded as ordinary medical treatment when it comes to insurance coverage, being viewed in the same way as all other effective therapies, yet it is placed in a special category when it comes to considering its commercialization.[32]

XENOGRAFTS

In 1992, a milestone in xenograft surgery, or cross-species transplantation, took place at the University of Pittsburgh Medical Center's Presbyterian Hospital under the direction of the pioneering transplant surgeon Thomas E. Starzl. A thirty-five-year-old man dying from hepatitis B became the world's first recipient of a baboon liver. Because he was suffering from hepatitis B, he was ineligible to receive a liver from another human;

idea that our bodies are temples and must be treated with the utmost respect. Many Indians are opposed to the buying and selling of kidneys because they fear it will lead to blatant commercialism, which will inevitably exploit the poor. Given the abject poverty in which countless Indians exist, such commercialism would be insidiously coercive.

On the other hand, quite a few Indian physicians support the purchase of kidneys for transplantation, particularly considering the absence of regular dialysis programs, cadaveric transplantation, and intensive care units to support organs from those who are brain dead.[33] Furthermore, on the basis of Hindu teachings regarding karma—the moral principle of cause and effect—the transaction of selling and buying a kidney could benefit both parties, especially if the transaction takes place with "rewarded gifting" as a feature. Rewarded gifting means that the recipient of the kidney pays the donor a substantial amount and also covers all follow-up medical costs that the donor incurs as a result of the donation. The recipient also rewards the transplant institution by covering related costs.

Some advocates of the purchase of kidneys encourage a system of "mandated philanthropy":

The kidney buyer should also provide something that is more specifically directed at gradually reducing the need for unrelated living donations, such as contributing to a cadaveric donor organ support facility; improving fresh water and sewage to the population sector from which the donor comes; providing a related living kidney donor transplant free of charge, with follow-up, to another member of that sector who might have renal failure; and/or combinations of the above.[34]

Supporters argue that in a country of dire poverty like India, where few options exist to address the need for kidney transplants, mandated giving may help restore some material and economic inequities. Nevertheless, India's context of woeful poverty gives rise to the constant risk that the sale of kidneys will lead to commercialization and exploitation. How India will safeguard against this danger is yet to be tried and tested.

the hepatitis B virus would have destroyed any human liver given to him. On June 29, while one surgical team was painstakingly excising his diseased liver, another team in a nearby surgical unit was carefully extracting the liver of a fifteen-year-old adult male baboon who was bred for the purpose of organ use at the Southwest Foundation in San Antonio, Texas. The patient lived for about seventy days following the transplant. The startling procedure evoked further wonder at the new "miracles" in medicine and also stirred up a storm of controversy.

Why was a baboon used? After all, chimpanzees are more closely matched to humans both genetically and anatomically. But chimpanzees are an endangered species, while baboons are not. Furthermore, a baboon liver is still anatomically compatible with that of a human. Thus, the success of this experiment would allow a future supply of organs from baboons bred for the purpose of supplying organs to humans.

This surgery was not the first xenograft. Since 1905, at least thirty-three xenografts had already been attempted, although none had been successful. The most famous of these was the case of Baby Fae, an infant who received a baboon heart at Loma Linda

Medical Center, California, on October 26, 1984. As mentioned in Chapter 6, Baby Fae died twenty days after the operation because she developed an antibody to the baboon's blood. At the time, she received the conventional anti-rejection agent cyclosporine, and herein lies one significant difference between Baby Fae and Dr. Starzl's liver recipient. The success of the transplant in Pittsburgh was attributed to the new experimental antirejection drug FK-506, discovered in Japan and developed in Pittsburgh. FK-506 prevented the human body's natural rejection of a foreign organ, while cyclosporine did not have this capacity.

Baby Fae's case drew worldwide attention. Born three weeks premature, she suffered from hypoplastic left heart syndrome, which meant that the left side of her heart was virtually helpless to pump blood. This condition is usually fatal. The chief pediatric surgeon at Loma Linda Medical Center, Leonard Bailey, proposed the possibility of a xenograft to the baby's parents. Following their approval, Baby Fae received a heart from Goobers, a female baboon less than ten months old.

The xenograft evoked strong reaction. A primary criticism was that the so-called donor, Goobers, was being exploited. Animal rights activists challenge the notion of using animal parts for humans, many of them arguing that animals possess moral status and using them as a source of organs is an abuse of their rights. Another criticism charged that Baby Fae was being exploited as well. Critics questioned whether the operation was truly in her best interests, since there were no grounds to believe that the experiment would produce any therapeutic benefit for her. Many felt that she was treated more as a research subject than as a patient. If so, she was essentially exploited for the benefit of the researchers. In addition, many challenged the legitimacy of her parents' consent on her behalf, feeling that they may not have been sufficiently informed of the risks.

Thomas Starzl, the transplant surgeon in Pittsburgh, had already become a legend in transplant surgery. In 1967, he had performed the world's first successful liver transplant. Liver transplantations have since become commonplace, with over 10,000 operations as of 1999. Starzl was also among the pioneers in performing xenografts. He transplanted baboon kidneys into humans six times in 1963, and the recipients lived from nineteen to ninety-eight days. Nearly seven months after the first baboon-to-human liver transplant, discussed above, a second xenograft was performed in Pittsburgh. The sixty-two-year-old patient survived less than one month, never regaining consciousness.

Research is being conducted on the use of pigs for transplantable organs in humans. In institutions such as Duke University, researchers are also studying the effects of transferring human genes into pigs in the hope of someday facilitating more viable transplantations. The article at the end of the chapter by the Working Group on Genetic Engineering in Nonhuman Life Forms focuses particularly on research on pigs' hearts being conducted at Cambridge University. In addition to describing the purpose behind the genetic modification of pigs, the group addresses some of the more critical issues regarding cross-species transplantation. We will next consider some of the arguments raised both in opposition to and in support of xenografts.

Arguments Against Xenografts

What constitutes "medical success" for an organ recipient? In the Pittsburgh case, Starzl reported that "our chances of succeeding are really quite good."[35] As we have seen, the first recipient of a baboon liver lived for nearly seventy days, whereas the second recipient lived for less than a month, never fully regaining consciousness. If patients experience marginal therapeutic benefit, are they being viewed as research subjects or as patients? Of additional concern is whether xenografts run the risk of transplanting an unknown baboon disease into the human recipient. According to Starzl, hundreds of experiments were conducted prior to his operation to ensure that this would not happen.

The most vocal opposition to xenografts comes from animal rights groups. Regarding the Pittsburgh operation, Sue Brebner, who works for People for the Ethical Treatment of Animals (PETA), stated, "Even though we have sympathy for the patient and his family, we believe that animals don't exist to provide spare parts for human beings."[36] Philosopher Tom Regan argues further that nonhuman animals must also be treated as persons; that is, they possess moral status and it is unethical to use them for human ends. In reference to the Baby Fae affair, he stated:

> Those people who seized [the baboon's] heart, even if they were motivated by their concern for Baby Fae, grievously violated Goobers's right to be treated with respect. That she could do nothing to protest, and that many of us failed to recognize the transplant for the injustice that it was, does not diminish the wrong, a wrong settled before Baby Fae's death.[37]

Further, how can we classify the baboon as a "donor" if the notion of consent is meaningless in this case?

Another argument is that the money spent in xenograft research could be spent in more useful ways, such as maternity care and cardiac disease prevention programs. A typical liver transplant costs around $275,000. Because the surgery in Pittsburgh was considered experimental, the University of Pittsburgh picked up all costs. Not only could these funds be better spent, but picking up the tab causes prices in other departments to rise.

Do xenografts allow genuine informed consent? There certainly was not informed consent on the part of Goobers. Whether potential recipients can give genuine informed consent in these situations is also questionable. Even though the Pittsburgh Medical Center's institutional review board approved the consent form and the protocol, what guarantee is there that the patients truly understood the procedure and its accompanying risks? As in the case of Christiaan Barnard, we might ask what conversations transpired between Starzl and other transplant team surgeons and the patient concerning the prospects for success. For instance, if the patient was told that he had a "50 percent chance of success," just what did that mean, especially given that the procedure was experimental?

Arguments in Favor of Xenografts

Supporters argue that xenografts are justifiable as long as there is proper consent, since this respects the autonomy of the patient. In the Pittsburgh case, the consent form was investigated by the university's institutional review board in order to ensure that proper protocol would be followed in obtaining genuine consent. The board recommended that the surgeons wait another twenty-four hours after the initial request for consent in order to open the door for a change of mind by the patient.

Supporters point out that xenografts would help reduce the catastrophic shortage of available organs for transplantation into humans. Currently, because of the critical shortage of donor organs, at least one person dies each day waiting for an organ. In many cases, there is no alternative. The thirty-five-year-old suffering from hepatitis B, for example, was expected to die within days. Such cases constitute a medical emergency. Healthcare professionals are committed to saving human lives, and that commitment, they believe, overrides the rights of nonhumans.

Some critics of animal rights claim that valuing nonhuman life equally with human life lessens the worth of human lives. This criticism is especially pertinent to the ongoing research into genetically engineering pigs to become a viable source of human organs in the future. Although some other cultures, such as Buddhism, emphasize that nonhuman animals and humans ought to be treated with equal respect, the United States has maintained a strong historical consensus that the rights and well-being of humans supersede those of nonhuman animals.

KEVIN O'ROURKE

Research with Fetal Tissue

Kevin O'Rourke is the former director of the Center for Health Care Ethics at St. Louis University. After describing how transplanting fetal tissue may benefit persons with conditions such as Alzheimer's disease and Parkinson's disease, he addresses the most critical ethical issues by first suggesting ways to prevent the promotion of elective abortion. He also reminds scientists of the link between professional and personal responsibility. Moreover, he questions the reliance on consent as well as the language used to depict the fetus. O'Rourke concludes that extreme caution must accompany fetal tissue research.

THE ISSUE

A new form of "Buck Rogers Research" is well underway. Living cells taken from aborted fetuses are being transplanted into other human beings with serious diseases. People with Alzheimer's Disease and Parkinson's Disease, for example, have received transplants of brain tissue from recently aborted fetuses. The thought underlying the research is that therapy might be developed for people with these and other debilitating diseases. Fetal tissue is more adaptable for research, and perhaps for therapy, because fetuses do not have a well-developed immune system. Thus the tissue garnered from fetuses is less likely to be rejected in another person's body and seems to grow faster than tissue taken from other sources. Researchers think that there is enough indication of eventual success to justify continuing the research.

Many scientists have expressed concern about ethical issues involved in this form of research because the raw material for research comes from fetuses which are killed in elective abortions. The best material for research seems to come from fetuses in the second trimester of life. As one scientist stated, "At the embryo stage, you're not just dealing with material, you're dealing with living human beings, emotions, and ethical issues; scien-

tists are scared they won't be able to do the necessary research." Observers of the research scene are even more outspoken; a columnist in *The Wall Street Journal,* for example, called for international control of trade in fetal tissue to limit unethical procedures. The following observations are offered as a framework for considering some of the ethical issues resulting from research with fetal tissue taken from aborted fetuses.

ETHICAL REFLECTIONS

(1) Clearly, the research in fetal tissue has not caused the legalization of elective abortions. All know that one and one-half million abortions per year were occurring in our country long before research with fetal tissue was initiated. For this reason, a group of lawyers, researchers, and ethicists in 1986 declared support for transplanting tissue taken from aborted fetuses. At the time they stated, "We're fully aware the issue will be clouded by association with abortion, but it is important to stress we are in no way making a comment or taking a stand on the morality or legality of abortion."

However, the foregoing statement does not solve all the ethical problems. While there is no intrinsic connection between research on fetal tissue and elective abortions, those involved in this form of research have an ethical responsibility to make sure that the distance between the two realities is kept clear. There should be no indication that researchers are *promoting* elective abortion. In order to accomplish this, two steps should be taken: (a) No monies should be paid for fetal tissue. Some researchers and scientists have commented that they see no difficulty in using the fetal tissue from elective abortions because such abortions are legal. However, they would not approve of women becoming pregnant with the intention of having an abortion and selling the fetal tissue. But experience attests that men and women in our society will do anything for money. If money can be made by becoming pregnant, then we can be assured that such a commerce will be developed. There are federal laws against the sale of organs for transplantation. It seems there should be federal laws prohibiting the sale of fetal tissue for research as well. (b) A second manner of disassociating with the destruction of living human beings is to foster the availability of fetal tissue derived from culture processes. The ethical issue resulting from the source of supply for fetal tissue might be solved if the source-material for the culture is derived from spontaneous as opposed to elective abortions.

(2) Though scientists are aware of the ethical issues resulting from research with fetal tissue, some consider that it is not their responsibility to grapple with these issues personally. Rather, they look to the federal government or some other agency to handle the ethical and legal issues while they continue their research. Making ethical decisions about one's work or profession is a personal responsibility. This responsibility cannot be transferred to a group of lawyers or ethicists. History demonstrates sad results when scientists renounce their personal responsibility of determining the ethical implications of their work.

(3) Some ethicists and scientists compare fetal research to organ transplants from cadavers. Thus they maintain that the use of aborted fetuses is acceptable if the mother gives consent. But further consideration belies this assumption. When a family surrenders through proxy consent organs from a cadaver for heart or liver transplant, they have not been involved in causing the death of the person in question. Hence, though there is no direct connection between researchers and abortion, let there be no confusion that informed consent solves the ethical issues resulting from the use of tissue from aborted fetuses.

(4) Some will object to the description of elective abortion as killing a human being. One ethicist said, "Please, call it removing fetal tissue." However, it is extremely important to be clear and honest about actions under ethical analysis. This is especially true when human beings are involved. Once a group of people is deprived of their humanity, then all forms of oppression may be justified. For example, reflect upon what happened to some human beings in World War II because they were designated as "non-Aryans"; think of the atrocities justified in Vietnam because Americans were fighting "Gooks"; or think about the lies and destruction of life in Central America justified because the people are identified as "Communists." If we are to reach valid ethical solutions in health care and research, we must be accurate in defining the issues. The fetal tissue in this form of research comes from fetuses well along in development. While all would not designate them as persons to be protected fully by the law, maintaining that fetuses are anything other than living beings and of the human species is scientifically untenable. People may differ as to whether there is any good which justifies ending a human life in its early stages of development. But, in view of the scientific evidence, one has a difficult time maintaining that a fetus is anything other than a human being.

CONCLUSION

Research therapy with human tissue has a promising future. But when assessing the ethical reasons in research and therapy, scientists must be concerned with more than the results. The act which produces the results must be evaluated ethically, as well as the implications which follow from the action and its effects.

1. While O'Rourke admits that there is no "intrinsic" link between fetal tissue research and abortion, he strongly advises that efforts be made to maintain a clear difference between the two. What steps does he recommend?
2. Do you agree or disagree with his recommendations? Explain your answer in detail.
3. How does O'Rourke address the analogy sometimes made between fetal research and transplants from cadavers? Do you agree or disagree with his response? Explain.
4. O'Rourke insists on describing the fetus as a living human being. Do you think his ethical analysis is sound? Explain.

TRACY E. MILLER

Multiple Listing for Organ Transplantation: Autonomy Unbounded*

Tracy E. Miller is a lawyer in New York who specializes in bioethics and served as executive director of the New York State Task Force on Life and Law. After giving a concise rendition of the development of organ transplant policies and a description of current U.S. policy, she cites reasons why multiple listing has proliferated, describing its advantages. She then discusses arguments for and against multiple listing and examines how policies have addressed the issue of multiple listing. Miller compares national policies with policies recently implemented in New York State. She concludes by pointing out how these issues raise more fundamental questions concerning access to healthcare.

Scarcity has marked organ transplantation since its inception. In the early stages of kidney, heart, and liver transplantation, transplant centers rigorously screened prospective patients, relying on medical and psychosocial criteria to select those most likely to survive (Fox and Swazey 1978, pp. 305–44). As

---

*Unless otherwise stated, the views expressed are those of the author and not of the New York State Task Force on Life and the Law.

the procedures crossed the threshold from experimental to therapeutic, two other factors limited access: the lack of universal coverage for heart and liver transplants, and the finite supply of donated organs.

The supply of donor organs continues to limit access to solid organ transplantation; the number of individuals waiting for kidney, heart, and liver transplants far outstrips the supply of donated organs (UNOS 1990b, p. 26). Indeed, as surgeons have broken new boundaries, transplanting patients who are older and sicker, as well as those who need multiple transplants, the number of patients considered medically eligible has swelled. The steady success of transplantation has ensured that hard choices about distributing organs persist.

Some of those hard choices have been confronted. A national registry of those awaiting transplantation has been established. Explicit policies for organ distribution have replaced informal agreements. Standards for screening donors have been set, and data collection may soon yield new insight into the relationship between donor characteristics and recipient outcome. In response to reports that wealthy foreign nationals had gained priority on waiting lists through large donations to transplant centers, policies for access by nonimmigrant aliens have been established.

Despite these changes, problems remain. Debate among policy makers has recently focused on one dimension of access to donor organs—whether prospective transplant recipients should be permitted to place themselves on lists at several transplant programs or organ procurement organizations. Patients engage in this practice of "multiple listing" to improve their chances of receiving a donated organ. For potential kidney recipients, multiple listing may shorten their wait or increase the odds of receiving a well-matched kidney. The stakes are higher for heart and liver transplants because some patients die while waiting for a donated organ.

The question of whether patients should be allowed to multiple list resonates beyond transplantation to the broader arena of access to health care. In national discussions, the debate about multiple listing has been framed as a need to balance the demands of justice and autonomy (UNOS 1988a, pp. 7–10). The equity of distribution has been pitted against the right of individuals to seek treatment in whatever fashion best meets their own needs.

Because of the federal government's role in paying for kidney transplants, questions about the nature and limits of individual entitlement to health care are also implicit, although not explicit, in the debate. The End-Stage Renal Disease (ESRD) Program gave those with end-stage renal disease special status: the federal government pays all costs arising from treatment, including the costs of evaluative tests. When patients multiple list, the government pays for the costly evaluative tests at each center where the patient seeks treatment.

This article examines multiple listing, focusing on the claims of justice and autonomy posed by the practice. It describes the policies embraced at the national level, and discusses the different approach taken by New York State. The article concludes by exploring the implications of the debate about multiple listing for national consideration of access to health care.

DISTRIBUTING ORGANS: NATIONAL POLICY

Organs are procured for transplantation by organizations called organ procurement organizations (OPOs). Some OPOs procure and distribute organs in a geographic area that encompasses just a few hospitals while others cover all hospitals in an entire state or region. Other OPOs are based in hospitals and serve only the needs of the transplant center at that hospital; organs procured are generally offered first to patients at that center, then to patients at other hospitals if no recipient at the center is identified. Kidneys must be shared on a national basis when a six antigen or "perfect" donor-recipient match appears on a national list of patients waiting (UNOS 1988c, sec. 3.3).

The federal government pays the costs of recovering kidneys through the ESRD Program, and is the primary source of funds for OPOs (Task Force on Organ Transplantation 1986, p. 55). The costs of procuring hearts, livers, and other organs are charged to recipients and paid by the individual or by third-party insurers that cover the transplant.

Prior to the development of national policies in 1987, each OPO devised its own criteria or process for distributing organs to transplant centers. Transplant centers, in turn, were free to distribute organs based on facility policy or on the judgments of individual surgeons. There were no publicly available records of the choices made by OPOs or by surgeons. The decisions were essentially private, and often based on agreements among transplant surgeons in a given region or hospital.

In 1984, the federal government initiated efforts to provide national policies for procuring and distributing organs. Congress passed the National Organ Transplant Act, creating a national task force on organ transplantation (National Organ Transplant Act 1984, 42 U.S.C., sec. 273). In its report, issued in 1986, the Task Force recommended numerous policies to promote equitable access to transplantation (Task Force on Organ Transplantation 1986, pp. 65–99).

The 1984 act also mandated the creation of a national organ procurement and transplantation network (the Network). In 1986, the Department of Health and Human Services (HHS) contracted with the United Network for Organ Sharing (UNOS), a private, not-for-profit entity, to establish and operate the Network. As a condition of receiving Medicare funds, hospitals, OPOs, and histocompatibility laboratories must be members of the Network. As of October 1990, 258 transplant centers, 51 independent procurement organizations, 43 tissue typing laboratories, 9 voluntary health organizations, 21 professional organizations, and 12 individuals representing the public were Network members (Johnson 1990, personal communication).[1]

Initially, all members of the Network were obligated to comply with policies established by UNOS. In December 1989, HHS redefined UNOS's authority, concluding that compliance with UNOS policies would be voluntary unless such policies are approved by HHS and promulgated as federal regulations (54 Fed. Reg. 51803 (1989)).

In authorizing creation of the Network, Congress sought to ensure the equitable distribution of organs for transplantation. As stated in the Senate report on the National Organ Transplant Act of 1984, "the conferees are particularly concerned that OPOs adopt medical criteria for the equitable allocation of donated organs among transplant centers and patients" (United States Senate 1984, p. 3992). In 1988, Congress amended the Act to clarify that OPOs must distribute organs equitably, not among transplant centers, but among patients

waiting (Health Omnibus Program Extension 1988, Title IV, sec. 402).[2]

In May 1987, UNOS established criteria for distributing kidneys and extrarenal organs such as the heart and liver (UNOS 1987, sec. 3). The criteria developed for each organ have been periodically reviewed and modified by UNOS since that time. After determinations based on blood type and organ size, the primary factors in distributing organs are the medical needs of the patient and the length of time the patient has been waiting. Criteria for distributing extrarenal organs give priority to medically urgent patients. Because patients waiting for a kidney transplant can be sustained on dialysis, the criteria for kidneys do not focus on medical urgency, but include consideration of the immunological compatibility of donors and recipients. The criteria apply to the distribution of organs by OPOs to transplant centers, and to the selection of patients by transplant centers from among patients on the center's waiting list (UNOS 1988c, secs. 3.5–3.6).[3]

MULTIPLE LISTING

Patients multiple list by seeking treatment at more than one transplant center. Depending on the arrangements between OPOs and local transplant centers, patients can multiple list by seeking treatment at several transplant centers in one region, or at several centers in different regions. For example, five OPOs may each serve a different geographic region. By seeking treatment at a transplant program in each of those five regions, a patient could be placed on all five OPO lists. Alternatively, where an OPO provides organs to several hospitals, each of which maintains its own waiting list, patients could multiple list by seeking treatment from numerous transplant centers in a single area, each of which would list the patient as a potential recipient.

Patients multiple list principally to gain better access to the limited supply of donated organs (UNOS 1988a, p. 8). Support for the practice derives primarily from the belief that patients should be free to maximize their access to treatment, including access to the scarce supply of donated organs. By multiple listing, patients gain access to one or more additional pools of organs. They also improve their chance of receiving an organ under national policies that give priority to patients on local lists or to patients at hospitals nearest to the transplant hospital where the donor is located. For example, under UNOS policies, one factor weighed in distributing hearts and livers is the proximity of the donor and the transplant center where the procedure will be performed (UNOS 1987, secs. 3.6–3.7).

Other less significant reasons for multiple listing have also been advanced. Multiple listing provides a convenience for patients who live part of the year in different locations and might otherwise have to travel on short notice to be transplanted (Owen 1988, p. 2). A significant percentage of the patients awaiting kidney transplantation are sensitized: they are hard to match with a donor kidney for immunological reasons. In regions that have no program to share kidneys for these patients, multiple listing gives them broader access to available donors, thereby increasing their chance of finding a kidney.

For patients who list at small centers, multiple listing provides additional assurance that a transplant team will be available if an organ is offered to them.[4] Finally, in national debates about multiple listing, proponents of the practice also suggested that a ban on multiple listing would hinder the growth of small transplant programs by making patients reluctant to list only at those programs (UNOS 1988b, p. 4). Some maintained that the public would need more information about outcomes and the performance of transplant centers if multiple listing were banned and patients were forced to choose only one center (UNOS 1988b, p. 4).

The predominant objection to multiple listing stems from a belief that the practice is inequitable, giving some patients an advantage over others (Childress 1989, p. 107; New York State Task Force on Life and the Law (NYTF) 1988, p. 93). In order to multiple list, patients must be informed about the advantages it offers and must have the time and financial resources to travel to different cen-

ters for the evaluative tests and follow-up care that must be provided. The UNOS Board of Directors in a 1988 policy statement observed that multiple listing favors "the wealthy patient over a less well-to-do patient" who may not be able to afford to travel for the initial work-up and follow-up treatment (UNOS 1988a, p. 9). The Board also concluded: "It seems clear that for every advantage afforded a transplant patient a commensurate disadvantage is created for other transplant patients thus creating inequality of opportunity to receive a donated organ" (UNOS 1988a, p. 8).

Other objections to multiple listing focus on the costs of duplicative clinical evaluation and testing for patients awaiting transplantation. For kidney transplantation, the laboratory charges alone for evaluative tests average $3,000 for the initial work-up and ongoing care.[5] In addition, once on a transplant list, many patients undergo expensive monthly or periodic panel reactive antibody tests so that the transplant center has current immunological information about the patient. Through the ESRD Program, the federal government pays the cost for both the initial evaluation and periodic tests at each center where the patient seeks treatment.

This duplication of costs for the medical work-up is also incurred for extrarenal transplants. As explained by representatives of a major cardiac transplant center:

> The preoperative medical workup which includes (for heart patients) both tissue typing, right heart catheterizations, psychological evaluations, oral surgery evaluations, social service evaluations, cardiology evaluations and the transplant surgeons' evaluations would all need to be repeated every time the patient went to another center. Our center would never accept the evaluation of a patient from another center. (Cavarocchi and Kolff 1988, p. 1)

It has also been argued that multiple listing diminishes the quality of patient care. The process of seeking treatment from several centers and physicians may disrupt the patient-physician relationship because patients do not consider any single person as their physician. In particular, the process of informed consent and preoperative education of recipients may be impaired when patients multiple list (Cavarocchi and Kolff 1988, p. 1). When patients are principally treated at one center and placed on waiting lists at other institutions, long-term cooperation between the transplant surgeon and the patient's internist may also be disrupted. As pointed out by the UNOS Board, multiple listing may also lead to variations in tissue typing results because sera samples are taken from potential transplant recipients by different transplant centers at different times.

DEVISING POLICIES ON MULTIPLE LISTING

National Policy

To date, policies on multiple listing have been adopted nationally and in New York State. National policy has been established by UNOS, although like other UNOS policies, the policy on multiple listing has been submitted for review to the Health Care Financing Administration. The UNOS Board of Directors voted to permit patients to be placed on more than one waiting list in August 1987, as part of UNOS's initial efforts to establish comprehensive policies for organ distribution. Several months after the new policies became effective, the UNOS Board reversed itself, voting at a January 1988 meeting to prohibit multiple listing. As articulated by the UNOS Board, the reversal rested on the belief that multiple listing had led to inequities in the distribution of organs (UNOS 1988b, p. 1). In a statement that weighed the arguments on both sides of the debate, the Board of Directors concluded that the inequities created by permitting multiple listing outweigh considerations supporting the practice (UNOS 1988a, p. 10).

Following adoption of its policy on multiple listing, the UNOS Board solicited public comments by sending the policy to individuals and organizations on the UNOS distribution list. At a public hearing held by UNOS on March 21, 1988, five individuals offered testimony. Others submitted written comments. Among the thirty-three written comments received was a form letter signed by sixty-three transplant patients opposing the prohibition against multiple listing. The most common basis for opposing the prohibition rested on claims that it would "intolerably infringe on individual rights" (UNOS 1988b, p. 2). Some patients argued that wealth determines access to other kinds of health care, and transplantation should not be distinguished (Abt Associates, Inc. 1990, p. 75). In statements submitted to UNOS, both the American Association of Kidney Patients and the National Kidney Foundation recognized the inequity created by multiple listing, but proposed that the ban should not be implemented until the needs of highly sensitized and medically urgent patients could be met through policies to improve organ sharing among regions and nationally (American Association of Kidney Patients 1988; Glassok 1988).

Following the public comment period, the UNOS Board changed its position. UNOS policies released in May 1988 expressly allow patients to multiple list (UNOS 1988c, sec. 3.2). In May 1990, UNOS adopted a policy to prohibit hospitals from listing a patient with more than one OPO, but left patients free to multiple list by seeking treatment at different hospitals (UNOS 1990a, sec. 3.2).[6]

New York State Policy

In July 1990, New York State became the first state in the country to pass a law banning multiple listing. The ban was enacted as part of a package of comprehensive policies to enhance the equitable distribution of organs for transplantation and to establish public standards for procuring and distributing organs and tissues throughout the state.

A 1988 report by the New York State Task Force on Life and the Law sparked consideration of multiple listing in New York State.[7] In response to a mandate to recommend policy on transplantation, the Task Force undertook a two-year study of the process in New York State for procuring and distributing donated organs and tissues. As part of that study, the Task Force sent a questionnaire to the directors of kidney transplant programs in the state. Ten of the twelve directors estimated that some of their patients were listed on three or more different hospital waiting lists (NYTF 1988, p. 93). At one transplant center, the director estimated that 50 percent of the patients enrolled in the program were also on waiting lists at one or more other programs.

In its recommendations, the Task Force urged that state initiatives to ensure equitable access remained crucial, despite the existence of national policies for organ procurement and distribution. As argued by the Task Force, the state has a clear obligation to its citizens as potential donors and recipients to ensure that donated organs and tissues are distributed by a system that is effective and fair. The state's required request law, mandating requests for organs and tissues from all suitable donors, had heightened that duty.[8]

The Task Force identified the fragmentation of waiting lists and multiple listing as significant barriers to equitable access. The two problems are interrelated; fragmented waiting lists in a single region increase the opportunities for and advantages of multiple listing. For example, in 1987, each of the six kidney transplant programs in the Greater New York Metropolitan Area had different rates of access to donor organs and maintained different waiting lists. Access to organs therefore depended on which hospital in the Metropolitan Area was treating the patient, rather than on patient-centered criteria such as which patient had waited longest or was medically best suited for the organ (NYTF 1988, pp. 90–96). The fragmented lists also enabled patients to increase their chances of receiving an organ each time they listed with a different hospital.

The Task Force proposed that waiting lists should be consolidated at the OPO level, rather than allow six transplant centers in a single metropolitan area to maintain separate lists.[9] The Task Force also advocated a ban on multiple listing. As stated by the Task Force, "Multiple waiting lists give a distinct advantage to persons who are more informed health care consumers and more assertive about seeking available treatment, characteristics that usually correlate strongly with higher socioeconomic status" (NYTF 1988, p. 93).

The Task Force's recommendation responded to the special needs of patients who multiple list because they are highly sensitized and need access to a large pool of potential donors.[10] The Organ Transplant Act of 1984 sought to address this problem by requiring the national Network to

> prepare and distribute, on a regionalized basis, samples of blood sera from individuals who are included in the list and whose immune system makes it difficult for them to receive organs to facilitate matching the compatibility of such individuals with donor organs. (National Organ Transplant Act 1984, 42 U.S.C., sec. 274)

No such system had been developed in New York State. The Task Force recommended that a council be created within the State, to assume, among other responsibilities, the task of devising plans and policies to develop a system of organ sharing to benefit the growing population of highly sensitized patients.

As enacted, New York's law on organ distribution prohibits patients from placing themselves on more than one waiting list maintained by any organ procurement organization designated to serve any part of New York State (N.Y. Public Health Law 1990, sec. 4363). The law also bars OPOs from placing patients on a list if the patient is already listed with another OPO. In addition, the law establishes a council on organ and tissue transplantation and empowers the Commissioner of Health, in consultation with the council, to develop standards for organ sharing among OPOs in the state to meet the needs of highly sensitized patients (N.Y. Public Health Law 1990, sec. 4361).

The Legislature chose to grandfather in those who were multiple listed as of the date the bill was signed into law, implicitly recognizing the sense of entitlement some patients might feel, but curtailing the practice as an ongoing pattern. The law covers OPO lists for OPOs designated by HHS to serve any part of New York State, recognizing that comprehensive national policy must await federal action or similar initiatives in other states.

DISCUSSION

Stripped to its essentials, the debate about multiple listing poses a choice between equity and autonomy. Arising within the overall context of the

American health care system, the debate is informed by the expectations and values that infuse our national health care policies.

The inequities of our current health care system, and the extent to which it allows ability to pay and market principles to determine access, have come under increasing scrutiny and attack. However, even when considered in light of our current health care system, the reasons to bar multiple listing are compelling. Those reasons stem, in part, from distinctive features of organ transplantation: the special status accorded ESRD treatment, the finite supply of organs, the technology's dependence on donated organs, and the life-saving nature of the treatment.

The crux of the argument supporting multiple listing rests on the notion that individuals should not be constrained in seeking medical treatment. Indeed, the past two decades in the United States have witnessed increasing support for patient autonomy—the right of patients to decide about treatment in accord with their own religious, personal, and moral convictions. This support has been accompanied by a growing body of case law recognizing a common law and constitutional right to decide about treatment.[11]

The right to multiple list, however, bears no relation to patient autonomy as generally understood and promoted. A ban on multiple listing would leave patients free to seek treatment from the physician and transplant center of their choice. The right to decide about the nature and course of treatment would also be undiminished.

Essentially, multiple listing entails a right to seek the same treatment at two, three or more transplant centers, and for kidney transplant recipients, to have the federal government pay for such duplicative care. Although the practice has been defended under the banner of individual "liberty," it approximates a liberty interest or right only if one understands patient rights in the context of a market model in which consumer choice and provider willingness to accommodate those choices are the only lodestars for policy.

Although market principles govern many aspects of health care delivery in the United States, the ESRD Program stands as one of the few unequivocal rejections of the market model. Seeking to avoid the agonizing responsibility of deciding who should live and who should die, Congress enacted the ESRD Program to give all persons with end-stage renal disease access to treatment without regard to ability to pay (Fox and Swazey 1978, pp. 347–48). One of the ironies of multiple listing is that it allows wealthier individuals to gain an advantage over others waiting, thereby undermining the principles that animated creation of the ESRD Program, and the special status granted all ESRD patients.

The ESRD Program covers only kidney transplants. Access to hearts, livers, and other solid organs still depends on ability to pay for the costly transplant procedure. Nonetheless, the voluntary donation of organs by the public, with the implicit understanding that organs will be distributed fairly, strains the libertarian principles that undergird the market approach.

Individuals are routinely asked to donate organs, either their own organs through an advance consent or the organs of their loved ones. The request for donation and the donation itself are premised on altruism; the donation symbolizes and reinforces a sense of community and connectedness. As explained by Thomas Murray (1987, p. 37), the meaning of this gift is significant for society, as well as for the donor and recipient:

> In the face of impersonal bureaucracies, gifts to "strangers" affirm a number of vital social values including our solidarity with others in our community, and our vision of human flourishing, individual and social, that require more than the thin relationships established by markets and contracts.

Proposals to allow the sale of organs, and shift to a market model for organ procurement and distribution, have never been accepted in the United States. Although the debate about "financial incentives" for organ donations, such as payment for funeral expenses, has recently been revived, current state and federal laws prohibit the sale of organs and tissues (Peters 1991, pp. 1304–5; Pellegrino 1991, pp. 1305–6; National Organ Transplant Act 1984, 42 U.S.C., sec. 274e).

Neither transplant surgeons nor OPOs that distribute organs "own" the organs; they hold the organs in trust and are bound by the understandings, implicit and explicit, that motivate the donation.[12] Central to those understandings is the expectation that organs will be distributed fairly.

The findings of a 1988 Gallup survey sponsored by UNOS underscore this public expectation (Evans and Manninen 1988, pp. 781–85). Seeking to determine whether the public believed that citizenship should be considered in distributing organs, the study found that fairness overall, not citizenship, was the public's foremost concern. Eighty-eight percent of the people surveyed were most concerned that organs be distributed fairly. In addition, 81.4 percent believed that "medical need, not social or economic factors, should be the only criteria used to select transplant recipients" (Evans and Manninen 1988, p. 782).

This public expectation, and the altruism which motivates the intensely personal gift of an organ, defeat any claim that market principles should govern access to organs. In fact, failure to match the public's expectation of fairness is likely to undermine public trust in the donation system, and threaten public willingness to donate. As stated by Arthur Caplan (1987, p. 18) in discussing the demands of equity in selecting heart transplant recipients, "Nothing is more threatening to the integrity of the present system for obtaining organs and tissues than the perception that bias and inequity prevail within the allocation process."

Apart from the values implicit in the ESRD Program and the donation of organs, any notion of a right to multiple list must also be weighed against the demands of distributive justice. Based on this analysis alone, multiple listing should be prohibited. Placed on the scales of liberty and justice, the right to multiple list pales by comparison to the interests of those who are disadvantaged by the practice because they are not savvy or wealthy enough to avail themselves of its benefits.

The asserted right to multiple list rests on a weak moral claim; even if the right is denied, patients would be free to choose their own doctor, hospital, and course of treatment. Just as important, the demands of justice are especially compelling because transplantation is life-saving for certain patients and because the supply of organs

is finite in an absolute sense. In our open-ended health care delivery system, decisions to provide treatment to one patient may have little, if any, bearing on the availability of resources for another patient. Due to the finite number of donated organs, transplantation is a clear exception. Giving an advantage to one patient necessarily harms another patient who is waiting.

Finally, as practiced now, multiple listing for kidney transplantation involves payment by the federal government for repeated tests and subsequent visits at each center where patients list for a transplant. This government subsidy makes the market model altogether inapposite to multiple listing for kidney transplants. In a nation where 37 million individuals lack access to basic care, payment for duplicative tests and a claim of entitlement to such payment also defy rational explanation.

Such claims do, however, provide a powerful example of the way in which economic factors shape medical practice and consumer expectation. In 1975, Judith Swazey and Renee Fox observed that Medicare funding for transplantation and dialysis led not only to the relaxation of psychosocial criteria used in the 1960s to screen patients, but also to the relaxation of biomedical contraindications. They asserted that it had become:

> difficult for physicians to "deselect" any patient in irreversible renal failure for a transplant (or dialysis), regardless of how little benefit he or she may be expected to derive from the treatment, how much added suffering it may entail, and what additional problems it may create for allocation of scarce resources. (Fox and Swazey 1978, p. 309)

As demonstrated by the debate on multiple listing, by 1988 the difficulties of deselection had spread to the provision of duplicative care and a relaxation of standards for equitable access. In the national debate on multiple listing, some patients asserted a right to multiple list as a basic entitlement, and changed the course of national policy. Implicit in that assertion is the right to gain an advantage over others who are waiting, and to have government pay the cost of duplicative care. It is a claim that recognizes no bonds or restraints of community. While perhaps not surprising as a general outlook in American society, it is striking when embraced by those who benefit from one of society's most powerful symbols of kinship and community: the donation of organs for transplantation.

CONCLUSION

In the national debate about access to health care, Daniel Callahan (1990, pp. 57–62) has maintained that the United States cannot seriously address the twin problems of access and rising health care costs unless it identifies limits to the notion of individual entitlement. The debate about multiple listing highlights the importance of a principled and coherent understanding of access and entitlement to health care.

It also suggests the pitfalls of allowing those most intensely interested in the outcome of access policies to dominate and define public debate. Patients who are multiply listed represent only a small segment of the public. Public policy must also respond to the interests of those who are not wealthy or assertive enough to multiple list. Ultimately, the voices of those seeking to multiple list must also be weighed against the wishes of those who provide the organs and pay for the practice—the American public. At a time of fiscal scarcity and government cutbacks, funding for multiple listing would undoubtedly strike an unresponsive or distinctly negative chord with the American public.

The distribution of organs for transplantation has posed profound and agonizing ethical dilemmas, tragic choices that present no satisfying resolution.[13] A policy to prohibit multiple listing is not a tragic choice—just a question of basic fairness and common sense.

The author wishes to thank Nancy Dubler and James Childress for their thoughtful comments on an earlier draft of the article.

NOTES

1. Professional non-profit organizations must be engaged in organ transplantation or donation or provision of services or support to transplant recipients to qualify as a UNOS member.

2. The requirement that OPOs equitably distribute organs to patients waiting implicitly binds the Network and UNOS as well.

3. OPOs and transplant centers are not obligated to follow these criteria if they obtain a "variance" from UNOS. As of August 1991, UNOS had granted 25 variances to OPOs serving 87 of the 254 (34 percent) transplant centers nationwide (Abt Associates, Inc. 1990, pp. 75, 91).

4. Testimony submitted to UNOS proposed that transplant centers could develop backup arrangements to compensate when the transplant team is occupied and an extrarenal organ becomes available (UNOS 1988b, p. 4). Other comments submitted suggested that transplant centers that could not provide such backup should reconsider whether they should perform extrarenal transplants (Cavarocchi and Kolff 1988, p. 2).

5. Charges for evaluative tests to place a patient on a waiting list at a transplant center range between $1,100.00–$1,200.00, with an on-going charge for antibody screening of approximately $150.00 for each month the patient remains on the waiting list (Medicare 1990). Between October 1, 1987 and December 31, 1989, the median waiting time for a kidney transplant was 396.9 days (UNOS 1990c).

6. A survey of UNOS members conducted in 1990 found that 63 percent of UNOS members support a policy that bars patients from listing at more than one transplant center (Abt Associates, Inc. 1990, p. 75).

7. Convened by Governor Cuomo in 1985, the Task Force has a broad mandate to recommend policies on issues raised by medical advances, including organ transplantation.

8. Thirty-three states have passed required request legislation. Congress adopted the required request approach in 1986, obligating all hospitals to develop request policies as a condition of receiving Medicare funds (Omnibus Reconciliation Act of 1986, PL No. 99-509).

9. A 1990 Report by the Inspector General at the Department of Health and Human Services concluded that the fragmentation of waiting lists, and the disparity in waiting times for patients at different transplant centers, were significant detriments to the attainment of equity nationally (Office of Inspector General 1990, p. 11). UNOS is currently reviewing its policy permitting each transplant center to maintain its own waiting list.

10. According to estimates by the directors of twelve kidney transplant centers in New York State, of 1,300 patients waiting for kidney transplants in September 1986, 622 or 45 percent were highly sensitized—with sensitization defined to mean patients with panel reactive antibodies greater than 46 percent (NYTF 1988, p. 139).

11. See, e.g., *Cruzan v. Director, Missouri Dept. of Health,* 497 U.S. ———, 110 S.Ct. 2841, 2846–2851 (1990); *Fosmire v. Nicoleau,* 75 N.Y.2d 218, 226, 551 N.E.2d 771 (1990).

12. In his article, "Gifts of the Body and the Needs of Strangers," Murray (1987, p. 32) argues that gifts create moral obligations for the recipient, including "grateful acceptance of the gift"—the concurrence of the recipient's will with the donor's and/or the recipient's consent to abide by that will.

13. The phrase "tragic choices" is drawn from the title of a book that focuses on the painful choices society must make when confronted with scarcity (Calabresi and Bobbitt 1978).

REFERENCES

Abt Associates, Inc. 1990. *Evaluation of the Organ Procurement and Transplantation Network: Final Report.*

American Association of Kidney Patients, Inc., Board of Directors. 1988. *Policy on Multiple Listing* (12 March).

Calabresi, Guido, and Bobbitt, Philip. 1978. *Tragic Choices.* New York: W. W. Norton Company.

Callahan, Daniel. 1990. *What Kind of Life: the Limits of Medical Progress.* New York: Simon and Schuster.

Caplan, Arthur. 1987. Equity in the Selection of Recipients for Cardiac Transplants. *Circulation* 75: 10–18.

Cavarocchi, Nicholas, and Kolff, Jacob. 1988. Letter to Walter K. Graham, Assistant Executive Director, UNOS, on behalf of Temple University Hospital (17 March).

Childress, James. 1989. Ethical Criteria for Procuring and Distributing Organs for Transplantation. *Journal of Health Politics, Policy and Law* 14 (1): 107.

Evans, R. W., and Manninen, D. L. 1988. U.S. Public Opinion Concerning the Procurement and Distribution of Donor Organs. *Transplantation Proceedings* 20: 781–85.

Fox, Renee, and Swazey, Judith. 1978. *The Courage to Fail.* Chicago: University of Chicago Press.

Glassok, Richard. 1988. Letter to Walter K. Graham, Assistant Executive Director, UNOS, on behalf of the National Kidney Foundation (14 March).

Johnson, Donna. 1990. Personal communication regarding UNOS by-laws (7 November).

Medicare. 1990. Histocompatibility Labs-Interim Reimbursement Rates (1 October).

Murray, Thomas H. 1987. Gifts of the Body and the Needs of Strangers. *Hastings Center Report* 17 (2): 30–38.

New York State Task Force on Life and the Law. 1986. *The Required Request Law.*

———. 1988. *Transplantation in New York State: The Procurement and Distribution of Organs and Tissues, New York State.*

Office of Inspector General. 1990. *The Distribution of Organs for Transplantation: Expectations and Practices.* Washington, D.C.: U.S. Department of Health and Human Services.

Owen, Jack W. 1988. Letter to Walter K. Graham, Assistant Executive Director, UNOS, on behalf of the American Hospital Association (17 March).

Pellegrino, Edmund D. 1991. Families' Self-Interest and the Cadaver's Organs: What Price Consent? *Journal of the American Medical Association* 265: 1305–6.

Peters, Thomas G. 1991. Life or Death: The Issue of Payment in Cadaveric Organ Donation. *Journal of the American Medical Association* 265: 1302–5.

Task Force on Organ Transplantation. 1986. Transplantation: Issues and Recommendations. Washington, D.C.: U.S. Department of Health and Human Services.

UNOS. 1987. *UNOS Policies* (September).

———. 1988a. *UNOS Policy Proposal Statement* (February).

———. 1988b. *UNOS Policy Proposal Statement Regarding the Listing of Patients on Multiple Transplant Waiting Lists: Public Hearing Background Statement* (March).

———. 1988c. *UNOS Policies* (May).

———. 1990a. *UNOS Policies* (January).

———. 1990b. *UNOS Update* 6 (5): 26.

———. 1990c. *OPTN Analysis: Activity and Median Waiting Times* (4 December).

United States Senate. 1984. Report No. 98-382, Committee on Labor and Human Resources.

QUESTIONS FOR COMPREHENSION AND REFLECTION

1. What are the most prominent arguments in support of multiple listing? What are the most common arguments against it?

2. What was the rationale behind New York's ban on multiple listing? Do you agree or disagree? Explain.

3. Prohibiting multiple listing places limits on the expression of individual autonomy. Miller argues that these limits are justified. Discuss her fundamental reasons for banning multiple listing. Do you agree or disagree? Support your answer.
4. Provide utilitarian and deontological support for positions that support and oppose multiple listing. Explain in detail.

ALVIN H. MOSS AND MARK SIEGLER

Should Alcoholics Compete Equally for Liver Transplantation?

Alvin H. Moss teaches at the Center for Health Ethics and Law at West Virginia University Health Sciences Center in Morgantown, West Virginia. Mark Siegler teaches at the Center for Clinical Ethics, University of Chicago Pritzker School of Medicine. They tackle the contentious issue of liver transplants for those suffering from alcohol-related end-stage liver disease. They first describe the uniqueness of liver transplantation, underscoring the extreme scarcity of donor livers. They then go on to argue that justice requires that patients who have end-stage liver disease and have not incurred it through their own actions should have priority over unrehabilitated alcoholics. They justify a prioritization scheme that rewards responsible behavior and rules out a policy of first-come, first-served.

Until recently, liver transplantation for patients with alcohol-related end-stage liver disease (ARESLD) was not considered a treatment option. Most physicians in the transplant community did not recommend it because of initial poor results in this population[1] and because of a predicted high recidivism rate that would preclude long-term survival.[2] In 1988, however, Starzl and colleagues[3] reported 1-year survival rates for patients with ARESLD comparable to results in patients with other causes of end-stage liver disease (ESLD). Although the patients in the Pittsburgh series may represent a carefully selected population,[3,4] the question is no longer Can we perform transplants in patients with alcoholic liver disease and obtain acceptable results? but Should we? This question is particularly timely since the Health Care Financing Administration (HCFA) has recommended that Medicare coverage for liver transplantation be offered to patients with alcoholic cirrhosis who are abstinent. The HCFA proposes that the same eligibility criteria be used for patients with ARESLD as are used for patients with other causes of ESLD, such as primary biliary cirrhosis and sclerosing cholangitis.[5]

SHOULD PATIENTS WITH ARESLD RECEIVE TRANSPLANTS?

At first glance, this question seems simple to answer. Generally, in medicine, a therapy is used if it works and saves lives. But the circumstances of liver transplantation differ from those of most other lifesaving therapies, including long-term mechanical ventilation and dialysis, in three important respects:

Nonrenewable Resource

First, although most lifesaving therapies are expensive, liver transplantation uses a nonrenewable, absolutely scarce resource—a donor liver. In contrast to patients with end-stage renal disease, who may receive either a transplant or dialysis therapy, every patient with ESLD who does not receive a liver transplant will die. This dire, absolute scarcity of donor livers would be greatly exacerbated by including patients with ARESLD as potential candidates for liver transplantation. In 1985, 63,737 deaths due to hepatic disease occurred in the United States, at least 36,000 of which were related to alcoholism, but fewer than 1000 liver transplants were performed.[6] Although patients with ARESLD represent more than 50% of the patients with ESLD, patients with ARESLD account for less than 10% of those receiving transplants (*New York Times*. April 3, 1990:B6[col 1]). If patients with ARESLD were accepted for liver transplantation on an equal basis, as suggested by the HCFA, there would potentially be more than 30,000 additional candidates each year. (No data exist to indicate how many patients in the late stages of ARESLD would meet transplantation eligibility criteria.) In 1987, only 1182 liver transplants were performed; in 1989, fewer than 2000 were done.[6] Even if all donor livers available were given to patients with ARESLD, it would not be feasible to provide transplants for even a small fraction of them. Thus, the dire, absolute nature of donor liver scarcity mandates that distribution be based on unusually rigorous standards—standards not required for the allocation of most other resources such as dialysis machines and ventilators, both of which are only *relatively* scarce.

Comparison with Cardiac Transplantation

Second, although a similar dire, absolute scarcity of donor hearts exists for cardiac transplantation, the allocational decisions for cardiac transplantation differ from those for liver transplantation. In liver transplantation, ARESLD causes more than 50% of the cases of ESLD; in cardiac transplantation, however, no one predominant disease or contributory factor is responsible. Even for patients with end-stage ischemic heart disease who smoked or who failed to adhere to dietary regimens, it is rarely clear that one particular behavior caused the disease. Also, unlike our proposed consideration for liver transplantation, a history of alcohol abuse is considered a contraindication and is a common reason for a patient with heart disease to be denied cardiac transplantation.[7,8] Thus, the allocational decisions for heart transplantation differ from those for liver transplantation in two ways: determining a cause for end-stage heart disease is less certain, and patients with a history of alcoholism are usually rejected from heart transplant programs.

Expensive Technology

Third, a unique aspect of liver transplantation is that it is an expensive technology that has become a target of cost containment in health care.[9] It is, therefore, essential to maintain the approbation and support of the public so that organs continue to be donated under appropriate clinical circumstances—even in spite of the high cost of transplantation.

General Guideline Proposed

In view of the distinctive circumstances surrounding liver transplantation, we propose as a general guideline that patients with ARESLD should not compete equally with other candidates for liver transplantation. We are *not* suggesting that patients with ARESLD should *never* receive liver transplants. Rather, we propose that a priority ranking be established for the use of this dire, absolutely scarce societal resource and that patients with ARESLD be lower on the list than others with ESLD.

OBJECTIONS TO PROPOSAL

We realize that our proposal may meet with two immediate objections: (1) Some may argue that since alcoholism is a disease, patients with

ARESLD should be considered equally for liver transplantation.[10] (2) Some will question why patients with ARESLD should be singled out for discrimination, when the medical profession treats many patients who engage in behavior that causes their diseases.[11] We will discuss these objections in turn.

Alcoholism: How Is It Similar to and Different from Other Diseases?

We do not dispute the reclassification of alcoholism as a disease.[12] Both hereditary and environmental factors contribute to alcoholism, and physiological, biochemical, and genetic markers have been associated with increased susceptibility.[13] Identifying alcoholism as a disease enables physicians to approach it as they do other medical problems and to differentiate it from bad habits, crimes, or moral weaknesses. More important, identifying alcoholism as a disease also legitimizes medical interventions to treat it.[14]

Alcoholism is a chronic disease,[14,15] for which treatment is available and effective. More than 1.43 million patients were treated in 5586 alcohol treatment units in the 12-month period ending October 30, 1987.[16] One comprehensive review concluded that more than two thirds of patients who accept therapy improve.[17] Another cited four studies in which at least 54% of patients were abstinent a minimum of 1 year after treatment.[18] A recent study of alcohol-impaired physicians reported a 100% abstinence rate an average of 33.4 months after therapy was initiated. In this study, physician-patients rated Alcoholics Anonymous, the largest organization of recovering alcoholics in the world, as the most important component of their therapy.[19]

Like other chronic diseases—such as type I diabetes mellitus, which requires the patient to administer insulin over a lifetime—alcoholism requires the patient to assume responsibility for participating in continuous treatment. Two key elements are required to successfully treat alcoholism: the patient must accept his or her diagnosis and must assume responsibility for treatment.[20,21] The high success rates of some alcoholism treatment programs indicate that many patients can accept responsibility for their treatment. ARESLD, one of the sequelae of alcoholism, results from 10 to 20 years of heavy alcohol consumption. The risk of ARESLD increases with the amount of alcohol consumed and with the duration of heavy consumption.[22] In view of the quantity of alcohol consumed, the years, even decades, required to develop ARESLD, and the availability of effective alcohol treatment, attributing personal responsibility for ARESLD to the patient seems all the more justified. We believe, therefore, that even though alcoholism is a chronic disease, alcoholics should be held responsible for seeking and obtaining treatment that could prevent the development of late-stage complications such as ARESLD. Our view is consistent with that of Alcoholics Anonymous: alcoholics are responsible for undertaking a program for recovery that will keep their disease of alcoholism in remission.[23]

Are We Discriminating Against Alcoholics?

Why should patients with ARESLD be singled out when a large number of patients have health problems that can be attributed to so-called voluntary health-risk behavior? Such patients include smokers with chronic lung disease; obese people who develop type II diabetes; some individuals who test positive for the human immunodeficiency virus; individuals with multiple behavioral risk factors (inattention to blood pressure, cholesterol, diet, and exercise) who develop coronary artery disease; and people such as skiers, motorcyclists, and football players who sustain activity-related injuries. We believe that the health care system should respond based on the actual medical needs of patients rather than on the factors (eg, genetic, infectious, or behavioral) that cause the problem. We also believe that individuals should bear some responsibility—such as increased insurance premiums—for medical problems associated with voluntary choices. The critical distinguishing factor for treatment of ARESLD is the scarcity of the resource needed to treat it. The resources needed to treat most of these other conditions are only moderately or relatively scarce, and patients with these diseases or injuries can receive a share of the resources (ie, money, personnel, and medication) roughly equivalent to their need. In contrast, there are insufficient donor livers to sustain the lives of all with ESLD who are in need.[24] This difference permits us to make some discriminating choices—or to establish priorities—in selecting candidates for liver transplantation based on notions of fairness. In addition, this reasoning enables us to offer patients with alcohol-related medical and surgical problems their fair share of relatively scarce resources, such as blood products, surgical care, and intensive care beds, while still maintaining that their claim on donor livers is less compelling than the claims of others.

REASONS PATIENTS WITH ARESLD SHOULD HAVE A LOWER PRIORITY ON TRANSPLANT WAITING LISTS

Two arguments support our proposal. The first argument is a moral one based on considerations of fairness. The second one is based on policy considerations and examines whether public support of liver transplantation can be maintained if, as a result of a first-come, first-served approach, patients with ARESLD receive more than half the available donor livers. Finally, we will consider further research necessary to determine which patients with ARESLD should be candidates for transplantation, albeit with a lower priority.

Fairness

Given a tragic shortage of donor livers, what is the fair or just way to allocate them? We suggest that patients who develop ESLD through no fault of their own (eg, those with congenital biliary atresia or primary biliary cirrhosis) should have a higher priority in receiving a liver transplant than those whose liver disease results from failure to obtain treatment for alcoholism. In view of the dire, absolute scarcity of donor livers, we believe it is fair to hold people responsible for their choices, including decisions to refuse alcoholism treatment, and to allocate organs on this basis.

It is unfortunate but not unfair to make this distinction.[25] When not enough donor livers are available for all who need one, choices have to be made, and they should be founded on one or more proposed principles of fairness for distributing scarce resources.[26,27] We shall consider four that are particularly relevant:

- *To each, an equal share of treatment.*
- *To each, similar treatment for similar cases.*
- *To each, treatment according to personal effort.*
- *To each, treatment according to ability to pay.*

It is not possible to give each patient with ESLD an *equal share,* or, in this case, a functioning liver. The problem created by the absolute scarcity of donor livers is that of inequality; some receive livers while others do not. But what is fair, need not be equal. Although a first-come, first-served approach has been suggested to provide each patient with an equal chance, we believe it is fairer to give a child dying of biliary atresia an opportunity for a *first* normal liver than it is to give a patient with ARESLD who was born with a normal liver a *second* one.

Because the goal of providing each person with an equal share of health care sometimes collides with the realities of finite medical resources, the principle of *similar treatment for similar cases* has been found to be helpful. Outka[26] stated it this way: "If we accept the case for equal access, but if we simply cannot, physically cannot, treat all who are in need, it seems more just to discriminate by virtue of categories of illness, rather than between rich ill and poor ill." This principle is derived from the principle of formal justice, which, roughly stated, says that people who are equal in relevant respects should be treated equally and that people who are unequal in relevant respects should be treated differently.[27] We believe that patients with ARESLD are unequal in a relevant respect to others with ESLD, since their liver failure was preventable; therefore, it is acceptable to treat them differently.

Our view also relies on the principle of *To each, treatment according to personal effort.* Although alcoholics cannot be held responsible for their disease, once their condition has been diagnosed they can be held responsible for seeking treatment and for preventing the complication of ARESLD. The standard of personal effort and responsibility we propose for alcoholics is the same as that held by

Alcoholics Anonymous. We are not suggesting that some lives and behaviors have greater value than others—an approach used and appropriately repudiated when dialysis machines were in short supply.[26-30] But we are holding people responsible for their personal effort.

Health policymakers have predicted that this principle will assume greater importance in the future. In the context of scarce health care resources, Blank[31] foresees a reevaluation of our health care priorities, with a shift toward individual responsibility and a renewed emphasis on the individual's obligation to society to maximize one's health. Similarly, more than a decade ago, Knowles[32] observed that prevention of disease requires effort. He envisioned that the next major advances in the health of the American people would be determined by what individuals are willing to do for themselves.

To each, treatment according to ability to pay has also been used as a principle of distributive justice. Since alcoholism is prevalent in all socioeconomic strata, it is not discrimination against the poor to deny liver transplantation to patients with alcoholic liver disease.[33] In fact, we believe that poor patients with ARESLD have a stronger claim for a donor liver than rich patients, precisely because many alcohol treatment programs are not available to patients lacking in substantial private resources or health insurance. Ironically, it is precisely this group of poor and uninsured patients who are most likely not to be eligible to receive a liver transplant because of their inability to pay. We agree with Outka's view of fairness that would discriminate according to categories of illness rather than according to wealth.

Policy Considerations Regarding Public Support for Liver Transplantation

Today, the main health policy concerns involve issues of financing, distributive justice, and rationing medical care.[34-37] Because of the many deficiencies in the US health care system—in maternal and child health, in the unmet needs of the elderly, and in the millions of Americans without health insurance—an increasing number of commentators are drawing attention to the trade-offs between basic health care for the many and expensive, albeit lifesaving care for the few.[9,25,38,39]

Because of its high unit cost, liver transplantation is often at the center of these discussions, as it has been in Oregon, where the legislature voted to eliminate Medicaid reimbursement for all transplants except kidneys and corneas.[9] In this era of health care cost containment, a sense of limits is emerging and allocational choices are being made. Oregon has already shown that elected officials and the public are prepared to face these issues.

In our democracy, it is appropriate that community mores and values be regarded seriously when deciding the most appropriate use of a scarce and nonrenewable organ symbolized as a "Gift of Life." As if to underscore this point, the report of the Task Force on Organ Transplantation recommended that each donated organ be considered a national resource for the public good and that the public must participate in decisions on how to use this resource to best serve the public's interests.[40]

Much of the initial success in securing public and political approval for liver transplantation was achieved by focusing media and political attention not on adults but on children dying of ESLD. The public may not support transplantation for patients with ARESLD in the same way that they have endorsed this procedure for babies born with biliary atresia. This assertion is bolstered not only by the events in Oregon but also by the results of a Louis Harris and Associates[41] national survey, which showed that lifesaving therapy for premature infants or for patients with cancer was given the highest health care priority by the public and that lifesaving therapy for patients with alcoholic liver disease was given the lowest. In this poll, the public's view of health care priorities was shared by leadership groups also polled: physicians, nurses, employers, and politicians.

Just because a majority of the public holds these views does not mean that they are right, but the moral intuition of the public, which is also shared by its leaders, reflects community values that must be seriously considered. Also indicative of community values are organizations such as Mothers Against Drunk Driving, Students Against Drunk

Driving, corporate employee assistance programs, and school student assistance programs. Their existence signals that many believe that a person's behavior can be modified so that the consequences of behavior such as alcoholism can be prevented.[42] Thus, giving donor livers to patients with ARESLD on an equal basis with other patients who have ESLD might lead to a decline in public support for liver transplantation.

SHOULD ANY ALCOHOLICS BE CONSIDERED FOR TRANSPLANTATION? NEED FOR FURTHER RESEARCH

Our proposal for giving lower priority for liver transplantation to patients with ARESLD does not completely rule out transplantation for this group. Patients with ARESLD who had not previously been offered therapy and who are now abstinent could be acceptable candidates. In addition, patients lower on the waiting list, such as patients with ARESLD who have been treated and are now abstinent, might be eligible for a donor liver in some regions because of the increased availability of donor organs there. Even if only because of these possible conditions for transplantation, further research is needed to determine which patients with ARESLD would have the best outcomes after liver transplantation.

Transplant programs have been reluctant to provide transplants to alcoholics because of concern about one unfavorable outcome: a high recidivism rate. Although the overall recidivism rate for the Pittsburgh patients was only 11.5%, in the patients who had been abstinent less than 6 months it was 43%.[2] Also, compared with the entire group in which 1-year survival was 74%, the survival rate in this subgroup was lower, at 64%.[2]

In the recently proposed Medicare criteria for coverage of liver transplantation, the HCFA acknowledged that the decision to insure patients with alcoholic cirrhosis "may be considered controversial by some."[5] As if to counter possible objections, the HCFA listed requirements for patients with alcoholic cirrhosis: patients must meet the transplant center's requirement for abstinence prior to liver transplantation and have documented evidence of sufficient social support to ensure both recovery from alcoholism and compliance with the regimen of immunosuppressive medication.

Further research should answer lingering questions about liver transplantation for ARESLD patients: Which characteristics of a patient with ARESLD can predict a successful outcome? How long is abstinence necessary to qualify for transplantation? What type of a social support system must a patient have to ensure good results? These questions are being addressed.[43] Until the answers are known, we propose that further transplantation for patients with ARESLD be limited to abstinent patients who had not previously been offered alcoholism treatment and to abstinent treated patients in regions of increased donor liver availability and that it be carried out as part of prospective research protocols at a few centers skilled in transplantation and alcohol research.

COMMENT

Should patients with ARESLD compete equally for liver transplants? In a setting in which there is a dire, absolute scarcity of donor livers, we believe the answer is no. Considerations of fairness suggest that a first-come, first-served approach for liver transplantation is not the most just approach. Although this decision is difficult, it is only fair that patients who have not assumed equal responsibility for maintaining their health or for accepting treatment for a chronic disease should be treated differently. Considerations of public values and mores suggest that the public may not support liver transplantation if patients with ARESLD routinely receive more than half of the available donor livers. We conclude that since not all can live, priorities must be established and that patients with ARESLD should be given a lower priority for liver transplantation than others with ESLD.

REFERENCES

1. Scharschmidt BF. Human liver transplantation: analysis of data on 540 patients from four centers. *Hepatology*. 1984;4:95S–101S.

2. Kumar S, Stauber RE, Gavaler JS, et al. Orthotopic liver transplantation for alcoholic liver disease. *Hepatology*. 1990;11:159–164.

3. Starzl TE, Van Thiel D, Tzakis AG, et al. Orthotopic liver transplantation for alcoholic cirrhosis. *JAMA*. 1988;260:2542–2544.

4. Olbrisch ME, Levenson JL. Liver transplantation for alcoholic cirrhosis. *JAMA*. 1989;261:2958.

5. Health Care Financing Administration. Medicare program: criteria for Medicare coverage of adult liver transplants. *Federal Register*. 1990;55:3545–3553.

6. Office of Health Technology Assessment, Agency for Health Care Policy Research. *Assessment of Liver Transplantation*. Rockville, Md: US Dept of Health and Human Services; 1990:3, 25.

7. Schroeder JS, Hunt S. Cardiac transplantation update 1987. *JAMA*. 1987;258:3142–3145.

8. Surman OS. Psychiatric aspects of organ transplantation. *Am J Psychiatry*. 1989;146:972–982.

9. Welch HG, Larson EB. Dealing with limited resources: the Oregon decision to curtail funding for organ transplantation. *N Engl J Med*. 1988; 319:171–173.

10. Flavin DK, Niven RG, Kelsey JE. Alcoholism and orthotopic liver transplantation. *JAMA*. 1988;259:1546–1547.

11. Atterbury CE. The alcoholic in the lifeboat: should drinkers be candidates for liver transplantation? *J Clin Gastroenterol*. 1986;8:1–4.

12. Mendelson JH, Mello NK. *The Diagnosis and Treatment of Alcoholism*. 2nd ed. New York, NY: McGraw-Hill International Book Co; 1985:1–20.

13. Blum K, Noble EP, Sheridan PJ, et al. Allelic association of human dopamine D_2 receptor gene in alcoholism. *JAMA*. 1990;263:2055–2060.

14. Aronson MD. Definition of alcoholism. In: Barnes HN, Aronson MD, Delbanco TL, eds. *Alcoholism: A Guide for the Primary Care Physician*. New York, NY: Springer-Verlag NY Inc; 1987:9–15.

15. Klerman GL. Treatment of alcoholism. *N Engl J Med*. 1989;320:394–395.

16. *Seventh Special Report to the US Congress on Alcohol and Health*. Washington, DC: US Dept of Health and Human Services; 1990. Publication 90-1656.

17. Saxe L. *The Effectiveness and Costs of Alcoholism Treatment: Health Technology Case Study No. 22*. Washington, DC: Congress of the United States, Office of Technology Assessment; 1983:3–6.

18. Nace EP. *The Treatment of Alcoholism*. New York, NY: Brunner/Mazel Publishers; 1987:43–46.

19. Galanter M, Talbott D, Gallegos K, Rubenstone E. Combined Alcoholics Anonymous and professional care for addicted physicians. *Am J Psychiatry*. 1990;147:64–68.

20. Johnson B, Clark W. Alcoholism: a challenging physician-patient encounter. *J Gen Intern Med*. 1989;4:445–452.

21. Bigby JA. Negotiating treatment and monitoring recovery. In: Barnes, HN, Aronson MD, Delbanco TL, eds. *Alcoholism: A Guide for the Primary Care Physician*. New York, NY: Springer-Verlag NY Inc; 1987:66–72.

22. Grant BF, Dufour MC, Harford TC. Epidemiology of alcoholic liver disease. *Sem Liver Dis*. 1988;8:12–25.

23. Thoreson RW, Budd FC. Self-help groups and other group procedures for treating alcohol problems. In: Cox WM, ed. *Treatment and Prevention of Alcohol Problems: A Resource Manual*. Orlando, Fla: Academic Press Inc; 1987:157–181.

24. Winslow GR. *Triage and Justice*. Berkeley: University of California Press; 1982:39–44, 133–150.

25. Engelhardt HT Jr. Shattuck Lecture: allocating scarce medical resources and the availability of organ transplantation. *N Engl J Med*. 1984;311:66–71.

26. Outka G. Social justice and equal access to health care. *J Religious Ethics*. 1974;2:11–32.

27. Beauchamp TL, Childress JF. *Principles of Biomedical Ethics*. 3rd ed. New York, NY: Oxford University Press; 1989:256–306.

28. Ramsey P. *The Patient as Person*. New Haven, Conn: Yale University Press; 1970:242–252.

29. Fox RC, Swazey JP. *The Courage to Fail*. 2nd ed. Chicago, Ill: University of Chicago Press; 1978:226–265.

30. Annas GJ. The prostitute, the playboy, and the poet: rationing schemes for organ transplantation. *Am J Public Health*. 1985;75:187–189.

31. Blank RH. *Rationing Medicine*. New York, NY: Columbia University Press; 1988:1–37, 189–252.

32. Knowles JH. Responsibility for health. *Science*. 1977;198:1103.

33. Moore RD, Bone LR, Geller G, Marmon JA, Stokes EJ, Levine DM. Prevalence, detection, and treatment of alcoholism in hospitalized patients. *JAMA*. 1989;261:403–407.

34. Fuchs VR. The 'rationing' of medical care. *N Engl J Med*. 1984;311:1572–1573.

35. Daniels N. Why saying no to patients in the United States is so hard: cost containment, justice, and provider autonomy. *N Engl J Med*. 1986;314: 1380–1383.

36. Callahan D. Allocating health resources. *Hastings Cent Rep*. 1988;18:14–20.

37. Evans RW. Health care technology and the inevitability of resource allocation and rationing decisions. *JAMA*. 1983;249:2047–2053, 2208–2219.

38. Thurow LC. Learning to say no. *N Engl J Med.* 1984;311:1569–1572.

39. Caper P. Solving the medical care dilemma. *N Engl J Med.* 1988;318:1535–1536.

40. Task Force on Organ Transplantation. *Organ Transplantation: Issues and Recommendations.* Washington, DC: US Dept of Health and Human Services; 1986:9.

41. Louis Harris and Associates. *Making Difficult Health Care Decisions.* Boston, Mass: The Loran Commission; 1987:73–89.

42. Fishman R. *Alcohol and Alcoholism.* New York, NY: Chelsea House Publishers: 1986:27–34.

43. Beresford TP, Turcotte JG, Merion R, et al. A rational approach to liver transplantation for the alcoholic patient. *Psychosomatics.* 1990;31:241–254.

QUESTIONS FOR COMPREHENSION AND REFLECTION

1. Moss and Siegler present two critical arguments against allowing alcoholics with end-stage liver disease to have equal status with other patients who have the same disease. First, they feel that personal responsibility must weigh in as a factor in determining priority for transplantation. Do you agree or disagree with their analysis? Support your answer.

2. Is the authors' analysis more utilitarian or deontological? Explain.

3. Moss and Siegler argue that public support for liver transplantation programs would decline if ARESLD patients were treated the same as other ESLD patients. Do you agree or disagree? Support your answer.

4. Do you think that ARESLD patients should be treated the same as other ESLD patients? Support your answer with both utilitarian and deontological premises.

CARL COHEN AND MARTIN BENJAMIN

Alcoholics and Liver Transplantation

Carl Cohen is a professor of philosophy at the University of Michigan, Ann Arbor. Martin Benjamin chaired the Ethics and Social Impact Committee at the Transplant and Health Policy Center and teaches philosophy at Michigan State University. Cohen and Benjamin disagree with the conclusion of Moss and Siegler. They find fundamental flaws in the major arguments Moss and Siegler have constructed to support a prioritization scheme, namely, that alcoholics are to blame for their own condition and will not demonstrate sufficient post-transplant survival and recovery. They conclude that no sound moral or medical arguments can sustain the position of not considering alcoholics as candidates for liver transplantation.

Alcoholic cirrhosis of the liver—severe scarring due to the heavy use of alcohol—is by far the major cause of end-stage liver disease.[1] For persons so afflicted, life may depend on receiving a new, transplanted liver. The number of alcoholics in the United States needing new livers is great, but the supply of available livers for transplantation is small. *Should those whose end-stage liver disease was caused by alcohol abuse be categorically excluded from candidacy for liver transplantation?* This question, partly medical and partly moral, must now be confronted forthrightly. Many lives are at stake.

Reasons of two kinds underlie a widespread unwillingness to transplant livers into alcoholics: First, there is a common conviction—explicit or tacit—that alcoholics are morally blameworthy, their condition the result of their own misconduct, and that such blameworthiness disqualifies alcoholics in unavoidable competition for organs with others equally sick but blameless. Second, there is a common belief that because of their habits, alcoholics will not exhibit satisfactory survival rates after transplantation, and that, therefore, good stewardship of a scarce lifesaving resource requires that alcoholics not be considered for liver transplantation. We examine both of these arguments.

THE MORAL ARGUMENT

A widespread condemnation of drunkenness and a revulsion for drunks lie at the heart of this public policy issue. Alcoholic cirrhosis—unlike other causes of end-stage liver disease—is brought on by a person's conduct, by heavy drinking. Yet if the dispute here were only about whether to treat someone who is seriously ill because of personal conduct, we would not say—as we do not in cases of other serious diseases resulting from personal conduct—that such conduct disqualifies a person from receiving desperately needed medical attention. Accident victims injured because they were not wearing seat belts are treated without hesitation; reformed smokers who become coronary bypass candidates partly because they disregarded their physicians' advice about tobacco, diet, and exercise are not turned away because of their bad habits. But new livers are a scarce resource, and transplanting a liver into an alcoholic may, therefore, result in death for a competing candidate whose liver disease was wholly beyond his or her control. Thus we seem driven, in this case unlike in others, to reflect on the weight given to the patient's personal conduct. And heavy drinking—unlike smoking, or overeating, or failing to wear a seat belt—is widely regarded as morally wrong.

Many contend that alcoholism is not a moral failing but a disease. Some authorities have recently reaffirmed this position, asserting that alcoholism is "best regarded as a chronic disease."[2] But this claim cannot be firmly established and is far from universally believed. Whether alcoholism is indeed a disease, or a moral failing, or both, remains a disputed matter surrounded by intense controversy.[3-9]

Even if it is true that alcoholics suffer from a somatic disorder, many people will argue that this disorder results in deadly liver disease only when coupled with a weakness of will—a weakness for which part of the blame must fall on the alcoholic. This consideration underlies the conviction that the alcoholic needing a transplanted liver, unlike a nonalcoholic competing for the same liver, is at least partly responsible for his or her need. Therefore, some conclude, the alcoholic's personal failing is rightly considered in deciding upon his or her entitlement to this very scarce resource.

Is this argument sound? We think it is not. Whether alcoholism is a moral failing, in whole or in part, remains uncertain. But even if we suppose that it is, it does not follow that we are justified in categorically denying liver transplants to those alcoholics suffering from end-stage cirrhosis. We could rightly preclude alcoholics from transplantation only if we assume that qualification for a new organ requires some level of moral virtue or is canceled by some level of moral vice. But there is absolutely no agreement—and there is likely to be none—about what constitutes moral virtue and vice and what rewards and penalties they deserve. The assumption that undergirds the moral argument for precluding alcoholics is thus unacceptable. Moreover, even if we could agree (which, in fact, we cannot) upon the kind of misconduct we would be looking for, the fair weighting of such a consideration would entail highly intrusive investigations into patients' moral habits—investigations universally thought repugnant. Moral evaluation is wisely and rightly excluded from all deliberations of who should be treated and how.

Indeed, we do exclude it. We do not seek to determine whether a particular transplant candidate is an abusive parent or a dutiful daughter, whether candidates cheat on their income taxes or their spouses, or whether potential recipients pay their parking tickets or routinely lie when they think it is in their best interests. We refrain from considering such judgments for several good reasons: (1) We have genuine and well-grounded doubts about comparative degrees of voluntariness and, therefore, *cannot pass judgment fairly.* (2) Even if we could assess degrees of voluntariness reliably, we *cannot know what penalties different degrees of misconduct deserve.* (3) *Judgments of this kind could not be made consistently in our medical system*—and a fundamental requirement of a fair system in allocating scarce resources is that it treat all in need of certain goods on the same standard, without unfair discrimination by group.

If alcoholics should be penalized because of their moral fault, then all others who are equally at fault in causing their own medical needs should be similarly penalized. To accomplish this, we would have to make vigorous and sustained efforts to find out whose conduct has been morally weak or sinful and to what degree. That inquiry, as a condition for medical care or for the receipt of goods in short supply, we certainly will not and should not undertake.

The unfairness of such moral judgments is compounded by other accidental factors that render moral assessment especially difficult in connection with alcoholism and liver disease. Some drinkers have a greater predisposition for alcohol abuse than others. And for some who drink to excess, the predisposition to cirrhosis is also greater; many grossly intemperate drinkers do not suffer grievously from liver disease. On the other hand, alcohol consumption that might be considered moderate for some may cause serious liver disease in others. It turns out, in fact, that the disastrous consequences of even low levels of alcohol consumption may be much more common in women than in men.[10] Therefore, penalizing cirrhotics by denying them transplant candidacy would have the effect of holding some groups arbitrarily to a higher standard than others and would probably hold women to a higher standard of conduct than men.

Moral judgments that eliminate alcoholics from candidacy thus prove unfair and unacceptable. The alleged (but disputed) moral misconduct of alcoholics with end-stage liver disease does not justify categorically excluding them as candidates for liver transplantation.

MEDICAL ARGUMENT

Reluctance to use available livers in treating alcoholics is due in some part to the conviction that, because alcoholics would do poorly after transplant as a result of their bad habits, good stewardship of organs in short supply requires that alcoholics be excluded from consideration.

This argument also fails, for two reasons: First, it fails because the premise—that the outcome for alcoholics will invariably be poor relative to other groups—is at least doubtful and probably false. Second, it fails because, even if the premise were true, it could serve as a good reason to exclude alcoholics only if it were an equally good reason to exclude other groups having a prognosis equally bad or worse. But equally low survival rates have not excluded other groups; fairness therefore requires that this group not be categorically excluded either.

In fact, the data regarding the post-transplant histories of alcoholics are not yet reliable. Evidence gathered in 1984 indicated that the 1-year survival rate for patients with alcoholic cirrhosis was well below the survival rate for other recipients of liver transplants, excluding those with cancer.[11] But a 1988 report, with a larger (but still small) sample number, shows remarkably good results in alcoholics receiving transplants: 1-year survival is 73.2%—and of 35 carefully selected (and possibly nonrepresentative) alcoholics who received transplants and lived 6 months or longer, only two relapsed into alcohol abuse.[12] Liver transplantation, it would appear, can be a very sobering experience. Whether this group continues to do as well as a comparable group of nonalcoholic liver recipients remains uncertain. But the data, although not supporting the broad inclusion of alcoholics, do suggest that medical considerations do not now justify categorically excluding alcoholics from liver transplantation.

A history of alcoholism is of great concern when considering liver transplantation, not only because of the impact of alcohol abuse upon the entire system of the recipient, but also because the life of an alcoholic tends to be beset by general disorder. Returning to heavy drinking could ruin a new liver, although probably not for years. But relapse into heavy drinking would quite likely entail the inability to maintain the routine of multiple medication, daily or twice-daily, essential for immunosuppression and survival. As a class, alcoholic cirrhotics may therefore prove to have substantially lower survival rates after receiving transplants. All such matters should be weighed, of course. But none of them gives any solid reason to exclude alcoholics from consideration categorically.

Moreover, even if survival rates for alcoholics selected were much lower than normal—a supposition now in substantial doubt—what could fairly be concluded from such data? Do we exclude from transplant candidacy members of other groups known to have low survival rates? In fact we do not. Other things being equal, we may prefer not to transplant organs in short supply into patients afflicted, say, with liver cell cancer, knowing that such cancer recurs not long after a new liver is implanted.[13,14] Yet in some individual cases we do it. Similarly, some transplant recipients have other malignant neoplasms or other conditions that suggest low survival probability. Such matters are weighed in selecting recipients, but they are insufficient grounds to categorically exclude an entire group. This shows that the argument for excluding alcoholics based on survival probability rates alone is simply not just.

THE ARGUMENTS DISTINGUISHED

In fact, the exclusion of alcoholics from transplant candidacy probably results from an intermingling, perhaps at times a confusion, of the moral and medical arguments. But if the moral argument indeed does not apply, no combination of it with probable survival rates can make it applicable. Survival data, carefully collected and analyzed, deserve to be weighed in selecting candidates. These data do not come close to precluding alcoholics from consideration. Judgments of blameworthiness, which ought to be excluded generally, certainly should be excluded when weighing the impact of those survival rates. Some people with a strong antipathy to alcohol abuse and abusers may, without realizing it, be relying on assumed unfavorable data to support a fixed moral judgment. The arguments must be untangled. Actual results with transplanted alcoholics must be considered without regard to moral antipathies.

The upshot is inescapable: there are no good grounds at present—moral or medical—to disqualify a patient with end-stage liver disease from consideration for liver transplantation simply because of a history of heavy drinking.

SCREENING AND SELECTION OF LIVER TRANSPLANT CANDIDATES

In the initial evaluation of candidates for any form of transplantation, the central questions are whether patients (1) are sick enough to need a new organ and (2) enjoy a high enough probability of benefiting from this limited resource. At this stage the criteria should be noncomparative.[15,16] Even the initial screening of patients must, however, be done individually and with great care.

The screening process for those suffering from alcoholic cirrhosis must be especially rigorous—not for moral reasons, but because of factors affecting survival, which are themselves influenced by a history of heavy drinking—and even more by its resumption. Responsible stewardship of scarce organs requires that the screening for candidacy take into consideration the manifold impact of heavy drinking on long-term transplant success. Cardiovascular problems brought on by alcoholism and other systematic contraindications must be looked for. Psychiatric and social evaluation is also in order, to determine whether patients understand and have come to terms with their condition and whether they have the social support essential for continuing immunosuppression and follow-up care.

Precisely which factors should be weighed in this screening process have not been firmly established. Some physicians have proposed a specified period of alcohol abstinence as an "objective" criterion for selection—but the data supporting such a criterion are far from conclusive, and the use of this criterion to exclude a prospective recipient is at present medically and morally arbitrary.[17,18]

Indeed, one important consequence of overcoming the strong presumption against considering alcoholics for liver transplantation is the research opportunity it presents and the encouragement it gives to the quest for more reliable predictors of medical success. As that search continues, some defensible guidelines for case-by-case determination have been devised, based on factors associated with sustained recovery from alcoholism and other considerations related to liver transplantation success in general. Such guidelines appropriately include (1) refined diagnosis by those trained in the treatment of alcoholism, (2) acknowledgment by the patient of a serious drinking problem, (3) social and familial stability, and (4) other factors experimentally associated with long-term sobriety.[19]

The experimental use of guidelines like these, and their gradual refinement over time, may lead to more reliable and more generally applicable predictors. But those more refined predictors will never be developed until prejudices against considering alcoholics for liver transplantation are overcome.

Patients who are sick because of alleged self-abuse ought not be grouped for discriminatory treatment—unless we are prepared to develop a detailed calculus of just deserts for health care based on good conduct. Lack of sympathy for those who bring serious disease upon themselves is understandable, but the temptation to institutionalize that emotional response must be tempered by our inability to apply such considerations justly and by our duty *not* to apply them unjustly. In the end, some patients with alcoholic cirrhosis may be judged, after careful evaluation, as good risks for a liver transplant.

OBJECTION AND REPLY

Providing alcoholics with transplants may present a special "political" problem for transplant centers. The public perception of alcoholics is generally negative. The already low rate of organ donation, it may be argued, will fall even lower when it becomes known that donated organs are going to alcoholics. Financial support from legislatures may also suffer. One can imagine the effect on transplantation if the public were to learn that the liver of a teenager killed by a drunken driver had been transplanted into an alcoholic patient. If selecting even a few alcoholics as transplant candidates reduces the number of lives saved overall, might that not be good reason to preclude alcoholics categorically?

No. The fear is understandable, but excluding alcoholics cannot be rationally defended on that basis. Irresponsible conduct attributable to alcohol abuse should not be defended. No excuses should be made for the deplorable consequences of drunken behavior, from highway slaughter to familial neglect and abuse. But alcoholism must be distinguished from those consequences; not all alcoholics are morally irresponsible, vicious, or neglectful drunks. If there is a general failure to make this distinction, we must strive to overcome that failure, not pander to it.

Public confidence in medical practice in general, and in organ transplantation in particular, depends on the scientific validity and moral integrity of the policies adopted. Sound policies will prove publicly defensible. Shaping present health care policy on the basis of distorted public perceptions or prejudices will, in the long run, do more harm than good to the process and to the reputation of all concerned.

Approximately one in every 10 Americans is a heavy drinker, and approximately one family in every three has at least one member at risk for alcoholic cirrhosis.[3] The care of alcoholics and the just treatment of them when their lives are at stake are matters a democratic polity may therefore be expected to act on with concern and reasonable judgment over the long run. The allocation of organs in short supply does present vexing moral problems; if thoughtless or shallow moralizing would cause some to respond very negatively to transplanting livers into alcoholic cirrhotics, that cannot serve as good reason to make such moralizing the measure of public policy.

We have argued that there is now no good reason, either moral or medical, to preclude alcoholics categorically from consideration for liver transplantation. We further conclude that it would therefore be unjust to implement that categorical preclusion simply because others might respond negatively if we do not.

REFERENCES

1. Consensus conference on liver transplantation, NIH. *JAMA.* 1983;250:2961–2964.
2. Klerman FL. Treatment of alcoholism. *N Engl J Med.* 1989;320:394–396.
3. Vaillant GE. *The Natural History of Alcoholism.* Cambridge, Mass: Harvard University Press; 1983.
4. Jellinek EM. *The Disease Concept of Alcoholism.* New Haven, Conn: College and University Press; 1960.
5. Rose RM, Barret JE, eds. *Alcoholism: Origins and Outcome.* New York, NY: Raven Press; 1988.
6. *Alcohol and Health: Sixth Special Report to the Congress.* Washington, DC: US Dept of Health and Human Services; 1987. DHHS publication ADM 87-1519.
7. Fingarette H. Alcoholism: the mythical disease. *Public Interest.* 1988;91:3–22.
8. Madsen W. Thin thinking about heavy drinking. *Public Interest.* 1989;95:112–118.
9. Fingarette H. A rejoinder to Madsen. *Public Interest.* 1989;95:118–121.
10. Berglund M. Mortality in alcoholics related to clinical state at first admission: a study of 537 deaths. *Acta Psychiatr Scand.* 1984;70:407–416.
11. Scharschmidt BF. Human liver transplantation: analysis of data on 540 patients from four centers. *Hepatology.* 1984;4:95–111.
12. Starzl TE, Van Thiel D, Tzakis AG, et al. Orthotopic liver transplantation for alcoholic cirrhosis. *JAMA.* 1988;260:2542–2544.
13. Gordon RD, Iwatsuki S, Tzakis AG, et al. The Denver-Pittsburgh Liver Transplant Series. In: Terasaki PI, ed. *Clinical Transplants.* Los Angeles, Calif: UCLA Tissue-Typing Laboratory; 1987:43–49.
14. Gordon RD, Iwatsuki S, Esquivel CO. Liver transplantation. In: Cerilli GJ, ed. *Organ Transplantation and Replacement.* Philadelphia, Pa: JB Lippincott; 1988:511–534.
15. Childress JF. Who shall live when not all can live? *Soundings.* 1970;53:339–362.
16. Starzl TE, Gordon RD, Tzakis S, et al. Equitable allocation of extrarenal organs: with special reference to the liver: *Transplant Proc.* 1988;20:131–138.
17. Schenker S, Perkins HS, Sorrell MF. Should patients with end-stage alcoholic liver disease have a new liver? *Hepatology.* 1990;11:314–319.
18. *Allen v Mansour A*, US District Court for the Eastern District of Michigan, Southern Division. 1986; 86-73429.
19. Beresford TP, Turcotte JG, Merion R, et al. A rational approach to liver transplantation for the alcoholic patient. *Psychosomatics.* 1990;31: 241–254.

QUESTIONS FOR COMPREHENSION AND REFLECTION

1. Cohen and Benjamin criticize the idea that personal moral accountability should play a role in the assessment of eligibility for liver transplantation. Do you agree or disagree with their analysis? Support your answer.
2. The authors also rebut the notion that treating alcoholics the same as other candidates for liver transplants will produce adverse long-term effects, both medically and publicly. Do you agree or disagree? Explain.
3. How would a utilitarian and a Kantian deal with this issue? Explain in detail.
4. How would a virtue theorist address this issue? Explain in detail.

The Ethics of Xenografting— Transplanting Animal Organs into Humans

The Working Group's report was part of a paper submitted to the Nuffield Council on Bioethics in June 1995. The report starts with a discussion of the Cambridge pig heart research and its promising application for use in humans, as well as its potential dangers. It then addresses various objections to this type of xenograft and research, paying special attention to theological objections based on Scripture. The discussion extends more broadly into theological considerations concerning the use of animals in research for human ends. The group's report concludes by recognizing some partial validity of the theological objections, along with the need to exercise some caution.

THE CHURCH OF SCOTLAND'S WORK RELATED TO XENOGRAFTING

Xenografting is, by nature, interfacial between animal and human bioethics, and there are thus both human and animal issues involved. The Church of Scotland's Board of Social Responsibility is the church's body primarily responsible for medical ethics, and produced a study group report on human transplants which was accepted by the General Assembly in 1990. This report has been submitted to you separately, and it discussed a number of important general issues on transplantation which are relevant to the present case, but it touched only briefly on xenografting as such, and mostly in connection with animal tissue and valve transplants. At that time there was little technical prospect of full animal organ transplants. Recent advances in the technology, however, have overtaken that situation, so that when the SRT [Society, Religion and Technology] working group was set up, it was felt that the time had now come to give a more detailed consideration of xenograft-

ing. In this, however, we have focussed primarily on the animal perspective. Although of course we have touched on the human aspects from time to time, for the major issues on transplantation in general, we would refer you to the Board of Social Responsibility's report.

The issues under discussion by our working group cover a very wide range. In some we are responding to an existing technology where there is already a commercial product (e.g. the "FlavrSavr" tomato). In others we are assessing a promising technology which is still under development (PPL's transgenic sheep producing alpha-1-antitripsin). In a few cases, we are looking at the potential implications of what is still at the level of more speculative research. The Cambridge xenografting research on genetically modified pigs' hearts for transplants represents an example of the latter. We have prepared a case study on this issue, even though strictly there is as yet no "case," in the sense of a proven technology. We considered it important to study precisely because of the need to be pro-active on the ethics of new technological developments, especially those with important implications and wide potential application. It has also already excited media and public attention and controversy, which therefore in that sense "makes it" an issue.

SUMMARY OF THE GENETICALLY MODIFIED PIG HEART TECHNOLOGY

Although we are aware of other research going on in this field, such as at Duke University, our knowledge is primarily that of the Cambridge pig heart research. This, however, raises many of the issues which would arise in other applications of the xenografting concept. This potential application arises because in recent years there has been an increase in the number of heart transplantations to the point that demand significantly exceeds any reasonable expectation of the routine "supply" of suitable hearts from cadavers. By definition, patients who would benefit from heart transplantation are critically ill. Hence the limitation in supply inevitably means that some people will die before a suitable organ becomes available. This suggests an ethical motive for this research.

Genetic manipulation has become involved as a possible way of preventing the hyperacute response whereby human antibodies act rapidly to reject the transplanted tissue as though responding to an infection. The Cambridge research is attempting to transfer the gene which directs the production of regulatory factors for human "complement" into pigs, so that the heart is no longer recognised as foreign. Conventional drug therapy is, however, still required to prevent rejection by response to the histocompatibility antigens, which react to the different tissue surface chemicals of an organ transplanted even within the same species.

The actual technique being used involves a single gene (it is presumed without a regulator). There appear to be several groups of people working on the technique and different groups appear to have chosen different genes to work with. The Cambridge group was still some way from applying the technology to human recipients. In early 1995, they were only at the stage of producing homozygous lines of transgenic pigs. Groups overseas have gone further in the genetic engineering aspects, but none are at a clinical trial stage.

Some believe that even if the hyperacute rejection problem could be solved in xenografting through one or other of these genetic manipulations, other problems may need to be solved which could mean that clinical application was still some years away. This in itself poses the problem, to which we shall return, that incautious reporting, publicity and media coverage can prematurely raise expectations of a "cure" amongst sufferers and those who care for them.

The most pragmatic question is whether the treatment would actually work. This is not in itself an ethical issue, but as we will see, its implications do raise some issues. It would seem that several formidable obstacles must all be overcome, including the effectiveness of the animal donor heart as a heart, matching the specific donor pig heart to a specific host human physiology, freedom of donor heart from carrying an animal-originated disease into the human being, the surgery and its aftermath, hyperacute rejection, and histocompatibility rejection.

One of the dangers which is inherent in this type of research is that it is not possible to predict the outcome of organ transplantation from such pigs. The first patients would face a very uncertain future. However, as they were already facing a high likelihood of death from their existing grave clinical condition, they might be content to gamble. The research so far has concentrated on overcoming the immunological difficulties. It might be asked if we would do better using preliminary stages such as transplanting veins from pigs as a less drastic way of assessing the rejection. Against this it could be argued that this would be creating an unnecessary new risk to a very sick person without treating their actual condition.

Problems may arise because of differences in physiology between humans and pigs. There are differences in life-span, heart rate blood pressure, and the structure of the regulatory hormones which maintain the basic physiological stability of the animal. It is not clear how an organ from one species would perform in another. It would be essential that the organ did not carry any infective agent able to harm a human. Hence it would be necessary to use animals from specialist disease free facilities, which raises some animal welfare questions.

POSSIBLE OBJECTIONS IN PRINCIPLE

Unnaturalness

The most common issue of principle is that xenografting could be seen as doing something "unnatural". In ethics, the concept of natural/unnatural is not straightforward, however. There is always a large element of human construction in the way we perceive our surroundings, even where appeal is made to some particular concept of naturalness as "given." What is perceived as "natural" or "unnatural" clearly depends on one's assumptions. There are many current and historical examples where both have been either romanticised or demonised. For these reasons we prefer not to discuss this issue primarily in terms of "unnaturalness," but we recognise that there is, nonetheless a significant perception underlying the idea. Put at its most basic it is the concern that, in making possible by human technology what is quite impossible among living creatures in nature, are we violating something of the given order of the natural world?

But what is it that is seen as "unnatural"? Several possibilities might include:

- Any sort of transplant, including a human to human transplant,

- The transplant of even a "normal" animal organ into a human being,

- The genetic engineering of an animal to produce an organ suitable for transplanting,

- The crossing of particular species boundaries—e.g. pig–human rather than another animal,

- Transplants involving certain organs, rather than others.

Some already object on principle to human–human transplants, but the particular significance of xenografting is the transfer of organs between different species. Does this represent breaking a barrier between the various natural species, and especially between human beings and animals? The issue is complicated by the possibility of an objection in principle to genetic modification of animals. Because of the problems of hyperacute rejection of organs or tissue from a different species, it seems likely that xenografting would always entail genetic modification on the part of the donor animal. Conceivably, it might also require some measure of genetic therapy on the human recipient as well. To unravel this complication, we would first pose the question of how people would react to the idea of a xenograft if the heart was from a normal pig rather than a transgenic one (supposing for a moment that the suppressors for the acute immune reaction could be supplied in some other way than genetic modification of the pig or human).

We would conclude that, whether or not one associates it with the sense of unnaturalness or a violation of the natural order, there is clearly something artificial about putting a pig's heart into a man or woman. The point is: does that matter?

Theological and Other Underlying Issues

The intermingling of distinct plant or animal kinds by cross breeding is specifically forbidden in the Hebrew Bible (the Old Testament) in Lev. 19:19. Moreover humans were especially forbidden to eat an animal until the blood had been drained from it, or to have sexual relations with animals. From this some Christians, and also, we would expect, some members of the Jewish and Islamic faith communities, would argue that the biological intermingling of human and animal is thus strictly condemned.

Others argue that none of these prohibitions exactly meets the case in point, since the intent of xenografting is not to interbreed humans and animals, and that the divine prohibition could not be against the exchange of genetic material as such, since at least at the level of micro-organisms, such exchange occurs routinely in nature. Moreover the normal Christian understanding is that human beings have been reconciled to God through the death and resurrection of Jesus Christ, fulfilling and superseding the numerous ceremonial regulations in the Old Testament, such as which animals may be eaten, and the way in which animals are slaughtered. It is a moot point whether the regulation against crossing animal or plant kinds falls into this category, or whether it reflects a wider moral teaching which would still be relevant.

It might be argued that there are many cases in nature where one living organism makes use of the metabolism of another by parasitic action on a host, or by co-operative (symbiotic) co-existence. These would seem, however, to be of a different order from physically cutting out an organ and implanting it in another organism.

The very concept of "species" is an attempt to rationalise and classify the biological diversity of the natural world, in ways that take due recognition of the similarities and differences that genuinely exist. The classification may be a human construct, but it is not without justification. The questions of whether this implies barriers between species is another matter, however. In terms of evolutionary biology, some might argue that, since the evolutionary grouping of a potential continuum of genetic possibilities into discrete nodes is in a state of continual, if slow, variation, then barriers are not relevant. This is especially true in the case of mammals, because so much of our genetic material is common.

Others, however, would point out that pigs and humans have nonetheless developed down different "branches" of the genetic tree, and are patently different, however much DNA they actually have in common. A pig's heart is ordered for a pig to live. The Old Testament distinction of "kinds", whether or not this should be linked to the biological notion of species, may be said to reflect the goodness and purposiveness of the Creator who had caused a cosmos to be generated so well suited to human life. For some this order represents a wisdom which humans are certainly invited and called on to use, but which they should not seek to alter radically, in the sense of altering aspects which are seen as inherent in the order itself. This is in part a matter of respect for the Creator, and part a reflection of the feeling of risk involved in fundamental changes to God's order by "mere" human beings, and proud human beings at that. Because human beings cannot know the full extent of the consequences of interventions at this level, we should not attempt to do so. Some argue that perhaps the Old Testament prohibition reflects divine knowledge of the risk to human health that would result from crossing living biological material from another kind. They ask how can we be sure that intermingling pig and human genes, say, will not give rise to new diseases which cannot be put back into the test-tube. This, however, leads the discussion into consequential issues. . . .

From the clear cultural distinction between humans and non-humans flow vital features of human moral and social life. Human life is uniquely valued, and the killing of humans is forbidden in ethical systems except as punishment or in time of war. If human life and animal life become intermingled, it might be argued that there is a danger of the distinctive moral claims ascribed to human life being undermined. It has been observed by some that the closer one moves animals, in concept, towards humans (so increasing one's duty of care to animals), the more ready is the danger of treating some humans merely "like animals". There are grounds for some caution on this point.

In summary, a case can be advanced for religious prohibition of intervention across the "kinds", on the basis of natural order of God's creation, and elements of this view could also be argued from some non-religious perspectives. Most of our group would not take this position. For many Christians (and others), it remains to be justified why a line should be drawn at this particular point rather than any other human intervention into nature or to God's created order, and why the Old Testament proscription should be read as universal and therefore valid in a Christian understanding.

Genetic Modification as a Principle

We have mentioned the possibility of an objection in principle to genetic modification of animals or (if it ever became appropriate in the treatment) humans. We would not object in principle on either of these, but, bearing in mind that a specific alteration to the fundamental genetic makeup of an animal is involved, we would need to consider the justification for this in the light of the consequences, both advantages and disadvantages.

Is the Heart Special?

Researchers are working on the possibility of using donor kidneys from pigs; would this be less controversial? For some it might be. In many cultures, the heart has a special resonance. In the English language, it is the seat of emotions (especially love), courage, enthusiasm and innermost thoughts. In many cultures the heart is similarly accorded a special place in human identity. Obviously this is culturally driven, and subject to change. (Oliver Cromwell used the metaphor the "bowels of Christ", which would seem strange today.) For some people, perhaps, the heart is seen as too vital to what it is to be human to allow substitution by an animal's heart, but this would not seem to be an overwhelming objection. From a biblical standpoint especially, we would not relate essential humanness to any one part of the body. Rather the human being is seen as a whole. One would require a very good reason to have a non-human heart, but it would not a priori violate one's humanness.

To put the xenografting case in the extreme, one might ask the theoretical question of how much of a person would have to be made up of animal organs, blood and tissues before that person would cease to be "human"? Pragmatically, one might answer that long before a stage had been reached where this question had much reality, the life would probably be non-viable. But on the underlying point, from a Christian perspective (and in most traditional societies), the person is indivisibly mind and body, and does not cease to be that, notwithstanding a wide range of physiological changes, disabilities and injuries.

Intuitive Repulsion—the "Yuk Factor"

A frequent reaction on first hearing of this type of research programme is a sense of repulsion, an intuitive "gut reaction", the so-called "yuk factor". Some dismiss this as mere emotion, inferior to rational argument, but this would seem to miss two important points. People do not make moral and ethical judgements as if they were simply a matter of cold logic; moral intuition may often play an important or even

decisive part, especially in recent years. Moreover, there has to be something we feel "yuk" about, even if it is hard to pin it down. The sense of repulsion is one way our culture makes judgements, but this is clearly something that is socially conditioned, particular to a certain time, certain groups, certain countries, and so on. Specific things focus our attention today which were not so important, say a generation ago—like our concept of the body and its boundaries and taboos, and our concerns about risk and hidden side-effects. The notion of introducing a pig's heart can thus raise connotations of polluting the body through breaking boundaries. In our opinion of most of our group, this does not make a decisive argument against xenografting, but helps put in context where the feelings of repulsion come from.

Much can depend on how the question is presented—say in the media, or by proponents or opponents of the technology. It can be presented in terms of here is a "miracle" that someone who has suffered a major trauma is now able to walk around because of this wonderful technological innovation. It might, on the other hand, be presented as yet another example of natural boundaries being abused by technology driven blindly, without sufficient care for the consequences to you and me, or to the rights and feelings of animals. The sense of suggestion, either way, is very powerful.

Some argue that this is primarily a case of unfamiliarity. On thinking through the issues, they conclude that there is little difference between killing an animal specifically to obtain one of its organs and killing it to eat it, but we are more familiar with one than the other. With many technological developments, unfamiliarity has been a barrier to the society to whom it was first announced. The next generation often grows up better informed and used to the idea, and often tends to look back on earlier attitudes with surprise or even condescension. Indeed, heart transplants are themselves an example of this effect. The sense of "yuk" has in this case been largely dispelled by familiarity. But education and familiarity are not always the answer to overcoming these intuitions; the case of nuclear power has to some extent worked the other way.

Issues of public perception in biotechnology are important and should be treated with respect, and not simply be dismissed because they may contain elements of ignorance, emotion and cultural conditioning. We are all members of the public.

Wrong Use of Animals in Principle

This represents the objection to human reliance on an animal to prolong human life, at the cost of the animal's. It is a particular case of the wider issue of the human use of animals. If it is seen as wrong in principle to use animals for any human use, or more specifically to take an animal's life, then even to save a human life by xenografting would be ruled out. We would not adopt such an "in principle" position. On Biblical grounds, appropriate human use of animals is part of the order of creation which God ordained. This is not carte blanche for any and every use, but it does allow for many valid uses, including the killing of animals for food.

Conclusion on Issues of Principle

One of our group affirms his objection to xenografting on principle, but as a whole the group are not convinced that either the various theological and other arguments of principle, or the sense of revulsion, present an overwhelming objection to xenografting. But we recognise that these issues reveal some valid concerns that need to be taken into account. In particular, they imply a need for caution against too instrumental a way of looking at the issue. It needs to be seen in the context of how we see our relationship to animals, not just their function to us. Xenografting raises "naturalness" and other questions because it extends the relationship between humans and animals. Non-vegetarians accept that humans can eat other animals to survive. If we now start using animals to supply spare parts, then we have changed the way in which we look at animals. . . .

QUESTIONS FOR COMPREHENSION AND REFLECTION

1. What is the essential purpose behind genetically modifying pigs, according to the authors? Do you think this practice is morally justifiable? Explain.
2. The authors address the question of the alleged "unnaturalness" of xenografting. Do you agree or disagree with their position? Explain.
3. The authors point out certain theological arguments opposing cross-species interventions. Discuss these arguments. Do you agree or disagree with them? Explain your answer.
4. Do you find the authors' position regarding the use of animals by human beings justifiable? Does it reflect a speciesist perspective? Explain.

✿ CASES FOR ANALYSIS*

1. Allen[38]

When Allen was seven years old, he was diagnosed with leukemia. His mother was single and unemployed. The boy's physician recommended a bone marrow transplant, which would be performed in a nearby state. Allen was admitted to the hospital for the procedure after his mother had made the appropriate contacts, applied for coverage through Medicaid, and been told that the operation and related costs would be paid for. However, the state legislature made an unanticipated decision to reallocate funding for bone marrow transplants to other medical services. Thus, the state could no longer pay for Allen's procedure. In addition, the hospital required a rather sizable

---

*Names and cases are fictitious unless noted otherwise.

down payment before it would even consider further treatment for Allen. A publicized media campaign to raise funds followed, but Allen died before sufficient funds could be raised.

DISCUSSION QUESTIONS

1. Was the reallocation of funds justified?
2. How do media campaigns tend to affect public views regarding transplants?
3. There are others besides Allen in need of bone marrow transplants. Under what conditions would they be considered as potential recipients ahead of Allen?

2. Sung Po

Quite a few desperate patients have traveled to China to obtain organs taken from executed prisoners. Although the commercial exploitation of organs is outlawed in China, it continues to be a highly organized business. Sung Po is a prisoner in China, and he is on death row. Not at all certain when he will be executed, he wants to compensate for his crime by giving money to his family before he dies. In order to do this, he has decided to sell one of his kidneys—and he will do so rather soon. He intends the money for his kidney to go to his family.

DISCUSSION QUESTIONS

1. Amnesty International, a human rights organization that criticizes the use of executed prisoners' organs for transplants, argues that universal principles such as non-maleficence apply. On the other hand, Sung Po desires to benefit his family through his transaction. Are there universally binding principles, as claimed by Amnesty International, or is Amnesty International forcing its Western values on the Chinese? Support your answer.
2. Does the Chinese government have the moral right to use executed prisoners as a source for organs? Why or why not? What if the prisoner and his or her family are opposed to the practice? Support your answers.
3. In the United States, buying and selling organs is illegal. If an American went to China and obtained an organ from an executed prisoner within the requirements of Chinese law, would the action be morally justifiable for the American?
4. What would a utilitarian think about the utility of using prisoners as organ donors? What would a Kantian think about this practice? Would the practice be consistent with the categorical imperative?

3. Mickey Mantle[39]

In 1995, sixty-three-year-old New York Yankee baseball star and Hall-of-Famer Mickey Mantle lay critically ill in a Dallas hospital. He was suffering from end-stage liver disease, the result of forty years of alcohol abuse. In the United States, most people who die from liver disease also suffer from alcoholism. With little time remaining, the only hope for Mantle was a liver transplant. Although donor livers are quite scarce, a suitable donor was found the night following Mantle's hospitalization. The former ballplayer was moved to the top of the waiting list and received the healthy liver; however, he died soon after.

DISCUSSION QUESTIONS

1. Since organs for transplants are scarce resources, should they be distributed on a first-come, first-served basis? Should fame or social contribution be a criterion in determining who gets an available organ? Should a person's life-style be a criterion? Should chronic alcoholics such as Mickey Mantle receive priority over candidates who suffer non-alcohol-related liver disease? Support your answers.
2. In 1991, the AMA proposed that patients with alcohol-related end-stage liver disease (ARESLD) should not compete equally with others in need of a liver. Is this a fair proposal? Should alcoholics who are rehabilitated be treated the same as nonrehabilitated alcoholics? Explain.
3. As with most liver transplants, the medical costs for Mickey Mantle's operation were rather high. Who should pay these costs? Studies show that the medical expenses of alcohol and tobacco users are much higher than those of nonusers. Who should cover these expenses? Should tobacco companies foot the bill for diseases caused by tobacco use? How would Aristotle approach this question? How would a utilitarian approach it? Explain your answers.

4. Jamal Hassan

Jamal Hassan came to the University of Pittsburgh Medical Center's Presbyterian Hospital from Saudi Arabia seeking a liver transplant. He had been on the waiting list for only a short while before he became a viable candidate for a transplant. Although his condition was serious, others on the same waiting list were in more serious condition. Many of them had been on the waiting list for a longer period. Mr. Hassan came from an extremely wealthy family. A good portion of his family accompanied him to Pittsburgh, and it was made quite clear that he would donate a sizable endowment to the university's transplant research program if he obtained a healthy liver. Within a week of his arrival at the center, he received a liver.

DISCUSSION QUESTIONS

1. The sale of organs is illegal in the United States. Is this case different from the sale of an organ? Why or why not?
2. Under what conditions should a patient on the waiting list for an organ transplant be assigned top priority? Was it justifiable that Jamal was given top priority? Support your answer.
3. How would a utilitarian view Jamal Hassan's status as a liver transplant candidate? How would a Kantian view it?
4. Should American citizens have priority over foreign nationals when it comes to obtaining organ transplants in America? Why or why not?

5. Xenotransplants[40]

In 1995, researchers at the University of California, San Francisco, injected an AIDS patient with bone marrow taken from a baboon. Baboons are resistant to HIV, and it was hoped that the baboon's marrow could be a suitable replacement for the patient's own damaged immune system. In that same year, researchers at Massachusetts's Lahey

Hitchcock Medical Center injected cells from fetal pig brains into patients suffering from Parkinson's disease.

DISCUSSION QUESTIONS

1. Many of those who oppose the use of baboons for xenotransplants have no objections to the use of pigs. Is the fact that pigs are slaughtered for food morally relevant? What about the fact that pigs are not primates? Are we being speciesist in making distinctions between baboons and pigs? Explain.
2. Because xenotransplants raise the possibility of bringing about new infectious diseases—retroviruses that could be potentially fatal in humans—should xenotransplants be banned? Does the possibility of contracting a disease from another species weaken the anthropocentric argument that humans are special? Support your answers.
3. Weigh the rights, if any, of nonhuman animals against those of humans who need organ transplants. Is it morally acceptable to sacrifice the life of nonhuman animals for humans whose organs are damaged due to a destructive life-style? Support your answers.

6. Fetal Tissue for Roland Armstrong

Roland Armstrong is a thirty-seven-year-old professor of philosophy at a small Catholic college in Rhode Island. He has recently been having trouble walking upright and often finds himself stooped over, unable to control his posture. He also has difficulty maintaining a steady pace while walking. He has begun to shuffle with short steps. Moreover, during his lectures his voice has become uncharacteristically monotone, quite a change from his normally vibrant teaching style.

After seeing a number of physician-specialists, Armstrong was diagnosed with Parkinson's disease. The disease involves a gradual progressive neurological disorder that significantly influences the nuclei of the brain stem. Dr. Alice Cassidy, a neurologist, recommended surgery. Armstrong, however, did not at all like the idea of surgery on his brain. When he asked Cassidy about other options, she mentioned the possibility of a procedure in which brain cells from a fetus could be implanted into Armstrong. She referred to several similar operations that had produced positive results. The procedure is still regarded as experimental.

The patient's wife, Jeanne, feels inclined toward obtaining fetal tissue for her husband. She proposes that she become pregnant and then have an abortion during her second trimester in order to enable the brain cells from the fetus to be transplanted into her husband. Armstrong himself feels drawn to this option because he dislikes the prospect of any other surgery. Both request the transplant.

DISCUSSION QUESTIONS

1. Is the request to transplant fetal tissue morally justifiable? Explain in detail.
2. Provide utilitarian grounds both for supporting the Armstrongs' request and for opposing it.
3. Provide deontological arguments both for supporting the fetal tissue transplant and for opposing it in this case.

4. What theological arguments enter in? Apply the analysis given by O'Rourke in his article. Do you agree or disagree with these arguments? Explain.

7. Nancy Arnold and Jennifer Behr

Twenty-four-year-old Nancy Arnold has been receiving kidney dialysis for the past four years. Arnold is a single woman enrolled at a college for nursing in Michigan. This regular treatment has placed many restrictions on her activities, particularly her schoolwork. Despite these burdens and the amount of time spent at the dialysis clinic, she has managed to do fairly well in her classes. She intends to graduate in another year.

This past summer, Arnold grew substantially weaker from the treatments. She had been placed on the waiting list for a kidney at a nearby transplant center in Detroit soon after starting her dialysis. At the end of the summer, she looked forward to the prospect of a kidney transplant and was confident that an organ would soon become available.

Thirty-three-year-old Jennifer Behr lives in the same town as Arnold. She has been undergoing dialysis for close to two years and was placed on the waiting list around the same time that she started dialysis. Behr is the mother of two children, ages five and eight. When she is not receiving her dialysis, she spends her time at home caring for her family. Behr was placed not only on the waiting list for the Detroit region, but also on a number of other lists.

Fortunately for Behr, a kidney became available that was a close match for her. The kidney also happened to be a close match for Arnold, since both Behr and Arnold were histocompatible. However, because Arnold was not registered in the organ district of the donor kidney, she was not eligible for it. Behr was registered in that district as well as in others, so she received the kidney.

DISCUSSION QUESTIONS

1. Arnold was on the waiting list for a longer time than Behr. Do you think it was unfair for Behr to receive the available kidney before Arnold? Explain your answer.
2. What do you think should be the most important criterion for selecting recipients of available organs? Age? Family responsibilities? Something else? Explain.
3. Provide utilitarian arguments that both support and oppose multiple listing.
4. Give deontological grounds for both supporting and opposing multiple listing.

8. Vijay Dhar

Vijay Dhar's ancestry can be traced all the way back to the upper class of Brahmanas in Hindu society. In traditional India, the Brahmana class was the highest in the strict caste system and consisted of priests and educators. It was also the wealthiest class. Forty-eight-year-old Vijay Dhar, his wife, Indira, and their four children still enjoy the inherited wealth of his lineage.

However, Dhar suffers from end-stage renal disease (ESRD) and is desperately in need of a kidney transplant. He is willing to pay a generous fee for a compatible kidney from a living donor. Not only will he give the donor a substantial sum of money, but he will also pay any needed healthcare costs incurred by the donor's family over a period of five years. He makes his proposal known to the transplant center in New Delhi.

DISCUSSION QUESTIONS

1. Is Dhar morally justified in his proposal to buy a kidney? Given the circumstances, would anyone be justified in selling his or her kidney to Dhar? Explain your answer.
2. Are there morally relevant circumstances in India that would allow the purchase of organs for transplantation? Explain.
3. What utilitarian and deontological grounds can be given for opposing and supporting the sale of organs in India?

Euthanasia
End-of-Life Decisions

Arthur and Cynthia Koestler had not been seen for days following their last social engagement, a Scrabble™ game at the home of friends. Arthur, a prolific intellectual and world-renowned writer, was suffering from leukemia and Parkinson's disease. Knowing that his condition would eventually get the better of him, he dreaded the loss of his mental skills. He had once vowed that should he no longer be able to play a decent game of Scrabble, it would signal for him a critical descent in his quality of life.

Arthur was a member of Exit, a British organization committed to empowering its members, all facing chronic and crippling medical conditions, to take control over their deaths in the quickest, most painless fashion and thus leave this life with some measure of personal dignity. Apparently, that time finally came for the seventy-seven-year-old Koestler as his condition grew worse. On March 3, 1983, the police broke into the Koestlers' London flat and found the couple in their living room. Both had taken an overdose of barbiturates. Near Mrs. Koestler's body was her suicide note, which declared that she could not live in this world without Arthur. She was in her fifties and did not suffer from any debilitating illness.

Their deaths rocked the literary world and unlocked a Pandora's box of far-reaching moral questions. Can the decision to commit suicide ever be rational? Do we have a moral right to end our lives? If so, is it an absolute right? Who is the ultimate arbiter of our quality of life? Is there such a thing as a life not worth living?

The Koestler incident occurred in 1983. Let us consider a more recent case, in which an individual obtained help in her suicide from a physician. Judith Curren was retired pathologist Jack Kevorkian's thirty-fifth assisted suicide. She suffered from chronic fatigue and unrelenting pain, which made everyday chores impossible. Thoroughly depressed, she became grossly overweight and even attempted suicide. These attempts were thwarted by her psychiatrist husband. She brought charges of abuse against her husband and insisted on getting the "aid" of Jack Kevorkian. In the fall of 1996, she and her husband made their last journey together as they drove to meet Dr. Kevorkian.

This case introduces a new twist: suicide assistance provided by a healthcare professional. The questions posed above now become even more complex. If we do have a moral right to end our own lives, do we also have a moral right to request the aid of another? If so, does another party have a moral duty to assist in our death? Physician-assisted suicide reaches deep into the heart of both the physician/patient relationship and the goal of medicine.

In a groundbreaking ruling on June 26, 1997, the U.S. Supreme Court unanimously upheld laws banning physician-assisted suicide in New York and Washington states, where these laws had been challenged. This ruling followed on the heels of earlier efforts to legalize physician-assisted suicide and active euthanasia. Washington's Initiative 119 in 1991 and California's Proposition 161 in 1992 had been defeated by only slight margins. In 1994, Oregon voters approved a ballot measure permitting physician-assisted suicide. The Oregon ruling soon came under federal court review and thus did not take effect. In November 1997, the issue was again put before Oregon's voters, who again approved the measure. Oregon became the first state to legally sanction physician-assisted suicide.

The signals are clear. There is a growing tide of support for the right of hopelessly ill patients to take active measures to bring about their own death. Witness the continued success of Derek Humphrey's *Final Exit*. This best-seller (also published in large print) by the founder of the Hemlock Society is a handbook of lethal drug combinations. To be sure, in the twenty-first century, these old issues will become even sharper as they assume new shapes. Let us now review the historic incident that ushered in these issues—the landmark case of Karen Quinlan.

On June 13, 1986, after more than ten years in a nursing home, Karen Quinlan died of pneumonia. She had first lapsed into an irreversible coma eleven years earlier, on April 15, 1975, after taking a combination of benzodiazepine (Valium), alcohol, and barbiturates during a friend's birthday party. Their combined effect on the dieting twenty-one-year-old induced anoxia, a lack of oxygen, in her brain. Since that time, Quinlan had remained in a **persistent vegetative state,** her brain irreparably damaged and her coma irreversible. She was sustained by a nasogastric feeding tube and a ventilator (respirator) at St. Clare's Hospital. Her family eventually consulted with their parish priest and requested that she be disconnected from her ventilator and allowed to die.

The Catholic Church, in Pope Pius XII's 1957 address "The Prolongation of Life," had officially endorsed the withholding and withdrawal of so-called "extraordinary treatment" under certain conditions. The article by Michael Brannigan at the end of this chapter discusses the distinction between extraordinary and ordinary treatments. The American Medical Association (AMA), however, maintained that once treatment had been started it could not be justifiably withdrawn. Quinlan's physicians, Robert Morse and Arshad Javed, refused to go along with the family's request. The Quinlans' lawyer, Paul Armstrong, sought to resolve the issue by appealing to Karen Quinlan's right to refuse treatment rather than seeking the legal path of least resistance and simply request her transfer to a facility that would comply with her family's wishes.

An intense legal skirmish took place over the next eight months. Instead of appointing Quinlan's father as her guardian *ad litem,* Judge Muir appointed lawyer Daniel Coburn. Coburn's task was to represent Quinlan's best interests. In November 1975, after hearing impassioned pleas concerning the sacredness of life, the harmful long-term consequences of violating this sacredness, and the fact that Karen was not totally brain dead, Judge Muir decided against disconnecting the respirator. With regard to Armstrong's appeal to the constitutional right to privacy, it was counterargued that this did not grant a "right to die."

AMERICAN MEDICAL ASSOCIATION STATEMENTS ON END-OF-LIFE ISSUES

- [A physician] ought not to abandon a patient because the case is deemed incurable; for [their] attendance may continue to be highly useful . . . even to the last period of a fatal malady, by alleviating pain and other symptoms, and by soothing mental anguish.

(AMA Code of Ethics, 1847)

- The intentional termination of the life of one human being by another—mercy killing—is contrary to that for which the medical profession stands. . . . The cessation of the employment of extraordinary means to prolong the life of the body when there is irrefutable evidence that biological death is imminent is the decision of the patient and/or his immediate family. The advice and judgment of the physicians should be freely available to the patient and/or his immediate family.

(House of Delegates of the AMA, 1973)

- For humane reasons, with informed consent, a physician may do what is medically necessary to alleviate severe pain, or ease or omit treatment to permit a terminally ill patient to die when death is imminent. . . . Even if death is not imminent but a patient is beyond doubt permanently unconscious . . . it is not unethical to discontinue all means of life-prolonging medical treatment . . . [which] includes medication and artificially or technologically supplied respiration, nutrition or hydration.

(AMA Council on Scientific Affairs and Council on Ethical and Judicial Affairs, 1990)

Within weeks, the New Jersey Supreme Court reviewed the case and raised these questions: How can the AMA reasonably support a distinction between withholding and withdrawing treatment? Why not simply transfer the patient to another facility? Also, evidence revealed that as an "unwritten standard" some physicians occasionally did allow patients to die. As for the right to privacy, the court felt that it included the right to refuse lifesaving treatment and that the family was extended that same right in deciding on behalf of a family member. This was the first supreme court to apply the right to privacy in a case involving end-of-life medical decisions. In January 1976, the court allowed Karen's father to be her official guardian and ruled in favor of the family's request.

But Karen did not die until ten years later. Why? St. Clare's administrators disagreed with the court's ruling. Instead of directly disconnecting the respirator, Morse and Javed took four months to slowly wean Karen off the respirator until she could breathe on her own. Because her brain stem was still functioning, she was able to breathe spontaneously. She was transferred to a nursing home a month later. Had her condition improved? Not at all. For the next ten years, she remained irreversibly comatose in a persistent vegetative state and curled up in a rigid fetal position. Who or what survived? Was it Karen, or was it just her body?

HOW DO WE DEFINE DEATH?

The Quinlan case reveals the complexity of defining death within the context of modern medicine. What constitutes death? What is legal death? What are the standards for clinical death? How does clinical or legal death relate to our more profound philosophical notions of personal death? Why do we feel compelled to reexamine our notions of death? First of all, we need to consider the staggering presence of life-saving medical technologies. Even an individual in an irreversible coma can have his or her cardiac and pulmonary functions maintained nearly indefinitely. Would this individual still be a living "person"? Second, our ability to transplant viable vital organs is a delicate matter of timing, but the heart and the liver can be removed from the donor only after death has been determined. Therefore, we need clear clinical and legal standards for ascertaining death. The state of the art of medicine has, not gently, forced us to rethink what death is and when it occurs.

Defining death is not a purely clinical affair. It presupposes deeper, philosophical currents. Ascertaining a person's death assumes some idea of what a "person" is. As we have seen regarding abortion, the heart of the matter is philosophical. What constitutes a person's essence? That is, what is it without which an entity is no longer a person? The three most common definitions of death, which we discuss below, have underlying philosophical notions regarding personhood.

Cardiopulmonary Death

Cardiopulmonary death, the most common definition of death, entails the irreversible cessation of heartbeat and respiration. Outside the context of life-saving medical technologies, this definition is not problematic. As for what constitutes a person, this definition assumes at least two possible meanings of *person*. First, since the cessation of heartbeat and respiration is strictly a biological criterion, the essence of personhood equates with biological existence: I am my body. Second, personhood involves a "higher," cognitive aspect, so the person is essentially a thinker with mental activity: I am my mind, and mind is distinct from brain activity. Both views of personhood resurrect the perennial philosophical questions concerning the relationship between mind and body.

Decerebrate Death

Individuals in irreversible comas can be kept alive with life support. Their physiological functions are still operative, but their cognitive functions are irreparably impaired. How can we determine death in this situation, since heartbeat and respiration can continue indefinitely?

Most states in the United States have ruled that total brain death, or decerebrate death, is an appropriate legal definition of the death of a person. At the risk of simplifying, consider the brain as having two primary components: the cortical region, which oversees our thought and level of awareness, and the brain stem, which controls the vital functions of pulse and respiration. If the brain stem is dysfunctional, we cannot breathe on our own. Total brain death entails the complete cessation of the functions of both the cortical region and the brain stem. In order to ascertain brain death, clini-

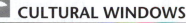

CULTURAL WINDOWS

PERSONHOOD AND AUTONOMY IN CHINA AND JAPAN

Cultural factors influence how the term *person* is defined. For instance, American culture tends to emphasize the person as a private, individual entity. In contrast, Chinese culture essentially defines personal identity in terms of significant social relationships, with the most important relationship being decidedly the family. For the Chinese, one's personal identity is intrinsically intertwined with familial ties and their accompanying obligations. Furthermore, membership within a family brings with it a moral duty to respect the family as a whole as well as each member of the family. This duty is part of the principle of **filial piety,** or filiality, one of the most important teachings in Confucianism. It explains why the patient's family members routinely make end-of-life decisions along with the patient's physician. The patient's family plays a critical role in decision making, since patients do not view themselves apart from the relational family web. This is not to say that the patient's own preferences are not given serious attention. In fact, there is evidence of a growing sense of individualized autonomy among the Chinese, not without serious consequences. For example, there have been more reported cases of terminally ill patients committing suicide after having their requests to stop life-sustaining treatment refused by their physicians.[1] Nevertheless, Chinese patients generally do not think of individual autonomy as being of paramount significance, and their own interests are weighed together with the interests of the entire family unit.

Similarly, the Japanese view the person essentially in relational ways. In fact, the Japanese term for "human," *ningen,* incorporates the idea of "in-betweenness." Humans are situated between other humans (comprising the social environment) as well as between things in the natural environment. Family members are commonly expected to intervene on behalf of the patient. In one of Japan's most publicized medical cases and the first of its kind, a terminally ill, comatose patient at Tokai University Hospital developed renal failure and multiple myeloma. His family members requested that his pain be quickly alleviated. At their request, the physician withdrew medical feeding. When he gave the patient an intravenous injection of potassium chloride, the patient soon died. The following year, the physician was charged with murder. Prosecutors argued that the family merely requested the alleviation of the patient's pain and did not intend the physician to bring about his death.[2] This case underscored the critical difference between alleviating pain and intending death. (Compare this to Rachels's discussion of the role of intention in his classic article at the end of this chapter.) The Tokai case did much to bring about public awareness of the difficulties surrounding active euthanasia. The case especially illustrates the powerful role the family plays in making end-of-life decisions.

This discussion does not imply that in China and Japan the decision-making process is uncompromisingly

continued on page 478

continued from page 477
shared between physicians and family members. Both cultures have a strong tradition of deference to physician authority. Rather, it points out that, as far as the relation between patient and family is concerned, the patient is not viewed in the same individualized, private sense of autonomy that Americans stress. This compels us to reassess our notion of autonomy. *Autonomy* literally means "self-rule," yet it is apparent that other cultures, such as China and Japan, attach somewhat different meanings to "self." A more communal notion of self, which seems to apply in both China and Japan, thus lends itself to a more communal interpretation of autonomy. Whereas North Americans tend to think of autonomy as self-determination in the sense that self is viewed as a privatized entity, China and Japan (and other cultures) think of autonomy as involving a more communal sense of self.

cal criteria have been proposed, the most prominent of which are the Harvard Ad Hoc Committee on brain death standards: no response to external stimuli, no reflexes, no bodily movement, and two nearly flat EEG (electroencephalogram) readings twenty-four hours apart.[3]

Thus, the patient in a coma who exhibits brain activity is still legally alive. The Quinlan case occurred before whole-brain statutes such as the Uniform Brain Death Act were enacted, but the fact that Quinlan continued to breathe on her own after she was weaned off the respirator indicates that she was not brain dead. This is the painful moral rub. Only after ten years entirely spent in a rigid fetal posture in a nursing home was Quinlan considered legally dead. Nonetheless, the law favors this cautious approach to death. Its assumptions concerning personhood are equally prudent, for it establishes that, at least legally, personhood comprises both physiological and cognitive functions. Yet not all cultures accept the total brain death standard. As we saw in Chapter 7 on organ transplantation, Japan, for example, is resistant to this standard.

Neocortical Death

Karen Quinlan, in an irreversible coma, remained in a persistent vegetative state (PVS). She was legally alive, but was she still the same person? It is estimated that from ten to twenty-five thousand adults and four to ten thousand children in the United States are being kept alive in persistent vegetative states.[4] PVS is an extreme clinical condition, with the appearance of wakefulness yet no real awareness and purely involuntary muscle movements. PVS is agonizing for family members, who often perceive these muscle movements as positive signs.

Many critics believe that such a state calls for a new definition of death—death of the higher brain, or neocortical death. This death occurs with irreversible cessation of cortical activity, amounting to permanent loss of consciousness. The individual no longer has the capacity for reasoning, remembering, imagining, and experiencing emotions, even though the brain stem continues to function. Proponents of this definition feel that individuals under such circumstances should be regarded as legally dead. They claim that the essence of personhood consists in our higher brain functions, that is, in thinking. This is how Arthur Koestler perceived his identity—in terms of his ability to reason.

Just what level of mental functioning is sufficient for personhood? As a gifted intellectual, Arthur Koestler may have set higher standards than many of us would. A neocortical definition, therefore, contains the potential for abuse and may result in arbitrary judgments of personhood based on subjective views of quality of life, which explains why no state has accepted this standard as an appropriate definition of death. Nevertheless, frequent anguishing scenarios like the Quinlan case continue to make attempts to define death and issues related to euthanasia all the more pressing.

TYPES OF EUTHANASIA

Euthanasia literally means "good death," from the Greek terms *eu* ("good") and *thanatos* ("death"). Just as there are different definitions of death, there are different types of a "good death." Let us look at two common sets of distinctions: active versus passive, and voluntary versus nonvoluntary.[5]

Active and Passive Euthanasia

Active euthanasia occurs when an agent performs an action that directly induces the death of the patient. For example, a physician gives a lethal injection that results in a patient's death. Any form of active euthanasia is illegal in all fifty states in the United States. Both the American Medical Association (AMA) and the British Medical Society condemn active euthanasia. Active euthanasia is at least technically distinct from **passive euthanasia,** which takes place when an agent either withholds or withdraws life-sustaining treatment, resulting in the patient's death. For example, a physician turns off a patient's ventilator, and death is the outcome.

Herein lies the most critical ethical issue in euthanasia: Is there a genuine moral difference between active and passive euthanasia? If so, where does the relevant moral distinction lie? If not, why not? Before we explore this critical issue more closely, let us sketch the second set of distinctions.

Voluntary and Nonvoluntary Euthanasia

The difference here rests on the degree of competency and volition that the patient manifests in an end-of-life decision. Since American culture highly esteems freedom of choice as a critical expression of personal autonomy, the difference is especially relevant to the morality of euthanasia in the United States.

Voluntary euthanasia occurs when the patient, in a sound and lucid state of mind, competently expresses his or her desire, preference, or value regarding the decision to end his or her life. It includes situations in which patients competently instruct others as to their wishes should they ever become incapable of expressing a request for euthanasia. Therefore, if I am in a clear state of mind and am not substantively affected by medication, pain, depression, or some other factor, my expression of my wishes regarding treatment is voluntary. My request is also voluntary if I formulate an advance directive and authorize others to act later according to my instructions.

The two sets of distinctions combine to form the following four types of euthanasia, all of which remain, to some degree, morally controversial:

1. *Voluntary active.* For example, a physician administers a lethal injection to a patient at the patient's competent request.

2. *Nonvoluntary active.* For example, a physician administers a lethal injection to a patient at the request of his spouse, and there is no certainty as to what the patient himself would have wanted. It is more morally problematic than voluntary active euthanasia, since there is uncertainty as to the patient's own wishes.

3. *Voluntary passive.* For example, at the patient's competent request, a physician turns off the ventilator. Under certain conditions, this practice has been legally sanctioned. Whether it is always morally appropriate remains in dispute.

4. *Nonvoluntary passive.* For example, a physician turns off the ventilator at a family member's request and without any certainty as to the patient's own wishes. Although this has been legally sanctioned on occasions, it still poses some moral problems, particularly since the patient's real wishes are unclear.

Nonvoluntary euthanasia, in contrast, occurs when persons are not able to express their preferences or desires and there is no clear indication of what they would decide, since they have not documented their wishes. In this case, another person, usually a family member, makes the decision for the patient. For instance, suppose that I have only vaguely alluded to what I would want should I ever become totally respirator-dependent and I am now in this predicament, unable to make my desire known. Someone else, my proxy decision-maker, will have to assume the burden of deciding what to do, a role that surely is morally taxing because the decision-maker must found his or her judgment on my own inferred values and preferences.

ACTIVE AND PASSIVE: IS THERE A GENUINE MORAL DIFFERENCE?

Having mapped out euthanasia's terrain, let us now examine some crucial ethical concerns. Since the Quinlan case, a legal consensus in the United States and most other Western nations has evolved endorsing passive euthanasia under certain conditions. Legal scholar Alan Meisel points out that this consensus involves the following points:

1. Competent patients have a legal right to refuse treatment, even treatment that is life-saving.

2. Incompetent patients possess the same legal rights as competent patients; however, incompetent patients require others to act on their behalf.

3. Just as no moral right is presumed to be absolute, neither can we presume a legal right as absolute; there are times when this right is limited by societal interests.

4. Both morally and legally, active euthanasia is clearly different from passive euthanasia.

In summary, this consensus is characterized by a qualified justification of passive euthanasia along with a thorough indictment of active euthanasia. In fact, other terms are often preferred over "passive euthanasia," such as "forgoing life support" or "withholding or withdrawing life-sustaining measures," in order to clearly differentiate these measures from active euthanasia, which is legally prohibited.[6]

This distinction takes us to the heart of the euthanasia debate. Is there a relevant moral difference between actively bringing about a patient's death and withholding or withdrawing life-sustaining treatment? Since our entire discussion hinges on whether we have a moral right to make end-of-life decisions for ourselves, we need to recall our earlier discussion regarding the nature of moral rights (see Chapter 1). One characteristic feature of moral rights is that they are not in and of themselves absolute, in the sense that they prevail over all other rights in every situation. Because U.S. culture stresses the primacy of self-determination, many Americans may presume a moral right to make their own end-of-life decisions. However, even if we do have this moral right, it is not necessarily absolute.

The Difference Position[7]

According to what we may call the difference position, there is a strict moral difference between active and passive euthanasia. This means that, even though passive forms may be ethically appropriate under certain conditions, active forms are never ethically justifiable, nor should active euthanasia be legalized. This position is represented by Beauchamp and Childress in their response to Rachels's article in which Rachels challenges the idea of a real moral difference between active and passive euthanasia. Two fundamental arguments support the difference position. The first concerns the issue of causation (the cause of the patient's death), and the second concerns intention (the intent behind the decision to end life).

The difference position argues that when one actively brings about the death of the patient (active euthanasia), the agent actually causes the death. Withholding or withdrawing life-sustaining treatment (passive euthanasia), on the other hand, simply allows the condition from which the patient suffers to finally overtake him or her. Thus, in the latter case, the condition itself causes the patient's death.

This argument can be stated in another way. There is a real moral difference between actively killing versus letting die. By virtue of the act of killing, the agent is the cause of the death. By virtue of letting die, some other factor acts as the cause of death. This difference is morally pertinent. At times, such as when the patient is experiencing interminable pain and suffering and the burdens of continued treatment far outweigh any benefits, it may be morally justifiable to allow the natural course of the disease or illness to overtake the patient. As discussed in Brannigan's article, the Catholic Church officially allows the forgoing of so-called "extraordinary" treatment for precisely this reason. When it comes to taking positive steps to end the patient's life, however, such as giving lethal medication to the patient, the agent is inappropriately interfering by causing the patient's death instead of allowing nature to take its course.

The second argument implies that an agent who actively brings about another's death intends that the patient die. In contrast, in withholding life support, the intent is to minimize the patient's suffering. There is a vast moral gap between intending death and intending to relieve suffering. This is where the principle of double effect again enters into our discussion (as it did in our discussion of abortion). Recall that double effect involves the subtle but crucial distinction between the primary intention and foreseen consequences. In other words, by withholding or withdrawing life support, we are fully aware that death will be the consequence; nonetheless, our primary intention is to minimize any further suffering, not to kill the patient. Supporters of the difference position argue that the same cannot be said regarding actively bringing about someone's death, since the action itself betrays its intent. The action is a direct means to an intended end, that end being the death of the patient.

The Nondifference Position

The nondifference position is diametrically opposed to the difference position and repudiates any relevant moral difference between active and passive euthanasia. In other words, it holds that whatever rationale morally supports passive euthanasia should justify active euthanasia as well. This is the thrust of Rachels's argument in his article. Defenders of this stance discredit the arguments of supporters of the difference position regarding causation and intention.

As for causation, consider the physician who turns off a ventilator, resulting in the patient's death. The patient's death is the effect. If we define *cause* as that without which a particular effect would not have occurred, it is evident that the physician who turns off the machine is just as much a cause of death as the condition from which the patient suffers. The difference position's argument is therefore conceptually weak. We can counter that the "real" cause is not necessarily that which chronologically precedes the effect, but we are still forced to recognize that the chain of causation is complex.[8]

As for intention, why would we assume that the primary intention of the physician who actively brings about the patient's death with a lethal injection is to end the patient's life? Isn't it possible for the physician to primarily intend that the patient's pain and suffering come to an end? An injection could be the most efficient, painless, and humane means to that end. Furthermore, isn't it also possible for a physician who withholds life-sustaining treatment to do so with the insidious primary intention of killing the patient? Given these possibilities, supporters of the nondifference position contend that relevant moral lines of distinction cannot be drawn between passive and active forms of euthanasia.

The issues are complex, as becomes even more evident when we add public policy concerns to the mix. A supporter of the difference position would most likely oppose legalizing any form of active euthanasia. On the other hand, a proponent of the nondifference position, while morally justifying certain forms of active euthanasia, might still resist legislative endorsement of them. We will focus next on nonvoluntary aspects of end-of-life decisions, since these tend to pose the more intensely difficult moral questions.

ACTIVE AND PASSIVE EUTHANASIA IN CHINA

In June 1988, the first National Conference on Social, Ethical, and Legal Issues Relating to Euthanasia was held in Shanghai. The following opinion of some of the participants reflects the growing consensus among the Chinese that euthanasia is ethically justifiable under certain circumstances.

Under the condition of expressing her or his will orally or written, previously or presently, patients who are terminally ill and not incompetent [may reasonably request euthanasia]. If no living will is left, the withholding or withdrawal of useless, painful, or burdensome treatment *or active measures to end his or her life painlessly* [italics added] may be taken out of compassion and a desire to be of assistance.[9]

The wording here appears to indicate little, if any, distinction between active and passive euthanasia. Even though both the general public and many physicians seem to advocate euthanasia, a number of lawyers still feel that it violates Chinese law and constitutes murder in light of two factors: motive and cause. These lawyers argue that the motive in euthanasia, whether passive or active, is to bring about the death of the patient. They also claim that the act, either passive or active, is such that it causes the patient's death.[10] Therefore, despite increasing public and medical support, euthanasia in China remains a controversial issue. Resolving the issue legally will require addressing the twin concerns of cause and intent.

DECISION MAKING FOR INCOMPETENT PATIENTS

On a cold, early Missouri morning in January 1983, twenty-four-year-old Nancy Cruzan was thrown from her car after it hit a patch of ice. By the time paramedics arrived, her brain had suffered anoxia for nearly fifteen minutes, resulting in irreversible damage to her cerebral cortex, that portion of the brain that accounts for our cognitive functions. Despite her cortical atrophy, her brain stem remained intact, so her pulse and respiration could function spontaneously, without mechanical assistance. For the next seven years until her death, Cruzan remained in this persistent vegetative state, kept alive by medical feeding.

During the first three years, her parents insisted on all possible measures to keep their daughter alive, including the insertion of a gastrostomy tube for feeding and hydration. Experts estimated that she could "live" this way for another thirty years.[11] Her parents remembered their daughter as free-spirited and independent and were convinced that she herself would not want to be kept alive in this state. Eventually realizing that she would probably never regain consciousness, they requested the removal of her feeding tube.

Because many on the hospital staff considered artificial feeding to be ordinary treatment and, therefore, morally obligatory, the hospital refused their request. The

Cruzans then took the case to court. Immediately after the lower probate court ruled in favor of the parents, the state's supreme court repealed the ruling, arguing that the state's first and foremost task is to protect the interests of the patient. Only clear and convincing evidence that the patient herself would refuse treatment was proper grounds for the removal of life support; and in Nancy Cruzan's case, apart from vague memories of past conversations, there was no such evidence.

In a landmark decision in June 1990 that attracted national attention, the U.S. Supreme Court reviewed this finding and confirmed the judgment of the Missouri Supreme Court. Moreover, it maintained the following. First, competent patients have a right to refuse even lifesaving medical treatment. This was the first time the U.S. Supreme Court had acknowledged this right. Second, artificial feeding does constitute medical treatment, so withdrawing feeding in some circumstances is equivalent to withdrawing measures such as respirators. Third, in the case of incompetent patients, each state has the right to require clear and convincing evidence of that patient's former wishes to decline such medical treatment, and each state may interpret for itself what constitutes clear and convincing evidence. Since the Cruzan case could not pass this test, the state's ruling was upheld, and Cruzan's medical feeding was continued.

Five months later, in an interesting twist of fate, Cruzan's friends offered new and convincing testimony to a lower court, which finally granted the removal of Cruzan's feeding tube. Prior to her accident, Cruzan had received a divorce, but she was still known to some of her friends as Nancy Davis. These friends later made the connection to this nationwide case. Cruzan died on December 14, 1990, as scores of protestors demonstrated in the hospital parking lot and even threatened to enter the hospital in order to reattach Cruzan's feeding tube.

The thorniest ethical issues arise when end-of-life decisions are made for incompetent patients. What moral guidelines exist for such cases? Legally, as a result of the Cruzan case, the courts now apply three distinct standards: advance directives, substituted judgment, and best interests. Although these standards are legal criteria and thereby distinct from moral criteria, they still provide us with some level of moral guidance.

Advance Directives

The courts first look for documented evidence of the patient's own wishes regarding life-sustaining treatment. This evidence is known as an advance directive. Ideally, it is an expression of the person's most cherished values concerning life and death and the decision to die. Advance directives typically take one of two forms: living wills and durable power of attorney.

Living Wills—the Ultimate Gamble   A **living will** is a future-oriented document that indicates what a person desires regarding life-sustaining treatment should that person ever be terminally or hopelessly ill and become unable to make a competent request. It goes into effect only when that person cannot express his or her own decision. (A sample of a living will is included in the Appendix.) The living will carries legal weight in most states, yet it is not without its problems.

The most critical problem concerns interpretation. How should we interpret key stipulations such as "hopeless," "irreversible," and even "terminal"? Should we adhere strictly to the letter of the document? Earlier types of living wills were general statements indicating the refusal of any further "life-sustaining measures." However, this statement became too vague due to different persons' interpretations of "life-sustaining." More recent living wills are much more detailed as to various treatments to be rejected or maintained, yet this shopping list approach faces a paramount hurdle in that some of the indicated treatments (respirators, medical feeding, and so on) may in certain circumstances be necessary as a temporary measure.

Whether a living will has the form of a general document or a shopping list, it is still subject to interpretation. Thus, the living will, in some respects, represents the gambler's gamble. In this exercise of our autonomy, the stakes are high. What do we risk? Due to possible misinterpretation, we risk either wrongful prolongation or wrongful termination of our life. Just as it is vital for us to know the risks of medical procedures in order to give our informed consent, we also need to seriously consider the risks of drawing up a living will.

Another, more philosophical, difficulty regarding the living will is the matter of predictability. There is no certainty that at a future point in time I will be the same person with the same set of values, desires, and preferences that I now have and would like to have in the future. Suppose I formulate a living will at point M in my life and it goes into effect at point Y. What certainty do I have that, at point Y, I will have the same values? This is the gamble I am willing to take in order to assert my autonomy. One way to minimize this uncertainty would be to regularly review and update the living will, at least once a year. Then if I reach point Y and my physician notes that my document was recently reviewed and updated, he or she could feel reassured that the document actually conveys my current wishes and values.

Durable Power of Attorney In the United States, all fifty states recognize a **durable power of attorney,** that is, someone legally appointed to make healthcare decisions for persons unable to make their own decisions. Some states have enacted a Durable Power of Attorney for Health Care, which operates along the same lines. The person appointed should be someone who can be fully trusted to make decisions in accordance with your own value system and wishes and someone with whom you have discussed various clinical scenarios.

One advantage of the durable power of attorney is that it obviates some of the problems of interpretation regarding a living will. Rather than relying on a stranger to decipher the document, a person with a durable power of attorney appoints his or her own proxy. More recent living wills include a clause that assigns durable power of attorney.

In order to recognize the rights of all patients, the Patient Self-Determination Act (PSDA) was passed in 1991 by the Health Care Financing Administration. This act requires all healthcare facilities receiving federal funding to notify all patients of their right to refuse treatment. Not only must these facilities document whether or not their patients have drawn up advance directives, but they must also inform patients about the nature and purpose of advance directives and any related institutional policies or state laws. The PSDA further urges these institutions to engage in efforts to educate its staff and the community about advance directives. Such a policy clearly emphasizes the importance of individual self-determination. At the same time, in view of our culture's escalating habit of pursuing medical litigation, the policy operates to ensure more clear and compelling evidence of the patient's wishes in order to minimize the need for litigation.

THE ARAB PATIENT:
Discussions Regarding Termination of Treatment

We should not assume that the importance of informing all persons about their right to make end-of-life decisions is a universally accepted principle. Consider the case of an Arab patient who was recently hospitalized in the United States.[12] Mr. Ahmed, born in Egypt, had just moved to the United States to join family members who had immigrated earlier. When his neck became seriously swollen and spotted with inflamed lymph nodes, he was immediately rushed to the emergency room of a nearby hospital. He appeared to have symptoms of Hodgkin's disease, and he was admitted to the same hospital for further treatment. He also needed to undergo assessment for chemotherapy. Neither he nor his family was conversant in English.

Because there was very little documentation of Ahmed's medical history, the staff questioned him regarding his own and his family's health history. However, from the start, he and his family were deeply offended by the hospital staff's efforts to inform him more thoroughly of his condition by inquiring into his personal health status. He did not respond to many of the nurses' questions, which he regarded as rude and intrusive. Furthermore, in the opinion of Ahmed and his family, both the nurses and the physicians appeared to lack sufficient professional competence because they asked so many questions. In Arab cultures, patients usually entrust themselves totally to the healthcare staff, who in turn direct few questions to patients.

When the staff insisted on the patient's signature on the written consent form, they were met with further resistance and distrust. The patient and his

---

In all this, we need to be circumspect. Advance directives are not a panacea or a magic bullet. Our problems run much deeper in that American culture, unlike that of India and China, for example, lacks a coherent philosophy of life's stages that gives intrinsic meaning to aging and to death. Americans generally have serious difficulty openly communicating issues pertaining to death, particularly with family members. Not only does American culture militate against an honest acceptance of our mortality, but discussion along these lines most often occurs in suboptimal settings—when the patient and family are already facing a volatile, acute-care situation. Dialogue about these issues should take place before we even enter the clinical setting, yet the absence of a consistent view of life and all its phases makes this all the more difficult.

Substituted Judgment

Despite all the talk about advance directives, the fact is that most Americans do not have them. In the absence of an advance directive, to what standard can we appeal regarding appropriate treatment of an incompetent patient? Consider the case of Brother Fox. In 1980, Brother Joseph Fox, an eighty-three-year-old member of a

family could not understand why anything in writing was necessary. Giving consent in writing is viewed in Arab cultures as aloof and impersonal. Arabs contend that a verbal agreement is personally and legally binding, and placing pressure on a patient to sign his or her consent can be construed by Arabs as an insult. It appears to doubt the patient's word, and the patient's word is his or her honor. For Ahmed and his family, honor, not the law, was at stake.

Matters became more complicated and certainly more serious when Ahmed needed to have a tracheostomy tube inserted after he choked while sipping soup. Inserting the tube was difficult, and the long time it took to do so resulted in anoxic encephalopathy. Ahmed suffered a severe loss of oxygen to his brain and from that time on remained in a coma. Not yet brain dead, his situation deteriorated. His family was extremely offended when approached by the medical staff regarding the possibility of forgoing treatment and was deeply suspicious of the staff's motives. Like most Arabs, they were Muslims and due to their devout and total trust in the will of Allah viewed any discussion concerning termination of treatment to be completely antithetical to this trust. According to Muslim teachings, absolute confidence in Allah is crucial, regardless of whether death or recovery occurs. The medical staff's sincere attempt to conduct an open discussion about possible death and treatment options signified to the family the medical staff's resignation and abandonment of hope.

Muslim perspectives no doubt challenge the cultural current in the United States, which assumes that informed consent, honest disclosure, and candid communication are of universal importance. As Ahmed's experience indicates, these components may be vital to Americans, but there is no substitute for making an earnest effort to be sensitive to all patients, including those from other cultures.

Catholic order known as the Society of Mary, suffered a severe cardiac arrest during an elective inguinal hernia operation. Despite attempts at resuscitation, extensive anoxia had occurred, and he remained respirator-dependent and in a persistent vegetative state. After it became clear that his brain was severely impaired and that he would remain respirator-dependent, his friend and Superior of the order, Father Eichner, requested that his respirator be disconnected. Eichner testified that Fox, after closely following the Quinlan case, had clearly made it known that he himself would not want to be kept alive in similar circumstances. Consistent with official Catholic teachings promulgated since the time of Pope Pius XII, he would refuse "extraordinary means."

Weighing the evidence, both the New York trial and appeals courts ruled in favor of the request. In the opinion of the court, there was enough "clear and convincing evidence" of the patient's wishes. The court not only reaffirmed the right of a competent adult to refuse lifesaving treatment but also extended this right to incompetent adults who, when previously competent, had given clear indication of this refusal. Brother Fox died during the court proceedings after spending a few months in the ICU. The court made its final decision much later, on March 31, 1981. This case points out the disturbing incongruity between the long, drawn-out judicial process and the urgency inherent

CULTURAL WINDOWS

LIFE'S STAGES IN INDIA AND CHINA

A rich facet of Hindu teaching is its philosophy of life's stages, which describes four stages in our journey through life, each with its own inherent value and each a necessary step to spiritual insight and self-discovery. Spiritual awakening, or moksha, is the supreme goal in Hinduism, and the four stages of life are paths toward this awakening. These stages are called **ashramas;** *ashrama,* or the English derivative *ashram,* literally means "rest-stops," that is, stops along the way to spiritual enlightenment.

First is the student stage, the time for total dedication to formal learning and training. The student is particularly committed to learning the most sacred Hindu texts, the Vedas and the Upanishads. From these texts, the student first becomes aware of an ultimate, spiritual reality, deeper than the material and more profound than what we ordinarily see. The student learns

that his or her entire life must be devoted to discovering this ultimate reality.

The second stage is the householder stage, the time when the student leaves the safety of school, grows more mature, and realizes that he or she must assume responsibilities that are more social in nature, especially responsibilities within the family. The householder is fully committed to serving others by embracing marriage, raising children, and providing for the needs of the entire family. All self-interests are put aside for the good of the family.

The third stage is that of the forest-dweller. This stage begins after familial responsibilities have been rendered and one's children have become more independent. This is the time for returning to private interests by reintegrating with one's own inner self as one grows older and closer to retire-

---

in clinical decision making. While he was alive, Fox's proxy request and his own previously expressed wishes were not granted.

In the absence of an advance directive, the courts use a standard known as substituted judgment, which addresses the question What would this particular patient choose to do if he or she could decide here and now? This standard requires gathering evidence from previous discussions, conversations with family and friends, and insights into the patient's character and values. Does sufficient evidence exist to reasonably assert that this patient would choose a particular course of action over another? Eichner persuaded the court on the basis of discussions he had had with the patient. However, as the case analysis of Mary O'Connor at the end of this chapter shows, different courts interpret "clear and convincing evidence" in different ways.

It is important to keep in mind that substituted judgment does not mean *projected* judgment, which occurs when we confuse the patient's values and desires with our own. Projected judgment surfaces in statements like "If that were me, I would . . . ." Although we may be inclined to identify with the suffering patient, projected judgment does not lend itself to a morally sound resolution, nor does it respect patient autonomy. Family

ment. The forest-dweller feels the need to reconnect with his or her spiritual self, to nourish the interior.

The fourth and last stage, the hermit stage, is the time to experience spiritual awakening in the deepest sense. This stage requires a detachment from all material concerns and is, indeed, a solitary journey. As Hindu philosopher Sarvepalli Radhakrishnan (1888–1975) reminds us, "The last part of life's road has to be walked in single file."

Note that, through all this, Hindu teachings convey the idea that aging has intrinsic value, for our acquired wisdom and experience bring us closer to self-discovery. By emphasizing these stages, Hindus in effect celebrate aging. Aging provides us the opportunity to reconnect with our true spiritual nature, our genuine self, or **atman.**

Aging is also endowed with an intrinsically positive meaning in China. An example of this value is the contrast between the death of an elderly person and the death of a newborn infant. The Chinese assign a much higher value to the elderly than to the newborn, because they place a high value on tradition and cherish the past. The older we grow, the more we inherit the past. The elderly are respected trustees of tradition. Because the elderly person represents a rich past, the death of an elderly person symbolizes the loss of this history, which, for the Chinese, inspires deep regret. The death of a newborn, on the other hand, though tragic, is viewed with less sadness than the death of an elderly person because the newborn is not yet a full person with a real history.

This perspective is the reverse of how life's stages are viewed in America. American culture is profoundly youth-oriented, and in this respect it is future-oriented as well. American culture does not exhibit the same ingrained respect for tradition as is shown in India and China. Therefore, Americans tend to view a newborn's death as more tragic than the death of an elderly person. The death of the newborn represents the loss of potential and, in a sense, the loss of the future.

members will sometimes reverse the patient's prior decision because they unknowingly project their own values onto the patient. Instead, we need to ask, What would this patient decide for him- or herself if he or she could make the decision?

As we have pointed out, our cultural aversion to discussing matters of death with family and others is a profound obstacle. Without more open dialogue concerning death and end-of-life issues, it will remain difficult to glean evidence of patients' wishes in order to apply substituted judgment.

Best Interests

What about situations in which the standard of substituted judgment cannot be applied? Consider the case of Joseph Saikewicz. In April 1976, Joseph Saikewicz was diagnosed with acute myeloblastic monocytic leukemia, a fatal condition. Although temporary remission was possible with chemotherapy, the side effects of infection and anemia were onerous, as was the remote chance of remission for adults over sixty. Saikewicz was sixty-seven. Mentally disabled since birth, he possessed an IQ of 10 with a mental age of around two and a half. A resident of Massachusetts's Belchertown State School, he was able neither to speak nor to respond to speech, communicating only through gestures.

The probate court appointed a guardian *ad litem* to offer an opinion on Saikewicz's behalf regarding his continued treatment. The guardian had the perplexing task of doing this without the benefit of any grounds for applying the principle of substituted judgment. After careful consideration, the guardian recommended forgoing chemotherapy and other treatment. What were his reasons? First, Saikewicz's leukemia was fatal. Second, even given the slim possibility that chemotherapy might bring about short-term remission, its side effects would be seriously burdensome for someone in Saikewicz's situation. Providing chemotherapy would run counter to his "best interests." The Massachusetts Supreme Judicial Court ruled in favor of forgoing treatment, rendering its judgment in November 1977. However, Saikewicz had died on September 4, 1976.

What should be done when there is no basis upon which to gather evidence concerning the patient's values, wishes, and preferences? How can we make end-of-life decisions for those who are severely mentally disabled or for young children or newborn infants? Because Saikewicz's prolonged impaired mental state offered no grounds to apply substituted judgment, the courts resorted to a **best interests principle,** which involves asking what any reasonable person would want to have done in the particular situation.

This standard is the most morally problematic of the three standards. What constitutes a "reasonable person"? How can we ascertain this reasonable person's choice in a specific situation, since each situation is unique? Resorting to this standard usually produces a more deliberately cautious approach in dealing with end-of-life decisions. Since we have no real basis for applying substituted judgment, given what is at stake it might make better moral sense to err on the side of life. At the same time, might we not unfairly penalize an individual such as Saikewicz on account of his or her condition? Resorting to the best interests standard often presents the most distressing and most morally tenuous choices. The agonizing predicament of severely impaired newborns is a case in point.

Seriously Ill Newborns

When Baby Doe was born in Bloomington, Indiana, on April 9, 1982, he suffered two stomach liabilities. First, he was born with tracheoesophageal fistula, a gap between the trachea and the stomach. However, the fistula, or gap, was relatively minor, and an immediate operation could enable food to reach the baby's stomach. Second, the baby was born with Down syndrome. The obstetrician, Walter Owens, felt that this condition would present rather extensive burdens and long-term difficulties for the baby and his family. After consultation, both parents declined surgery for the fistula.

The decision ignited an immediate, negative response from the hospital administration. At an emergency court hearing, both Owens and the baby's father testified to what they considered an extremely dismal quality of life for children with Down syndrome, with Baby Doe being no exception. Judge Baker ruled in favor of the parents' right to make their own decision on behalf of their baby. Two consecutive appeals, to the county circuit court and to the Indiana Supreme Court, failed. The courts maintained that the parents were the final authority in making the decision for their child. Surgery was not performed. Just before the U.S. Supreme Court took up the case, six days after his birth, Baby Doe died of starvation.

The parents later had another child, this one healthy. Would this child have been born if they had kept alive and cared for Baby Doe? Several families had offered to adopt Baby Doe. That the baby had Down syndrome ultimately swayed their refusal to operate, a quality-of-life assessment that is highly questionable. Should the state have taken a more active role in appointing a guardian *ad litem* on behalf of the baby and his best interests?

One of the most heartrending examples of the difficulty in applying the best interests principle is the case of seriously ill newborns. Down syndrome, for example, is not necessarily a serious illness. Motivated by the Baby Doe case, the U.S. government formulated the Baby Doe Rules, which stipulate that lifesaving treatment must always be provided to the infant unless the infant is in an irreversible coma or the treatment itself is essentially futile. This rule also helped further refine the best interests standard by advocating a determination of the overall benefits of treatment versus the burdens, an approach known in theology as the **principle of proportionality**.[13] In other words, we ask the question What is the proportion between benefits and burdens for this particular patient? For example, what were the burdens for Baby Doe, given that adoption was available?

In weighing benefits and burdens, however, quality-of-life evaluations are inescapable. According to the proportionality principle, the most cautious route would be to forgo treatment only if the burdens clearly outweigh any benefits. What the parents of Baby Doe perceived to be the burdensome prospects associated with Down syndrome (not always supported by empirical studies) surely played a role in their final, anguishing decision about their son.

Should the notion of "burden" extend to significant others, such as family members? This is even more germane today given our uneasiness about healthcare costs, particularly with most families facing the constraints associated with managed care. Who can blame parents for considering the overall benefits and burdens for their family, financial as well as emotional?

On the other hand, many argue that extending the notion of "burden" to include considerations such as finances introduces a more discriminatory aspect, in that euthanasia can then be used on marginalized populations such as persons with handicaps, infants, and women. At the same time, various cultures may view these groups in different ways. Many argue further that the sole consideration should be the infant's moral status as equal to that of adults, so that any decision is based exclusively on the infant's best interests. This position appears to be consistent with modern medicine's vitalist ethos, which is to save life at all costs regardless of the burdens placed on others.

Recall from our discussion of abortion that not everyone believes that newborn infants are persons in the same sense as adults. However, even if we admit that newborns are not persons and therefore do not possess moral status, this does not necessarily sanction a decision that will result in their death. Again, we return to the key question: With respect to a person's best interests, what morally relevant role do quality-of-life assessments play? In the case of Baby Doe, was quality of life the issue, or did quality of life cloak a bias against handicapped persons? We will next address a topic that directly confronts the issue of quality-of-life assessment: physician-assisted suicide.

INDIA, NEPAL, AND SRI LANKA:
What Constitutes Burdens?

India, Nepal, and Sri Lanka are three countries that illustrate how economic, religious, philosophical, social, and cultural factors play a major role in determining health outcomes. In this respect, they exemplify how burdens (as opposed to benefits) necessarily include the toll placed on the family, particularly parents. All three countries give special weight to having children, since it is expected that children will later provide security and support for their aging parents. At the same time, all three countries have taken active measures to regulate family planning, primarily because of severe shortages of medical and economic resources.

In these three countries, many newborns are at risk due to poor hygiene, lack of proper healthcare facilities, insufficient health education, inadequate nutrition, and a shortage of healthcare providers and medicine.[14] The reality of scarce personal, material, and medical resources in these countries means that economic burdens weigh heavily, along with emotional burdens. Calculating quality of life must therefore involve consideration of the consequences on the most important collective entity—the family. K. N. Siva Subramanian comments:

Quality-of-life considerations play a significant role in decision making concerning the imperiled or very ill newborn. If the physician advises that any intervention is not in the best interests of the infant, the parents usually accept this decision. The quality-of-life decision may include, in addition to medical factors, the family makeup, the family's ability to obtain further care, and cost considerations. Also considered are limited resources that could be utilized more beneficially on another patient with the potential for an outcome described as a "good" quality of life. The definition of quality of life is left to the individual physician and the family. *If one dies, it is destined* [italics added]; if a child or infant, especially one who is impaired, dies,

PHYSICIAN-ASSISTED SUICIDE (PAS)

Willy Barth, a young fashion magazine editor in Manhattan, was dying of AIDS. Since 1994, he had been treated aggressively for complications such as parasitic infections, fevers, and skin lesions from Kaposi's sarcoma. His family showed constant support. However, after two years, he decided to forgo any further treatment other than painkillers. He had had enough. He asked his physician, Howard Grossman, to prescribe a lethal drug so that he could end his life. Grossman's hands were tied, however, for he was currently involved, with two other physicians, in contesting New York's ban against the prescription of lethal drugs for terminally ill patients. If he violated the law on behalf of Barth, it would jeopardize his case and impact on other patients making similar requests. Barth's family watched helplessly as he slowly died over about eight weeks. He died in November 1996.[17]

Two months later, a New York lower court overturned the long-standing prohibition against physician-assisted suicide. Earlier, a similar ban had been thrown out in a

it is felt that this is predetermined and we as mere mortals cannot do anything about it. Quality of life rather than sanctity of life is a consideration because of a strong belief in rebirth.[15]

Note the emphasis on rebirth in relation to karma. While India and Nepal are largely Hindu, Sri Lanka has a majority of Buddhists, with a significant Hindu minority. Nevertheless, all three countries share a belief in rebirth and karma, and while these notions are viewed differently in some respects by Hindus and Buddhists, the views share some common elements. The belief in karma is key. Karma is the principle of moral causality, the idea that specific deeds and thoughts produce their effects, if not in this life, then in future lives. According to Subramanian, the Hindu belief in karma tends to take on more fatalistic overtones, with illnesses and diseases being passively construed in terms of a "destiny" that Hindus are taught to accept. Acceptance of this destiny and acknowledgment of the severe scarcity of resources together preclude an all-out effort to rescue the dying.

It is important to recognize a distinction between Buddhist and Hindu views of karma. One Buddhist criticism has been that the Hindu interpretation of karma may be too literal in that it could incline the believer to too fatalistic an attitude. The Buddhist understands karma as less predetermined, which partly explains Buddhism's denunciation of the rigidity of the Hindu caste system. Furthermore, the Buddhist notion of karma can be used as an argument against euthanasia. If the original Buddhist teachings sustain the premise of the absolute inviolability of life, then defiling one's own sacredness through euthanasia would surely reap negative karma. According to the Dalai Lama:

Your suffering is due to your own karma, and you have to bear the fruit of that karma anyway in this life or another, unless you can find some way of purifying it. In that case, it is considered to be better to experience the karma in this life of a human where you have more abilities to bear it in a better way, than, for example, an animal who is helpless and can suffer even more because of that.[16]

Washington state court. Nevertheless, on June 26, 1997, the U.S. Supreme Court rendered a pivotal decision reaffirming the legal ban against physician-assisted suicide. Even though the court's judgment appeared somewhat tentative, allowing for the possibility of states' coming up with their own ruling, its decision no doubt will have a sweeping effect on nearly all end-of-life decisions.

What Do We Mean by Suicide?

In Brian Clark's Broadway hit *Whose Life Is It Anyway?* sculptor Ken Harrison is paralyzed from the neck down after a car accident. After months in the hospital, he desires to forgo lifesaving dialysis and return home to die. Based on the nature of his request, his physician, Dr. Emerson, challenges Harrison's competency and claims that he is suffering from clinical depression. He argues further that Harrison's desire to die is comparable to suicide.

Is forgoing lifesaving treatment the same as suicide? In the Conroy case, described in Brannigan's article, the New Jersey Supreme Court in 1985 suggested a clear

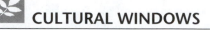

CULTURAL WINDOWS

AQUINAS AND HUME ON SUICIDE

Thomas Aquinas (1225–1274)

Murder is a sin, not only because it is contrary to justice, but also because it is opposed to charity which a man should have towards himself: in this respect suicide is a sin in relation to oneself. In relation to the community and to God, it is sinful, by reason also of its opposition to justice.

. . . One who exercises public authority may lawfully put to death an evildoer, since he can pass judgment on him. But no man is judge of himself. Wherefore it is not lawful for one who exercises public authority to put himself to death for any sin whatever: although he may lawfully commit himself to the judgment of others.

. . . Man is made master of himself through his free-will: wherefore he can lawfully dispose of himself as to those matters which pertain to this life which is ruled by man's free-will. But the passage from this life to another and happier one is subject not to man's free-will but to the power of God. Hence it is not lawful for man to take his own life that he may pass to a hap-

pier life, nor that he may escape any unhappiness whatsoever of the present life, because the ultimate and most fearsome evil of this life is death, as the Philosopher [Aristotle] states (*Ethic.* iii.6). Therefore to bring death upon oneself in order to escape the other afflictions of this life, is to adopt a greater evil in order to avoid a lesser. . . .

. . . It belongs to fortitude that a man does not shrink from being slain by another, for the sake of the good of virtue, and that he may avoid sin. But that a man takes his own life in order to avoid penal evils has indeed an appearance of fortitude . . . yet it is not true fortitude, but rather a weakness of soul unable to bear penal evils, as the Philosopher (*Ethic.* iii.7) and Augustine (*De Civitate Dei* I.22, 23) declare.

(From Thomas Aquinas, *Summa Theologica*, Part II-II, Question 64, Article 5, trans. Benziger Brothers, 1925)

David Hume (1711–1776)

Shall we assert that the Almighty has reserved to himself in any peculiar manner the disposal of the lives of

difference between harboring a "specific intent to die" and desiring to live "free of unwanted medical technology, surgery, or drugs, and without protracted suffering."[18] Similarly, we can point out the difference between desires and preferences. Harrison did not genuinely desire to die. If there had been any other option that would have allowed him to live the way he wanted, he would have chosen it. But given his dismal prognosis and his utter dependency on others, he preferred not to be kept alive.

Is this a valid distinction? Consider someone who, in a competent state of mind, decides to kill himself because he judges his present life and circumstances to be so overwhelmingly burdensome that his life is no longer worth living. Is he not also preferring to die rather than truly desiring to die? If his circumstances were to improve, would he not choose to stay alive? In other words, does a person who commits suicide necessarily, above all else, genuinely desire to die?

men, and has not submitted that event, in common with others, to the general laws by which the universe is governed? This is plainly false; the lives of men depend upon the same laws as the lives of all other elements; and these are subjected to the general laws of matter and motion. . . . Since therefore the lives of men are for ever dependent on the general laws of matter and motion, is a man's disposing of his life criminal, because in every case it is criminal to encroach upon these laws, or disturb their operation? But this seems absurd; all animals are entrusted to their own Prudence and skill for their conduct in the world, and have full authority, as far as their power extends, to alter all the operations of nature. Without the exercise of this authority they could not subsist a moment; every action, every motion of a man, innovates on the order of some parts of matter, and diverts from their ordinary course the general laws of motion. Putting together, therefore, these conclusions, we find that human life depends upon the general laws of matter and motion, and that it is no encroachment on the office of providence to disturb or alter these general laws: Has not everyone, of consequence, the free disposal of his own will? And may he not lawfully employ that power with which nature has endowed him? In order to destroy the evidence of this conclusion, we must show a reason why this particular case is excepted; is it because human life is of so great importance, that 'tis a presumption for human prudence to dispose of it? But the life of a man is of no greater importance to the universe than that of an oyster. And were it of ever so great importance, the order of nature has actually submitted it to human prudence, and reduced us to a necessity in every incident of determining concerning it. Were the disposal of human life so much reserved as the peculiar province of the Almighty that it were an encroachment of his right for men to dispose of their own lives, it would be equally criminal to act for the preservation of life as for its destruction. If I turn aside a stone which is falling upon my head, I disturb the course of nature, and I invade the peculiar province of the Almighty by lengthening out my life beyond the period which by the general laws of matter and motion he had assigned it.

(From David Hume, *Of Suicide*, Edinburgh, Scotland, 1777)

What is at issue is the meaning of *suicide*. On the broadest level, suicide is any self-destructive act. However, there is a difference between a suicidal act and suicidal intent. Furthermore, because many allegedly suicidal persons are actually ambivalent about their desire to die, attempted suicides are most often cries to be rescued. Because the meaning of *suicide* seems to be unclear, some commentators prefer the label "physician aid-in-dying" over "physician-assisted suicide," not only out of concern for life-insurance compensation, but also because of the social stigma attached to the term *suicide* in our culture, a stigma unfairly borne by family members.

To return to our earlier question, are instances of forgoing life support, as in voluntary passive euthanasia, the same as suicide? The answer must be a qualified no. Much depends on what we mean by suicide, taking into account the intent as well as the act. Are instances of voluntary active euthanasia comparable to suicide? Surely, active euthanasia employs more direct means, yet intention remains a primary factor. Whether the means are direct or indirect, we still need to weigh the intent behind the act. Thus, we cannot simply equate all forms of voluntary active euthanasia with suicide, even though physician-assisted suicide may at times be an expression of voluntary active euthanasia.

Is PAS Ever Morally Justified?

We can at least establish this: If suicide is morally justifiable, it can be so only if it is the result of a competent decision. Competency is a necessary, though not sufficient, condition of moral justifiability. Let us now more closely examine the key features of assessing the morality of physician-assisted suicide (PAS).

Recall our earlier discussion about the nature of the difference between active and passive euthanasia. Suppose we insist on the difference position and hold that there is and will always be a clear-cut moral difference such that passive euthanasia is sometimes justifiable but active euthanasia never is. This being the case, PAS would also never be justified, because, even though not all instances of voluntary active euthanasia are suicide, PAS is always an expression of voluntary active euthanasia. Suppose, on the other hand, that we support the nondifference position and hold that the same rationale that justifies passive forms of termination also justifies active forms. This position could allow for the possibility of morally justifying PAS, depending on the circumstances.

There are two layers of concern. The first is a matter of personal conscience. Are there specific situations in which PAS is morally appropriate? The answer depends in large measure on how we view active euthanasia, as well as on whether we consider suicide morally justifiable. How much priority do we assign to individual autonomy? If we insist that we have the moral right to refuse life-sustaining medical treatment, does this right encompass bringing about our own death? Does it include a moral right to request the assistance of a physician? If so, do physicians have a moral duty to assist in our death? What impact does this have on the role of the healthcare professional? It is contradictory to claim that healthcare professionals have a moral obligation to do that which violates their own moral conscience. Therefore, we have no moral right to demand the assistance of a physician. Nonetheless, if we do have a moral right to actively bring about our own death, then this right entails a right to request the aid of another.

The second layer of concern relates to public policy. If we rigorously oppose PAS, we might equally well oppose it as a public policy, but not necessarily. A person can find PAS morally repugnant while at the same time granting that others should be officially allowed to make their own choices. Alternatively, someone who admits that in certain instances PAS is morally justified may not necessarily endorse the legalizing of PAS. What are the most common arguments for and against PAS? Battin gives a succinct summary of the leading arguments in her article at the end of this chapter, along with objections and counterobjections. We will summarize these arguments here.

Supporting Arguments　(1) PAS recognizes the centrality of autonomy and respects each person's moral agency. The request for PAS can be autonomous only if it is the result of a competent decision. (However, as we will see, this argument upholding autonomy cuts both ways in that it can also be used as an argument against PAS.) (2) According to the cherished medical principle of nonmaleficence, the physician is both

BUDDHIST VIEWS ON EUTHANASIA AND SUICIDE

There are currently more than 500 million Buddhists. Without a doubt, Buddhist teachings continue to leave a profound, indelible imprint on cultures within and beyond Asia. At the same time, Buddhism is extremely complex, consisting of numerous subschools and sects. Its two major schools are Theravada and Mahayana. **Theravada Buddhism,** the older, more conservative and traditional Buddhism, is found throughout Southeast Asia in countries such as Cambodia, Laos, Thailand, and Indonesia. **Mahayana Buddhism,** the later, more liberal branch of Buddhism, has spread throughout Tibet, China, Korea, and Japan.

As complex and varied as they may appear, the core of Buddhist teachings remains universal among all Buddhists, regardless of school. For instance, all Buddhists believe in the **Four Noble Truths:** (1) Suffering is universal; (2) the source of suffering is desire and attachment; (3) we can free ourselves from suffering; (4) liberation from suffering comes from following the prescriptions laid down in the Eightfold Path. These truths constitute the heart of the Buddha's teachings, known in general as the dharma.

Not all scholars, however, agree on interpretations of more refined aspects of the dharma, particularly on how these teachings may apply to questions regarding euthanasia and suicide. For instance, many scholars maintain that Buddhist teachings advocate a strict sanctity-of-life ethic. They base their argument on teachings found within the Buddhist monastic rules, or *Vinaya*, rules concerning monastic discipline, devotion, and service. These scholars ground their interpretation on the older, traditional Buddhist school of Theravada. In this respect, Buddhism seems to share common ground with Christianity.[19] This argument is supported by Buddhist teachings regarding noninjury, or ahimsa. This notion of ahimsa originated in Hindu teachings. Applied to euthanasia, ahimsa means that even if one is suffering from the most debilitating condition, it is generally forbidden to end that suffering by taking one's life. Such suicide is viewed as acting essentially out of self-centeredness, and any act—or even thought—of self-centeredness violates dharma. Another teaching concerns karma, the principle of cause and effect in determining moral and immoral behavior. Illnesses and diseases are often believed to be the result of past negative karma, as is the suffering that accompanies them. Deliberately interfering with this karma through euthanasia or suicide is prohibited and can produce further negative karma.[20] This notion is reinforced by Buddhist teachings regarding compassion, known as **karuna.** Buddhists believe that we must express compassion for all living creatures by avoiding acting as the cause of injury or violence to others. Ahimsa, karma, and karuna are key Buddhist ideas. Compassion is perhaps the most important of all Buddhist virtues. For this reason, this group of scholars claims that Buddhism is unequivocally and staunchly opposed to suicide and euthanasia.

continued on page 498

continued from page 497

Other scholars, however, take issue with this conclusion. They challenge the claim that there is a consensus regarding the illegitimacy of either suicide or euthanasia among Buddhist teachings. They point out that the numerous divisions and sects inevitably give rise to striking differences of interpretation within these same schools.[21] For instance, concerning the Buddhist virtue of compassion, can taking one's own life in order to save another be an act of compassion? Compassion requires a degree of selflessness, and selflessness is an integral teaching in Buddhism (as well as in most major religious traditions). Are there instances when suicide may be justified? Suppose a patient chooses to end his or her life in order to alleviate the suffering of his or her family?

Scholars who find a consensus within all of Buddhism prohibiting euthanasia and suicide tend to rely on interpretations based on the traditional Theravada system. On the other hand, scholars who underscore differences among the various schools and interpretations tend to give more weight to the Mahayana school. In any case, it is clear that as Buddhism entered various countries throughout Asia its teachings underwent modifications and shifting emphases. Thus, we need to be aware of both the existence of a core body of Buddhist teachings and Buddhism's complexities.

professionally and morally obliged to alleviate suffering. PAS humanely ends the unavoidable suffering associated with debilitating and hopeless conditions. Pain management may well work to relieve pain, but personal suffering runs deeper. (3) A major fear patients face is losing control. As an available option, PAS offers patients the prospect of having some measure of control over their life and a more dignified way of dying. (4) Rigorous guidelines, as in Holland and Australia, can and should be enacted in order to prevent abuse. (5) Legalizing PAS permits physicians to assist in a patient's suicide without fear of prosecution yet in no way requires physicians to act against their own values.

Opposing Arguments   (1) PAS can never be the result of a competent decision, because any decision to commit suicide is itself irrational. Since we can genuinely express our autonomy only if we are rational and competent, PAS actually violates the centrality of autonomy. Kant's prohibition of suicide represents this position. (2) PAS runs contrary to what the medical profession is all about. Physicians have a professional and moral duty to preserve their patients' lives. (3) Because of the potential for abuse of the physician's power and privilege, sanctioning PAS would be another step toward eroding the cherished relationship between physician and patient, a relationship founded on trust. (4) In this age of cost-cutting, medical efficiency, and managed care, more vulnerable groups such as the terminally ill, the elderly, and the severely disabled stand to suffer from the abuse of euthanasia legislation. (5) The legalization of PAS runs counter to the U.S. culture's time-honored belief in the preservation of life and the protection of the defenseless. (6) Alternatives for caring for hopelessly ill and dying patients, such as hospice, must be seriously considered. (7) PAS will lead us down the slippery slope of insidious social harms. Even with stringent guidelines, there is no guarantee that violations will not occur. Where will physicians draw the line? What if patients are simply tired of living? What if they feel that they are a monetary burden on their family? (8) Feminist critics (such as Susan Wolf in her article at the end of this chapter) point out that legislation permitting PAS would reinforce prevailing cultural biases toward women and further exploit women and other vulnerable groups when it comes to healthcare delivery.

Hospice Care   The **hospice** movement began in England in 1967 through the pioneering efforts of physician Cicely Saunders.[22] She founded the first hospice, St. Christopher's in London. The movement eventually came to the United States, where the first program was started in 1974. On visiting St. Christopher's in London, the visitor is immediately struck by the level of activity. Children are playing, entire families are visiting patients, and even pets are welcome. There are no strict visiting hours, and family members can stay overnight with their loved ones.

One way to get a sense of the meaning behind hospice is to observe something unique about the patients' rooms. The windows go from floor to ceiling. Even the patient who is bedridden can still somehow participate in life outside the walls of the hospice. The philosophy behind hospice is straightforward, simple, and yet profound: to enable terminally ill patients to live until they die. According to Saunders:

> We are not so poor a society that we cannot afford time and trouble and money to help people live until they die. We owe it to all those for whom we can kill the pain which traps them in fear and bitterness. To do this we do not have to kill them. . . . To make voluntary [active] euthanasia lawful would be an irresponsible act, hindering help, pressuring the vulnerable, abrogating our true respect and responsibility to the frail and the old, the disabled and dying.[23]

Hospice care addresses the two greatest fears of those who are dying: experiencing intense, ongoing pain, and dying alone. Hospice care seeks to control pain while still enabling the patient to maintain a lucid state of mind. In this way, there is pain control without over-sedation of the patient. Next, hospice care offers human comfort and companionship to the dying. Hospice patients are not abandoned or isolated in segregated wards. Through these two avenues—pain control and human companionship—hospice care offers hope to the terminally ill in that they can genuinely live out their final months, weeks, and days.

In these respects, hospice offers a reasonable alternative to forms of euthanasia. Critics of euthanasia fear that many dying patients may not sufficiently consider hospice a sensible option to a so-called "good death," thus hastening their death prematurely. Moreover, these critics point out, legalizing active euthanasia would fundamentally undermine the philosophy of hospice and would instead offer a reckless shortcut for resolving dying patients' fears.

A Closer Look at the Slippery Slope   The slippery slope argument is the most pronounced criticism of PAS and active euthanasia. (It is the leading argument raised by Beauchamp and Childress in their critique of Rachels.) Throughout the text, this slippery slope criticism occupies a conspicuous place in medical ethics controversies. Nevertheless, there is a flaw in the argument. Critics often compare the current trend in euthanasia to the Nazi euthanasia program, which started out from small, innocuous

DECRIMINALIZING ACTIVE EUTHANASIA:
Holland and Australia

In 1993, the Dutch Supreme Court officially legislated earlier proposals to decriminalize active euthanasia, which had actually been taking place in Holland for the past twenty-five years. The 1993 ruling protects physicians who assist in any form of active euthanasia, including PAS, from legal prosecution. However, they must follow strict guidelines, including the following:

- Only the patient can make the request.

- The request must be reviewed, discussed, and repeated.

- The request must be the result of sound, informed consent, meaning that the patient is sufficiently informed, the petition is voluntary, and the patient is competent.

- The patient's suffering, both mental and physical, must be severe.

- All other options must have been exhausted and discussed.

- There must not be any pressure, manipulation, or coercion.

- Only physicians may engage in euthanasia.

- The physician must consult with and obtain confirmation from another physician regarding the patient's prognosis.

Despite these safeguards, critics point to abuses of the guidelines. They claim that in some instances physicians have assumed a more active role in encouraging PAS. They also claim that cases of physician-assisted suicide have been underreported in Holland and fear that the legal requirements will be difficult to enforce. Furthermore, there appears to be no real consensus among Dutch physicians as to the moral justifiability of active euthanasia. Defenders, on the other hand, claim that alleged abuses are exaggerated and argue that the safeguards have worked to ensure that those who are hopelessly debilitated have the reassuring option of dying with some modicum of control. Whether we criticize or defend the Dutch practice, we need to critically observe its development.

We should also closely observe Australia, the first country in the world (apart from Nazi Germany) to legalize active euthanasia. Australia's Rights of the Terminally Ill Act was put into effect in 1996 for its Northern Territory. The act permits, under strict conditions, physician-assisted suicide and active euthanasia. It goes beyond a 1994 proposal to legislate physician-assisted suicide. As in Holland, the new law requires that the patient be the one who initiates discussion regarding PAS. The patient must also repeat the request frequently. The law allows physicians to refuse to honor the request on the basis of their conscience.

Learning lessons from abroad requires that we refrain from literally adopting the same policies, since the healthcare and cultural context in the United States differs from that in Holland, Australia, and elsewhere. For instance, as Margaret Pabst Battin points out in her article, cost considerations are not a relevant factor in the PAS debate in Holland, since all Dutch citizens have medical coverage and therefore do not face the same economic pressures as do Americans, particularly regarding life-sustaining treatment.

beginnings, allowing those who were terminally ill to forgo life support. It soon raged out of control, and certain individuals made quality-of-life judgments for vulnerable groups such as the feeble, the elderly, and non-Aryans.

Is this a good analogy? It is worth examining. Our contemporary ideological and social context is, in some respects, different from that of Nazi Germany. The key sustaining principle throughout the Third Reich—the *Volk,* or welfare of the state—swallowed up all individual rights and privileges. Lines were drawn between upholders and enemies of the Volk, resulting in perverse quality-of-life verdicts being pronounced on enemies of the state, who were viewed as subhuman and lacking in moral status. The theoretical and cultural context in the United States today is quite different because of its emphasis on the value of individual autonomy. The entire patients' rights movement is an embodiment of the importance placed on personal self-determination. However, the United States still remains a very hierarchical society, prone to marginalizing people such as the mentally ill and the elderly.

On the other hand, the underlying temper of the slippery slope criticism warrants serious attention. Indeed, an essential feature of both individual and collective responsibility is the measure of our accountability for the immediate and long-range consequences of our actions. As we have seen in our discussion of developments in genetic engineering, we need to be judicious concerning the wide-ranging results and implications of medical research. In Europe in April 1996, the first drug patent for the sole purpose of euthanizing nonhuman animals was granted. The drug was developed by Michigan State University with funds from the German chemical firm Hoechst AG. Although the drug's use is purportedly for euthanizing nonhuman animals, critics fear its potential human use for a European nation's legalizing active euthanasia. The implications, particularly incentives for marketing the drug, are indeed serious and deserve our attention.

Any knowledge should be accompanied by responsible use of that knowledge. Knowledge and moral responsibility go hand in hand. Whatever we decide concerning PAS and active euthanasia, whether personally or with regard to public policy, moral responsibility demands that we sensibly consider the short- and long-term risks and benefits for all of us, now and in future generations.

In the Matter of Kevorkian and Quill

No single individual in the United States has evoked more public fury and sympathy over the issue of physician-assisted suicide than Jack Kevorkian. Consider the case of Janet Adkins. When her husband and three sons accompanied her from Oregon to Michigan to visit Jack Kevorkian, a sixty-three-year-old retired pathologist, they purchased a round-trip ticket for her, hoping that she would change her mind about her decision to die. Their hopes were eclipsed soon after they arrived in Michigan on June 3, 1990. After Kevorkian and his two sisters interviewed her, they determined that Adkins's request to die seemed to be the result of a rational and lucid state of mind. That night, both families shared a last meal together.

Adkins was fifty-four years old and in the early stages of Alzheimer's. She was well aware that her condition would eventually get worse, with irreversible neural cell deterioration leading to an irreparable loss of memory. For Adkins, who lived an active life both physically and mentally and often hiked and played tennis, this outlook was devastating. She had already begun to experience the intense frustration of some memory loss, and for her, a member of the Hemlock Society, nothing was worse than the slow ebbing of her mental faculties. Having heard of Kevorkian and his views advocating physician-assisted suicide, she had decided it was time to meet with him.

On June 4, Adkins went alone to meet Kevorkian, and together they drove to a nearby public park where, inside his 1968 Volkswagen van, he connected her via an intravenous line to a device that first supplied her with a saline solution. By pushing a switch, she stopped the saline, released the sedative thiopental, and engaged a timer that soon dispensed potassium chloride. Within minutes, Janet Adkins was dead. Shortly afterward, Kevorkian was indicted for murder, yet, because he had not violated any law (Michigan at that time had no legal ban against physician-assisted suicide), the charges were dropped.

In November 1998, things changed for Kevorkian, however, when he incited Michigan legal authorities by taping the assisted suicide of fifty-two-year-old Thomas Youk, who suffered from ALS. Kevorkian then sent the tape to CBS. On November 22, 1998, the tape aired on *60 Minutes* and showed Kevorkian delivering a lethal injection to Youk. Three days later, Kevorkian was arrested and charged with murder. As a result, on April 13, 1999, he was sentenced to serve ten to twenty-five years in prison for the second-degree murder of Youk and for using a controlled substance, a lethal drug, without a license. By that time, Michigan had passed a law (in September 1998) making physician-assisted suicide illegal. Although Kevorkian was also charged with violation of that statute, the assisted-suicide charge was later dropped. On November 16, 1999, Kevorkian filed an appeal, hoping to overturn his murder conviction. As of this writing, the appeals court has not yet ruled on the conviction. He is currently at the medium-security Kinross Correctional Facility in Kincheloe, Michigan.

Jack Kevorkian has now assisted in more than 100 known "suicides" and has been acquitted of murder charges three times. By stumping the Michigan courts, he has exposed the legal limbo in the United States regarding PAS. Also, there seems to be a rising tide of public support for physician-assisted suicide. For instance, in Michigan, former Ann Arbor mayor and retired physician Edward Pierce spearheaded a 1998 ballot measure to legalize PAS for competent adults even though this met with no success.[24] Yet some rather poignant criticisms of Kevorkian's approach have been put forth. To begin with, quite a number of his "patients" were not even terminally ill. Janet Adkins, though in the early stages of Alzheimer's, was otherwise healthy. She had beaten her thirty-three-year-old son in tennis two weeks before she died. Also, Kevorkian's relationships with his patients have been short-term, enabling him neither to know them well enough nor to critically appraise their psychological mechanisms and the motives behind their request. Thirty-nine-year-old Rebecca Badger claimed to be suffering from multiple sclerosis. Although she was certainly clinically depressed, her autopsy revealed no signs of MS.[25] Judith Curren, whose case we discussed at the beginning of this chapter, experienced ongoing pain and suffering that evidently contributed to her obesity. She may also have been the victim of domestic violence. Her thinking may well have been severely clouded by her sense of helplessness.

Many physicians criticize Kevorkian's methods. For instance, Austin Bastable, a fifty-four-year-old Canadian suffering from chronic multiple sclerosis, met with Kevorkian after corresponding with Janet Good, who uses e-mail to link people with Kevorkian. Bastable died in May 1996 by inhaling carbon monoxide, a method rejected by nearly all physicians as a medically accepted treatment to alleviate pain. This use of e-mail in the practice of PAS poses another set of questions. People can now log on to the Internet to purchase, for $30, a so-called "Customized Exit Bag," trademarked by the Right to Die Society of Canada and used by Bastable. John Hofsess, who runs the Internet "service," makes the hard-to-argue claim that it is "a considerable improvement over a garbage bag."[26]

A further critique is that Kevorkian sees himself as a personal crusader on a mission to sanction PAS. Much of this inflated image may be attributed to the efforts of his former outspoken lawyer, Geoffrey Fieger, who deftly used the media on behalf of Kevorkian and his crusade. Contrast this image with that of Dr. Timothy Quill, less of a celebrity than Kevorkian though more respected within the medical community. Quill achieved professional notoriety when he published an article in the respected *New England Journal of Medicine* describing his experience with his patient "Diane," a forty-five-year-old with acute myelomonocytic leukemia who refused chemotherapy.[27] At her apparent request, he instead provided the dosage of barbiturates needed for her to end her life. Although he was later prosecuted for murder, the grand jury in New York did not indict him. (See Case Analysis 2.)

Quill was not alone in having this type of experience. Other physicians soon admitted to having similarly aided their patients. In fact, a recent study reported that some physicians did not even involve their patients in the decision to end their lives.[28] There are differences, however, between Quill's actions and those of Kevorkian. Quill insists on a long-standing and honest relationship with the patient, suggesting that the principle of patient autonomy is not an absolute principle that trumps all other principles. The absoluteness of patient autonomy is a position Kevorkian seems to assume. For Quill, the integrity of the physician/patient relationship is uppermost. However, this particular difference between Kevorkian and Quill may be peripheral to the issue. After all, both still condone PAS, an act vigorously censured by professionals and laypersons alike.

PAS and Women in the United States

It is interesting to note that most examples of both euthanasia and PAS in the literature and in the media involve women. The PAS and euthanasia debate has basically ignored this fact. The debate, therefore, needs to more seriously explore gender-related issues. Wolf's article, for example, situates the controversy within the context of a long-standing Western cultural bias that views women as essentially self-sacrificing. In the United States, this bias is further fueled by the fact that women in general are more often than not second-class citizens when it comes to healthcare delivery. Most women continue to be subject to the priorities and policies formulated by a predominantly male medical profession.[29]

Women, on the whole, are disvalued all the more by a cultural milieu that has made a virtue of bodily beauty. In the United States, women especially are objectified and judged on the basis of their physical allure. Add to this the fact that U.S. culture typically glorifies youth and places little value on the elderly, and it becomes clear why for many women growing old constitutes a profound source of depression and diminished self-esteem.

Critics of PAS point out that women's subordinate status in U.S. healthcare delivery, along with the U.S. tendency to value self-sacrifice and associate it with women, would likely produce gender-related consequences if PAS were legalized. This is the point raised by Susan Wolf in her article. Not only would there be a higher incidence of

CULTURAL WINDOWS

AGING IN AMERICA

The nineteenth-century American reformer Eliza Farnham was indeed ahead of her time when she reflected on the plight of older American women who assimilated their culture's view of a "diminished instead of an expanded self-hood." Describing an older woman facing the "gates" of her future, Farnham wrote:

No wonder that she looks upon these gates, as the condemned upon the door which is next to open the way to his scaffold—that she counts sadly every step which brings her nearer to them—that she would fain convince herself and the world that she is yet far off; thirty-five instead of forty-five; fresh with youth instead of cosmetics; gay from happiness instead of simulation. For that awful future! Wherein it is not mysterious it is worse; *insulting, neglectful, chilling.*[30] (italics added)

American culture is fixated on the stages of youth and young adulthood and obsessed with the appearance of youthfulness, misconstruing it to be equivalent to health. The rising success of the multibillion-dollar cosmetic industry in the United States is evidence of this. American culture further associates youth and young adulthood with productivity, and, in an American milieu so strongly pragmatic, productivity is equated with progress. The downside is that in the United States such pragmatism bestows no inherent value on aging in and of itself. There is no unified, consistent philosophy that connects all of life's stages. Therefore, growing old lacks intrinsic meaning, with the result that, in the words of

Erik Erikson in his *Insight and Responsibility* (1964), "our lives are to be one-way streets to success—and sudden oblivion."

Such a pragmatic context spells hardship for the elderly. On the whole, many Americans can make little sense of aging. Older persons inhabit the margins of American society, no longer regarded as valuable and productive citizens. They are stereotyped in ways that make the inevitable—aging—an object of dread. Just as the court jester taunts the aged King Lear and calls him a "Zero without a figure," Americans have little use for the elderly. Consider the brutal predicament of nursing homes in which the elderly are shuffled off to spend their remaining days alone with others. Australian writer Ellen Newton describes this situation in *This Bed My Centre:*

Because there is so little coming and going from outside, and no communication worth mentioning inside, living in a nursing home is an odd kind of segregation. It's like being lost in a fog that closes down more heavily, just as you think you can see your way out.

Bed as a residence is not a thing to cultivate.[31] (italics added)

This unmerciful ageism in the United States cannot help but influence how Americans view euthanasia. If the elderly are among those stereotyped as intrinsically less worthwhile, then we can more easily cross a dangerous line and cast them as likely candidates for a so-called merciful end, for a "good death."

women requesting PAS, but their reasons for making such requests would likely be different from those of men. For instance, due to women's inferior healthcare, relevant factors would include pain relief, depression, and poverty, all of which would affect how physicians respond to women's euthanasia and assisted suicide requests. Consider Jack Kevorkian. His first eight "patients" were women, and whether he paid adequate attention to each woman's own personal context regarding her request remains highly suspect. We need to seriously weight the personal, social, and cultural backdrops against which such requests are made.

Together with the elderly, the disabled, and minorities, women continue to be among the more vulnerable groups in the United States. Therefore, their requests for euthanasia and assisted suicide need to be evaluated within the broader U.S. cultural context, with its perceptions and attitudes toward marginalized groups.

HOW FAR DOES AUTONOMY GO? THE ISSUE OF FUTILITY

The Case of Helga Wanglie

Hospital ethics committees often address cases that involve intense conflict between the medical staff's providing of futile treatment and patient and/or family requests. Consider the highly publicized case of Helga Wanglie. After slipping on a rug and breaking her hip, eighty-five-year-old Wanglie faced several medical complications. She was hospitalized on New Year's Day 1990 and, due to dyspnea, or labored breathing, received emergency tracheal intubation and was placed on a respirator. For months, her physicians at Hennepin County Medical Center in Minneapolis, Minnesota, tried unsuccessfully to wean her from the respirator. Though conscious, she was unable to communicate clearly, particularly when asked about continuing treatment.

In May, she was transferred to another facility. During a further attempt to wean her from the respirator, she experienced cardiac arrest and, although resuscitated, never regained consciousness. After it became apparent that Wanglie would remain in a vegetative state and that any life-sustaining measures would be medically futile, physicians approached the family—her husband, son, and daughter—about considering the withdrawal of ventilator support.

Not only did her family refuse, but they transferred her back to Hennepin County Medical Center, where physicians also advised withdrawing the respirator. For Wanglie's family, this was tantamount to playing God, and they believed that, since God gave life, only God could take it away (known in theology as the stewardship position). What Wanglie herself would have wanted remained unclear, although during later court testimony her husband insisted that she would have wanted her treatment continued. Even after the ethics committee recommended removal of treatment, the family still insisted that the treatment stay on course. Kept alive by a ventilator and medical feeding, Wanglie suffered irreversible damage to her cortex, and her recovery was hopeless due to severe anoxic encephalopathy. It was the unanimous opinion of the hospital staff that no reasonable possibility of recovery existed.

In a tense legal battle over Wanglie's fate, hospital attorneys urged her husband to transfer her to another facility. When he refused, the hospital counsel advised that he obtain a court order if he persisted in maintaining life support for his wife. Again he refused, and the medical center took the case to court. Hospital attorneys, trying to dismiss the husband completely from the case, requested that the court appoint a guardian for Wanglie. Her husband, himself an attorney, then petitioned to be named as her guardian. The court granted his request on July 1, 1991. The hospital now had little choice but to continue life support for Wanglie, since the hospital's legal obligation to provide medically futile treatment was unclear. Wanglie died a few days later, on July 4, after septicemia led to organ failures.

In this scenario, the question is whether or not the medical staff should render medically futile treatment in the face of family requests. Wanglie's husband felt that keeping his wife alive was congruous with her own and her family's values. Should physicians respect patients' autonomy even if it means providing futile treatment? Should physicians simply discontinue treatment that they perceive as medically futile? What if family members act contrary to the expressed wishes of the patient and insist on futile treatment? What about possible conflicts of interest? For example, if the Wanglies had moved Helga to a nursing home, her care could easily have swallowed up her resources, including any funds left for her family.[32]

This brings us full circle to the importance we assign to patient autonomy. Does autonomy have limits? Earlier we asked whether patients and their surrogates have a moral right to forgo life support. Now our questions are these: Do patients and their representatives have a moral right to insist on medically futile life support? Do physicians have a moral duty to provide futile treatment?

Defining "Medical Futility"

What do we mean by **medical futility?** Some claim that any medical treatment that keeps the body alive cannot be considered futile. Others go even further and declare that any medical treatment that sustains a bodily organ, not necessarily the entire body, is not futile. The problem with both claims is that they seem to assume a purely physiological conception of the individual and dismiss the patient's personal viewpoint and values. Others suggest that futility rests mostly on the patient's own desires and his or her exercise of autonomy. The problem with this position is that it ignores any difference between genuine healthcare needs and health-related desires. (See Chapter 10 on healthcare reform.) Patient-centered medicine does not mean that the scope of medicine should be defined strictly by patients. Still others use a proportionality standard, proposing that medical futility pertains to treatments whose medical burdens far outweigh any medical benefits. A bodybuilder who frequently takes anabolic steroids will most likely see an increase in strength, but the long-term effects can be devastating. In this case, steroid use would be futile.[33]

While the appeal to proportionality makes sense, others challenge it for being too restrictive. Ethicists Lawrence Schneiderman and Nancy Jecker argue that the sole standard for determining futility is simply whether there are "significant medical benefits" from the treatment in that specific situation for that patient. Anabolic steroids are futile not because they lead to overall harm, but because they clearly provide no real medical benefit, since enhancing an already normal condition is not a medical goal. They define medical futility as "any effort to provide a benefit to a patient that is highly likely to fail and whose rare exceptions cannot be systematically produced."[34] Furthermore, they recommend that physicians should be *required* to forgo futile treatment, underscoring the fact that the healthcare provider, along with the patient, is a moral agent. Respecting the physician's moral agency entails recognizing (not necessarily agreeing with) his or her professional and personal values, obligations, and concerns. To respect only the moral agency of the patient seriously minimizes the vital nature of the physician/patient relationship.

Regarding the term *benefit* in Schneiderman and Jecker's definition, a physiological effect is not necessarily a benefit. The respirator is keeping Helga Wanglie alive, but is it providing her with any medical benefit? One possible response is that staying alive is itself a benefit, yet this chapter indicates that this position is not universally held. We again are faced with a core question: What are the goals and purposes of medicine?

Medicine is not a science of certainty, and medical uncertainty clashes with the public's expectations. Consider Baby K, who was born in a Virginia hospital with **anencephaly,** the absence of a major portion of her brain and skull. She had no cognitive functions, nor would she ever be conscious. The entire medical staff felt that all measures other than hydration and comfort were futile, yet the baby's mother insisted on all-out efforts regarding life support. After a month, Baby K continued to survive through life-sustaining measures such as mechanical ventilation, but the treatments provided no medical benefit. After the hospital ethics committee failed to resolve the quandary of what to do, the hospital brought the case to court. The U.S. Court of Appeals ruled in favor of the mother's request for continued life support.[35]

When the media tout new medical technologies, they add fuel to the fire. The era of managed care will spawn more medical advertisements, which surely fill a public service in informing people of new advancements in healthcare. At the same time, however, they inflate the public's hopes concerning medical treatments and prospects for medical "miracles." It is not surprising that family members often change their minds about forgoing life support for the patient, hoping for some eleventh-hour reprieve.

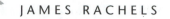

JAMES RACHELS

Active and Passive Euthanasia

James Rachels is University Professor of Philosophy at the University of Alabama at Birmingham. His article, one of the classics in the literature on euthanasia, challenges the notion that there is a clear moral difference between active and passive euthanasia. Using arguments from humaneness and from the absence of any distinction between killing and letting die, he concludes that, in certain cases, active euthanasia may be morally preferable to passive euthanasia. The moral justifiability of euthanasia rests on circumstances and intentions. He concludes that no moral weight ought to be assigned to the legal distinction already drawn between active and passive euthanasia and expressed in the American Medical Association policy.

The distinction between active and passive euthanasia is thought to be crucial for medical ethics. The idea is that it is permissible, at least in some cases, to withhold treatment and allow a patient to die, but it is never permissible to take any direct action designed to kill the patient. This doctrine seems to be accepted by most doctors, and it is endorsed in a statement adopted by the House of Delegates of the American Medical Association on December 4, 1973:

> The intentional termination of the life of one human being by another—mercy killing—is contrary to that for which the medical profession stands and is contrary to the policy of the American Medical Association.
>
> The cessation of the employment of extraordinary means to prolong the life of the body when there is irrefutable evidence that biological death is imminent is the decision of the patient and/or his immediate family. The advice and judgment of the physician should be freely available to the patient and/or his immediate family.

However, a strong case can be made against this doctrine. In what follows I will set out some of the relevant arguments, and urge doctors to reconsider their views on this matter.

To begin with a familiar type of situation, a patient who is dying of incurable cancer of the throat is in terrible pain, which can no longer be satisfactorily alleviated. He is certain to die within a few days, even if present treatment is continued, but he does not want to go on living for those days since the pain is unbearable. So he asks the doctor for an end to it, and his family joins in the request.

Suppose the doctor agrees to withhold treatment, as the conventional doctrine says he may. The justification for his doing so is that the patient is in terrible agony, and since he is going to die anyway, it would be wrong to prolong his suffering needlessly. But now notice this. If one simply withholds treatment, it may take the patient longer to die, and so he may suffer more than he would if more direct action were taken and a lethal injection given. This fact provides strong reason for thinking that, once the initial decision not to prolong his agony has been made, active euthanasia is actually preferable to passive euthanasia, rather than the reverse. To say otherwise is to endorse the option that leads to more suffering rather than less, and is contrary to the humanitarian impulse that prompts the decision not to prolong his life in the first place.

Part of my point is that the process of being "allowed to die" can be relatively slow and painful, whereas being given a lethal injection is relatively quick and painless. Let me give a different sort of example. In the United States about one in 600 babies is born with Down's syndrome. Most of these babies are otherwise healthy—that is, with only the usual pediatric care, they will proceed to an otherwise normal infancy. Some, however, are born with congenital defects such as intestinal obstructions that require operations if they are to live. Sometimes, the parents and the doctor will decide not to operate, and let the infant die. Anthony Shaw describes what happens then:

> . . . When surgery is denied [the doctor] must try to keep the infant from suffering while natural forces sap the baby's life away. As a surgeon whose natural inclination is to use the scalpel to fight off death, standing by and watching a salvageable baby die is the most emotionally exhausting experience I know. It is easy at a conference, in a theoretical discussion, to decide that such infants should be allowed to die. It is altogether different to stand by in the nursery and watch as dehydration and infection wither a tiny being over hours and days. This is a terrible ordeal for me and the hospital staff— much more so than for the parents who never set foot in the nursery.[1]

I can understand why some people are opposed to all euthanasia, and insist that such infants must be allowed to live. I think I can also understand why other people favor destroying these babies quickly and painlessly. But why should anyone favor letting "dehydration and infection wither a tiny being over hours and days"? The doctrine that says that a baby may be allowed to dehydrate and wither, but may not be given an injection that would end its life without suffering, seems so patently cruel as to require no further refutation. The strong language is not intended to offend, but only to put the point in the clearest possible way.

My second argument is that the conventional doctrine leads to decisions concerning life and death made on irrelevant grounds.

---

[1]A. Shaw, "Doctor, Do We Have a Choice?" *New York Times Magazine,* January 30, 1972, p. 54.

Consider again the case of the infants with Down's syndrome who need operations for congenital defects unrelated to the syndrome to live. Sometimes there is no operation, and the baby dies, but when there is no such defect, the baby lives on. Now, an operation such as that to remove an intestinal obstruction is not prohibitively difficult. The reason why such operations are not performed in these cases is, clearly, that the child has Down's syndrome and the parents and doctor judge that because of that fact it is better for the child to die.

But notice that this situation is absurd, no matter what view one takes of the lives and potential of such babies. If the life of such an infant is worth preserving, what does it matter if it needs a simple operation? Or, if one thinks it better that such a baby should not live on, what difference does it make that it happens to have an unobstructed intestinal tract? In either case, the matter of life and death is being decided on irrelevant grounds. It is the Down's syndrome, and not the intestines, that is the issue. The matter should be decided, if at all, on that basis, and not be allowed to depend on the essentially irrelevant question of whether the intestinal tract is blocked.

What makes this situation possible, of course, is the idea that when there is an intestinal blockage, one can "let the baby die," but when there is no such defect there is nothing that can be done, for one must not "kill" it. The fact that this idea leads to such results as deciding life or death on irrelevant grounds is another good reason why the doctrine should be rejected.

One reason why so many people think that there is an important moral difference between active and passive euthanasia is that they think killing someone is morally worse than letting someone die. But is it? Is killing, in itself, worse than letting die? To investigate this issue, two cases may be considered that are exactly alike except that one involves killing whereas the other involves letting someone die. Then, it can be asked whether this difference makes any difference to the moral assessments. It is important that the cases be exactly alike, except for this one difference, since otherwise one cannot be confident that it is this difference and not some other that accounts for any variation in the assessments of the two cases. So, let us consider this pair of cases:

In the first, Smith stands to gain a large inheritance if anything should happen to his six-year-old cousin. One evening while the child is taking his bath, Smith sneaks into the bathroom and drowns the child, and then arranges things so that it will look like an accident.

In the second, Jones also stands to gain if anything should happen to his six-year-old cousin. Like Smith, Jones sneaks in planning to drown the child in his bath. However, just as he enters the bathroom Jones sees the child slip and hit his head, and fall face down in the water. Jones is delighted; he stands by, ready to push the child's head back under if it is necessary, but it is not necessary. With only a little thrashing about, the child drowns all by himself, "accidentally," as Jones watches and does nothing.

Now Smith killed the child, whereas Jones "merely" let the child die. That is the only difference between them. Did either man behave better, from a moral point of view? If the difference between killing and letting die were in itself a morally important matter, one should say that Jones's behavior was less reprehensible than Smith's. But does one really want to say that? I think not. In the first place, both men acted from the same motive, personal gain, and both had exactly the same end in view when they acted. It may be inferred from Smith's conduct that he is a bad man, although that judgment may be withdrawn or modified if certain further facts are learned about him—for example, that he is mentally deranged. But would not the very same thing be inferred about Jones from his conduct? And would not the same further considerations also be relevant to any modification of this judgment? Moreover, suppose Jones pleaded, in his own defense, "After all, I didn't do anything except just stand there and watch the child drown. I didn't kill him; I only let him die." Again, if letting die were in itself less bad than killing, this defense should have at least some weight. But it does not. Such a "defense" can only be regarded as a grotesque perversion of moral reasoning. Morally speaking, it is no defense at all.

Now, it may be pointed out, quite properly, that the cases of euthanasia with which doctors are concerned are not like this at all. They do not involve personal gain or the destruction of normal, healthy children. Doctors are concerned only with cases in which the patient's life is of no further use to him, or in which the patient's life has become or will soon become a terrible burden. However, the point is the same in these cases: The bare difference between killing and letting die does not, in itself, make a moral difference. If a doctor lets a patient die, for humane reasons, he is in the same moral position as if he had given the patient a lethal injection for humane reasons. If his decision was wrong—if, for example, the patient's illness was in fact curable—the decision would be equally regrettable no matter which method was used to carry it out. And if the doctor's decision was the right one, the method used is not in itself important.

The AMA policy statement isolates the crucial issue very well; the crucial issue is "the intentional termination of the life of one human being by another." But after identifying this issue, and forbidding "mercy killing," the statement goes on to deny that the cessation of treatment is the intentional termination of a life. This is where the mistake comes in, for what is the cessation of treatment, in these circumstances, if it is not "the intentional termination of the life of one human being by another"? Of course it is exactly that, and if it were not, there would be no point to it.

Many people will find this judgment hard to accept. One reason, I think, is that it is very easy to conflate the question of whether killing is, in itself, worse than letting die, with the very different question of whether most actual cases of killing are more reprehensible than most actual cases of letting die. Most actual cases of killing are clearly terrible (think, for example, of all the murders reported in the newspapers), and one hears of such cases every day. On the other hand, one hardly ever hears of a case of letting die, except for the actions of doctors who are motivated by humanitarian reasons. So one learns to think of killing in a much worse light than of letting die, for it is not the bare difference between killing and letting die that makes the difference in these cases. Rather, the other factors—the murderer's motive of personal gain, for example, contrasted with the doctor's humanitarian motivation—account for different reactions to the different cases.

I have argued that killing is not in itself any worse than letting die; if my contention is right, it follows that active euthanasia is not any worse than passive euthanasia. What arguments can be given on the other side? The most common, I believe, is the following:

"The important difference between active and passive euthanasia is that, in passive euthanasia, the doctor does not do anything to bring about the patient's death. The doctor does nothing, and the patient dies of whatever ills already afflict him. In active euthanasia, however, the doctor does something to bring about the patient's death: He kills him. The doctor who gives the patient with cancer a lethal injection has himself caused his patient's death; whereas if he merely ceases treatment, the cancer is the cause of the death."

A number of points need to be made here. The first is that it is not exactly correct to say that in passive euthanasia the doctor does nothing, for he does do one thing that is very important: He lets the patient die. "Letting someone die" is certainly different in some respects, from other types of action—mainly in that it is a kind of action that one may perform by way of not performing certain other actions. For example, one may let a patient die by way of not giving medication, just as one may insult someone by way of not shaking his hand. But for any purpose of moral assessment, it is a type of action nonetheless. The decision to let a patient die is subject to moral appraisal in the same way that a decision to kill him would be subject to moral appraisal: It may be assessed as wise or unwise, compassionate or sadistic, right or wrong. If a doctor deliberately let a patient die who was suffering from a routinely curable illness, the doctor would certainly be to blame for what he had done, just as he would be to blame if he had needlessly killed the patient. Charges against him would then be appropriate. If so, it would be no defense at all for him to insist that he didn't "do anything." He would have done something very serious indeed, for he let his patient die.

Fixing the cause of death may be very important from a legal point of view, for it may determine whether criminal charges are brought against the doctor. But I do not think that this notion can be used to show a moral difference between active and passive euthanasia. The reason why it is considered bad to be the cause of someone's death is that death is regarded as a great evil—and so it is. However, if it had been decided that euthanasia—even passive euthanasia—is desirable in a given case, it has also been decided that in this instance death is no greater an evil than the patient's continued existence. And if this is true, the usual reason for not wanting to be the cause of someone's death simply does not apply.

Finally, doctors may think that all of this is only of academic interest—the sort of thing that philosophers may worry about but that has no practical bearing on their own work. After all, doctors must be concerned about the legal consequences of what they do, and active euthanasia is clearly forbidden by the law. But even so, doctors should also be concerned with the fact that the law is forcing upon them a moral doctrine that may well be indefensible and has a considerable effect on their practices. Of course, most doctors are not now in the position of being coerced in this matter, for they do not regard themselves as merely going along with what the law requires. Rather, in statements such as the AMA policy statement that I have quoted, they are endorsing this doctrine as a central point of medical ethics. In that statement, active euthanasia is condemned not merely as illegal but as "contrary to that for which the medical profession stands," whereas passive euthanasia is approved. However, the preceding considerations suggest that there is really no moral difference between the two, considered in themselves (there may be important moral differences in some cases in their *consequences*, but, as I pointed out, these differences may make active euthanasia, and not passive euthanasia, the morally preferable option). So, whereas doctors may have to discriminate between active and passive euthanasia to satisfy the law, they should not do any more than that. In particular, they should not give the distinction any added authority and weight by writing it into official statements of medical ethics.

1. According to Rachels, how would the alleviation of suffering be grounds for challenging the traditional distinction between active and passive euthanasia and for justifying, at times, active euthanasia?
2. Rachels's position opens the door to making end-of-life decisions based on quality-of-life assessments. Is this a dangerous turn? Is it sensible? Explain your answers.
3. Is killing worse than letting die? Do you agree with Rachels's analysis? Are his examples appropriate when applied to the area of euthanasia? Support your answers.
4. In challenging the traditional distinction between active and passive euthanasia as well as the wording in the AMA policy statement, Rachels underscores a pair of critical factors: intention and causation. His position reflects the nondifference position discussed in the text. Is his reasoning regarding intention and causation sound? Support your answer.

TOM L. BEAUCHAMP AND JAMES F. CHILDRESS

Rachels on Active and Passive Euthanasia

Tom L. Beauchamp is a professor of philosophy at Georgetown University and Senior Research Scholar at Georgetown University's Kennedy Institute of Ethics. James F. Childress is Edwin B. Kyle Professor of Religious Studies and a professor of medical education at the University of Virginia. Although Beauchamp and Childress agree with certain aspects of Rachels's argument, they insist that there is a genuine moral difference between active and passive euthanasia. They point out that Rachels leaves some critical considerations out of his equation, namely, social consequences. They discuss slippery slope concerns about the broader social context and the necessity of maintaining that active and passive euthanasia are morally set apart. In doing so, they defend the current AMA policy.

James Rachels contends that killing is not, in itself, worse than letting die; the "bare difference" between acts of killing and acts of letting die is not in itself a morally relevant difference. We agree with Rachels that the acts in his two cases are equally reprehensible because of the agents' motives and actions, and we agree that killing as a type of act is in itself no different *morally* than allowing to die as a type of act. However, we do not accept his conclusion that his examples and arguments show that the distinction between killing and letting die and passive and active euthanasia are morally irrelevant in the formulation of public policy. We also do not agree that his cases demonstrate what he claims.

PROBLEMS IN RACHELS'S ANALYSIS

First, Rachels's cases and the cessations of treatment envisioned by the AMA are so markedly disanalogous that Rachels's argument is misdirected. In some cases of unjustified acts, including both of Rachels's examples, we are not interested in moral distinctions between killing and letting die (per se). As Richard Trammell points out, some examples have a "masking" or "sledgehammer" effect; the fact that "one cannot distinguish the taste of two wines when both are mixed with green persimmon juice, does not imply that there is no distinction between the wines."[1] Because Rachels's examples involve two morally unjustified acts by agents whose motives and intentions are despicable, it is not surprising that some other features of their situations, such as killing and letting die, are not morally compelling considerations in the circumstances.

Second, Smith and Jones are morally responsible and morally blameworthy for the deaths of their respective cousins, even if Jones, who allowed his cousin to drown, is not causally responsible. The law might find only Smith, who killed his cousin, guilty of homicide (because of the law's theory of proximate cause), but morality condemns both actions alike because of the agents' commissions and omissions. We find Jones's actions reprehensible because he should have rescued the child. Even if he had no other special duties to the child, there is an affirmative obligation of beneficence in such a case.

Third, the point of the range of cases envisioned by the AMA is consistent with Rachels's arguments, though he thinks them inconsistent. The AMA's central claim is that the physician is always morally prohibited from killing patients but is not morally bound to preserve life in all cases. According to the AMA, the physician has a right and perhaps a duty to stop treatment if and only if three conditions are met: (1) the life of the body is being preserved by extraordinary means, (2) there is irrefutable evidence that biological death is imminent, and (3) the patient or the family consents. Whereas Rachels's cases involve two unjustified actions, one of killing and the other of letting die, the AMA statement distinguishes cases of unjusti-

fied killing from cases of justified letting die. The AMA statement does not claim that the moral difference is entirely predicated on the distinction between killing and letting die. It also does not imply that the bare difference between (passive) letting die and (active) killing is the major difference or a morally sufficient difference to distinguish the justified from the unjustified cases. The point is only that the justified actions in medicine are confined to letting die (passive euthanasia).

The AMA statement holds that "mercy killing" in medicine is unjustified in all circumstances, but it holds neither that letting die is right in all circumstances nor that killing outside medicine is always wrong. For an act that results in an earlier death for the patient to be justified, it is necessary that it be an act of letting die, but this condition is not sufficient to justify the act; nor is the bare fact of an act's being a killing sufficient to make the act wrong. This AMA declaration is meant to control conduct exclusively in the context of the physician-patient relationship. The rationale for the prohibition is not stated, but the scope of the prohibition is quite clear.

Even if the distinction between killing and letting die is morally irrelevant in many cases, it does not follow that it is morally irrelevant in all contexts. Although we quite agree that Rachels does effectively undermine all attempts to rest moral judgments about ending life on the "bare difference" between killing and letting die, his target may nonetheless be made of straw. Many philosophers and theologians have argued that there are independent moral, religious, and other reasons both for defending the distinction and for prohibiting killing while authorizing allowing to die in some circumstances or based on some motives.

One theologian has argued, for example, that we can discern the moral significance of the distinction between killing and letting die by "placing it in the religious context out of which it grew."[2] That context is the biblical story of God's actions toward his creatures. In that context it makes sense to talk about "placing patients in God's hands," just as it is important not to usurp God's prerogatives by desperately struggling to prolong life when the patient is irreversibly dying. But even if the distinction between killing and letting die originated within a religious context, and even if it makes more sense in that context than in some others, it can be defended on nontheological grounds without being reduced to a claim about a "bare difference." We turn next to this defense of the distinction.

HOW AND WHERE TO DEFEND THE DISTINCTION BETWEEN KILLING AND LETTING DIE

Even if there are sufficient reasons in some cases to warrant mercy killing, there may also be good reasons to retain the distinction between killing and letting die and to maintain our current practices and policies against killing *in medicine*, albeit with some clarifications and modifications.

Acts and Practices

The most important arguments for the distinction between killing and letting die depend on a distinction between acts and practices. It is one thing to justify an act; it is another to justify a general practice. Many beliefs about principles and consequences are applied to rules rather than directly to acts. For example, we might justify a rule of confidentiality because it encourages people to seek therapy and because it promotes respect for persons and their privacy, although such a rule might lead to undesirable results in particular cases where confidentiality should not be maintained.

Similarly, a rule that prohibits "active killing" while permitting some "allowed deaths" may be justifiable, even if it excludes some particular acts of killing that in themselves are justifiable. For example, the rule would not permit us to kill a patient who suffers from terrible pain, who will probably die within three weeks, and who rationally asks for a merciful-assisted death. In order to maintain a viable practice that expresses our principles and avoids seriously undesirable consequences, it may be necessary to prohibit some acts that are not otherwise wrong and in some cases may be morally justified. Thus, although particular *acts* of killing may be humane and compassionate, a *policy* or *practice* that authorizes killing in medicine—in even a few cases—might create a grave

risk of harm in many cases and a risk that we find it unjustified to assume.

The prohibition of killing even for "mercy" expresses principles and supports practices that provide a basis of trust between patients and health-care professionals. When we trust these professionals, we expect them to ask our consent and to do us no harm without a prospect of correlative benefit. The prohibition of killing is an attempt to promote a solid basis for trust in the role of caring for patients and protecting them from harm. This prohibition is both instrumentally and symbolically important, and its removal could weaken a set of practices and restraints that we cannot easily replace.

Wedge or Slippery Slope Arguments

This last argument—an incipient wedge or slippery slope argument—is plausible but needs to be stated carefully. Because of the widespread misuses of such arguments in biomedical ethics, there is a tendency to dismiss them whenever they are offered. However, as expressions of the principle of nonmaleficence, they are defensible in some cases. They also force us to consider whether unacceptable harms may result from attractive and apparently innocent first steps. Legitimation of acts such as active voluntary euthanasia run the risk of leading to other acts or practices that are morally objectionable even if some individual acts of this type are acceptable in themselves. The claim made by those who defend these arguments is that accepting the act in question would cross a line that has already been drawn against killing; and once that line has been crossed, it will not be possible to draw it again to preclude unacceptable acts or practices.

However, wedge arguments of some types may not be as damaging as they may seem at first. . . . In other words, the counterreply is that relevant distinctions can be drawn, and we are not subject to uncontrollable implications from general principles. Some versions of the wedge argument, therefore, do not assist supporters of the distinction between killing and letting die as much as they might suppose.

Indeed, the argument can be used against them: If it is rational and morally defensible to allow patients to die under conditions X, Y, and Z, then it is rational and morally defensible to kill them under those same conditions. If it is in their best interests to die, it is (*prima facie*) irrelevant how death is brought about. Rachels makes a similar point when he argues that reliance on the distinction between killing and letting die may lead to decisions about life and death made on irrelevant grounds—such as whether the patient will or will not die without certain forms of treatment—instead of being made in terms of the patient's best interests.

In the now famous Johns Hopkins Hospital case, an infant with Down syndrome and duodenal atresia was placed in a back room and died eleven days later of dehydration and starvation. This process of dying, which senior physicians had recommended against, was extremely difficult for all the parties involved, particularly the nurses. If decision makers legitimately determine that a patient would be better off dead (we think the parties mistakenly came to this conclusion in this case), how could an act of killing violate the patient's interests if the patient will not die when artificial treatment is discontinued? A morally irrelevant factor would be allowed to dictate the outcome.

The lack of empirical evidence to determine the adequacy of slippery slope arguments is unfortunate, but it is not a sufficient reason to reject them. Some arguments of this form should be taken with the utmost seriousness. They force us to think carefully about whether unacceptable harm is likely to result from attractive and apparently innocent first steps.

NOTES

1. Richard L. Trammell. "Saving Life and Taking Life," *Journal of Philosophy* 72 (1975):131–137.
2. Gilbert Meilaender. "The Distinction between Killing and Allowing to Die," *Theological Studies* 37 (1976): 467–470.

QUESTIONS FOR COMPREHENSION AND REFLECTION

1. What problems do Beauchamp and Childress find with Rachels's analysis?
2. Is their counterargument against Rachels more utilitarian or deontological in approach? Explain.
3. Beauchamp and Childress insist on maintaining a necessary distinction between killing and letting die. They therefore support what the text refers to as the difference position regarding active and passive euthanasia, particularly because of the negative social consequences if the distinction is eradicated. Discuss their slippery slope objection further.
4. Do you believe that the authors' slippery slope objection to euthanasia has merit? Is it sound? Explain your response in detail.

MICHAEL C. BRANNIGAN

Re-assessing the Ordinary/Extraordinary Distinction in Withholding/Withdrawing Nutrition and Hydration

Michael Brannigan is professor and chair of the philosophy department and executive director of the Center for the Study of Ethics at La Roche College in Pittsburgh. After discussing the origin of the traditional distinction between ordinary and extraordinary treatment, he goes on to describe how the meaning behind the distinction has veered away from its original intent. Then, using a phenomenological approach, he argues that the distinction is generally misleading and no longer defensible. Any appeal to the distinction makes sense only within a phenomenological framework. Brannigan concludes that the withholding and withdrawing of artificial nutrition and hydration are justified in certain contexts.

Karen Ann Quinlan has undoubtedly become a familiar name in the public memory. Yet, in the annals of medical litigation, the case of Claire Conroy is just as significant, even though it has garnered comparatively little media attention. When the New Jersey Supreme Court rendered its final decision concerning Ms. Conroy, it set a legal precedent for the state and the country. The court established that the artificial provision of food and fluids through the nasogastric tube was medical treatment which, under the constitutional law of privacy, an individual has a right to refuse.

Born in 1900, Ms. Conroy apparently lived a semicloistered existence in Belleville, New Jersey, where she shared a house with her three sisters, all of whom had died before she herself was placed in a nursing home in Bloomfield. Her only surviving blood relative, nephew Thomas Wittemore, was also her legal guardian. When admitted to the home, she was suffering from an organic brain syndrome, that is, "a diffuse or local impairment of brain tissue, manifested by alteration of orienta-tion, memory, comprehension, judgment."[1] Her physical condition soon became worse as she grew increasingly dependent and no longer able to communicate. After suffering a urinary tract infection and dehydration, necrotic gangrenous ulcers were discovered on her left foot. During her second hospital stay, she was fed by a nasogastric tube which, when it was removed for a trial period, was soon replaced after it became obvious that she could not sustain herself through eating. She returned to the nursing home with the nasogastric tube in place and another trial period proved to be futile. It was at this point that her nephew requested removal of her tube. Upon the refusal of her physician, Dr. Kazemi, Wittemore sought a court order. Ms. Conroy's condition was described as:

> . . . bed-bound in a semi-fetal position, suffering from hypertension, diabetes, and arteriosclerotic heart disease; with extensive bed-sores (decubitis ulcers) on her left-foot, leg, and hip, and her left-foot gangrenous to the knee; no bowel or bladder control, with a urinary catheter.[2]

Furthermore, her behavior and ability to respond to her environment was interpreted differently by the two physicians who testified at the court hearing. One, Dr. Davidoff, found her unable to respond and "severely demented without higher functioning or consciousness." On the other hand, Dr. Kazemi felt that, "although unaware and confused, she was able to respond." And, directly relevant to our topic, Davidoff characterized the feeding tube as extraordinary and optional treatment, contrary to Kazemi who was entirely opposed to withdrawal of the tube, convinced that it would constitute a violation of professional ethics. Rev. Kukura, a Roman Catholic priest, testified and described the distinction between ordinary and extraordinary treatment in Catholic doctrine and supported Davidoff's contention that the tube was extraordinary treatment and could justifiably be withdrawn.[3]

Given all this testimony, Judge Station issued an order allowing the removal of the feeding tube on February 2, 1983. However, the order was stayed pending appeal. In the meantime, the patient died with the tube in place. After a three-judge intermediate court of appeals overturned the initial ruling, on January 17, 1985, the New Jersey Supreme Court reversed the Appeals court in a 6–1 decision. The court referred to both the individual's right to privacy and a criterion whereby the tube may be removed if it imposes a "great burden to the patient" while "offering no hope of benefit or cure to the ailment that the individual is suffering."[4]

There are a host of ethical issues involved in this one case, ones which typically arise in situations where the withholding or withdrawing of life-sustaining treatment is requested, by either competent patients or by proxy decision-makers on behalf of incompetent patients. Some of these issues are:

- What moral distinctions, if any, exist between killing and allowing to die, or between commission and omission?
- How do we morally signify the "cause" of death, or define intent, or "aiming" at death?
- What constitutes "humane" treatment for terminally ill patients?

- Is withholding treatment ethically different from withdrawing treatment?
- What moral distinctions exist, if any, between so-called "ordinary" and "extraordinary" treatment?
- If patients are incompetent, what criteria exist for ethically sound proxy decision-making?
- How does one define competency?
- Can we regard medical nutrition and hydration as "medical treatment," subject to the same right of refusal as other treatments (dialysis, respirators, etc.)?
- Is medical nutrition and hydration to be regarded as "ordinary" treatment?
- What is the symbolic nature of feeding, and what role should it play in ethical decision-making?

These are only a few of the serious questions. My paper will focus upon the traditional distinction between ordinary and extraordinary treatment, and will do so for a number of reasons: (1) it has recently been the subject of critical debate, (2) it plays a significant role in cases involving the withholding/withdrawing of nutrition and hydration. This was clearly seen in Conroy when, at the appellate level, the courts did seek to affirm this traditional distinction in order to differentiate right from wrong actions. However, the Supreme Court, in overriding the appellate court's ruling, also proceeded in erasing this distinction. In the opinion of an attorney who was rather active at both appellate and Supreme Court levels, "Perhaps the most significant aspect of Conroy is the rejection of such treatment labels as 'ordinary' versus 'extraordinary' or 'artificial' versus 'natural.' The court noted that such terms confuse the issue and stand in the way of clear analysis."[5]

Throughout the remainder of my study, examination of the distinction will occur within a phenomenological framework. I suggested in an earlier work that phenomenology offered a feasible basis along with a more humanistic approach to medical-ethical issues.[6] Phenomenology arose as a reaction against the split between reason and experience in modern philosophy and recognizes the primacy of common experience in everyday life. It is thereby a method to help us understand an experience and, more specifically, the patient's own experience of an illness. After all, the patient is the center of concern in medicine. The methodology I am suggesting requires the suspension of the natural attitude so that illness can no longer be objectified, as done previously in both rationalist and empiricist approaches. In phenomenology, one cannot separate the illness from the patient's own experience and understanding of that illness. Therefore, we need to "bracket" the scientific-technical aspects of an illness so that we can view it, as best we can, from the perspective of the patient. The primary commitment of the health professional is to the patient as person. This demands transcending the mere technicism of medicine; not only is illness involved but, more importantly, a person who experiences that illness. Therefore, a phenomenological approach, in my opinion, offers a sound framework for approaching ethical issues in that the entire context of the illness is considered. In attempting to ascertain morally relevant factors in an ethically difficult situation, the patient's overall condition and preferences must be considered, and not merely the treatment modality itself.

We have briefly seen how the traditional distinction between ordinary and extraordinary treatment was appealed to in the Conroy case and played a major role in that it was eventually discredited by the Supreme Court decision. This distinction has become common parlance for both health professionals and ethicists. It has also been a significant factor in policy statements, for example, when the House of Delegates of the American Medical Association claimed that:

> The cessation of the employment of extraordinary means to prolong the life of the body when there is irrefutable evidence that biological death is imminent is the decision of the patient and/or his immediate family.[7]

Many recent court decisions, most notably Quinlan and Saikewicz, have also referred to the distinction.

Any re-examination of this traditional distinction must consider its origin and evolution. Its beginning is found within Catholic theology and its language has remained "staple fare" in the Catholic tradition of medical ethics. The terms were introduced by Banez in 1595 with reference to efforts to save a person's life by radical measures such as surgery. Due to lack of anaesthesia, surgery obviously entailed unbearable pain and Banez utilized the terms to designate means which were accompanied by either "negligible" or else "agonizing and unbearable" pain. In other words, the distinction was not proposed in view of patients for whom treatment would be essentially useless.[8] The original distinction referred to patients whose lives could be preserved and saved, and not those whose deaths would be prolonged. The early moralists held that one is not bound to preserve life if the anguish and suffering is extraordinarily disproportionate to any advantages. Therefore, the distinction between ordinary and extraordinarily marked a further distinction between obligatory and non-obligatory. What was considered either ordinary or extraordinary depended upon the total condition of the patient and the proportion or disproportion of benefits and burdens as viewed by that patient.

This original notion of proportionality in the Catholic tradition was actually maintained up until the first part of the 1900s as was expressed by Pope Pius XII in his 1957 address:

> But normally one is held to use only ordinary means—according to circumstances of persons, places, times and culture—means that do not involve any grave burdens for oneself or another.[9]

This, in turn, led Gerald Kelly, a leading authority on Catholic moral theology, to render his classic definition of the terms:

> *Ordinary* means of preserving life are all medicines, treatments, and operations, which offer a reasonable hope of benefit for the patient and which can be obtained and used without excessive expense, pain, or other inconvenience.

> *Extraordinary* means of preserving life . . . (are) all medicines, treatments, and operations, which cannot be obtained or used without excessive expense, pain, or other inconvenience, or which,

if used, would not offer a reasonable hope of benefit.[10]

This reflects the Catholic moral position prior to Vatican II and—more importantly—before the period of modern technological medicine. Kelly's definition demonstrates a terminology which is both descriptive and evaluative; that is, ordinary means morally obligated, or mandatory, whereas extraordinary means morally permissible, or elective. At the same time, the distinction is viewed in light of the total conditions of benefit (usefulness) and burden (inconvenience) to the patient.

Rather than present a long, tedious historical survey of the utilization of these terms, suffice it to say that these same terms have remained in use. However, and this is most critical, the science and art of medicine has radically changed. With the dramatic increase in medical technology, this original, more phenomenological understanding of ordinary and extraordinary underwent drastic modifications. Just as medical technology became more increasingly sophisticated, the *art* of medicine gave way to the *science* of medicine. Emphasis upon the technical aspects of illness sacrificed the centrality of that patient. The understanding of ordinary and extraordinary became more routinized and referred solely to the underlying technology. Ordinary and extraordinary means became just that, a categorization of the techniques being utilized. For example, there is the testimony of one physician concerning a 76-year-old man dying of amyotrophic lateral sclerosis who requested to stop his respirator. His attending physician stated:

> I deal with respirators every day of my life. To me this is not heroic. This is standard procedure . . . I have other patients who have run large corporations who have been on portable respirators. Other people who have been on them and have done quite well for as long as possible.[11]

The physician in this Florida case is defining ordinary means (the respirator) as that which is standard procedure, regardless of the condition of the patient, regardless of the proportionality or lack of as to benefits and burdens. Similarly, others have defined extraordinary in the same mechanical way, such as the trial judge in this same case who remarked:

> Certainly there is no question legally that putting a hole in a man's trachea and inserting a mechanical respirator is extraordinary life-preserving means.[12]

Here, as with the physician's remark, attention is paid solely to characteristics of the technology involved, apart from the patient's overall condition.

There have recently been a number of proposals to designate features in a given situation which would be relevant in categorizing a treatment modality as either ordinary or extraordinary. These features all depict, however, an emphasis upon the technology of the treatment and little, if any, regard for the patient's condition. Such features are:

- treatment which is simple as opposed to complex
- treatment which is usual, or standard, versus unusual
- treatment which is natural versus artificial
- treatment which is inexpensive as opposed to costly.

Perceived phenomenologically, it is obvious that, taken by themselves in isolation, none of these features are morally relevant because they focus solely upon the technique. It is precisely this type of scientism which phenomenology reacts against. For instance, if we were to employ the standard versus unusual treatment condition as categorizing whether that treatment is either ordinary or extraordinary, it becomes evident that this is quite insufficient: antibiotics are standard treatment, but if they are utilized for a patient who is close to death and who develops pneumonia, it is quite possible that he may view the treatment as prolonging his own death. In the same vein, the utilization of "natural" versus "artificial" as the criterion for categorizing treatment as either ordinary or extraordinary is also insufficient. Simply put, there is no real consensus among the medical community of experts as to what constitutes natural and artificial. This was especially highlighted in one study conducted after the Natural Death Act was legislated in California. From the study, it appears that the overall view of most physicians was that respirators, dialysis machines, and resuscitators were considered as artificial treatment means. However, when it came to intravenous feeding, they were divided. Moreover, more than half felt that insulin, antibiotics, and chemotherapy were natural.[13]

Interpretations of treatment as natural and artificial, and therefore as ordinary and extraordinary, remain morally irrelevant unless other factors are taken into consideration, namely factors which transcend the mere technicalism of treatment, factors which directly address the patient's interests and preferences. This underscores the need for a more phenomenological framework in reassessing the traditional distinction since such a framework naturally considers the entire context in which illness occurs.

Fortunately, other criteria have been suggested as features for the categorization of treatment as ordinary or extraordinary and these additional features come closer to recognizing the significance of the patient's condition, namely:

- treatment regarded as non-invasive versus invasive; even though this still depicts treatment measures, it does so with respect to effects upon the patient.

- likelihood for success versus little change of success.

- proportion and disproportion of benefits and burdens.

These last two clearly approach a phenomenological orientation since the condition of the patient, his interests and preferences are strongly implied.

To summarize, the past decade has witnessed a medical-technical understanding of ordinary/extraordinary rather than the phenomenological one which was attested to in its original use in Catholic moral theology. What I am suggesting is that by veering away from its original, more phenomenological construction, health professionals have substituted a technological understanding of the distinction, and, as Ramsey warns us, "A routinized understanding of 'ordinary'/'extraordinary' is the security blanket of some physicians—who nevertheless have been known to call some ethicists 'absolutists.'"[14]

Furthermore, while overemphasizing the technical aspects of ordinary/extraordinary, many have, at the same time, confused the medical meaning of the terms with their moral meaning; that is, a normative content has been unduly attached to the technology—if ordinary/extraordinary is to be reduced to its medical function, then moral weight must also be kept distinct. This has not been the case in practice. Ramsey indicates how this medical-moral confusion takes place by the different ways in which physicians and ethicists use the terms: while physicians speak of ordinary and extraordinary in terms of the "state of the art" of medicine and thereby of the practice of medicine, ethicists tend to use the terms in view of the "state of the person," and in this way the total context of the patient must be considered, meaning additional significant, nonmedical factors.[15] Confusing what is medically ordinary (that is, appealing to the earlier proposed criteria such as standard versus unusual, natural versus artificial, etc.) with what is ethically ordinary (that is, obligatory or mandatory) can have dangerous consequences since different meanings result from and depend upon differentiation in usage. There is an obvious need for clarity concerning the terms, both medically and ethically.

A phenomenological orientation to this task of clarification considers that a treatment is ethically ordinary, or obligatory, if it is essentially useful to the patient, beneficial, and does not add substantially to the burdens of the patient. This same orientation considers how that individual patient views the treatment, and respects his values and preferences. The net benefits must, therefore, outweigh the burdens for the patient. Features such as simple versus complex, or usual versus unusual, are *in themselves* morally irrelevant since they focus solely upon the means. A treatment which is rare, complex, artificial, and invasive may, at the same time, be ethically obligatory if it has a good chance of providing reasonable benefits for the patient without adding to her burdens.

The language of ordinary/extraordinary has become vague and unilluminating at best. The recent *Declaration on Euthanasia* (1980) by the Vatican proposes substituting the terms "proportionate" and "disproportionate" for the more traditional but misleading "ordinary" and "extraordinary." I suggest that these terms proposed by the Vatican are preferable in that they accord more weight to the context of the individual patient and consider net benefits and burdens. Of course, this phenomenological re-assessment only brings us to the starting-line in the controversy, since further examination of what constitutes "benefits" and "burdens" must ensue. Yet any serious analysis of this, if approached phenomenologically as I believe it should, must first of all respect the best interests of the patient in light of the patient's own values and preferences.

Let us now conclude by applying our analysis to the specific area of withholding/withdrawing nutrition and hydration, illustrated in the Conroy case. Employing the distinction between ordinary and extraordinary can become rather unfruitful in the area of nutrition and hydration, simply because of the undue emphasis upon technique along with the accompanying confusion between medical and moral. If we examine nutrition and hydration as medical artificial treatment in a phenomenological perspective, the ethical question of whether treatment can be justifiably withdrawn, or whether it is mandatory to continue treatment must rely heavily upon considerations of the patient's condition, interests, and preferences as being morally relevant factors in addition to the treatment modality itself. Lynn and Childress have described for us three specific situations whereby nutrition and hydration may be justifiably withdrawn:

> 1) the procedures that would be required are so unlikely to achieve improved nutritional and fluid levels that they could correctly be considered futile; 2) the improvement in nutritional and fluid balance, though achievable, could be of no benefit to the patient; 3) the burdens of receiving the treatment may outweigh the benefit.[16]

In light of considerations of futility, lack of benefit, and the presence of excessive burdens, it appears obvious that the language of ordinary/extraordinary is misleading if it pulls us away from the total context of illness. Language of proportionality makes more ethical sense. The current language of ordinary/extraordinary makes little sense, furthermore, if it *obscures* the very principles which

are fundamental in decisions concerning the withholding/withdrawing of life-sustaining treatment. These fundamental principles are two, and the ethical justifiability of the utilization of all treatment modalities must bear these in mind:

1) the principle of beneficence: what is in the best interests of the patient?

2) respect for persons: fashioned as the principle of autonomy, or self-determination.[17]

The language of ordinary/extraordinary is misleading when it emphasizes standard medical practice at the expense of disregarding these fundamental first principles, when it stresses *tekne,* when morality becomes attached to technology and the patient is not fully acknowledged.

With regard to nutrition and hydration, it is the attitude of many health professionals that such treatment is "ordinary" treatment. This was the claim of the nurse in the trial of the two California physicians Nejdl and Barber, who discontinued intravenous feeding to a patient with severe brain damage: "Food is an ordinary means. And everyone has a right to ordinary treatment."[18] Treatment needs to be considered within its entire context and in view of the fundamental principles of beneficence and autonomy. If treatment is beneficial, and the preference of the patient, then it is obligatory. If it is useless, burdensome, or contrary to the wishes of a competent patient (or incompetent if desires are known with some degree of certainty), then medicine is under no obligation to provide such treatment.

The distinction between ordinary and extraordinary has become misleading, and appealing to any intrinsic moral significance in this distinction adds nothing to the analysis except confusion. Although the original meaning of ordinary and extraordinary conveyed the ideal of proportionality of benefits and burdens, focus recently shifted to a more technological understanding, due to the increasing sophistication in medicine, and at the expense of the patient. Ordinary/extraordinary only makes sense if we can adopt a phenomenological perspective which will hope to resuscitate a genuine understanding of the terms. I believe that the terminology of proportionate and disproportionate is preferable, since resorting to the traditional distinction still evokes distorted meanings. The weakness of the traditional distinction is illustrated by the test case of withholding/withdrawing nutrition and hydration, where a phenomenological approach is critical in order to perceive and be sensitive to morally relevant features. The withholding/withdrawing of nutrition and hydration appears justified if the fundamental principles of beneficence and autonomy are upheld, and when the patient's condition and preferences are respected.

NOTES

1. *In re* Conroy, 190 N. J. Super, 453, 464, A.2d 303, 304 n. 1 (App. Div. 1983).
2. Jeff Stryker, "In re Conroy: History and Setting of the Case," in *By No Extraordinary Means*, ed. by Joanne Lynne (Bloomington: Indiana University Press, 1986), p. 230.
3. Ibid., pp. 231–232.
4. William Strasser, "The Conroy Case: An Overview," in *By No Extraordinary Means*, p. 247.
5. Joseph Rodriguez, Jr., "Role of the Public Advocate," in *By No Extraordinary Means*, p. 258.
6. Michael Brannigan, "A Phenomenological Orientation to Illness and Ethical Implications," *Contemporary Philosophy* X, 8 (Spring 1985), 6–8.
7. Cited in Benedict M. Ashley and Kevin D. O'Rourke, *Health Care Ethics: A Theological Analysis* (St. Louis: The Catholic Hospital Association, 1978), p. 390.
8. James J. McCartney, "The Development of the Doctrine of Ordinary and Extraordinary Means of Preserving Life in Catholic Moral Theology Before the Karen Quinlan Case," *Linacre Quarterly* 47 (August 1980), 216.
9. Pope Pius XII, "The Prolongation of Life," *AAS* 49 (1957), 1031–1032.
10. Gerald Kelly, *Medico-Moral Problems* (St. Louis: The Catholic Hospital Association, 1958), p. 129.
11. Cited in *Deciding to Forego Life-Sustaining Treatment*, President's Commission for the Study of Ethical Problems in Medicine and Biomedical and Behavioral Research (March 1983), p. 83.
12. Ibid.
13. Cited in James F. Childress, "When Is It Morally Justifiable to Discontinue Medical Nutrition and Hydration?" in *By No Extraordinary Means*, p. 71.
14. Paul Ramsey, *Ethics At the Edges of Life* (New Haven: Yale University Press, 1978), p. 159.
15. Paul Ramsey, *The Patient as Person* (New Haven: Yale University Press, 1970), pp. 118ff.
16. Joanne Lynn and James Childress, "Must Patients Always Be Given Food and Water?" *Hastings Center Report* 13 (October 1983), pp. 18–19.
17. Childress, "When Is It Morally Justifiable?", p. 69.
18. Cited in Ibid., p. 72.

QUESTIONS FOR COMPREHENSION AND REFLECTION

1. According to Brannigan, how does a phenomenological approach to illness provide a basis for challenging the traditional distinction between ordinary and extraordinary treatment? Explain your answer.
2. Discuss the author's account of the origin and evolution of the terms *ordinary* and *extraordinary* when applied to medical treatment.
3. Brannigan suggests that the development of the distinction between ordinary and extraordinary treatment has been influenced by our increasing (and misdirected) emphasis on medical technologies and techniques rather than on the personal context of patients. According to Brannigan, how has our current usage of the terms veered away from their original meanings? Do you agree or disagree? Explain.
4. In view of the originally intended context regarding the ordinary/extraordinary distinction, how could medical feeding at times be viewed as extraordinary? Is Brannigan's analysis sound or weak? Support your answers.

MARGARET PABST BATTIN

Physician-Assisted Suicide

Margaret Pabst Battin is a professor of philosophy and adjunct professor of internal medicine in the Division of Medical Ethics, University of Utah. After presenting arguments both favoring and opposing physician-assisted suicide, Battin delves into the most critical ethical issues. She treats religious perspectives as well as social issues, alluding to the experience in Holland where physician-assisted suicide is sanctioned. She concludes by offering reasons for her support of voluntary measures in physician-assisted suicide.

THE STRUCTURE OF THE DEBATE OVER PHYSICIAN-ASSISTED SUICIDE

Despite the many contexts in which dispute over the legalization of physician-assisted suicide occurs, the public debate tends to be played out with just a handful of basic arguments. Much of the same argumentation is also used in the associated debates about euthanasia, though since it is suicide that is our focus here, and since it is, I believe, physician-assisted suicide rather than voluntary active euthanasia that is more likely to be legalized or legally tolerated in the United States I will attend just to arguments about it here. They include:

THE DEBATE OVER PHYSICIAN-ASSISTED SUICIDE

Principal Arguments for Physician-Assisted Suicide	*Principal Arguments Against Physician-Assisted Suicide*
■ The argument from autonomy ■ The argument from mercy	■ The argument from the wrongness of killing ■ The slippery-slope argument ■ The argument concerning the physician's role

---

Each argument is then met by objections, counterobjections, and, in turn, countercounterobjections, and of course each of the principal lines of argument appears in a variety of different guises. For the sake of efficiency they are stated here in schematic form—the principal arguments and their principal objections and counterobjections . . .

Arguments Favoring Physician-Assisted Suicide

The argument from autonomy

Just as a person has the right to determine as much as possible the course of his or her own life, a person also has the right to determine as much as possible the course of his or her own dying. If a terminally ill person seeks assistance in suicide from a physician, the physician ought to provide it, provided the request is made freely and rationally.

Objection:

True autonomy is rarely possible, especially for someone who is dying, since not only are most choices socially formed, but in terminal illness depression and other psychiatric disturbances are likely to be a factor.

Counterobjection:

Even if many choices are socially shaped, they must be respected as autonomous.

Counterobjection:

Rational suicide is possible, and it is possible for patients to make choices about dying without distortion by depression.

Objection:

One cannot obligate another to do what is morally wrong, even if one's choice is made freely and rationally. Since suicide is wrong, the physician can have no obligation to assist in it.

Counterobjection:

No adequate moral argument shows that suicide in circumstances of terminal illness is morally wrong.

The argument from mercy

No person should have to endure pointless terminal suffering. If the physician is unable to relieve the patient's suffering in other ways and the only way to avoid such suffering is by death, then the physician ought to bring death about.

Objection:

Thanks to techniques of pain management developed by Hospice and others, it is possible to treat virtually all pain and to relieve virtually all suffering. Thus the dying process can be valuable as a positive, transformative experience of new intimacy and spiritual growth.

Counterobjection:

"Virtually all" is not "all"; if some pain or suffering cannot be treated, there will still sometimes be a need to avoid them by death.

Countercounterobjection:

Complete sedation can be used where pain cannot be controlled.

Countercountercounterobjection:

Complete sedation means complete obtundation, and because the patient can no longer communicate or perceive, is equivalent to causing death. If these are permitted, why not more direct methods of bringing about death?

Counterobjection:

There can be no guarantee of a positive, transformative experience.

Arguments Opposing Physician-Assisted Suicide

The argument from the intrinsic wrongness of killing

The taking of a human life is simply wrong; this is evident in the commandment "Thou shalt not kill."

Objection:

But killing is socially and legally accepted in self-defense, war, capital punishment, and other situations, and so it should be socially and legally accepted when it is the choice of the person who would be killed.

Counterobjection:

In self-defense, war, and capital punishment, the person killed is guilty; in assisted suicide the person killed is innocent.

The slippery-slope argument

Permitting physicians to assist in suicide, even in sympathetic cases, would lead to situations in which patients were killed against their will.

Objection:

A basis for these predictions must be demonstrated before they can be used to suppress personal choices and individual rights.

Counterobjection:

The basis for these predictions is increasing cost pressures, as well as greed, laziness, insensitivity, and other factors affecting physicians and their institutions.

Countercounterobjection:

It is possible, with careful design, to erect effective protections against abuse by doctors or institutions.

The argument concerning the physician's role

Doctors should not kill; this is prohibited by the Hippocratic Oath. The physician is bound to save life, not take it.

Objection:

In its original version the Hippocratic Oath also prohibits doctors from performing surgery, providing abortifacients, or taking fees for teaching medicine. If these can be permitted within the physician's role, why not assistance in suicide, where the patient is dying anyway and seeks the physician's help?

> *Counterobjection:*
> To permit physicians to kill patients would undermine the patient's trust in the physician.
>
> > *Countercounterobjection:*
> > Patients trust their physicians more when they know that their physicians will help them, not desert them as they die.

Clearly these arguments can all be extended and developed to a much greater degree.

None of the formulations presented here is canonical, and they occur in an enormous range of varieties. Indeed these arguments and counterarguments have appeared repeatedly throughout the public debate, and have been anticipated and addressed in many ways in the background philosophical issues we have been exploring. However, as we've said, in the public arena these debates are often conducted at a comparatively superficial level—often simply by reciting the above arguments in nearly equally schematic form, or by pitting cases like Janet Adkins and Dr. Kevorkian against others like Dr. Quill and Diane, when in fact such cases exhibit both similarities and differences. It is important for this reason to look more closely at the underlying philosophical issues.

THE BASIC ETHICAL ISSUES IN PHYSICIAN-ASSISTED SUICIDE

[To understand what lies beneath this debate], we can explore the basic ethical issues underlying the current public discussion of physician-assisted suicide. Though ethical theory is not their primary concern, . . . religious, social, and value-of-life arguments reflect three types of background normative positions, based in divine-command, utilitarian, and deontological ethical theories respectively. I shall be making a central assumption in exploring these issues: Physician-assisted suicide is a practice the purpose of which is to help a patient in need avoid what he or she perceives as a far worse death, or avoid continued existence in a state he or she perceives worse than death.

Religious Views of Physician-Assisted Suicide

Christian religious arguments, almost always employed to oppose both the legalization and practice of physician-assisted suicide, variously insist that it would violate the biblical commandment "Thou shalt not kill"; that it would violate the gratitude one owes God for the "gift of life," the obligation one has to "remain at one's post," or the trust one ought to have in one's heavenly father . . . and that it would run contrary to natural law. The variety of religiously based argumentation against physician-assisted suicide is enormous. To be sure, there have been some religious voices on the other side of the public debate: For example, some liberal Protestant churches have supported legalization initiatives in Washington, California, and Oregon, but most religious groups—especially the Catholic Church—have been opposed to legalization and would no doubt be opposed to the practice even if it were legalized.

In this political dispute, however, a number of much more basic issues are often overlooked. The first group are those associated with the fact that, as we've seen, Western religious views of an individual's role in his or her own dying developed during historical periods when death was likely to occur of infectious or parasitic disease, often comparatively suddenly and at any age. Thus these religious views may not be appropriate for late twentieth-century medical circumstances in the developed world, where the vast majority of people no longer die young or suddenly but predictably later in life of diseases with long, downhill deteriorative declines. The major religious traditions all developed during the "Age of Pestilence and Famine," which lasted from the beginning of human existence to about 1850; but the developed nations have all now passed through the various stages of the epidemiological transition to the "Age of Delayed Degenerative Diseases." Modern life in these nations presents an entirely different environment for dying.

This new epidemiological pattern may affect a number of the common religiously based arguments. For example, the argument from mercy, concerning the role of pain, may require modification to take account of the fact that the new pattern of death from degenerative diseases may lengthen and intensify the degree of suffering a dying person undergoes, even with modern pain-control techniques. The late twentieth-century first-world trajectories of death, with their extensive medicalization and long downhill courses, have the capacity even with modern pain-control techniques to prolong terminal suffering far beyond what would have been likely in any earlier historical period. After all, prior to the development of antibiotics in the 1940s, a person who became bedridden was likely to succumb to pneumonia not long afterward, and the prospect of an extended period of medical deterioration, with or without high-tech medical treatment such as intravenous feeding or machine-assisted respiration, did not arise. Nor did people with severe disabilities or illnesses, such as quadriplegia or ALS, survive very long, and issues about the quality of life in these conditions could not arise. It is sometimes even rather crudely remarked that, in terms of physical pain alone, the contemporary terminal-illness patient may endure more sustained pain over a longer period of time than the central figure of sacrifice in the Christian tradition, a first-century crucifixion victim, so that exhortations to emulate that central occasion of voluntary suffering cannot require the contemporary patient to continue on to the end.

This new picture may also affect some of the traditional religiously based arguments. For instance, the argument that "life is a gift from God and therefore wrong to destroy" may have looked quite different in eras during which the average life expectancy was around 30 or 35 than when it is 72. Throughout almost the entire history of humankind, people died—on average—in early or middle adulthood; in the advanced industrial nations it is now the *norm* that people die in *old* age. In the latter circumstances, it may be tempting to argue, to take just one of the traditional religious arguments against suicide, that the gift of life has already been welcomed—a full life has already been lived—so that ending it in suicide would not be to reject the gift in the same way that ending a life only half complete might represent. Then, too, since physician-assisted suicide would be occurring primarily in the context of terminal illness, it

might plausibly be claimed that bringing about death somewhat earlier cannot violate natural law for someone who is already in the process of dying: If the human being's natural end would be subverted by death, that will occur in any case, and if not, then there can be little objection to suicide on these grounds.

Most conspicuous, though, in current religious argumentation about physician-assisted suicide is the absence of attention to what I have called the religious "invitation" to suicide. The Christian tradition . . . incorporates five major inducements to suicide; two of them may be particularly relevant in the terminal-illness situations associated with physician-assisted suicide. One of these is the promise of reunion with the deceased: In the traditional Christian belief system, although the person facing death will be separated from loved ones who are now alive, he or she may hope for reunion with those who have already died. For the person dying of terminal illness, it may be particularly important that these loved ones who have already died are likely to be parents or older family members—persons who might provide comfort—since in terminal illness the dying person may slip into increasingly childlike, dependent conditions where care by a loved, long-missed elder would be especially desired. The pull of such an invitation can hardly be underestimated when the belief in a personal afterlife is strong.

The other promise within the Christian tradition perhaps constituting the strongest invitation to suicide in conditions of terminal illness is that of release of the soul. Given a traditional metaphysic in which the perishable body is viewed as distinct from the immortal soul, the prospect of release of the soul may seem especially alluring when the body is undergoing the deteriorative, degenerative processes associated with terminal illness. The body fails, in this view, but the soul lives on; and when the body's failing is prolonged and painful, it may seem especially inviting to liberate the soul earlier and more easily in this long downhill course. After all, death in this view is not really dying; it is a transition to another, better state in the afterlife to come.

These two invitations to suicide within the Christian tradition may seem, thus, much stronger when death is approaching in any case, and may be particularly inviting for a person undergoing a period of extended terminal decline accompanied by sustained, untreatable suffering or continuous pain, that is, in the very circumstances that would make physician-assisted suicide seem most plausible. The challenge for the traditional religious view is to come to full grips with the realities of modern dying, and to reexamine traditional claims about the purpose of suffering in the face of extended deteriorative illness.

To be sure, much of this has already been accomplished in the context of withdrawing or withholding treatment. As early as 1958 . . . Pope Pius XII held that it is not obligatory to use "extraordinary means" to prolong the lives of the dying, if it is "such a burden for the family that one cannot in conscience impose it on them."[1] But many of the same arguments apply in self-caused or self-authorized death as well; facing this parallel is what the traditional religious groups—perhaps because of the stigma attached to the very word 'suicide'—have often avoided. By and large, traditional religious groups have not really explored the issues of suicide or physician-assisted suicide in terminal illness, and have tended to reject it virtually unexplored.[2]

Finally, of course, exploration of these issues will direct attention to a question arising from the epidemiological shift as well as from the notion of invitation to death: Does the fact that contemporary medical treatment is now able to prolong life beyond the point at which the patient would earlier have died—beyond, some might like to say, its formerly "natural" endpoint—entail that views about the termination of life must be revised? If it is not wrong for a patient to decline further treatment, how can it be wrong to wish a more directly caused death for the same reasons and at the same time? If the traditional religious groups do explore these issues more carefully, they may see a way to play a major *supportive* role in aiding terminally ill persons who seek to bring their lives to a close in a responsible, dignified way—something we shall return to later in this chapter.

Of course traditional Christianity's two implicit invitations to suicide especially relevant in terminal illness are not now generally explicitly recognized by those committed to the Christian view. A more conventional account of traditional religious attitudes would no doubt emphasize the centrality of obedience, submission to God's will, the voluntary acceptance of suffering, and hope in an afterlife. But it is important to recognize all the ways—explicit and submerged—in which religious considerations bear on the issue of physician-assisted suicide in terminal illness.

Social Arguments and Physician-Assisted Suicide

. . . [T]he social arguments so frequently used to oppose suicide—that the suicide of a person would harm his or her family, community, or society, or that the suicide would deprive society of his or her contribution to that society—backfire whenever the suicide of a person would benefit rather than harm these other parties. Suicide . . . can mean the removal of social burdens, including the psychological, emotional, and/or financial burdens imposed by a person who is abusive, criminal, sociopathic, or chronically or terminally ill. This is an argument first associated with Plato, we have seen, but because it runs so strongly counter to the traditional taboo against suicide, and because it would yield such profoundly unsettling consequences for accepted social policies concerning suicide and suicide prevention, it is very, very rarely raised in contemporary discussion. The social-burdens argument is particularly problematic in the circumstances associated with physician-assisted suicide—terminal illness, and perhaps severe chronic illness, severe disability, and extreme old age—since the costs of medical treatment, hospitalization, palliation, rehabilitative treatment, domestic assistance, and other terminal and chronic care can be enormous. This is the root of the slippery-slope argument, that permitting some cases of physician-assisted suicide would lead to a situation in which patients are killed against their will. The social-burdens argument against suicide invites an argument about cost savings that is extremely sensitive and problematic, but which cannot be avoided if we are to look more closely at the underlying philosophical issues.

Almost no one involved in the current debates over the legalization of physician-assisted suicide and euthanasia dares to raise such issues publicly, and especially not the issue of cost savings in medical care. Yet, I think, there is a widespread assumption operative in these debates: Permitting physician-assisted suicide and euthanasia would mean huge savings at the end of life. This is not a partisan assumption; it is shared, I believe, by both those favoring legalization and those opposed to it. Those supporting legalization assume, I suspect, that the projected cost savings from euthanasia and assisted suicide are an additional reason favoring legalization, and consequently that in this special case, patients' rights of autonomous choice coincide with the demands of justice by permitting fairer distribution of health care resources. This is a view compatible with the utilitarian background of these arguments: Even though some losses might be borne by a few, the imposition of these losses would produce the greater good for the greater number. On this argument, however, when the talk is of *voluntary* suicide in terminal illness, the case is even stronger, since we cannot assume that the person who chooses death in preference to deteriorative terminal illness regards it as a loss.

Those opposing legalization seem to accept the same underlying assumption, that the practice of assisted suicide in terminal illness would mean huge cost savings, but draw from it a different conclusion: They fear that the prospect of huge savings, both in financial costs for institutions and in other psychological and emotional costs for family members, would lead physicians and the cost managers who influence them, as well as family members who bear the burdens of care, to manipulate or force terminally ill patients into such choices, thus effectively greasing the slippery slope.

Thus, although the social arguments concerning suicide are, as we have seen, almost always explicitly employed only in their negative form—that is, as slippery-slope arguments against suicide on the grounds that it would harm family, community, and society—I think that the corresponding positive version of these arguments—concerning potential benefits to society, especially in the form of cost savings—plays an extraordinary covert role

in contemporary thinking about physician-assisted suicide.

In view of this, I think both sides in the public debate over physician-assisted suicide are obligated to identify the roles these covert arguments play, examine them critically, and minimize the covert and unexamined influence they currently have. A preliminary calculation suggests that the actual cost savings of euthanasia and physician-assisted suicide, if practiced in the United States at the same rate and in the same conditions as in the one country in which they are effectively legal, the Netherlands, would be *very* much smaller than what is usually tacitly assumed. While euthanasia and physician-assisted suicide are widely approved in the Netherlands (by about 80% of the population) and universally known to be an option in terminal care, only a small fraction of Dutch actually choose these forms of dying, and when they do so they typically forgo only a few weeks of life. Two thirds of all requests for assisted suicide or euthanasia are turned down, and [about 3.4%] of all Dutch patients who die in a given year do so in this way.[3] Thus, although the majority of these Dutch patients have cancer and cancer is the most expensive terminal condition to treat, savings from this practice cannot be assumed to be great, and do not play a role in Dutch policy or practice at all. While in the United States it is sometimes assumed that permitting physician-assisted suicide or euthanasia would save a huge proportion of health care costs—as much, one sometimes hears, as a third or a fourth of all costs—more careful calculations suggest that the actual savings would be [less than 0.07% of total health care expenditures].[4] The smallness of this figure ought to silence talk of costs in discussions of the morality of physician-assisted suicide and euthanasia and return discussion to the ethical issues at hand, but it is important to recognize that tacit unfounded assumptions concerning costs are very widely made.

But the matter is not that simple. Under the social-burdens arguments we are considering here, all benefits and burdens must be accounted for. The cost of medical treatment in a terminal illness does not reflect ancillary financial expenses like home assistance or lost income of family members who serve as caretakers; and it does not include emotional or psychological costs at all. A true computation of all of the costs saved by a terminally or chronically ill person's suicide might be enormous (one need only consider the burden sustained by a spouse caring for a person with Alzheimer's over a period of up to ten years or more, and remember that in the age group 85 and older, the risks of Alzheimer's are as high as 1:4 or higher), even if this computation were somehow adjusted to compensate for the emotional and psychological gains of, say, greater family intimacy and understanding. This is a very problematic fact, of course. Calculating such costs has in the past invited the involuntary killing of the terminally ill, along with the chronically ill and the developmentally disabled; Nazi Germany's early T4 euthanasia program is no doubt the most horrifying example. But the discussion here is not about *involuntary* killing, or the kinds of practices that would not only produce endemic fear in a society but impose the incalculable cost of depriving people who wished to continue them of their lives; the issue in physician-assisted suicide concerns *voluntary* self-killing, consentingly performed by one's physician and accepted by one's family, community, and society. Under the sort of calculus the social arguments concerning suicide invites, ... physician-assisted suicide may seem to produce, on balance, benefits rather than harms. That is what makes these arguments so particularly problematic in these contexts, and makes the slippery-slope objection to accepting physician-assisted suicide such a powerful one.

Social-burdens arguments, covert or explicit, ought also to be examined in relation to classical utilitarian theory. . . . It will be evident, I believe, that like the justice objection, these social-burdens arguments concerning suicide constitute another major objection to utilitarian theory across the board. Utilitarian theory in its classical form, we saw, appears to welcome the exit not only of any person whose care represents a cost to others, but also of any person whose misery reduces the average or aggregate level of happiness or utility. Thus, even apart from costs, the earlier exit of those suffering in terminal illnesses is to be encouraged—

or, rather, on this theory, is morally required, rather than acknowledged as an option open to the voluntary request or refusal of those who are terminally ill. Only if the degree of distress to people under such expectations were greater than the burdens lifted from others would this not be the case, but—given the enormous objective burdens an extended deteriorative illness like Alzheimer's, Huntington's, or ALS can constitute—this is hardly likely. Yet this result—that utilitarian theory would encourage or require suicide, perhaps socially urged or recommended by the physician, is a result that is difficult to accept. Indeed this result is so difficult to accept, in fact, that it should be explored as a potential counterobjection to classical utilitarian theory as a whole and to the kinds of computations of losses and gains that give the arguments considered here such problematic pull. It would be irresponsible not to acknowledge that these arguments work covertly in the background of the public discussions; but it would be equally irresponsible not to examine them with a severely critical eye.

Physician-Assisted Suicide and the Value of Life

In current ferment over the issue of physician-assisted suicide, appeal is often made—almost always by those opposed to legalization—to the concept of the value of life. Life is of absolute, intrinsic value, it is often asserted, and hence it is always wrong to put it to an end. . . . [T]he principle of the value of life is usually modified to apply only or primarily to human life and to permit certain exceptions, such as killing in self-defense, war, and capital punishment, but it is not usually held to permit suicide.

Indeed it might seem that physician-assisted suicide in terminal illness would not be licensed by any of these limitations on the principle of the value of life. Physician-assisted suicide involves the killing of a human being; and, except in an extended sense, it cannot be said to be killing in self-defense, war, or capital punishment. Of course it is sometimes argued that suicide in circumstances of terminal illness is analogous to killing in self-defense, but if so, it is clearly not any ordinary form of self-defense: There is no aggressor against whom one defends oneself (though some have argued that the disease plays this role), and in any case one does not kill the aggressor but oneself, the person presumably to be defended.

Furthermore, although the notion of "quality of life" is often substituted for that of "value of life" in discussions of end-of-life medical practices about when it would be appropriate to withdraw life-sustaining support, such as a respirator or artificial nutrition and hydration, from a patient, physician-assisted suicide cannot involve ending a life that has fallen below a certain minimum quality. . . . [T]he standards for withdrawing life support are sometimes fixed quite narrowly at irreversible coma or at brain death; sometimes they are set at intermediate levels to include capacity for reflex response or minimal EEG activity; and sometimes they are set comparatively high, to require some degree of emotional response, reflection, and reasoning activity. But *suicide,* as we said, would seem to presuppose life that meets or exceeds the highest minimum standards, since anyone capable of making a decision to commit suicide—and to request the physician for assistance in doing so—must be able to think, intend, at least to some extent to forsee the future otherwise in store, and, in general, reason in a deliberative way. All recent and current legislative proposals put forward in the United States would permit physician-assisted suicide only for mentally competent persons, and, since these proposals have covered only *voluntary* active euthanasia, have made the same requirement for physician-performed euthanasia as well.

Of course this conclusion—that under the principle of the value of life, physician-assisted suicide could not be permitted, since it would mean the self-killing of a life of sufficient quality to meet standards of mental competency and voluntariness in making this choice—is open to further challenges. For example, a person forseeing that his or her life is about to drop below a specified level—that is, that he or she is about to slip below an acceptable quality of life—might use an advance directive to instruct the physician to perform the termination of life after it drops below a specified

level (though it would then be counted as euthanasia). Alternatively this person might choose to commit suicide in a preemptive way, by ending his or her life before the foreseen deterioration begins.

This latter notion poses a substantial challenge to the value-of-life position against physician-assisted suicide. It has been a central ingredient of many of the most conspicuous physician-assisted suicide cases—including Jack Kevorkian's use of his "suicide machine" for Janet Adkins and Timothy Quill's writing a prescription for a lethal dose of barbiturates for his patient Diane. Janet Adkins sought Dr. Kevorkian's assistance very early in the downhill course of Alzheimer's disease, while she still possessed nearly her full mental skills as well as her physical abilities, while she could still see clearly what lay ahead, and while she could discuss her choice with her husband, her physician, and with Dr. Kevorkian. Similarly Dr. Quill's patient Diane preferred suicide to undertaking the very difficult treatment for her leukemia, recognizing that it had only a low chance of success, but remained quite functional virtually up until the time she took the lethal drug. To be sure, Janet Adkins' suicide was timed further in advance than Diane's of the onset of the condition each wished to avoid; indeed Adkins understood that she would have to plan her suicide and carry it out well in advance, since there would be no chance of doing so later on, while Diane could wait until symptoms of her illness began to be pronounced. Yet in neither case did the patient's *current* quality of life fall below any reasonable threshold.

The underlying issue here is what C. G. Prado has introduced as the question of *preemptive* suicide: suicide undertaken not out of current suffering, illness, or extreme old age, but to avoid what is otherwise predictably a part of terminal decline—"a sensible alternative to demeaning deterioration and stultifying dependency."[5] Preemptive suicide is not the same as surcease suicide, . . . an escape from current suffering; it is suicide that takes place *before* the predictable suffering or deterioration begins, as with Janet Adkins, or at least, as with Diane, before it has progressed very far. Some legislative proposals, however, appear to have addressed only what would be surcease suicide: They permit such choices just when the patient is already enduring, in the language of the Dutch guidelines, "intolerable suffering," though, like the Dutch, they may permit the patient to determine what counts as intolerable. Other proposals, including most of those in the United States, require that the patient be terminally ill, usually defined as within six months of death. If the terminal course is likely to be longer, these proposals would nevertheless prohibit assistance in suicide even if terminal course is likely to involve more suffering over a longer period of time. A 1994 proposal published in the *New England Journal of Medicine* by Dr. Quill and others would not limit physician-assisted suicide to terminally ill persons—and so would include "incurable and debilitating" conditions like ALS—but insists that lethal treatment be made available "only as a last resort for unrelievable suffering."[6] None of these proposals would clearly permit doctors to honor the choice of person who has been diagnosed with a terminal illness but is still comparatively healthy to avoid the whole course of terminal decline. Preemptive suicide of this sort does involve trading the good time left for the certainty of avoiding an extended decline and a bad death; it is this choice, Prado says, that our present culture largely denies us.[7]

Preemptive choices will become, I suspect, an increasingly central issue as physician-assisted suicide is legalized or grows increasingly widely accepted in practice. How great a tradeoff is to be permitted between current still-good life, and the certainty of avoiding a very much worse future? This, of course, is a prudential problem for anyone considering suicide to avoid any feared future that has not yet materialized; but it is a particular problem in physician-assisted suicide. After all, in cases where physician-assisted suicide is relevant, it is typically the physician who provides information about the future to be expected, and it is typically the physician who answers patients' questions about what lies ahead for them: what it will be like to have Alzheimer's, whether it will be possible to control cancer pain, whether communication will be at all possible in advanced ALS. It is also the physician who would play a large role in mitigating the worst effects of that feared future, whether it is a future of Alzheimer's, cancer, or ALS, or perhaps in exacerbating them. The underlying question here is one about the value of life—not just about assessing it, but about comparing the value of life now and the value or disvalue of life in the future, as the patient sees it, where the difficulty of making this comparison is exacerbated by the physician's role both in predicting what the characteristics of life in the future will be and in treating and altering them. The issue of the value of life is difficult enough in suicide issues generally; it is made far more complex by the physician's role in mediating perceptions in the context of treatment or medically assisted suicide. . . .

NOTES

1. See Pius XII, "The Prolongation of Life" [V/34].
2. Of course, there are exceptions. See, for example, Kenneth L. Vaux, *Death Ethics: Religious and Cultural Values in Prolonging and Ending Life*. Philadelphia: Trinity Press, 1992.
3. *New England Journal of Medicine* 335 (1996): 1699–1705. Data on the practice of euthanasia and physician-assisted suicide in the Netherlands is available in Paul J. van der Mass, Johannes J. M. van Delden, and Loes Pijnenborg, "Euthanasia and Other Medical Decisions Concerning the End of Life: An Investigation Performed upon Request of the Commission of Inquiry into the Medical Practice Concerning Euthanasia," published in full in English as a special issue of *Health Policy* 22, nos. 1 and 2 (1992), and, with Caspar W. N. Looman, in summary in *The Lancet* 338 (Sept. 14, 1991): 669–74.
4. Ezekiel J. Emanuel and Margaret P. Battin, "What Are the Potential Cost Savings from Legalizing Physician-Assisted Suicide?" *New England Journal of Medicine* 339, no. 3 (July 16, 1998):167–72.
5. C. G. Prado, *The Last Choice: Preemptive Suicide in Advanced Age*. Westport, Conn.: Greenwood Press, 1990, p. 5.
6. Franklin G. Miller, Timothy E. Quill, Howard Brody, John C. Fletcher, Lawrence O. Gostin, and Diane E. Meier, "Regulating Physician-Assisted Death," *New England Journal of Medicine* 331(2):119–23 (July 14, 1994).
7. Ibid., p. 7.

1. Battin lays out the arguments for and against physician-assisted suicide. Which position do you think is more defensible? Support your answer.
2. Battin minimizes the relevance of cost factors as an issue in assessing the legitimacy of physician-assisted suicide. In what way does her comparison of the Dutch and the U.S. experiences support this?
3. Discuss Battin's account of the difference between "preemptive" suicide and "surcease" suicide.
4. Why does Battin claim that preemptive suicide will eventually become more central in the debate over physician-assisted suicide? Do you agree or disagree? Explain.

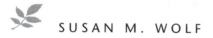

SUSAN M. WOLF

A Feminist Critique of Physician-Assisted Suicide

Susan M. Wolf is an associate at the University of Minnesota's Center for Biomedical Ethics. She is also an associate professor of law and medicine at the University of Minnesota Law School. Wolf contends that the practices surrounding euthanasia are biased with respect to gender. That is, the U.S. culture still assumes a view of women as self-sacrificing, and this traditional perspective exerts subtle pressures on women, more so than on men, to request varying forms of euthanasia. This perspective also expresses itself in the male physician/female patient relationship in that male physicians will be more likely to comply with a female patient's euthanasia request. Wolf argues that women would be more directly affected by any legalization of euthanasia. Opposing rights-based arguments for euthanasia, she concludes that euthanasia should remain illegal.

The debate in the United States over whether to legitimate physician-assisted suicide and active euthanasia has reached new levels of intensity. . . .

Yet the debate over whether to legitimate physician-assisted suicide and euthanasia (which I mean active euthanasia, as opposed to the termination of life-sustaining treatment) is most often about a patient who does not exist—a patient with no gender, race, or insurance status. This is the same generic patient featured in most bioethics debates.

Little discussion has focused on how differences between patients might alter the equation.

Even though the debate has largely ignored this question, there is ample reason to suspect that gender, among other factors, deserves analysis. The cases prominent in the American debate mostly feature women patients. This occurs against a backdrop of a long history of cultural images revering women's sacrifice and self-sacrifice. Moreover, dimensions of health status and health care that may affect a patient's vulnerability to considering physician-assisted suicide and euthanasia—including depression, poor pain relief, and difficulty obtaining good health care—differentially plague women. And suicide patterns themselves show a strong gender effect: women less often complete suicide, but more often attempt it.[1] These and other factors raise the question of whether the dynamics surrounding physician-assisted suicide and euthanasia may vary by gender.

Indeed, it would be surprising if gender had no influence. Women in America still live in a society marred by sexism, a society that particularly disvalues women with illness, disability, or merely advanced age. It would be hard to explain if health care, suicide, and fundamental dimensions of American society showed marked differences by gender, but gender suddenly dropped out of the human equation when people became desperate enough to seek a physician's help in ending their lives.

What sort of gender effects might we expect? There are four different possibilities. First, we might anticipate a higher incidence of women than men dying by physician-assisted suicide and euthanasia in this country. This is an empirical claim that we cannot yet test; we currently lack good data in the face of the illegality of the practices in most states and the condemnation of the organized medical profession. . . .

There may, however, be a second gender effect. Gender differences may translate into women seeking physician-assisted suicide and euthanasia for somewhat different reasons than men. Problems we know to be correlated with gender—difficulty getting good medical care generally, poor pain relief, a higher incidence of depression, and a higher rate of poverty—may figure more prominently in women's motivation. Society's persisting sexism may figure as well. And the long history of valorizing women's self-sacrifice may be expressed in women's requesting assisted suicide or euthanasia.

The well-recognized gender differences in suicide statistics also suggest that women's requests for physician-assisted suicide and euthanasia may more often than men's requests be an effort to change an oppressive situation rather than a literal request for death. Thus some suicidologists interpret men's predominance among suicide "completers" and women's among suicide "attempters" to mean that women more often engage in suicidal behavior with a goal other than "completion."[2] The relationship between suicide and the practices of physician-assisted suicide and euthanasia itself deserves further study; not all suicides are even motivated by terminal disease or other factors relevant to the latter practices. But the marked gender differences in suicidal behavior are suggestive.

Third, gender differences may also come to the fore in physicians' decisions about whether to grant or refuse requests for assisted suicide or euthanasia. The same historical valorization of women's self-sacrifice and the same background sexism that may affect women's readiness to request may also affect physicians' responses. Physicians may be susceptible to affirming women's negative self-judgments. This might or might not result in physicians agreeing to assist; other gender-related judgments (such as that women are too emotionally labile, or that their choices would not be taken seriously) may intervene.[3] But the point is that gender may affect not just patient but physician.

Finally, gender may affect the broad public debate. The prominent U.S. cases so far and related historical imagery suggest that in debating physician-assisted suicide and euthanasia, many in our culture may envision a woman patient. Although the AIDS epidemic has called attention to physician-assisted suicide and euthanasia in men, the cases that have dominated the news accounts and scholarly journals in the recent renewal of debate have featured women patients. Thus we have reason to be concerned that at least some advocacy for these practices may build on the sense that these stories of women's deaths are somehow "right." If there is a felt correctness to these accounts, that may be playing a hidden and undesirable part in catalyzing support of the practices' legitimation.

Thus we have cause to worry whether the debate about and practice of physician-assisted suicide and euthanasia in this country are gendered in a number of respects. Serious attention to gender therefore seems essential. Before we license physicians to kill their patients or to assist patients in killing themselves, we had better understand the dynamic at work in that encounter, why the practice seems so alluring that we would court its dangers, and what dangers are likely to manifest. After all, the consequences of permitting killing or assistance in private encounters are serious, indeed fatal. . . .

The debate over physician-assisted suicide and euthanasia so starkly raises questions of rights, caring, and context that at this point it would take determination *not* to bring to bear a literature that has been devoted to understanding those notions. Indeed, the work of Lawrence Kolhberg bears witness to what an obvious candidate this debate is for such analysis. It was Kohlberg's work on moral development, of course, that provoked Carol Gilligan's *In A Different Voice*, criticizing Kohlhberg's vision of progressive stages of moral maturation as one that was partial and gendered. Gilligan proposed that there were really two different approaches to moral problems, one that emphasized generalized rights and universal principles, and the other that instead emphasized contextualized caring and the maintenance of particular human relationships. She suggested that although women and men could use both approaches, women tended to use the latter and men the former. Both approaches, however, were important to moral maturity. Though Gilligan's and others' work on the ethics of care has been much debated and criticized, a number of bioethicists and health care professionals have found particular pertinence to questions of physician caregiving.

Embedded in Kohlberg's work, one finds proof that the euthanasia debate in particular calls for analysis in the very terms that he employs, and that Gilligan then critiques, enlarges, and reformulates. For one of the nine moral dilemmas Kohlberg used to gauge subjects' stage of moral development was a euthanasia problem. "Dilemma IV" features "a woman" with "very bad cancer" and "in terrible pain." Her physician, Dr. Jefferson, knows she has "only about six months to live." Between periods in which she is "delirious and almost crazy with pain," she asks the doctor to kill her with morphine. The question is what he should do.[4]

The euthanasia debate thus demands analysis along the care, rights, and context axes that the Kohlberg–Gilligan debate has identified. Kohlberg himself used this problem to reveal how well respondents were doing in elevating general principles over the idiosyncrasies of relationship and context. It is no stretch, then, to apply the fruits of more than a decade of feminist critique. . . .

GENDER IN CASES, IMAGES, AND PRACTICE

The tremendous upsurge in American debate over whether to legitimate physician-assisted suicide and euthanasia in recent years has been fueled by a series of cases featuring women. The case that seems to have begun this series is that of Debbie, published in 1988 by the *Journal of the American Medical Association (JAMA)*.[5] JAMA published this now infamous, first-person, and anonymous account by a resident in obstetrics and gynecology of performing euthanasia. Some subsequently queried whether the account was fiction. Yet it successfully catalyzed an enormous response.

The narrator of the piece tells us that Debbie is a young woman suffering from ovarian cancer. The resident has no prior relationship with her, but is called to her bedside late one night while on call and exhausted. Entering Debbie's room, the resident finds an older woman with her, but never pauses to find out who that second woman is and what relational context Debbie acts within. Instead, the resident responds to the patient's clear discomfort and to her words. Debbie says only one sentence, "Let's get this over with." It is unclear whether she thinks the resident is there to draw blood and wants that over with, or means something else. But on the strength of that one sentence, the resident retreats to the nursing station, prepares a lethal injection, returns to the room, and administers it. The story relates this as an act of mercy under the title, "It's Over, Debbie," as if in caring response to the patient's words.

The lack of relationship to the patient; the failure to attend to her own history, relationships, and resources; the failure to explore beyond the patient's presented words and engage her in conversation; the sense that the cancer diagnosis plus the patient's words demand death; and the construal of that response as an act of mercy are all themes that recur in later cases. The equally infamous Dr. Jack Kevorkian has provided a slew of them.

They begin with Janet Adkins, a 54-year-old Oregon woman diagnosed with Alzheimer's disease. Again, on the basis of almost no relationship with Ms. Adkins, on the basis of a diagnosis by exclusion that Kevorkian could not verify, prompted by a professed desire to die that is a predictable stage in response to a number of dire diagnoses, Kevorkian rigs her up to his "Mercitron" machine in a parking lot outside of Detroit in what he presents as an act of mercy.

Then there is Marjorie Wantz, a 58-year-old woman without even a diagnosis. Instead, she has pelvic pain whose source remains undetermined. By the time Kevorkian reaches Ms. Wantz, he is making little pretense of focusing on her needs in the context of a therapeutic relationship. Instead, he tells the press that he is determined to create a new medical specialty of "obitiatry." Ms. Wantz is among the first six potential patients with whom he is conferring. When Kevorkian presides over her death there is another woman who dies as well, Sherry Miller. Miller, 43, has multiple sclerosis. Thus neither woman is terminal.

The subsequent cases reiterate the basic themes. And it is not until the ninth "patient" that Kevorkian finally presides over the death of a man. By this time, published criticism of the predominance of women had begun to appear.

Kevorkian's actions might be dismissed as the bizarre behavior of one man. But the public and press response has been enormous, attesting to the power of these accounts. Many people have treated these cases as important to the debate over physician-assisted suicide and euthanasia. Nor are Kevorkian's cases so aberrant—they pick up all the themes that emerge in "Debbie." . . .

Prevailing values have imbued women's deaths with a specific meaning. Indeed, Carol Gilligan builds on images of women's suicides and sacrifice in novels and drama, as well as on her own data, in finding a psychology and even an ethic of self-sacrifice among women. Gilligan finds one of the "conventions of femininity" to be "the moral equa-

tion of goodness with self-sacrifice."[6] "[V]irtue for women lies in self-sacrifice. . . ."[7]

Given this history of images and the valorization of women's self-sacrifice, it should come as no surprise that the early cases dominating the debate about self-sacrifice through physician-assisted suicide and euthanasia have been cases of women. In Greek tragedy only women were ever candidates for sacrifice and self-sacrifice, and to this day self-sacrifice is usually regarded as a feminine not masculine virtue.

This lineage has implications. It means that even while we debate physician-assisted suicide and euthanasia rationally, we may be animated by unacknowledged images that give the practices a certain gendered logic and felt correctness. In some deep way it makes sense to us to see these women dying, it seems right. It fits an old piece into a familiar, ancient puzzle. Moreover, these acts seem good, they are born of virtue. We may not recognize that the virtues in question—female sacrifice and self-sacrifice—are ones now widely questioned and deliberately rejected. Instead, our subconscious may harken back to older forms, reembracing those ancient virtues, and thus lauding these women's deaths.

Analyzing the early cases against the background of this history also suggests hidden gender dynamics to be discovered by attending to the facts found in the accounts of these cases, or more properly the facts not found. What is most important in these accounts is what is left out, how truncated they are. We see a failure to attend to the patient's context, a readiness on the part of these physicians to facilitate death, a seeming lack of concern over why these women turn to these doctors for deliverance. A clue about why we should be concerned about each of these omissions is telegraphed by data from exit polls on the day Californians defeated a referendum measure to legalize active euthanasia. Those polls showed support for the measure lowest among women, older people, Asians, and African Americans, and highest among younger men with postgraduate education and incomes over $75,000 per year.[8] The *New York Times* analysis was that people from more vulnerable groups were more worried about allowing physicians to actively take life. This may suggest concern not only that physicians may be too ready to take their lives, but also that these patients may be markedly vulnerable to seeking such relief. Why would women, in particular, feel this?

Women are at greater risk for inadequate pain relief.[9] Indeed, fear of pain is one of the reasons most frequently cited by Americans for supporting legislation to legalize euthanasia.[10] Women are also at greater risk for depression.[11] And depression appears to underlie numerous requests for physician-assisted suicide and euthanasia.[12] These factors suggest that women may be differentially driven to consider requesting both practices.

That possibility is further supported by data showing systematic problems for women in relationship to physicians. As an American Medical Association report on gender disparities recounts, women receive more care even for the same illness, but the care is generally worse. Women are less likely to receive dialysis, kidney transplants, cardiac catheterization, and diagnostic testing for lung cancer. The report urges physicians to uproot "social or cultural biases that could affect medical care" and "presumptions about the relative worth of certain social roles."[13]

This all occurs against the background of a deeply flawed health care system that ties health insurance to employment. Men are differentially represented in the ranks of those with private health insurance, women in the ranks of the others—those either on government entitlement programs or uninsured.[14] In the U.S. two-tier health care system, men dominate in the higher-quality tier, women in the lower.

Moreover, women are differentially represented among the ranks of the poor. Many may feel they lack the resources to cope with disabilities or disease. To cope with Alzheimer's, breast cancer, multiple sclerosis, ALS, and a host of other diseases takes resources. It takes not only the financial resource of health insurance, but also access to stable working relationships with clinicians expert in these conditions, in the psychological issues involved, and in palliative care and pain relief. It may take access to home care, eventually residential care, and rehabilitation services. These are services often hard to get even for those with adequate resources, and almost impossible for those without. And who are those without in this country? Disproportionately they are women, people of color, the elderly, and children.

Women may also be driven to consider physician-assisted suicide and euthanasia out of fear of otherwise burdening their families. The dynamic at work in a family in which an ill member chooses suicide or active euthanasia is worrisome. This worry should increase when it is a woman who seeks to "avoid being a burden," or otherwise solve the problem she feels she poses, by opting for her own sacrifice. The history and persistence of family patterns in this country in which women are expected to adopt self-sacrificing behavior for the sake of the family may pave the way too for the patient's request for death. Women requesting death may also be sometimes seeking something other than death. The dominance of women among those attempting but not completing suicide in this country suggests that women may differentially engage in death-seeking behavior with a goal other than death. Instead, they may be seeking to change their relationships or circumstances. A psychiatrist at Harvard has speculated about why those women among Kevorkian's "patients" who were still capable of killing themselves instead sought Kevorkian's help. After all, suicide has been decriminalized in this country, and step-by-step instructions are readily available. The psychiatrist was apparently prompted to speculate by interviewing about twenty physicians who assisted patients' deaths and discovering that two-thirds to three-quarters of the patients had been women. The psychiatrist wondered whether turning to Kevorkian was a way to seek a relationship.[15] The women also found a supposed "expert" to rely upon, someone to whom they could yield control. But then we must wonder what circumstances, what relational context, led them to this point.

What I am suggesting is that there are issues relating to gender left out of all accounts of the early prominent cases of physician-assisted suicide and euthanasia or left unexplored that may well be driving or limiting the choices of these women. I am not suggesting that we should denigrate these choices or regard them as irrational. Rather, it is the opposite—that we should assume these decisions to be rational and grounded in a context. That forces us to attend to the background failures in that context. . . .

In analyzing why women may request physician-assisted suicide and euthanasia, and why indeed the California polls indicate that women may feel more vulnerable to and wary of making that request, we have insights to bring to bear from other realms. Those insights render suspect an analysis that merely asserts women are choosing physician-assisted suicide and active euthanasia, without asking why they make that choice. The analogy to other forms of violence against women behind closed doors demands that we ask why the woman is there, what features of her context brought her there, and why she may feel there is no better place to be. Finally, an analogy [to domestic violence] counsels us that the patient's consent does not resolve the question of whether the physician acts properly in deliberately taking her life through physician-assisted suicide or active euthanasia. The two people are separate moral and legal agents.

This leads us from consideration of why women patients may feel vulnerable to these practices, to the question of whether physicians may be vulnerable to regarding women's requests for physician-assisted suicide and euthanasia somewhat differently from men's. There may indeed be gender-linked reasons for physicians in this country to say "yes" to women seeking assistance in suicide or active euthanasia. In assessing whether the patient's life has become "meaningless," or a "burden," or otherwise what some might regard as suitable for extinguishing at her request, it would be remarkable if the physician's background views did not come into play on what makes a woman's life meaningful or how much of a burden on her family is too much.[16]

Second, there is a dynamic many have written about operating between the powerful expert physician and the woman surrendering to his care. It is no accident that bioethics has focused on the problem of physician paternalism. Instead of an egalitarianism or what Susan Sherwin calls "amicalism,"[17] we see a vertically hierarchical arrangement built on domination and subordination. When the patient is female and the doctor male, as is true in most medical encounters, the problem is likely to be exacerbated by the background realities and history of male dominance and female subjugation in the broader society. Then a set of psychological dynamics are likely to make the male physician vulnerable to acceding to the woman patient's request for active assistance in dying. These may be a complex combination of rescue fantasies and the desire to annihilate. Robert Burt talks about the pervasiveness of this ambivalence, quite apart from gender: "Rules governing doctor-patient relations must rest on the premise that anyone's wish to help a desperately pained, apparently helpless person is intertwined with a wish to hurt that person, to obliterate him from sight."[18] When the physician is from a dominant social group and the patient from a subordinate one, we should expect the ambivalence to be heightened. When the "help" requested *is* obliteration, the temptation to enact both parts of the ambivalence in a single act may be great. . . .

FEMINISM AND THE ARGUMENTS

Shifting from the images and stories that animate debate and the dynamics operating in practice to analysis of the arguments over physician-assisted suicide and euthanasia takes us further into the concerns of feminist theory. Arguments in favor of these practices have often depended on rights claims. More recently, some authors have grounded their arguments instead on ethical concepts of caring. Yet both argumentative strategies have been flawed in ways that feminist work can illuminate. What is missing is an analysis that integrates notions of physician caring with principled boundaries to physician action, while also attending to the patient's broader context and the community's wider concerns. Such an analysis would pay careful attention to the dangers posed by these practices to the historically most vulnerable populations, including women.

Advocacy of physician-assisted suicide and euthanasia has hinged to a great extent on rights claims. The argument is that the patient has a right to self-determination or autonomy that entitles her to assistance in suicide or euthanasia. The strategy is to extend the argument that self-determination entitles the patient to refuse unwanted life-sustaining treatment by maintaining that the same rationale supports patient entitlement to more active physician assistance in death. Indeed, it is sometimes argued that there is no principled difference between the termination of life-sustaining treatment and the more active practices.

The narrowness and mechanical quality of this rights thinking, however, is shown by its application to the stories recounted above. That application suggests that the physicians in these stories are dealing with a simple equation: given an eligible rights bearer and her assertion of the right, the correct result is death. What makes a person an eligible rights bearer? Kevorkian seems to require neither a terminal disease nor thorough evaluation of whether the patient has non-fatal alternatives. Indeed, the Wantz case shows he does not even require a diagnosis. Nor does the Oregon physician-assisted suicide statute require evaluation or exhaustion of non-fatal alternatives; a patient could be driven by untreated pain, and still receive physician-assisted suicide. And what counts as an assertion of rights? For Debbie's doctor, merely "Let's get this over with." Disease plus demand requires death. . . .

Feminist critiques suggest three different sorts of problems with the rights equation offered to justify physician-assisted suicide and euthanasia. First, it ignores context, both the patient's present context and her history. The prior and surrounding failures in her intimate relationships, in her resources to cope with illness and pain, and even in the adequacy of care being offered by the very same physician fade into invisibility next to the bright light of a rights bearer and her demand. In fact, her choices may be severely constrained. . . .

Second, in ignoring context and relationship, the rights equation extols the vision of a rights bearer as an isolated monad and denigrates actual dependencies. Thus it may be seen as improper to ask what family, social, economic, and medical supports she is or is not getting; this insults her individual self-governance. Nor may it be seen as

proper to investigate alternatives to acceding to her request for death; this too dilutes self-rule. Yet feminists have reminded us of the actual embeddedness of persons and the descriptive falseness of a vision of each as an isolated individual. In addition, they have argued normatively that a society comprised of isolated individuals, without the pervasive connections and dependencies that we see, would be undesirable.[19] Indeed, the very meaning of the patient's request for death is socially constructed; that is the point of the prior section's review of the images animating the debate. If we construe the patient's request as a rights bearer's assertion of a right and deem that sufficient grounds on which the physician may proceed, it is because we choose to regard background failures as irrelevant even if they are differentially motivating the requests of the most vulnerable. We thereby avoid real scrutiny of the social arrangements, governmental failures, and health coverage exclusions that may underlie these requests. We also ignore the fact that these patients may be seeking improved circumstances more than death. We elect a myopia that makes the patient's request and death seem proper. We construct a story that clothes the patient's terrible despair in the glorious mantle of "rights."

Formulaic application of the rights equation in this realm thus exalts an Enlightenment vision of autonomy as self-governance and the exclusion of interfering others. Yet as feminists such as Jennifer Nedelsky have argued, this is not the only vision of autonomy available.[20] She argues that a superior vision of autonomy is to be found by rejecting "the pathological conception of autonomy as boundaries against others," a conception that takes the exclusion of others from one's property as its central symbol. . . .

In fact, there are substantial problems with grounding advocacy for the specific practices of physician-assisted suicide and euthanasia in a rights analysis, even if one accepts the general importance of rights and self-determination. I have elsewhere argued repeatedly for an absolute or near-absolute moral and legal right to be free of unwanted life-sustaining treatment. Yet the negative right to be free of unwanted bodily invasion does not imply an affirmative right to obtain bodily invasion (or assistance with bodily invasion) for the purpose of ending your own life.

Moreover, the former right is clearly grounded in fundamental entitlements to liberty, bodily privacy, and freedom from unconsented touching; in contrast there is no clear "right" to kill yourself or be killed. Suicide has been widely decriminalized, but decriminalizing an act does not mean that you have a positive right to do it and to command the help of others. Indeed, if a friend were to tell me that she wished to kill herself, I would not be lauded for giving her the tools. In fact, that act of assistance has *not* been decriminalized. That continued condemnation shows that whatever my friend's relation to the act of suicide (a "liberty," "right," or neither), it does not create a right in her sufficient to command or even permit my aid.

There is even less ground for concluding that there is a right to be killed deliberately on request, that is, for euthanasia. There are reasons why a victim's consent has traditionally been no defense to an accusation of homicide. One reason is suggested by analogy to Mill's famous argument that one cannot consent to one's own enslavement: "The reason for not interfering . . . with a person's voluntary acts, is consideration for his liberty. . . . But by selling himself for a slave, he abdicates his liberty, he forgoes any future use of it. . . ."[21] Similarly, acceding to a patient's request to be killed wipes out the possibility of her future exercise of her liberty. The capacity to command or permit another to take your life deliberately, then, would seem beyond the bounds of those things [to] which you have a right grounded in notions of liberty. We lack the capacity to bless another's enslavement of us or direct killing of us. How is this compatible then with a right to refuse life-sustaining treatment? That right is not grounded in any so-called "right to die," however frequently the phrase appears in the general press. Instead, it is grounded in rights to be free of unwanted bodily invasion, rights so fundamental that they prevail even when the foreseeable consequence is likely to be death.

Finally, the rights argument in favor of physician-assisted suicide and euthanasia confuses two separate questions: what the patient may do, and what the physician may do. After all, the real question in these debates is not what patients may request or even do. It is not at all infrequent for patients to talk about suicide and request assurance that the physician will help or actively bring on death when the patient wants; that is an expected part of reaction to serious disease and discomfort. The real question is what the doctor may do in response to this predictable occurrence. That question is not answered by talk of what patients may ask; patients may and should be encouraged to reveal everything on their minds. Nor is it answered by the fact that decriminalization of suicide permits the patient to take her own life. The physician and patient are separate moral agents. Those who assert that what a patient may say or do determines the same for the physician, ignore the physician's separate moral and legal agency. They also ignore the fact that she is a professional, bound to act in keeping with a professional role and obligations. They thereby avoid a necessary argument over whether the historic obligations of the physician to "do no harm" and "give no deadly drug even if asked" should be abandoned. Assertion of what the patient may do does not resolve that argument.

The inadequacy of rights arguments to legitimate physician-assisted suicide and euthanasia has led to a different approach, grounded on physicians' duties of beneficence. This might seem to be quite in keeping with feminists' development of an ethics of care.[22] Yet the beneficence argument in the euthanasia context is a strange one, because it asserts that the physician's obligation to relieve suffering permits or even commands her to annihilate the person who is experiencing the suffering. Indeed, at the end of this act of beneficence, no patient is left to experience its supposed benefits. Moreover, this argument ignores widespread agreement that fears of patient addiction in these cases should be discarded, physicians may sedate to unconsciousness, and the principle of double effect permits giving pain relief and palliative care in doses that risk inducing respiratory depression thereby hastening death. Given all of that, it is far from clear what patients remain in the category of those whose pain or discomfort can only be relieved by killing them.

Thus the argument that a physician should provide so much "care" that she kills the patient is deeply flawed. . . .

The inadequacies of rights arguments to establish patient entitlement to assisted suicide and euthanasia are linked to the inadequacies of a "top-down" or deductive bioethics driven by principles, abstract theories, or rules. They share certain flaws: both seem overly to ignore context and nuances of cases; their simple abstractions overlook real power differentials in society and historic subordination; and they avoid the facts that these principles, rules, abstractions, and rights are themselves a product of historically oppressive social arrangements. Similarly, the inadequacies of beneficence and compassion arguments are linked to some of the problems with a "bottom-up" or inductive bioethics built on cases, ethnography, and detailed description. In both instances it is difficult to see where the normative boundaries lie, and where to get a normative keel for the finely described ship.

What does feminism have to offer these debates? Feminists too have struggled extensively with the question of method, with how to integrate detailed attention to individual cases with rights, justice, and principles. Thus in criticizing Kohlberg and going beyond his vision of moral development, Carol Gilligan argued that human beings should be able to utilize both an ethics of justice and an ethics of care. "To understand how the tension between responsibilities and rights sustains the dialectic of human development is to see the integrity of two disparate modes of experience that are in the end connected. . . . In the representation of maturity, both perspectives converge. . . ."[23] What was less clear was precisely how the two should fit together. And unfortunately for our purposes, Gilligan never took up Kohlberg's mercy killing case to illuminate a care perspective or even more importantly, how the two perspectives might properly be interwoven in that case. . . .

Here we find the beginning of an answer to our dilemma. It appears that we must attend to both context and abstraction, peering through the lens of both care and justice. Yet our approach to each will be affected by its mate. Our apprehension and understanding of context or cases inevitably involves categories, while our categories and principles should be refined over time to apply some contexts and not others. Similarly, our understanding of what caring requires in a particular case will grow in part from our understanding of what sort of case this is and what limits principles set to our expressions of caring; while our principles should be scrutinized and amended according to their impact on real lives, especially the lives of those historically excluded from the process of generating principles. . . .

This notion of principled caring captures the need for limits and standards, whether technically stated as principles or some other form of generalization. Those principles or generalizations will articulate limits and obligations in a provisional way, subject to reconsideration and possible amendment in light of actual cases. Both individual cases and patterns of cases may specifically reveal that generalizations we have embraced are infected by sexism or other bias, either as those generalizations are formulated or as they function in the world. Indeed, given that both medicine and bioethics are cultural practices in a society riddled by such bias and that we have only begun to look carefully for such bias in our bioethical principles and practices, we should expect to find it.

Against this background, arguments for physician-assisted suicide and euthanasia—whether grounded on rights or beneficence—are automatically suspect when they fail to attend to the vulnerability of women and other groups. If our cases, cultural images, and perhaps practice differentially feature the deaths of women, we cannot ignore that. It is one thing to argue for these practices for the patient who is not so vulnerable, the wealthy white male living on Park Avenue in Manhattan who wants to add yet another means of control to his arsenal. It is quite another to suggest that the woman of color with no health insurance or continuous physician relationship, who is given a dire diagnosis in the city hospital's emergency room, needs then to be offered direct killing.

To institute physician-assisted suicide and euthanasia at this point in this country—in which many millions are denied the resources to cope with serious illness, in which pain relief and palliative care are by all accounts woefully mishandled, and in which we have a long way to go to make proclaimed rights to refuse life-sustaining treatment and to use advanced directives working realities in clinical settings—seems, at the very least, to be premature. Were we actually to fix those other problems, we have no idea what demand would remain for these more drastic practices and in what category of patients. . . .

The required interweaving of principles and caring, combined with attention to the heightened vulnerability of women and others, suggests that the right answer to the debate over legitimating these practices is at least "not yet" in this grossly imperfect society and perhaps a flat "no." Beneficence and caring indeed impose positive duties upon physicians, especially with patients who are suffering, despairing, or in pain. Physicians must work with these patients intensively; provide first-rate pain relief, palliative care, and symptomatic relief; and honor patients' exercise of their rights to refuse life-sustaining treatment and use advance directives. Never should the patient's illness, deterioration, or despair occasion physician abandonment. Whatever concerns the patient has should be heard and explored, including thoughts of suicide, or requests for aid or euthanasia.

Such requests should redouble the physician's efforts, prompt consultation with those more expert in pain relief or support care, suggest exploration of the details of the patient's circumstances, and a host of other efforts. What such requests should not do is prompt our collective legitimation of the physician's saying "yes" and actively taking the patient's life. The mandates of caring fail to bless killing the person for whom one cares. Any such practice in the United States will inevitably reflect enormous background inequities and persisting societal biases. And there are special reasons to expect gender bias to play a role.

The principles bounding medical practice are not written in stone. They are subject to reconsideration and societal negotiation over time. Thus the ancient prohibitions against physicians assisting suicide and performing euthanasia do not magically defeat proposals for change. (Nor do mere assertions that "patients want it" mandate change, as I have argued above.) But we ought to have compelling reasons for changing something as serious as the limits on physician killing, and to be rather confident that change will not mire physicians in a practice that is finally untenable.

By situating assisted suicide and euthanasia in a history of women's deaths, by suggesting the social meanings that over time have attached to and justified women's deaths, by revealing background conditions that may motivate women's requests, and by stating the obvious—that medicine does not somehow sit outside society, exempt from all of this—I have argued that we cannot have that confidence. Moreover, in the real society in which we live, with its actual and for some groups fearful history, there are compelling reasons not to allow doctors to kill. We cannot ignore that such practice would allow for what now remains an elite and predominately male profession to take the lives of the "other." We cannot explain how we will train the young physicians both to care for the patient through difficult straits and to kill. We cannot protect the most vulnerable.

CONCLUSION

Some will find it puzzling that elsewhere we seek to have women's voices heard and moral agency respected, yet here I am urging that physicians not accede to the request for assisted suicide and euthanasia. Indeed, as noted above, I have elsewhere maintained that physicians must honor patients' requests to be free of unwanted life-sustaining treatment. In fact, attention to gender and feminist argument would urge some caution in both realms. As Jay Katz has suggested, any patient request or decision of consequence merits conversation and exploration. And analysis by Steven Miles and Alison August suggests that gender bias may be operating in the realm of the termination of life-sustaining treatment too. Yet finally there is a difference between the two domains. As I have argued above, there is a strong right to be free of unwanted bodily invasion. Indeed, for women, a long history of being harmed specially through unwanted bodily invasion such as rape presents particularly compelling reasons for honoring a woman's refusal of invasion and effort to maintain bodily intactness. When it comes to the question of whether women's suicides should be aided, however, or whether women should be actively killed, there is no right to command physician assistance, the dangers of permitting assistance are immense, and the history of women's subordination cuts the other way. Women have historically been seen as fit objects for bodily invasion, self-sacrifice, and death at the hands of others. The task before us is to challenge all three.

Certainly some women, including feminists, will see this problem differently. That may be especially true of women who feel in control of their lives, are less subject to subordination by age or race or wealth, and seek yet another option to add to their many. I am not arguing that women should lose control of their lives and selves. Instead, I am arguing that when women request to be put to death or ask help in taking their own lives, they become part of a broader social dynamic of which we have properly learned to be extremely wary. These are fatal practices. We can no longer ignore questions of gender or the insights of feminist argument.

NOTES

1. See Howard I. Kushner, "Women and Suicide in Historical Perspective," in Joyce McCarl Nielsen, ed., *Feminist Research Methods: Exemplary Readings in the Social Sciences* (Boulder, CO: Westview Press, 1990), 193–206, 198–200.
2. See generally Howard I. Kushner, "Women and Suicidal Behavior: Epidemiology, Gender, and Lethality in Historical Perspective," in Silvia Sara Canetto and David Lester, eds., *Women and Suicidal Behavior* (New York, NY: Springer, 1995).
3. Compare Jecker, "Physician-Assisted Death," 676, on reasons physicians might differentially refuse women's requests.
4. See Kohlberg, *The Psychology of Moral Development*, 644–47.
5. See "It's Over, Debbie," *Journal of the American Medical Association* 259 (1988): 272.
6. Gilligan, *In A Different Voice*, 70.
7. Ibid., 13–19.
8. See Peter Steinfels, "Help for Helping Hands in Death," *New York Times*, February 14, 1993, sec. 4, pp. 1, 6
9. See Charles S. Cleeland et al., "Pain and Its Treatment in Outpatients with Metastatic Cancer," *New England Journal of Medicine* 330 (1994): 592–96.
10. See Robert J. Blendon, U. S. Szalay, and R. A. Knox, "Should Physicians Aid Their Patients in Dying?" *Journal of the American Medical Association* 267 (1992): 2658–62.
11. See William Coryell, Jean Endicott, and Martin B. Keller, "Major Depression in a Non-Clinical Sample of Demographic and Clinical Risk Factors for First Onset," *Archives of General Psychiatry* 49 (1992): 117–25.
12. See Susan D. Block and J. Andrew Billings, "Patient Requests to Hasten Death: Evaluation and Management in Terminal Care," *Archives of Internal Medicine* 154 (1994): 2039–47.
13. Council on Ethical and Judicial Affairs, American Medical Association, "Gender Disparities in Clinical Decision Making," *Journal of the American Medical Association* 266 (1991): 559–62, 561–62.
14. See Nancy S. Jecker, "Can an Employer-Based Health Insurance System Be Just?" *Journal of Health Politics, Policy & Law* 18 (1993): 657–73, Employee Benefit Research Institute (EBRI), *Sources of Health Insurance and Characteristics of the Uninsured: Analysis of the March 1992 Current Population Survey*, EBRI Issue Brief No. 133 (Jan. 1993).
15. See Cohen, "Gender Question in Assisted Suicides."
16. As noted above, though, Nancy Jecker speculates that a physician's tendency to discount women's choices may also come into play. See Jecker, "Physician-Assisted Death," 676. Compare Silvia Sara Canetto, "Elderly Women and Suicidal Behavior," in Canetto and Lester, eds., *Women and Suicidal Behavior*, 215–33, 228, asking whether physicians are more willing to accept women's suicides.
17. Sherwin, *No Longer Patient*, 157.
18. Robert A. Burt, *Taking Care of Strangers* (New York, NY: Free Press, 1979), vi. See also Steven H. Miles, "Physicians and Their Patients' Suicides," *Journal of the American Medical Association* 271 (1994): 1786–88. I discuss the significance of the ambivalence in euthanasia context in Wolf, "Holding the Line on Euthanasia."
19. See, for example, Naomi Scheman, "Individualism and the Objects of Psychology," in Sandra Harding and Merrill B. Hintikka, eds., *Discovering Reality: Feminist Perspectives on Epistemology, Metaphysics, Methodology, and the Philosophy of Science* (Boston, MA: D. Reidel, 1983), 225–40, 240.
20. See Jennifer Nedelsky, "Recovering Autonomy: Sources, Thoughts and Possibilities," *Yale Journal of Law and Feminism* 1 (1989): 7–36.

21. See John Stuart Mill, "On Liberty," in Marshall Cohen, ed., *The Philosophy of John Stuart Mill: Ethical, Political and Religious* (New York, NY: Random House, 1961), 185–319, 304.

22. See Leslie Bender, "A Feminist Analysis of Physician-Assisted Dying and Voluntary Active Euthanasia," *Tennessee Law Review* 59 (1992):519–46, making a "caring" argument in favor of "physician-assisted death."

23. See Gilligan, *In A Different Voice*, 174. Lawrence Blum points out that Kohlberg himself stated that "the final, most mature stage of moral reasoning involves an 'integration of justice and care that forms a single moral principle,'" but that Kohlberg, too, never spelled out what the integration would be. See Lawrence A. Blum, "Gilligan and Kohlberg: Implications for Moral Theory," *Ethics* 98 (1988):472–91, 482–83 (footnote with citation omitted).

QUESTIONS FOR COMPREHENSION AND REFLECTION

1. What does Wolf mean when she refers to the Western cultural bias toward women as self-sacrificing? How might this bias impact on the euthanasia and physician-assisted suicide controversy?

2. In Wolf's opinion, what would be the likely gender-related results if physician-assisted suicide were legalized? Do you agree or disagree? Support your answer.

3. According to Wolf, what are the problems associated with addressing requests for physician-assisted suicide from both a solely rights-based and a solely care-based approach?

4. What does Wolf mean by "peering through the lenses of both care and justice" in dealing with such requests? Elaborate.

🌿 CASES FOR ANALYSIS*

1. Mary O'Connor[36]

Mary O'Connor worked as a nurse for twenty years and had personally cared for her dying stepmother, father, and two brothers. At the age of seventy-seven, she became paralyzed and demented following a series of severe strokes. When she was given a nasogastric feeding tube at Westchester County Medical Center, New York, her daughters requested that her tube be removed. They insisted that their mother had repeatedly declared that she would not want to be kept alive in this way. Despite their testimony and her own clinical background, the New York Court of Appeals ruled that there were no "clear and convincing" grounds that this was what O'Connor genuinely wanted. The court decision was not unanimous, and Judge Simons strongly opposed. Judge Wachtler wrote the majority opinion and appealed to the sanctity-of-life principle as well as to slippery slope arguments. In any case, the evidence presented by O'Connor's family was not enough to convince the court that she herself would want the treatment stopped.

DISCUSSION QUESTIONS

1. How would substituted judgment apply concerning the daughters' refusal of medical treatment on their mother's behalf? Explain.

---

*Names and cases are fictitious unless noted otherwise.

2. Compare the daughters' refusal of treatment to the role of the family in decision making in China.

3. In view of Brannigan's discussion of the original distinction between ordinary and extraordinary treatment, what would medical feeding in this case represent? How does the principle of proportionality apply? Explain.

4. Should physicians be required to provide their patients with what they believe to be medically futile treatment? Discuss.

2. "Diane"[37]

In 1990, forty-five-year-old "Diane" developed acute myelomonocytic leukemia, a devastating condition. She would have only a modest chance of survival as long as she underwent a strict treatment regimen of inductive chemotherapy, consolidation chemotherapy, and finally bone-marrow transplantation. The side effects would be nausea, loss of hair, and the probability of infection. Without this treatment, death was imminent—perhaps within a matter of weeks.

Diane had been under Dr. Timothy Quill's care for the past three years for her leukemia. Despite the hospital staff's eagerness to initiate treatment as soon as possible, Diane weighed the 25 percent survival rate against the harmful effects and the slim chance of later finding a well-matched bone-marrow donor. She chose to forgo any chemotherapy, judging the burdens to far outweigh any possible benefits. Days later, she realized that withholding treatment at this stage would neither diminish her suffering nor hasten her death.

Much to Quill's dismay, she asked him for barbiturates so that she could take a fatal overdose when she felt ready. Only after he was convinced that her state of mind was rational and lucid did he give her a prescription, informing her of the dosage needed for death. After three trying months, Diane sensed that she was near the end. She faced the choice of either enduring increasing debilitation and discomfort or ending her life. She herself took the fatal overdose of barbiturates, and she died alone.

DISCUSSION QUESTIONS

1. Does Diane have a moral right to take her own life? Support your answer.

2. Does Diane have a moral right to request the aid of her physician in the taking of her own life? How would Battin's arguments regarding the benefits of physician-assisted suicide apply here? Support your answers.

3. In light of the Islamic emphasis on trust in Allah, what do you think would be the Islamic view regarding this case? Explain.

3. Edward Kirwin

Edward Kirwin wrote out his living will in 1997. In it he specified that, should he ever become completely dependent on medical feeding to keep him alive, he would want to have the feeding withdrawn. In 2001, Kirwin's worst nightmare came about; due to a terrible automobile accident that left him virtually paralyzed, he was being maintained on artificial feeding. Though lucid for about three months in this condition, he eventually slipped into a coma. His wife then requested the removal of his feeding tubes according to his advance directive.

Upon examining Kirwin's advance directive, the attending physician noted that it had last been reviewed and dated in 1999, two years before the accident. He was therefore wary about whether the patient would still have wanted the removal of medical feeding. Furthermore, when Kirwin's daughter and son, both in their thirties, arrived from Florida, they made it quite clear to the physician that their father was to be kept alive at all costs. When the physician referred to their father's living will, they claimed that the request was not really what he would have wanted.

DISCUSSION QUESTIONS

1. Does the physician have an absolute duty to honor Kirwin's living will? How relevant is the reviewing of the advance directive? Explain in detail.
2. Should family members have a say in healthcare decisions involving another family member?
3. How would the role of the family in this case compare to the role of the family in other cultures?
4. Under what circumstances would you feel the physician has no duty to honor Kirwin's living will? Explain.

4. Donald Cowart[38]

In 1973, twenty-six-year-old jet pilot Donald Cowart was rocked by a violent explosion caused by leaking gas. His father was killed. Donald was engulfed by flames, and when a farmer found him burns covered over 65 percent of his body. Cowart begged the farmer for a gun so he could shoot himself, but the farmer refused. When paramedics arrived, Cowart asked to be left in the field to die. Instead, they administered lifesaving measures and took him to the hospital.

At the hospital, Cowart received daily baths in chlorine in order to clean his sores. He lost both his eyes and all his fingers. He underwent several skin graft operations, as well as amputations. Cowart constantly requested that he be given a lethal injection. After he was finally released from the hospital, he attempted suicide on a number of occasions. Cowart has now completed a law degree and speaks frequently at conferences on the issue of euthanasia. He still maintains that those at the hospital who treated him for his burns violated his right to self-determination by keeping him alive.

DISCUSSION QUESTIONS

1. Were the paramedics morally right in treating Cowart, even though he requested that they leave him alone? Support your answer.
2. Discuss the relevant moral principles and concerns in this case.
3. Suppose you are Cowart's best friend and you, instead of the farmer, come upon him at the scene. What would you do? Is the fact that you are his friend morally relevant? What if you were a stranger or a medical professional? Support your answers.
4. Imagine that the hospital administration, distressed over Cowart's repeated requests to die, called in a Buddhist monk to counsel Cowart. Role-play the conversation between the monk and Cowart.

5. Ngoc Ly[39]

Ngoc Ly was pronounced clinically brain dead at a Los Angeles trauma center after he was hit by a car while riding his bicycle. The twenty-five-year-old Vietnamese man was then placed on life support until his family could be informed. When his wife and parents arrived at the center, an interpreter told them of his condition. They soon left the center, and Ly remained on the ventilator because the staff neurosurgeon, who would have pronounced Ly officially dead, was involved in surgery.

Soon afterward, the family returned to the center and met with Dr. Isaacs and the interpreter. They told him that they had consulted an expert who indicated to them that "this was not the right time for Ngoc to die." This "expert" was an "astrologer who had read Ly's lunar chart" and "advised that his death be postponed until a more auspicious date." Fearing legal consequences, Isaacs agreed to keep Ly on life support. Nearly a week later, the family informed him that, according to their "expert," Ly could now die. He was then removed from the ventilator.

DISCUSSION QUESTIONS

1. Why would an astrologer be viewed as a "specialist" in this case? Explain why an understanding of Vietnamese culture is important.
2. Discuss how this case reflects the interaction between cultural beliefs and views about health and healing.
3. Explain how sensitivity to another cultural belief may enable us to understand why it was important for Ly's family to insist that he die at the right time. When an important decision is to be made, many Vietnamese and other Asians will consult a *bomoh* or *duken* to interpret the astrological charts. Although most people cannot predict or control the date of their death, simply knowing when someone has died can be helpful in terms of knowing what fate has in store for the deceased's descendants. If a person dies at the "proper" time, his or her children will be rewarded with good health and goodwill. If the time is inauspicious, the children will suffer financial losses, unhappy marriages, or similar negative fates. A *bomoh* can tell people what the future holds for them so they can be prepared.[40]

6. Sammy Linares[41]

In 1988, six-month-old Sammy Linares choked on a deflated balloon at a birthday party. By the time anyone noticed, he had turned blue. His father, Rudy Linares, carried Sammy in his arms and ran to the nearest fire station, nearly a block away. Sammy was then taken immediately to the McNeil Hospital's emergency room. By the time he was resuscitated, close to twenty minutes had passed between the time he became unconscious and the moment his heartbeat was restored. Sammy never regained consciousness. He remained totally dependent on a ventilator despite attempts to wean him away.

The ventilator kept him alive, and he remained in this state for nine months at Rush Presbyterian St. Luke's Medical Center. In the opinion of many on the medical staff, Sammy's coma was irreversible. This led Rudy Linares to request that the ventilator be withdrawn, yet his request was denied by the hospital administration at the recommendation of the hospital's attorney.

Linares persisted in his request, to no avail. The hospital's security guards even had to stop him once when he tried to disconnect his son's ventilator. Finally, during their regular visit to the intensive care unit, Rudy Linares told his wife to leave. After she had left, he took out a gun, held the ICU staff at bay after allowing them to remove other patients from the room, and disconnected the ventilator from Sammy. After his son died, he gave himself up to the police.

DISCUSSION QUESTIONS

1. The Linares family was a low-income family on welfare, and the expense of keeping Sammy alive had so far cost Medicaid over $500,000. Do you think this circumstance may have played a role in the hospital's refusal to withdraw Sammy's ventilator? Explain.
2. The ventilator had kept Sammy alive. Do you think the treatment was medically futile, or was it medically effective? Explain your response.
3. Assess this case from both the utilitarian and the deontological perspective. Provide grounds for both opposing and supporting the withdrawal of the ventilator.

7. Hans van der Wal

Hans van der Wal was a forty-seven-year-old civil engineer residing in Holland with his wife and their two children, ages eleven and nineteen. For some time, he had been diagnosed as having amyotrophic lateral sclerosis (ALS), also known as Lou Gehrig's disease, but he had not yet displayed any serious symptoms. Over six months ago, his Dutch company sent him to the United States to collaborate with an American firm on a project at Disney World in Orlando, Florida. He went there with his family. Soon after the van der Wals arrived in Florida, Hans began to evidence more serious difficulty walking and speaking. He entered the hospital at Orlando, and his physician told him that his ALS was getting worse and he could expect severe deterioration. His wife urged him to return to Holland. However, he insisted on staying in Florida. His family had long desired to travel to America, and this was a golden opportunity for them. He assured his company that matters would not become serious before the project was completed.

Over the next five months, although he did experience more distress in swallowing, he was able to conduct his business, albeit with increasing difficulty. However, in the sixth month, matters suddenly became much worse, and he was hospitalized. He could barely move his body at will and needed to be placed on a ventilator in order to breathe. He also needed to be fed medically. He was too weak to be moved, although his wife requested that they return to Holland.

Although his body had deteriorated rapidly, van der Wal was still mentally alert. He had determined that his own quality of living was minimal at best. He also wanted to decide the manner in which he would die. He discussed this with his wife, and together they requested that he be given a lethal mixture of drugs so that he could die quickly and painlessly. He was physically unable to take the drugs on his own, and they requested the aid of his physician. The physician refused their request. They persisted, explaining that their request would have been honored in Holland. The hospital continued to refuse.

DISCUSSION QUESTIONS

1. Would the fact that van der Wal is a Dutch citizen and that Holland sanctions some requests for physician-assisted suicide be relevant here? Explain.
2. Provide reasons for supporting the physician's refusal to assist in van der Wal's death.
3. Provide reasons for opposing the physician's refusal to assist the patient in his death.
4. To what extent should the values of patients from other cultures play a determining role in deciding what to do when it comes to requests for physician-assisted suicide?

8. Baby S[42]

Soon after Baby S was born five weeks prematurely, she had an apneic episode; that is, she stopped breathing and immediately needed oxygen. She was rushed to the nearest neonatal ICU. Upon displaying very little spontaneous motor activity, she was diagnosed as having trisomy 18, a chromosome aberration resulting in mental retardation and abnormal physical features. Baby S continued to have apneic episodes during the next twenty-four hours and eventually required a ventilator for sustained oxygen. A heart murmur also indicated that she had a serious heart condition. Her parents were informed that their baby had multiple birth defects along with extreme retardation. Both a pediatrician and a geneticist told the parents that Baby S's prognosis was rather bleak. There was a high likelihood that she would die within twelve months.

DISCUSSION QUESTIONS

1. Should resuscitative and other efforts be made in order to keep Baby S alive? Support your answer.
2. Using both utilitarian and deontological arguments, provide a case for keeping Baby S alive as long as possible.
3. Using both utilitarian and deontological grounds, provide a case for deliberately ending Baby S's life.
4. There can be a vast gap between textbook perspectives on such issues and real-life confrontations, especially regarding newborns. Putting yourself in the place of Baby S's parents, what would you do? Explain.

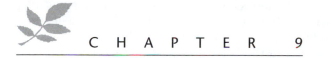

C H A P T E R   9

HIV and AIDS
Prejudice and Policies

Nushawn Williams, a twenty-one-year-old drug dealer from Brooklyn, New York, was arrested in November 1997. He was the first person in the United States to be criminally charged with deliberately and maliciously transmitting the AIDS virus. The prosecutor of Chautauqua County, in upstate New York, charged Williams with reckless endangerment and even attempted murder. Since being diagnosed as HIV positive in September 1996, Williams had knowingly infected six women with AIDS, one of them a thirteen-year-old. The victims claim that Williams never told them of his infection. In fact, splitting his time between New York City and Jamestown, New York, he may have exposed more than one hundred people to HIV through unprotected sex and drug abuse.

In February 1999, Nushawn Williams pleaded guilty to charges of statutory rape and reckless endangerment in exposing women to the HIV virus. On April 6 that same year, he was sentenced to four to twelve years in prison. His sentence may have been reduced because a number of his alleged victims had refused to cooperate with the prosecution.

Acquired immunodeficiency syndrome, or **AIDS,** continues to be one of the most devastating of all epidemics on a global scale. In June 1981, the U.S. Centers for Disease Control (CDC) reported the first cases of a mysterious, devastating, and lethal condition known initially as gay-related immune disorder (GRID). The condition was discovered after five young gay men in Los Angeles were diagnosed with pneumocystis carinii pneumonia, an infection of the lungs; about a month later, cases were reported in New York City of gay men diagnosed with Kaposi's sarcoma. All these cases appeared to share common etiologies, or causes for the disorders. The CDC realized that the condition, which later received the name acquired immunodeficiency syndrome, was extremely lethal.

In 1984, the viral agent responsible for the condition was discovered to be the **human immunodeficiency virus (HIV).** It is important to keep in mind that being infected with HIV does not automatically equate to having AIDS. HIV and AIDS are not identical. If a person is infected with HIV, however, there is a high probability that the virus will eventually affect the immune system in such a way that AIDS results. By the time HIV was discovered, AIDS was recognized as a grave epidemic in the United States and was particularly prevalent among gay men, intravenous drug users and their sexual partners, and many who had received transfusions of contaminated blood. By the end of 1990, the CDC reported more than 160,000 cases of AIDS, and well over half of the victims had died from the condition. Hundreds of thousands more cases were predicted, along with as many deaths. The CDC also estimated that in 1990 10,000 to 35,000 college students in the United States were infected with the AIDS virus.[1] In 1994, AIDS was the sixth-leading cause of death for Americans age fifteen to twenty-four.[2] By 1995, deaths from AIDS surpassed deaths from injuries and accidents for Americans age twenty-five to forty-four.[3] More recent figures from the CDC show that, as of June 1999, 687,313 persons in the U.S. were diagnosed with AIDS and 111,801 persons were infected with HIV.[4] Alarming numbers of AIDS cases were also reported worldwide, with millions of deaths resulting from the condition. According to recent figures from the UNAIDS Joint United Nations Programme on HIV/AIDS, as of December 1998, the total number of people throughout the world infected with HIV was 5.8 million, the total number of those living with HIV/AIDS was 33.4 million, the total number of AIDS deaths in 1998 was 2.5 million, and the total number of AIDS deaths since the beginning of the epidemic was 13.9 million.[5] More cases outside the United States occurred in patients who were heterosexual.

Because most of the reported deaths in the United States were among male homosexuals, male bisexuals, and intravenous drug users and their partners, AIDS was for quite some time associated with these groups. This perception affected public policy debates regarding measures to contain the epidemic, especially since the outbreak occurred just as gay rights groups were pressing for abolishment of discriminatory practices.

The death from AIDS of celebrities such as Rock Hudson, Liberace, Roy Cohn, and Perry Ellis, and famous athletes such as Jerry Smith and Arthur Ashe has certainly stirred up media attention to the AIDS epidemic. In the 1990s, hundreds of thousands of cases of AIDS in the United States were reported among heterosexuals, and it was finally recognized that AIDS could be transmitted through heterosexual sexual behavior. Moreover, the millions of cases among heterosexuals that continue to be reported worldwide have helped change the dimensions of how the AIDS threat is viewed. Nevertheless, a high proportion of AIDS cases are still linked to the groups mentioned above.

Scientists have reached a consensus that HIV infection is transmitted through three channels: blood, semen, and breast milk. The exchange of blood from an infected person to an uninfected person is particularly precarious. In this respect, the intravenous use of drugs is especially high risk, since it is the most conspicuous form of blood-to-blood contact. Contrary to popular myth, HIV cannot be contracted through simple bodily contact such as shaking hands or kissing. However, HIV can be transmitted by an exchange whereby HIV-infected semen manages to enter the bloodstream of another person. Thus, anal intercourse is high-risk behavior, as is vaginal intercourse when there are sores and tears in the uterine lining. Thus, condom use is always a sensible precaution. Even though scientists are learning more about the process of HIV transmission, as medical ethicist Gregory Pence points out, some puzzles still remain regarding heterosexual transmission.

What is most certain is that women who receive fluids from HIV-infected males can be infected, but how easy it is for an HIV-infected female to transmit the virus to an

GLOBAL WINDOW ON AIDS

The AIDS epidemic rages globally. According to a November 1997 United Nations report, more than 30 million people throughout the world are infected with AIDS and HIV. In fact, the epidemic is growing worse. It is estimated that, globally, one in every 100 sexually active adults under age forty-nine is infected with HIV, the virus that causes AIDS. Of those who are infected, one in every ten knows it. It is estimated that by the year 2000, 40 million people will be infected with HIV.

The table below shows the estimated number of persons with HIV infection and AIDS at the end of 1997, along with the increase or decrease in cases (in parentheses) since late 1996:[6]

As the table shows, sub-Saharan Africa alone experienced an increase of nearly 7 million AIDS cases in 1997. There was also a radical rise in AIDS in Eastern Europe and Central Asia in 1997, with much of this increase due to increasing drug use. India, in South Asia, had the most HIV and AIDS cases, with from 3 to 5 million people infected. This global portrait helps us put things into a more realistic, wider perspective. Although Americans may feel that the AIDS crisis is diminishing in the United States, it is in fact getting worse throughout most of the world.

North America	860,000 (+110,000)
Caribbean and Latin America	1.61 million (+40,000)
Western Europe	530,000 (+20,000)
Eastern Europe and Central Asia	150,000 (+100,000)
North Africa and the Middle East	210,000 (+10,000)
Sub-Saharan Africa	20.8 million (+6.8 million)
South and Southeast Asia	6 million (+800,000)
East Asia and the Pacific	440,000 (+340,000)
Australia and New Zealand	12,000 (−1,000)
Global total:	*30.6 million (+8 million)*

uninfected male during sex is uncertain; and some people who seemingly were infected during heterosexual intercourse may actually have contracted HIV nonsexually, in a directly blood-borne way such as IV drugs or transfusion.[7]

Like the bubonic plague in thirteenth-century Europe, AIDS reaches into nearly all social and medical corners. The issues it raises continue to evoke a good deal of visceral reaction. For instance, the women infected by Nushawn Williams and their families are outraged that the law offers little protection against the deliberate spread of the AIDS virus. Many scientists believe that we are not likely to see the end of the AIDS epidemic for some time. Moreover, they claim that pandemics of other diseases seem likely. Philosopher Albert Camus's incisive literary work *The Plague* seems prophetic. His fictional account of a modern-day plague that infects the Algerian town of Oran reveals a universal condition. Camus's characters reflect differing responses to the epidemic, similar to the varying reactions to the outbreak of the AIDS crisis. Our response to the plight of AIDS can enlighten us in our dealings with future crises.

AIDS EXCEPTIONALISM

The biggest ongoing challenge in public-health policy is to bring about a fair balance between benefiting the general populace and respecting individual rights and liberties. In the case of infectious diseases, public-health measures involve testing individuals, reporting the results of these tests, tracing others who may be infected, and notifying these contacts. In the past, these steps have been applied for infectious diseases such as diphtheria and tuberculosis. They continue to be applied for sexually transmitted diseases (STDs). However, these orthodox measures have not been consistently utilized for AIDS and HIV. This phenomenon is referred to as **AIDS exceptionalism.** It has been justified by several considerations, the most significant being the perceived need to protect HIV carriers and high-risk groups from further insult and discrimination.

AIDS and Gay Men

Soon after the first cases of AIDS appeared in early 1981, AIDS was perceived mainly as a male homosexual disease. Homosexuals were already facing a considerable social stigma. According to the U.S. Department of Justice, 13 percent of hate crimes reported to the FBI in 1995 stemmed from attitudes hostile to homosexual orientation.[8] On college campuses, four times the normal rate of assaults were perpetrated against gay and lesbian college students.[9] Gay rights groups such as the National Gay Task Force struggled to ensure that gay men would not be further targeted and disadvantaged by prejudice. When HIV was discovered to be the clinical cause of AIDS, gay rights groups opposed any measure to screen and identify individuals as HIV positive. In response to this pressure, the U.S. Food and Drug Administration (FDA) and the CDC took a tempered approach, stipulating that the HIV test could be used only to screen donated blood. In addition, screening of individuals would be purely voluntary.

Although the privacy rights of HIV-positive individuals were upheld by such measures, little was done to stem the spread of AIDS. Nevertheless, AIDS exceptionalism was and continues to be supported, for the following reasons:

1. The disease is strongly associated by many with male homosexuality.
2. Due to the stigma of male homosexuality, the confidentiality of those infected is likely to be violated.
3. Given the large numbers of infected sex partners, tracing those who are infected would be nearly impossible as well as useless.
4. Since there is neither a cure nor effective treatment for AIDS, it is pointless to report HIV-positive cases.

Critics of AIDS exceptionalism claim that these reasons are unfounded. According to commentator and journalist Chandler Burr, a prominent marker or associated illness condition for male homosexuality is rectal gonorrhea, and such cases have effec-

AIDS EXCEPTIONALISM IN AUSTRALIA, DENMARK, AND HOLLAND

In Australia, one of the biggest issues regarding public-policy measures has to do with whether AIDS should be treated differently from all other threats to public well-being. AIDS rights groups have spoken out in favor of an exceptionalist approach. Nevertheless, at a 1988 AIDS National Conference, politicians spoke out strongly against an exceptionalist policy. Their opposition, along with the outspoken opposition of many representatives in the medical profession, led to a 1989 national strategy that stressed that AIDS should no longer be viewed or treated as exceptional in any sense. As a result of this national strategy, efforts were made to mainstream AIDS treatment programs into the general health-promotion programs in Australia. However, whether exceptionalism or mainstreaming is currently practiced continues to be debated.

AIDS exceptionalism still appears to apply in Denmark, where it is part of the wider sphere of exceptionalism concerning sexually transmitted diseases. For instance, if a Danish citizen is discovered to have a sexually transmitted disease, the general practitioner is not even informed unless the person gives his or her consent. Similarly, a person who tests positive for HIV will not have this information relayed to what is referred to as the hospital's "red system," a computerized data bank that contains information about all patients. In other words, in the case of sexually transmitted diseases, and all the more so with regard to AIDS, exceptionalism prevails in Denmark.

Amsterdam has a number of gay bathhouses and is reputed to attract large numbers of gay tourists from all over the world, particularly from Europe and America. Most other major cities in Holland have gay bathhouses as well. Mainstream public-policy measures normally would have required the closure of these facilities, since they evidently provide a common setting for sexual relations among some gay men. However, there was no strong effort in the Netherlands to close down the bathhouses. This lack of effort reflects an exceptionalist policy. Instead, all-out efforts were made to inform and educate the gay community. As a result, there continues to be a more cooperative spirit in Holland regarding the prevention of AIDS, quite different from the more confrontational spirit in some U.S. cities, such as San Francisco.[10]

tively been reported. Furthermore, in 1999, twenty-six states required confidential reporting, and breaches of confidentiality have been rare. Two states, Minnesota and Colorado, have required confidential reporting since 1985, and there has been no reported breach of confidentiality. With regard to the likelihood of further discrimination, the American Disabilities Act (ADA), passed in 1990, forbids any discrimination based on HIV status. As to the task of tracing potential sex partners, other sexually transmitted diseases such as syphilis have involved extensive numbers of sex partners, yet reporting them has not created any real problems. As for the argument that there is

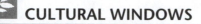

CULTURAL WINDOWS

ROMAN CATHOLIC TEACHINGS AND ISLAMIC APOLOGETICS

When AIDS first appeared as an epidemic of monumental proportions, some religious groups labeled the epidemic as a sign of God's wrath and judgment upon the perceived "sins" of homosexuality and drug addiction. To some degree, this way of thinking still exists, even though lesbians are at a very low risk for AIDS since they do not often engage in high-risk behavior. In any case, the fact that most lesbians do not contract HIV infection raises a question regarding the notion of God's curse on homosexuals. Most religions took a less harsh approach and viewed the AIDS crisis as an opportunity to express genuine compassion for fellow sufferers. Following is a statement by Roman Catholic archbishop John Roach of St. Paul and Minneapolis:

AIDS is not leprosy. Rather, I should like to see the persons with AIDS compared with the story of the Good Samaritan who found the dying man by the roadside and took him in and cared for him, and paid for his care. The curse of AIDS is not God's wrath. The curse of AIDS, it seems to me, would be our refusal to meet AIDS sufferers and their families with simple Christlike charity and love. AIDS is not God's curse, it is a human problem, but it is a problem that tests our ties to God. As dangerous as the disease is, the tragedy would be if we would be so small of heart and mind that we would shrink from reaching out to our sisters and brothers with AIDS.[11]

Islamic commentators, on the other hand, appear to take a harder line. They often point out that the underlying cause of the spread of AIDS involves the sexual promiscuity and rampant drug addiction that is more common in America and Europe. Muslims utilize the AIDS epidemic as a way to defend and bolster Islamic teachings. In other words, had more people embraced Islamic teachings, AIDS would not have reached such epidemic proportions worldwide. The best antidote to AIDS is to live according to faith in Allah as expressed through his prophet Muhammad.

Living according to Islamic teachings means shunning sexual perversion. The term for sexual perversion is **liwat,** which refers to homosexuality. Muslims also consider adulterous relationships, or **zina,** a type of sexual perversion. In fact, both homosexuality and adultery are capital offenses in Islam, and often both are punishable by death. One primary reason why they are serious offenses is that Muslims believe that both homosexuality and adultery ruin social stability and order. Thus, avoiding homosexuality and adultery and living according to Islamic teachings remain the cure for the AIDS epidemic.

still no cure for those individuals infected, there is the real possibility of lessening the risk of infection for potential partners through education and counseling, and such counseling can occur only after reporting has taken place.

New therapies such as protease inhibitors that apply to all who are HIV positive, not just gay men, have been shown to slow down the course of progression from HIV to full-blown AIDS, thus offering all the more reason to seek early testing. An infected person needs to receive these treatments in the early stages of infection, when the count of T4 lymphocytes (or T cells, a type of white blood cell) is higher.[12] White blood cells are an integral part of the human immune system and can help fight off bacterial and viral infections. When the number of T4 lymphocytes drops, the immune system is threatened.[13]

Finally, as Bernard Rabinowitz points out in his article at the end of this chapter, as important as concerns such as confidentiality are, they must take a subordinate position when the public welfare is at stake.[14] That is, principles that reflect privacy rights, the most significant in this case being the confidentiality of the person who is HIV infected, are not by their nature absolute principles. Other principles, such as those that protect public well-being, can under certain circumstances trump confidentiality. Many argue that the prevention of the spread of AIDS is one such circumstance.

AIDS and Women

Is AIDS a male homosexual disease, or is this belief a myth? Because AIDS was initially linked with male homosexuality in the United States, it came to be erroneously viewed as a male disease. Such a characterization is far from the truth. In December 1992, there were 27,485 women with AIDS in the United States, and 80,000 more were estimated to be HIV positive.[15] Two years later, 58,428 cases of women and adolescent girls with AIDS were reported. A total of around 123,000 women were infected by 1994.[16] The number of women with AIDS is increasing at a rapid pace.

A caveat is in order. We need to make a distinction between so-called high-risk groups and high-risk behaviors. Statistics clearly indicate that certain groups, such as intravenous drug users and gay men, tend to be at higher risk of HIV infection. However, this in no way means that all drug users and all gay men are at high risk. The reason these groups are more disposed to HIV infection is that quite a few individuals in these groups are more likely to engage in the high-risk behaviors of intravenous drug use and anal intercourse. By the same token, many gay men do not engage in high-risk behaviors, and many heterosexuals expose themselves to high risk when they engage in high-risk behavior. This distinction is critical, for it cautions us against stereotyping groups of people, such as male homosexuals, as being inherently promiscuous. It should also make us circumspect when we discuss women and AIDS.

Statistically, most HIV-positive women represent minority groups, particularly African American and Latin American. African-American women represent the fastest-growing population of people infected with the AIDS virus. Most of these women are in their late twenties. What is especially alarming is that the age at which women acquire HIV infection is steadily dropping. Between 1987 and 1991, 25 percent of women newly infected with HIV were under the age of twenty-two. Most of these women and adolescent girls were living in conditions of rather extreme poverty. Because most are poor and because many also engage in heavy drug use, they tend to make less use of the healthcare services available.[17] Their circumstances have diminished their access to the regular channels of healthcare. When they do have access to healthcare, they usually seek medical assistance only when they are already well beyond the early stages of infection. In the case of HIV infection, seeking medical assistance in later stages does little to slow down the onset of AIDS.

One of the most pernicious biases regarding AIDS and women is that women who are victimized by AIDS or HIV tend to be viewed primarily in terms of their roles as mothers and/or sexual partners. In other words, they are mistakenly perceived more as transmitters of the AIDS virus to their children or to their sexual or drug partners than as individuals who have had the AIDS virus transmitted to them. This bias, along with the misperception that AIDS is more a male disease, is not without its consequences. For instance, women in general have been omitted from research on AIDS, and more women than men have been underdiagnosed for AIDS and HIV infection. The delay in diagnosing women with AIDS and HIV infection has led to dangerous delays in treatment. This cluster of issues specific to women and adolescent girls points out the obvious need to rectify the inequalities of treatment experienced by women with AIDS through measures such as expanding access to primary care for women and girls, particularly those who are poor.

SHOULD HIV SCREENING BE ROUTINE?

Although cases of AIDS must be legally reported in all fifty states, problems arise when persons who know themselves to be HIV infected continue to engage in sex without informing their sexual partners of their HIV status. For example, Jeffrey Hanlon, an AIDS patient from New York, was extradited to Michigan in 1991 and charged with not disclosing his HIV status to his sexual partner, Kevin Leiffers, who lives in Michigan. Michigan is one of twenty states that require those who are HIV positive to inform their sexual partners of their status.[18] Ohio, another state that requires disclosure of HIV status, is considering a bill that would make intentional nondisclosure a felony. Offenders would be penalized under the law, facing two to eight years in prison along with a maximum fine of $15,000.[19]

According to CDC estimates, by 1997 as many as 900,000 Americans were infected with HIV. (An earlier CDC estimate found that in 1990 between 10,000 and 35,000 college students were HIV positive.[20]) Of these students, half were not aware of their condition.[21] This brings us to the sensitive issue of screening, or testing, for HIV infection. Whether, when, and how to disclose HIV-positive status is perhaps the most critical ethical issue in the complex drama surrounding AIDS and HIV. Within the intimate relationship of, for example, husband and wife, honest and open disclosure is, no doubt, the ethically right thing. However, what should public policy be outside of such relationships? HIV testing is required of immigrants, military personnel, and inmates in federal prisons. For the rest of the American population, it remains voluntary for the most part. Should screening be routine and mandatory? Should certain high-risk groups be targeted for routine screening? Keep in mind the distinction we made earlier between high-risk groups and high-risk behaviors. Targeting high-risk groups could be unfair for individuals in those groups who do not engage in high-risk behavior, and many individuals who do not belong to high-risk groups behave in ways that put them at high risk for HIV infection.

This concern is critical, since those who are at high risk for HIV infection are more likely to intentionally avoid screening. Moreover, the incubation period for HIV can sometimes last up to ten years, during which time the infected individual can unintentionally infect numerous others. The least problematic scenario regarding testing involves blood donations. Since donating blood is voluntary and can therefore be avoided if desired, it makes sense to require that blood donors be tested for HIV. After all, the goal of blood donation is to benefit the recipient, and testing reduces the possi-

HIV SCREENING POLICIES IN OTHER COUNTRIES

Australia's Commonwealth Minister for Health Neal Blewett convened a national meeting in July 1986 to discuss official strategies for dealing with AIDS. Adhering to the consensus of many other countries, the leading participants in the meeting agreed that screening should not be mandatory since it opened the door to possible discriminatory practices. Furthermore, many experts felt that an effective treatment for AIDS was not foreseeable in the near future. As a result, the meeting put forth the official policy of urging voluntary screening with the informed consent of parties. This policy was later reiterated by the Australian government's official White Paper in August 1989. The White Paper stressed the need for thorough educational programs, changes in individuals' behavior, and personal responsibility.

Australia's White Paper was presented despite strong lobbying efforts by medical professionals who advocated the mandatory screening of patients who could place healthcare professionals at risk of contracting HIV infection. Many surgeons were opposed to Blewett's policy, and an intense debate ensued regarding the compulsory testing of patients. Nevertheless, Blewett's position of voluntary screening remained in place.

Mandatory testing was strongly recommended by some groups in the United Kingdom for purposes of obtaining more accurate statistics regarding the incidence of AIDS. These groups urged mandatory testing that would be at the same time anonymous, without any effort at contact tracing,

that is, notification of sexual and drug partners. However, Britain's Department of Health argued that testing should be voluntary since there was a danger of discrimination. As a result, the government adopted a voluntary screening policy in January 1990. The government was less intrusive with regard to guidelines for contact tracing, allowing policies to be adopted by individual professional groups.

In Canada, no official attempt was made to shut down gay bathhouses, a reflection of Canada's official policy of opposing mandatory screening schemes. As elsewhere, official policy was very much influenced by AIDS activist groups who strongly contested mandatory measures. Furthermore, community groups felt that anonymous voluntary testing would encourage those at risk to be tested without fear of discriminatory repercussions. According to public opinion polls, most Canadians are aware of the dangers of discrimination against HIV-infected persons and are opposed to mandatory screening.[22] Therefore, the general official policy of voluntary screening seems compatible with popular opinion on the matter.

When AIDS became viewed as a public threat in Japan despite the relatively low incidence of cases, the Ministry of Health and Welfare took steps such as urging anonymous screening, and many Japanese were voluntarily tested for HIV. Despite the official insistence on anonymity, many Japanese were still suspicious of whether the testing would remain confidential, due to

continued on page 558

continued from page 557

reports of violated confidentiality in the United States and other countries. Suspicions were also heightened because physicians were required by law to report, anonymously, incidences of HIV infection as well as to penalize HIV-infected patients who did not comply with prevention regimens. The ministry also banned birth control pills and urged condom use in their place, believing that condom use was a more effective measure against AIDS.

When Philips, a major multinational electronics company based in the Netherlands, adopted the practice of some U.S. companies of screening job applicants for HIV infection, the policy created an uproar throughout the Netherlands. Under tremendous political, media, and public pressure, Philips revoked its policy.[23] This reaction to HIV screening reflects the consensus among the Dutch that issues regarding testing are less important than issues surrounding individual changes in sexual behavior. The official policy in the Netherlands stresses personal sexual responsibility by emphasizing the importance of working to change risky sexual behavior. It also stresses the critical need to obtain informed consent for testing—and for the testing to be voluntary. In contrast to policy measures in the United States, policies in the Netherlands place little emphasis on the role of screening.

bility of harm. As it stood in 1999, all cases of AIDS must be reported in all states. However, only twenty-six states required the (confidential) reporting of HIV-positive cases, and the two states with the largest populations of AIDS patients—New York and California—did not require the reporting of HIV infection.

Arguments Supporting Routine Testing

Perhaps the most common argument in support of routine, or mandatory, HIV testing is that routine testing is conducted in many other situations. Pregnant women are routinely tested for hepatitis B, newborns are tested for certain conditions such as hypothyroidism, and hospital patients are regularly given blood tests for various conditions. Why make an exception for HIV? Bernard Rabinowitz makes a strong and compelling case for this argument in his article "The Great Hijack," in which he argues that the rationale for a policy of AIDS exceptionalism has no medical or ethical grounds.

Second, it is argued that knowing who is infected with HIV will help deter the further spread of the virus to others. Identifying those infected with other sexually transmitted diseases has clearly helped prevent their further transmission. The problem is compounded, however, by the fact that some states do not classify HIV infection as a sexually transmitted disease (STD). While twelve states view AIDS and HIV infection as STDs, sixteen states view them as communicable diseases, and the remaining states view them as a separate category of disease. Because there is no clear, uniform classification of AIDS and HIV, the result is separate and often divergent policies and procedures for dealing with AIDS and HIV.

Third, supporters of routine testing point out that new treatments seem to show promise. For instance, early treatment of HIV-positive pregnant women with **azi-**

dothymidine (**AZT,** also known as zidovudine) has been shown to diminish the prospect of transmitting the virus to infants. Other new treatments include **protease inhibitors.** Because of the emergence of these treatments, the American Medical Association (AMA) recommends mandatory testing for pregnant women. New treatments for HIV infection may eventually make it a chronic illness. Its potential medical manageability further supports routine testing and early notification.

Thus, from a utilitarian perspective, routine testing would produce the greatest good for the greatest number of people because more lives would be saved and more people would be prevented from contracting HIV. A recent study of 14,000 subjects indicated that 38 percent of homosexuals had not been tested for HIV in the past five years. Moreover, 47 percent of IV drug users had not been tested within the past year, and 60 percent of those with multiple sex partners had not been tested.[24] Routine testing would thus help diminish the spread of HIV by alerting carriers to their status.

Arguments Against Routine Testing

There are powerful arguments in support of mandatory HIV testing; however, we need to critically weigh them against arguments opposed to mandatory testing. First, if HIV testing becomes routine, critics fear that AIDS will go underground; that is, those who are most prone to high risk will probably avoid anything related to the healthcare system. Routine screening thus may prove counterproductive.

Second, it is argued that routine screening carries a high potential for abuse. Medical coverage and employment might be adversely affected by an HIV-positive status. Mandatory screening might lead to employment discrimination, and insurance carriers might develop discriminatory policies. In the October 1992 case *McCann v. H and H Music Co.,* for example, the courts allowed the H and H Music Company to deny insurance coverage for employees with AIDS.

Third, certain technical problems related to HIV testing make routine testing less than totally effective. The usual testing procedure first utilizes an **ELISA (enzyme-linked immunosorbent assay)** test. If this test results in a positive finding, another test is performed, this time by the Western blot method, which is more accurate as well as more expensive. Yet these tests are not 100 percent accurate. They can result in numerous false positives and false negatives. Furthermore, a person who is HIV positive may not actually produce antibodies for up to a year, which means that a person may test negative while actually being positive. Thus, mandatory testing programs would be ineffective for those most recently infected.

Fourth, some argue that routine mandatory testing, even if it saves lives, will do so at the cost of violating some basic rights, especially the right to privacy. After all, what is the benefit of testing if the rule of confidentiality is always sustained? Philosopher Gregory Pence claims that routine testing would actually lead to a twofold violation of privacy: "first, by testing us against our will, and then by reporting positive results."[28]

Fifth, many fear that routine screening would result in further discrimination against homosexuals. Some laws already discriminate against homosexuals. In 1992, a bill was proposed in Colorado that would have prohibited legislation forbidding discrimination against homosexuals in matters of housing and employment. This bill was overturned, but the bias against homosexuals continues throughout much of the United States. Mandatory testing would likely further promulgate a discriminatory mindset.

CULTURAL WINDOWS

HIV TREATMENT IN AFRICA, THE HARDEST-HIT CONTINENT

In the summer of 1998, AIDS experts worldwide gathered in Geneva for the twelfth World AIDS Conference. Much of the discussion focused on the hardest-hit continent of AIDS victims, Africa, where one out of every four adults is infected with HIV. Of all the regions, sub-Saharan Africa is the hardest hit, with close to 21 million infected people. Of the 30.6 million people in the world with HIV or AIDS, over 65 percent live in sub-Saharan Africa. The ratios of AIDS cases in specific countries there are shocking. For example, in Botswana nearly 30 percent of the population is infected with HIV. In Zimbabwe, AIDS cases are expected to severely drive up the infant mortality rate by the year 2010.[24]

How is Africa dealing with the AIDS crisis? Due to the paucity of medical centers, there is less availability of treatments such as AZT. Nevertheless, according to a recent report from the CDC, Ugandan officials have announced that free drug treatments, consisting of AZT, will be offered to pregnant women who are HIV positive. These treatments began in spring 1999 and are supplied by the British pharmaceutical company Glaxo Wellcome. These treatments are expected to help significantly reduce the transmission of HIV from mothers to infants. In Zimbabwe, officials are reporting efforts to exert more control over the testing of imported condoms, amid widespread fears that defective condoms imported from India to South Africa have been smuggled into Zimbabwe.[25]

Certain sites in Africa that have been hit the hardest with AIDS have

Sixth, critics claim that the costs of testing are exorbitant in proportion to perceived benefits. If we were to test the general population, the costs of detecting persons with HIV who were previously undetected would be enormous. Even if only high-risk groups were tested, the costs would still remain high. Does testing for AIDS justify the dollars spent, particularly when the monies could be used in other ways?

Finally, if we allow routine testing for HIV infection, where do we draw the line? Routine testing may be seen as justified for other conditions such as alcoholism or drug abuse.

African Americans and the Pink Elephant of AIDS

What stands out in many of the objections to routine testing is that AIDS is still very much associated with marginalized groups in the United States, particularly gay men, who are seen as exceptionally promiscuous. This association is evident, for example, in the way the AIDS crisis has been dealt with—at least officially—by some African Americans. The two most prominent civil rights groups for African Americans are the National Association for the Advancement of Colored People (NAACP) and the Urban League. In the summer of 1998, both groups held their annual conventions. The subject of AIDS was not addressed at either convention.

become the locus of research funded by the United States, with many sites being targeted for AIDS vaccine trials. Many researchers find it easier to conduct vaccine trials in Africa than elsewhere, for a variety of reasons. For one thing, standards of permissible testing seem to be less stringent. Furthermore, the epidemiologic and scientific factors of HIV infection in Africa, where the AIDS epidemic has made its strongest imprint, make the setting more conducive to these vaccine trials. However, the fact that testing may be easier in Africa does not necessarily justify it.[26]

Will African subjects be treated as guinea pigs and in effect bear the burden of risks while not experiencing the benefits of an effective vaccine? Although on the surface African subjects appear to stand to gain from AIDS vaccine trials, should an effective vaccine come about will they really benefit? This concern is particularly pressing, because the subjects' economic stratum may not enable them to reap the rewards of the vaccine. In other words, they may not be able to afford the treatment for which they are being tested.

Can we appropriately apply our Western idea of informed consent to Africans? Americans think in terms of obtaining consent from the individual subject, while in African countries the person is viewed in more relational terms. A community leader or family member may be the proxy consenter for the human subject. Is this ethically acceptable? Also, can African subjects be properly informed of benefits and risks? For instance, are they able to comprehend the idea of randomized trials? Whether there is an absence of coercion is another issue. What may appear to the Westerner as coercive may be viewed and understood more as cooperative by an African.

Why is this situation surprising? Numbers strongly indicate that AIDS is very much an epidemic among black Americans. According to statistics from the CDC, black Americans constitute around 57 percent of those who are newly infected with HIV. Blacks account for 63 percent of young people between thirteen and twenty-four infected with HIV.[29] For black Americans between the ages of twenty-five and forty-four, AIDS continues to be the number-one cause of death. Yet some of the leading black organizations appear to have chosen to remain rather silent on this monumental issue.

The silence is not confined to civil rights groups. Many black churches have also chosen to avoid the topic of AIDS. One reason appears to be the common association of AIDS with homosexuality. Homosexuality remains a taboo topic within many churches that endorse a prohibition against it. Rev. Kwabena Rainey Cheeks, pastor of the Inner Light Fellowship Church in New York City, who is HIV positive, does address the issue yet admits that AIDS "is like the pink elephant that nobody wants to talk about."[30]

Even more troublesome is that many African-American victims of AIDS also choose to remain silent. Again, much of this reluctance to come forward is due to the association of AIDS with homosexuality and drug addiction, despite the fact that studies show the association of AIDS with homosexuality and drug use to be misplaced. The most common route of transmission among black Americans, for example, appears to be heterosexual sex. African-American women account for about 56 percent of the AIDS

CULTURAL WINDOWS

AIDS STRATEGIES IN MEXICO AND CUBA

Since 1992, seven of Mexico's thirty-two autonomous states have required HIV testing as a requirement for obtaining a marriage license. A two-year study was recently conducted that examined mandatory testing and its results in the state of Coahuila, located in northern Mexico on the U.S. border.[31] Coahuila has a population of more than 2 million. The study revealed that, in the two-year period from January 1992 through December 1993, 9,014 premarital HIV tests were performed. Of those tested, three were revealed to be HIV positive, and of these three, two had already known of their HIV status. This means that in the two-year period of testing, with all the cost incurred, there was only one newly discovered diagnosis of HIV. That single case, by the way, was denied a marriage license in Coahuila. Nevertheless, that same person married in a nearby state where the HIV test was not required.

Authors of the study, who are directly involved with Mexico's Consejo Nacional de Prevencion y Control del SIDA (CONASIDA, the National AIDS Council), believe that mandatory HIV testing is a violation of human rights. From their findings, they also concluded that mandatory testing was cost-inefficient and neither deterred further sexual activity nor prevented infected persons from marrying. In summary, mandatory testing did nothing to reduce the spread of AIDS while incurring high costs at the expense of the states.

After the results of the study were publicized, mandatory HIV testing was revoked in the state of Coahuila. It could well be that this serious study had an impact on public policy. Soon afterward, legislators and experts put together a statement, the Norma Oficial Mexicana (Mexican Official Regulation) "For the Prevention and Control of Infection with the Human Immunodeficiency Virus," that became effective in January 1995. It states:

HIV testing will not be a prerequisite to engage in any activity, have access to goods or services, get married, get a job, enroll in school, receive healthcare, revoke a labor contract, get expelled from school, be evicted, or interfere with entry or exit from our country.[32]

Since 1986, Cuba has legislated the quarantine of individuals with AIDS and those who are HIV positive. Cuba also requires HIV testing for all members of high-risk populations such as drug addicts, homosexuals, and prostitutes. Those who test positive are informed of the results, and their families and coworkers are also notified. Infected individuals are sent to special sanatoriums where they may remain nearly indefinitely. By U.S. standards, these measures seem drastic; however, in Cuba they appear to be effective. Recently, fewer than 300 Cubans tested positive out of a population of 3 million. However, quarantine as a strategy would seem to be logistically impossible in the United States. One of the strongest arguments against quarantining HIV-infected persons in the United States is its alleged violation of individual privacy and liberties. However, in the past, the United States has quarantined persons with tuberculosis.

cases among all women. Along with many white American women, they do not usually discover their HIV status until they are tested for HIV upon becoming pregnant, and most are able to rule out transmission through drug use. In any case, because homosexuality and drug addiction are mistakenly linked within the black community with AIDS, silence seems to be the chosen option. A basic distrust of the healthcare profession and a dire lack of medical coverage also contribute to the strong resistance to HIV testing among blacks.

One thing seems clear: If we could somehow diminish the level of homophobia and discrimination against homosexuals, there would be an added impetus to continue with voluntary testing. Voluntary testing could then become more effective, and there would be less need for mandatory testing. It is imperative that we work to dismantle unfair stereotypes of AIDS patients as a marginalized group. Susan Sontag, in *Illness as a Metaphor,* discusses how perceptions of certain illnesses and diseases can become thoroughly distorted due to a lack of certainty regarding their etiology. This distortion causes unfair myths and stigmas to be linked with the condition. Such has indeed been the case with AIDS. The way to diminish this distortion is to encourage ongoing efforts at public and professional education regarding the nature of AIDS and its transmission. In addition, we need to devise useful public health measures that will benefit the victims of AIDS and not reinforce discrimination against high-risk groups.

STRATEGIES AFTER TESTING

After testing for HIV, whether mandatory or voluntary, what specific strategies should be pursued? What would be the most reasonable and ethically sound way to deal with the testing results? After all, testing makes sense only if there is a reasonable and fair follow-up plan.

Treatment

An entire range of remedies has been proposed to treat AIDS, from conventional drug therapies to more exotic measures. For instance, Michio Kushi, director of the East-West Foundation, located in Brookline, Massachusetts, is one of the key leaders of a movement called macrobiotics. **Macrobiotics** is a special type of vegetarian diet that purportedly has deep-rooted religious and philosophical premises. The most prominent premise in macrobiotics is that our life-style and diet constitute the real cause of diseases.

Kushi contends that this is the case with AIDS. He argues that, since AIDS has its origin in life-style and diet, there is a viable treatment for AIDS—a special type of macrobiotic diet. He has been experimenting with this diet among New York City's gay community and has shared his research with the microbiology department at Boston University. Members of the department have admitted that the macrobiotic diet did seem to extend the life of some AIDS patients. Some might object that, even if true, this result does not necessarily validate his claims regarding the origins of AIDS. Kushi is now championing his approach in Zaire, where AIDS cases are numerous.

An obvious strategy for treating AIDS involves therapy for those who test positive. In 1987, the antiviral agent azidothymidine (AZT) was shown to slow down the effects of HIV. The positive effects of AZT were challenged in 1994 by a European investigation called the Concorde Study. Nevertheless, American physicians still claim that AZT has some value, though perhaps not in the earlier optimistic terms. AZT appeared to diminish AIDS symptoms in some patients, and, as stated earlier, there is mounting evidence that AZT significantly lessens the likelihood of a pregnant woman transmitting HIV to her fetus. Required testing of pregnant women may be defensible, since it provides an opportunity to stem the possibility of infection; however, critics of mandatory testing of pregnant women point out that it violates women's rights. At the same time, there is concern over the possible toxic effect of AZT on fetuses, since it has been shown to be toxic for some HIV-positive patients.

In its article at the end of this chapter, the Working Group on HIV Testing of Pregnant Women and Newborns opposes mandatory HIV testing. Instead, it recommends measures that will raise levels of awareness through efforts to inform and advise pregnant women concerning HIV and testing. At the same time, it opposes targeting the prevention of the vertical transmission of HIV (that is, transmission from the mother to the fetus) as a primary policy goal, because doing so conflicts with women's reproductive rights. Mandatory testing of pregnant women has been criticized for other reasons as well. Even though daily treatment with AZT appears to reduce the likelihood of vertical transmission of AIDS, the long-range effects of AZT are yet to be determined. Ronald Bayer, in his article at the end of this chapter, also points out that mandatory testing would essentially be a violation of women's right to informed consent.[33]

A critically important component in the treatment of AIDS is genuine caring. Of course, caring is useful in all aspects of healthcare delivery, but it is especially meaningful for AIDS patients. Ronald Nakasone writes about caring for AIDS patients in a Zen community, and he delineates some fundamental Buddhist teachings that are the basis for genuine caring.[34] These Buddhist precepts are compassion (*karuna*), interdependence (*pratityasamutpada*), and wisdom (*prajna*). These three precepts formed the basis for the institution of the Maitri Hospice in 1988 by the Hartford Street Zen Center, located in San Francisco's Castro District. The hospice was especially designed to care for AIDS patients, regardless of their drug history or sexual orientation. Nakasone points out that caring for these patients in the most humane fashion embodies core Buddhist teachings, the most essential being compassion.

In 1999, there were more than a million practicing Buddhists living on the West Coast. The Buddhist community has organized efforts to alleviate the suffering of persons with AIDS. One organized response was the establishment of the Buddhist AIDS Project in 1986, of which the Hartford Street Zen Center was an expression. It is based on Buddhist teachings that underscore the importance of alleviating suffering through the promotion of compassion. The project has been able to institute hospices for persons with AIDS and is politically engaged in opposition to any legislation that proposes mandatory testing and reporting of HIV infection.

Voluntary Abstention

Besides offering treatment, an additional strategy for those who test positive is to encourage the infected person to voluntarily refrain from any further activities that could jeopardize others. This strategy relies on the responsibility and good judgment of those who are HIV infected. Is this a realistic option? Do most people act responsibly when it comes to sexual behavior? Consider the case of Ozel Tendzin. The head of the order of

Vajradhatu, the largest Tibetan Buddhist group in the United States, Tendzin openly admitted his homosexuality. This admission stirred little reaction among the Buddhist community in North America, but when he tested positive for HIV in 1989 it became a major issue. The concern had less to do with his having the AIDS virus than with the fact that, even after knowing his condition, he showed a glaring indifference to human life and certainly violated Buddhist precepts by continuing to engage in sexual relations without informing his partners of his HIV status. Some of his partners in turn became infected with the virus.

Are all persons capable of modifying their sexual or drug-dependent behavior? Even counseling does not guarantee the modification or alteration of ingrained habits. How can we realistically expect voluntary and responsible follow-up if the testing itself was initially mandatory?

An interesting illustration of an attempt to modify drug behavior is the **Needle Exchange Program,** with 120 programs operating throughout the United States. A mobile home that acts as a center for the program will occasionally pull up to a drug site and provide drug users at that site with clean needles. Even before the AIDS outbreak, similar needle exchange programs were put into place in the Netherlands in order to prevent the spread of hepatitis B, and these programs appeared to be effective. The Dutch programs have also been effective in controlling the spread of AIDS. Both the Dutch government and the general public supported the idea of needle exchanges as a form of disease prevention.

However, in the United States, the Clinton administration announced that the federal government would not financially support the program, because in a sense it legitimizes the use of illicit drugs. Moreover, the administration questioned whether the program was effective. Many drug users continue to share dirty needles as well as trade drugs for sex. Trading drugs for sex makes the AIDS virus even more susceptible to transmission through heterosexual intercourse and other sexual networks. HIV infection thus reaches out its deadly arm to those not even involved in drugs. Supporters of the Needle Exchange Program disagree with the rationale of the Clinton prohibition, arguing that the program is one effective way to control as well as reduce the spread of AIDS, particularly among the black community, where the rate of transmission is high.

The critical need for educational programs regarding the nature of AIDS, HIV, and its transmission cannot be overstated. The adoption of safer sex practices would help reduce the spread of AIDS among the population as a whole. After many years of federal AIDS funding being channeled into the larger, more visible AIDS organizations, it is encouraging to see more monies being given to groups that focus on AIDS education among minorities.[35]

Contact Tracing

There would appear to be an urgent need to notify the sexual and drug partners of a person who is infected with HIV. Contact tracing could occur through two avenues. One way is through patient referral, whereby infected persons themselves notify their partners. However, like the strategy of voluntary abstention, which relies on the personal responsibility of the infected person, patient referral programs do not tend to be very effective. A second way to notify sexual or drug partners is through provider referral, in which the contacting and notifying are done by physicians or other healthcare

GREENLAND'S INUIT AND HETEROSEXUAL TRANSMISSION OF HIV

The Inuit of Greenland number around 50,000, yet an AIDS epidemic threatens to eradicate the entire population. This possibility is stunning, since only two cases of HIV were reported in Greenland in 1993. Many AIDS cases report to Queen Ingrid's Hospital in Nuuk, the capital of Greenland—the same place where cases of tuberculosis filled the hallways in the past. A physician who practices at Queen Ingrid's has studied the rapid growth of HIV infection in Greenland and has discovered that the growth rate is three times that in Europe, at 25 per 100,000[36] Moreover, within this population HIV infection has become full-blown AIDS in a much shorter span of time. What is striking about the AIDS crisis in Greenland is that it is almost entirely confined to transmission among heterosexuals. Greenland reportedly does not have a gay community, since most homosexuals formerly living in Greenland have moved to Denmark, particularly Copenhagen. Women account for 45 percent of reported cases.

It seems clear that notification and contact tracing are essential in order to stave off the spread of the disease. However, notification and contact tracing present a nearly insurmountable barrier in this circumstance. There is a high degree of alcohol consumption, and Greenlanders are sometimes noted for their hedonism, which can be viewed in this case as an indirect form of self-destruction. As for direct forms of self-destruction, the Inuit have an alarmingly increasing rate of suicide, due greatly to the difficult transition from a traditional hunting life-style to modernity. With regard to hedonism, health official Mikaela Englee states, "This is a cultural trait. We are guided by instant gratification."[37] This trait, combined with an overly casual approach to sex and multiple sex partners, intensifies the prospects of HIV transmission. A casual approach to sex is reflected in the reported abortion rate of 50 percent of all pregnancies, with condom use extremely rare. Although testing for HIV has become nearly routine and counseling is offered for individuals, many males scoff at the idea of counseling, since in their culture it is considered unmanly to disclose and discuss feelings with strangers. An aggressive educational campaign, augmented by telephone help lines, free counseling, and free condoms, is being undertaken in order to combat the spread of HIV among Greenland's Inuit.

officials who make the effort to confidentially contact partners of infected persons. Thirty-three states allow provider referral, but only four (Arkansas, North Carolina, South Carolina, and Oregon) actually require it.

A number of attempts have been made to legislate provider referral in the United States. In 1995, New York Democratic congressman Gary Ackerman proposed a bill to modify the CDC program that tested newborn infants for HIV. The purpose of the testing was to monitor HIV infection rates in pregnant women. Using blood samples from

CULTURAL WINDOWS

AFRICA:
Human Rights and HIV/AIDS

There is an definite link among the AIDS crisis, cultural customs, and the notion of human rights. For instance, the most somber aspect in many less developed countries plagued with AIDS is impoverishment. Another burden is the inferior status of women, which almost approaches repression in that they seem to have little control over their life. In countries such as the United States, which emphasize equality between the sexes, it is reasonable to suppose that responsible changes in sexual behavior can have an impact on the spread of AIDS. However, in countries where women face fewer choices, to speak of rehabilitative and responsible sexual behavior is practically meaningless. Lawyer Julie Hamblin, who visited countries in Africa, states:

There is nothing more poignant than talking to an African woman who knows all about HIV . . . but who says: I know my husband has other women but what can I do? If I suggest that he use a condom, he will assume that I must have had other lovers and tell me to leave. There is nowhere else for my children and me to go.[38]

Unless women become more empowered to have control over their sexual lives, such repression will continue to lead to an increase in the number of AIDS cases. Not only their lives are at stake, but also the lives and well-being of their children and families. Consider the situation of Safuyati Kawuda in Uganda. In the ten years since Safuyati Kawuda married at the age of twenty-eight, she has rarely seen her husband, Kadiri Mpyanku. He lives in the town of Jinja, 70 miles away, and partitions his time among his three wives and thirteen children. Safuyati belongs to the Bisoga tribe, which endorses polygamy, estimated to be practiced in at least half the marriages in Uganda.[39] Like most women in rural Africa, Safuyati, who lives in Namutumba, Uganda, spends most of her time performing farm labor, much of it backbreaking according to our standards. And although Safuyati and almost all other women do most of the physical labor in African countries, they do not seem to reap the benefits. For example, most women are not allowed to own land, and in some places it is not uncommon for husbands to beat their wives. Women are also discouraged from obtaining formal education. Women and children make up 77 percent of the population in ten African countries.[40]

Safuyati also supports her five children while remaining dependent on her husband for money and clothes. Life in her village is a struggle, and most women barely eke out an adequate existence for their families. In addition to the apparent inequalities inherent in the treatment of women, many, including Safuyati, have to confront the unsettling possibility that their husband may take other women as wives or engage in extramarital affairs, particularly since having many children is considered to be a sort of safety net for aging parents and also increases the labor force within families.

continued on page 568

continued from page 567
Safuyati and many other women are not familiar with condoms. Therefore, there is a growing fear of transmission of the AIDS virus through heterosexual intercourse. The possibility that her husband may be having affairs with various women increases the likelihood of HIV transmission to his wives. However, because Mpyanku provides clothing and money—and because he is the male—his affairs are not questioned.

newborn infants in forty-five states, CDC researchers were blind-testing infants for HIV, so their identities were not known. Thus, infants who tested positive were not identified, and mothers were not informed of their infants' status. Ackerman proposed to annul the mode of blind-testing so that infants who did test positive for HIV could be identified and their mothers informed.

The bill met with immediate resistance from AIDS activists, gay rights groups, and the American Civil Liberties Union (ACLU). They argued that such identification and notification would violate individual privacy. Richard Mohr, in his article at the end of this chapter, emphatically underscores the importance of individual rights and autonomy. He contends that AIDS policies, though often perceived by government as a legitimate form of legal paternalism, threaten this autonomy. Mohr's approach to the issue is rights-centered, stressing the value Americans as a culture place on individual freedoms. From this perspective, coercion can be justified only if harms are such that they in turn violate others' rights. Other critics of the bill argued that identification and notification would be ineffectual in preventing transmission from mothers to infants. Furthermore, it was argued that passing the Ackerman bill would intimidate pregnant women and keep them from seeking medical care in the first place.[41]

Pressured by these groups, the CDC threatened to suspend further infant testing unless Ackerman withdrew his proposal. Instead, Ackerman joined forces with Oklahoma Republican congressman Tom Coburn to draft the Baby AIDS Compromise, which would require healthcare professionals to offer voluntary HIV testing and counseling to pregnant women. This compromise was included as part of a larger bill, the Ryan White CARE Reauthorization Act.

In 1997, Coburn proposed a bill that would require the reporting of all HIV cases and notification of all relevant partners. This bill, the HIV Prevention Act of 1997, would also require patients about to undergo invasive surgery to be tested for HIV and urge states to criminalize those who intentionally infect others with HIV. All provisions presume the strict rule of confidentiality. The HIV Prevention Act of 1997 met with severe opposition. The AIDS Action Council vehemently opposed the bill, claiming that it essentially stigmatized those with HIV and AIDS by subjecting them to unfair federal paternalism and intervention.

Bonnie Steinbock, in her article at the end of this chapter, applies Mill's harm principle to legal paternalism in regard to AIDS and argues that such paternalism is justified when others may be adversely affected. She also contends that government intervention is justified if the intervention is effective and if it poses the least amount of restriction on others' rights. This argument raises serious questions. If contacts have a right to relevant knowledge in order to make informed choices regarding their sexual activity, is contact notification justifiable? Does the right to know outweigh the right of the AIDS victim to privacy and protection from discrimination?

DISCLOSURE OF HIV STATUS OF PATIENTS AND HEALTHCARE PROFESSIONALS

> AIDS has slowly destroyed me. Unless a cure is found, I will be another one of your statistics soon.
>
> . . . Who do I blame? Do I blame myself? I sure don't. I never used IV drugs, never slept with anyone and never had a blood transfusion. I blame Dr. Acer and every single one of you bastards. Anyone who knew Dr. Acer was infected and had full-blown AIDS and stood by not doing a damn thing about it. . . . You are all just as guilty as he was. . . .
>
> P.S. If laws are not formed to provide protection, then my suffering and death are in vain.
>
> I'm dying guys. Goodbye.[42]

This is part of a letter that twenty-two-year-old Kimberly Bergalis wrote to a health-service official just eight months before she died of AIDS complications in December 1991. Bergalis, who had graduated two years earlier from the University of Florida, contracted the AIDS virus from an HIV-infected dentist she had gone to see four years earlier in order to have two molars extracted. The dentist, David Acer, was referred to her through CIGNA, her family's medical plan.

Fifteen months after visiting Acer, she began to develop symptoms of HIV infection. At first, there was a shroud of mystery surrounding how she became infected. On July 27, 1990, the family watched Jane Pauley's report on *NBC Nightly News* about a dentist, Acer, who was HIV positive and yet still treating his patients, confirming their earlier suspicions that he had been the one who infected her. For some time, her family had suspected that Acer was the contact source, yet, despite the persistence of Bergalis and her family, public health officials did not take any steps to remove Acer from his practice.

Acer, a bisexual, admitted treating numerous patients without informing them of his HIV status. In July 1989, he gave up his practice and destroyed most of his records, including the names of his former patients. Less than two months after the news report aired, he died at the age of forty. The issue has still not been resolved. Questions abound concerning the exact source of Bergalis's infection. For instance, a *60 Minutes* television exposé suggested that Bergalis had been sexually active with a drug user. The same report further hinted that some of Acer's other patients were also engaged in high-risk behavior.

An Anatomy of Risk

What constitutes a legitimate risk? A real risk? A serious risk? We face many risks in our lives. AIDS is extreme, since it tends to be fatal, yet it does not mark the first time healthcare professionals have faced the risk of incurring some fatal or near-fatal disease. Healthcare workers have had to weather the risks involved in past epidemics, such as the Justinian plague in the sixth century (540–590) and the Black Death in the fourteenth century, which wiped out nearly 30 percent of Europe's population. Physicians and nurses surely faced the risk of death when they dealt with yellow fever, typhoid, and tuberculosis. Healthcare professionals clearly assume certain degrees of risk in virtue of their profession. The American Dental Association and the American Medical Association encourage their members to assume these risks as part of their professional obligation. What about the risk of AIDS? Should patients be tested for HIV? Should healthcare professionals disclose their HIV-positive status to their patients?

CULTURAL WINDOWS

AMA CODE OF ETHICS: HIV-INFECTED PATIENTS AND PHYSICIANS

A physician may not ethically refuse to treat a patient whose condition is within the physician's current realm of competence solely because the patient is seropositive for HIV. Persons who are seropositive should not be subjected to discrimination based on fear or prejudice.

When physicians are unable to provide the services required by an HIV-infected patient, they should make appropriate referrals to those physicians or facilities equipped to provide such services.

A physician who knows that he or she is seropositive should not engage in any activity that creates an identified risk of transmission of the disease to others. A physician who has HIV disease or who is seropositive should consult colleagues as to which activities the physician can pursue without creating a risk to patients.[43]

(From American Medical Association, *Code of Medical Ethics,* updated June 1996.)

In this section, we address the calculation of risk to both healthcare professionals and patients. Risks can be assessed in two ways. First, how *real* is the risk; that is, what is the probability of the harm actually occurring? The more likely the harm, the more real the risk. Second, how *serious* is the risk; that is, how dangerous or lethal is the harm? In the case of HIV infection, the risk may not be real, yet it is certainly serious since it can be fatal. Risks need to be assessed in light of these two standards—likelihood and seriousness—in order to ascertain whether there is a *significant* risk.

Many will argue that we also need to weigh the proportion of the risk being taken with the benefits that can come about. In the case of AIDS patients, even though AIDS has become more manageable, there is still no cure. Thus, there is no likelihood of restoring the patient to a sound state of health. Nevertheless, there is every obligation on the part of the healthcare professional to bring about some measure of comfort or palliative care. Providing comfort care is just as important as saving a patient's life. Even if the situation is hopeless in that the patient will eventually die, it is not genuinely hopeless as long as caring individuals see to it that the patient is not abandoned and is treated with the most humane and compassionate care available.

Hospital guidelines in the United States in 2000 stipulate universal precautions, for example, gloves and waterproof gowns, in order to lessen exposure to patients' bodily fluids. Despite these guidelines, there are healthcare professionals with AIDS who, through their practice, may pose a significant risk to their patients. At the same time, healthcare professionals are often unknowingly exposed to patients with AIDS.

Given the seriousness of the risk, doesn't it make sense simply to require disclosure of one's AIDS or HIV status? Granted, the likelihood of transmitting the AIDS virus may be quite small, yet the consequences of becoming infected are devastating, and accidents do happen. For example, in one hospital the same cotton swabs that were used on an HIV-infected patient were inadvertently used again on a woman during her annual pelvic examination.[44] In another bizarre incident, an organ donor was HIV positive, but his status was unknown to many of the healthcare professionals working with him. Three recipients of his organs died of AIDS. As many as fifty-nine other recipients of organs and various tissue grafts from this same donor may also be infected with the virus.[45]

In an ideal world, voluntary testing for healthcare professionals and patients seems reasonable, since such a world assumes good, sound judgment as well as a caring and sensitive response from the general public. Yet the reality is far from the ideal. Not all healthcare professionals and patients are conscientious. In fact, some healthcare professionals may even choose to put patients at risk rather than jeopardize their practice. For example, in New Jersey, it took a court order for one surgeon who had AIDS to inform his patients of his status before operating on them.[46]

Due to the gravity of the risks involved, in 1991 the CDC submitted guidelines for healthcare professionals. These guidelines urged that physicians who are customarily exposed to patients' fluids and blood be tested for HIV. The CDC then recommended that any healthcare professionals who tested positive withdraw from further invasive procedures until sanctioned by a review panel. The reaction to these guidelines was intense, with stern criticism being generated along the following lines:

- Just what is meant by an "invasive" procedure remained unclear.
- There is an extremely low risk of transmission of the AIDS virus from healthcare professional to patient. This low risk militates against disclosure.
- Any disclosure of the healthcare professional's status would jeopardize the professional's career and financial well-being.

A later study by the CDC revealed that through March 1993 there were 10,122 healthcare professionals with AIDS in the United States.[47] One of these was Dr. Neal Rzepkowski.

Thirty-nine-year-old Neal Rzepkowski was under no legal obligation to reveal his medical status. Nevertheless, in July 1991, he voluntarily disclosed his HIV-positive status to his patients and to administrators at Brooks Memorial Hospital in upstate New York, where he worked. Public fears regarding the transmission of the virus were already running at fever pitch, especially after the Dr. Acer incident in Florida. Later that month, due to public and professional pressures and widespread fear and antagonism, Rzepkowski was forced to resign. He was the first healthcare professional to resign since publication of the CDC's 1991 guidelines.

Arguments Supporting Disclosure

There are some rather strong arguments in favor of the disclosure of HIV-positive status for both healthcare professionals and patients. First, the anxiety over acquiring the virus is not unfounded. Indeed, the anxiety of patients, as well as the general public, over possibly contracting the virus from healthcare professionals is real, especially in surgical and dental contexts. By the same token, healthcare professionals have a legitimate worry of transmission from their patients. Given AIDS lethal status, there are serious risks involved.

Second, the public has a moral as well as a legal right to be protected from infected healthcare professionals, just as healthcare professionals have the right to be safeguarded against infected patients. This is a mutual appeal to rights between healthcare providers and patients.

Arguments Against Disclosure

The arguments for disclosure need to be weighed against the arguments against disclosure. First, if proper universal precautions are taken, the risk of becoming infected in a clinical setting remains exceptionally slight. Public policy should not be grounded on such a small likelihood of risk.

Second, because of the ongoing stigma attached to AIDS cases, disclosure could result in social, economic, familial, and professional ostracism due to irrational fear as well as misunderstanding regarding HIV infection. The possibility of discrimination continues to be a real threat, all the more so given the lack of support from professional organizations and society at large for those who honestly disclose their HIV-positive status.

Third, the real burdens involved in testing, identifying, reporting, and notifying healthcare professionals outweigh the perceived benefits of preventing possible harm to patients. To illustrate, once a healthcare professional tests positive, what steps are appropriate? Should the patients of that physician or dentist be notified? Notification may be counterproductive, since notifying patients would likely result in a diminishment or even loss of the professional's practice, leading healthcare professionals to resist being tested to begin with. Moreover, the financial costs of testing healthcare professionals would be extremely high and disproportionate to the perceived benefits. According to one report, testing all healthcare professionals in the United States just once would cost around $1.5 billion.[48] Is this a fair use of resources that could be used in other ways?

Resolving the Argument

Many feel that the more sound policy is to inform patients and healthcare professionals that, should some sort of accidental exposure occur, a test for HIV would be necessary. They would then have the option of either being informed or not being informed of the results. The case of Neal Rzepkowski might inspire professional organizations to think of ways to reward rather than punish those who disclose their HIV-infected status. Bioethicist A.R. Jonsen suggests that this reward could take the form of financial aid to replace loss of income when disclosure is made.[49] Jonsen comments:

> The HIV-positive providers must be responsible persons in responsible communities; they must know that their colleagues will support their responsibility in tangible ways.[50]

At the same time, just as we should reward disclosers, according to Jonsen, we should also be prepared to discipline discriminators.

Is there any way to resolve the conflict between the public's right to know and the individual's right to privacy? Thomasma and Marshall recommend the following practical guidelines:

1. Educational strategies aimed at informing health care workers of the importance of universal precautions should be developed and rigorously applied. Concurrently, possible strategies to reinforce compliance with universal precautions should be explored.
2. Invasive dental and medical procedures that might place individuals at risk for contracting the AIDS virus should be documented, investigated, and categorized. Since none has yet been proven to place patients at risk, there is no need for proposals to limit the ability of physicians to perform any procedures.

3. Strict enforcement of antidiscrimination laws and regulations designed to protect persons with AIDS is necessary.
4. An effective means of financing the health-related costs of HIV infection for all individuals who test positive for the AIDS virus and for institutions that treat AIDS patients should be developed and implemented. . . . Creative approaches to ensure the financial solvency of hospitals must be explored.
5. Financial reimbursement mechanisms should be developed and implemented by professional organizations to compensate for the loss of income incurred by HIV-positive health care workers who must or voluntarily do end their practice. In addition, alternative forms of insurance that might be purchased by HIV-positive health care providers to protect their families should loss of income result from the AIDS infection should be developed.
6. Expert panels should decide on a case-by-case basis whether to restrict or curtail an individual's practice.[51]

In the absence of a clear and genuine need to know, for instance, an exposure to infected blood, mandatory testing remains heavily criticized by many. However, due in part to the intense pressure and publicity resulting from the Bergalis case, in January 1991 both the American Medical Association and the American Dental Association stipulated new guidelines indicating that their members who are HIV positive should disclose this fact to their patients. If they do not disclose their status, they should not perform any invasive procedures.

What remains clear through all of this is that there needs to be a recognition of mutual rights and obligations between healthcare providers and patients. For example, it is morally appropriate for healthcare professionals to procure informed consent from patients for an invasive procedure. This means that a surgeon who is HIV infected must indicate this status to the patient so that the patient is well aware of the risk involved, even though the harm is not likely to occur. At the same time, respecting the patient's informed consent requires that patients, in turn, respect the well-being of the healthcare professional. This means that infected patients need to inform healthcare professionals of their HIV status, since it carries an accompanying and significant risk. There is a shared responsibility to ensure that the chances of transmitting the virus are diminished.

In summary, AIDS, with all the threat it poses and the images it evokes, challenges our view of a just and compassionate society. It forces us to ask whether we will be able to rise above the prejudices and stereotypes. It also forces us to ask whether we are able to enact policies that, in the long run, are in the best interests of all members of the community. Even more important, it challenges us to find the fortitude to include within our moral community those most at risk from AIDS—in essence, to determine to what extent we are in fact a truly caring community.

BERNARD RABINOWITZ

The Great Hijack

Bernard Rabinowitz is a retired surgeon in Johannesburg, South Africa. He argues that the concern in the United States for defending the rights of HIV-infected patients has overshadowed the more critical concern for the prevention of the spread of AIDS and the well-being of the wider community. He states that the movement to protect the rights of AIDS patients has been counterproductive. Rabinowitz strongly urges that testing, labeling, and contacting be required. Physicians, especially, must be free to test and label and must have access to medical records.

It is over 40 years since I qualified as a doctor and 35 since I was awarded the fellowship of the Royal College of Surgeons of England. As a student I read with enthusiasm about the revolution wrought by Pasteur, Jenner, and Lister. Later I was stirred as polio was defeated, diphtheria became a rarity, and smallpox vanished. We were taught and in turn passed on to our students the principles so decisively developed by these great men.

Any epidemic imposes obligations on the doctor. We must diagnose, isolate, localise, and treat. An overriding concern is the protection of the un-infected. That is the modern and proved way to limit and end an outbreak of an infectious disease. Indeed, it is a catechism for even our junior students.

In the early 1980s some hundred or more people who were immunocompromised came to light in the homosexual community in the United States. A diagnostic test was developed and an infecting agent was identified. Then modern medicine was made to run for cover. A positive test labelled the carrier as a homosexual. That community, generally erudite, articulate, and eloquent, was prominent in the arts, the media, and often in public life. The fear of possible labelling was real and immediate. It hit interested parties in the administration, which handed down speedy and even panicky legislation mandating secrecy and confidentiality and prohibiting testing without consent.

The medical profession remained obediently silent as this disease emerged as a lethal, spreadable infection. We, the doctors, were told that the standard approaches to an infectious disease would land us in court. Our professional bodies raced, with politically correct zeal, to endorse the criminalising of normal diagnostic protocols. With heavy ethical breathing we had endorsed the first legally protected epidemic in medical history.

Some of the jargon then and now bears looking at as we balance on the wobbly ethical platform. The sanctity of confidentiality is a prime example. We have never respected confidentiality at the expense of the common good. The profession has never permitted the rights of an individual to compromise the community. Would any doctor who sees a patient known to have epilepsy driving a school bus keep quiet? Would a person with angina be allowed to pilot an airliner? Doctors employed by insurance and building societies have never felt constrained to protect the secrecy of the person with tuberculosis or hypertension who is now refused a mortgage loan. Yet with AIDS the rights to secrecy of a tiny minority were deemed ethically more important than the rights of the huge uninfected majority.

The medical voices raised in protest at our feeble acquiescence were blasted with the labels of callous, unethical, and not compassionate. Our profession forgot its heritage and its duty. It abandoned its science and its obligation to apply it. As the years passed, young people died in their hundreds, then thousands, and soon, as heterosexual contacts spread, the figures will be millions. Secrecy and confidentiality have served the epidemic well.

What might we have achieved had we identified, labelled, and campaigned? The epidemic would not have been stopped, but millions of people who now have HIV would not have contracted the virus. Homosexuals and carriers identified as such would have had to live with whatever exposure ensued. The HIV infected developing world is, like the developed West, battling with the ethical nonsense formed in the United States 15 years ago. Earnest doctors, people who know better, are shackled by fear of prosecution if they identify a person with HIV. Yet ethical debates have never arisen on cholera, tuberculosis, or lassa fever. We even indulge the indefensible practice of anonymous testing without consent to gain statistics. Those identified as positive are not informed.

Medical law endorses the patient's right to refuse a test for HIV—a test that could be vital in an emergency or other cases. The law demands that the surgeon should proceed or risk prosecution. Can you envisage a scenario where a patient presents for, say, a hip replacement, or a partial gastrectomy and tells the surgeon that he or she cannot take an x ray examination of the chest or do renal functions but must do the operation anyway?

In years to come the profession may well label these past years as the great hijack. As doctors we can still save millions. We must be free to test, diagnose, and label. Families, lovers, and contacts must not be denied information. Obligatory tests for HIV, as in other countries for other diseases, should precede marriage and pregnancy. All patients; blood, organ, and sperm donors; schoolchildren; medical students; surgeons; boxers; rugby players; and anyone in an occupation where blood can be shed should be freely tested as and when indicated with no specific consent required. The person with AIDS will become an accepted feature of society. The hijackers have facilitated a worldwide disaster; I would urge that we speedily do what we can to minimise it.

QUESTIONS FOR COMPREHENSION AND REFLECTION

1. In what respects is AIDS the "first legally protected epidemic in medical history," according to Rabinowitz?
2. Rabinowitz takes strong exception to the policy of AIDS exceptionalism, for a variety of reasons. Do you find his arguments compelling? Explain your response.
3. Does Rabinowitz's position reflect more a utilitarian or a deontological approach? Do you think his line of reasoning is valid and sound? Support your answers.
4. Rabinowitz advocates, in certain instances, testing without informed consent. Do you believe that the rule of informed consent can ever be justifiably overridden? Support your answer.

RICHARD D. MOHR

AIDS, Gays, and State Coercion

Richard D. Mohr is a professor of philosophy at the University of Illinois, Urbana-Champaign. In contrast to Rabinowitz, Mohr contends that the values of individual autonomy need to be protected unless the public well-being is directly threatened. He argues against government intervention, since he believes that the harms are not apparent—even in the case of so-called indirect harm, that is, higher costs to the public in the form of taxes and insurance rates. In conclusion, he holds that acts of state paternalism in the case of AIDS are not justifiable.

ALARUMS AND EXCURSIONS

Of those dead and dying from AIDS three-quarters are gay men. Government funding for AIDS research was at best sluggish till the disease appeared to the dominant non-gay culture as a threat. That perceived threat has spawned state-mandated discrimination against groups at risk for AIDS in employment and access to services, allegedly on medical grounds but in pointed contradiction to the judgments of the very medical institutions to which society has entrusted the determination of such grounds (the US Department of Health and Human Services, the Centers for Disease Control, and the National Institutes of Health).[1]

Government's disregard for medical opinion and for the lives of gays strongly suggests that prejudicial forces are at work. There is of course nothing new in this, but the stakes here are high. The armed forces have already established quarantines of those at risk for AIDS on some bases (*The Washington Post*, 19 October 1985, A12; *The Advocate*, #442, 18 March 1986, p. 14). With state-mandated discriminations installed and calls for civilian quarantines circulating, it is clear that the AIDS crisis is going to test the country's mettle. Not since the Supreme Court affirmed the internments of Japanese-Americans in World War II has so live a danger existed to America's traditional commitment to civil liberties. And again the danger is created by hysteria and not a reasoned necessity.

The hysteria, when not simply an expression of old anti-gay prejudices, is based on the presumption that the disease is spread indiscriminately. This presumption permitted Jeane Kirkpatrick to begin a syndicated column by using AIDS as a metaphor for international terrorism—"it can affect anyone"—in the serene belief that her audience, educated America, already thought this about AIDS and might even be ready for extreme measures (*The Washington Post,* 13 October 1985, B8).

ALLEGED HARMS TO OTHERS

For public policy purposes, the most important fact about AIDS is not that it is deadly but that it, like hepatitis B, is caused by a blood-transmitted virus. For the disease to spread, body fluids of someone with the virus must *directly enter the bloodstream of another.* . . . But not just any bodily fluid will do. Only blood and semen have been implicated in the transmission of the virus (*MMWR* 34: 45, p. 682).

That the virus is blood transmitted means first and foremost that, in countries with reasonable sanitation, groups at risk for the disease are clearly definable—more so than for virtually any other disease known—with 96 per cent of cases having clearly demarcated modes of transmission and cause. And now that blood supplies are screened with a test for antibodies to the AIDS virus, the number of these groups is indeed dropping. Hemophiliacs not already exposed and blood transfusion recipients are now no longer groups at risk. . . .

The July 1985 cover of *Life* informed the nation in three-inch red letters that "NOW NO ONE IS SAFE FROM AIDS." The magazine used as its allegedly compelling example a seemingly typical Pennsylvania family all but one of whose members has the disease. But it turns out that all those members with the disease were indeed in high risk groups. The father was a hemophiliac, his wife had sex with him, and she conveyed the virus to a child in the process of giving birth. No one got the disease either mysteriously or through casual contact. The family example in fact was evidence *against* the article's generic contagion thesis. Equally irresponsible journalists, lobbyists, and elected officials have compared AIDS to air-borne viral disease like influenza and the common cold.

The case for general contagion cannot be made. In consequence government policy which is based on that fear is unwarranted. The extraordinary measures—including the suspension of civil liberties—which government might justifiably take, as in war, to prevent wholesale slaughter simply do not apply here. In particular, quarantining the class of AIDS-exposed persons in order to protect society from indiscriminate harm is unwarranted.

HARM TO SELF

The disease's mode of contagion assures that those at risk are those whose actions contribute to their risk of infection, chiefly through intimate sexual contact and shared hypodermic needles. In the transmission of AIDS, it is the general feature of self-exposure to contagion that makes direct coercive acts by government—like bathhouse closings—particularly inappropriate as efforts to abate the disease.

If independence—the ability to guide one's life by one's own rights to an extent compatible with a like ability on the part of others—is, as it is, a major value, one cannot respect that value while preventing people from putting themselves at risk through voluntary associations. Voluntary associations are star cases of people acting in accordance with the principle of independence, for mutual consent guarantees that the "compatible extent" proviso of the principle is fulfilled. But the state and even the courts have not been very sensitive to the distinction between one harming oneself and one harming another—nor has the medical establishment. It appears to all of them that a harm is a harm, a disease a disease, however caused or described. The moral difference, however, is enormous. Preventing a person from harming another is required by the principle of independence, but preventing someone from harming himself is incompatible with it. While no further from others, a rather powerful justification is needed if the state is to be warranted in protecting a person from himself.

In the absence of such a justification, the state sometimes tries to split the moral difference and argues that state coercion *may* be used when the harm to others is remote and indirect. Such an argument from indirect harms runs to the effect that state-coerced use of, say, seatbelts and motorcycle helmets is warranted, for helmetless motorcycle crashes and seatbeltless car accidents harm even those not involved in the accidents, by raising everyone's insurance costs and burdening the public purse when victims end up in county hospitals. Here state coercion comes in through the backdoor.

This line of argument has been used with increasing frequency even by self-described liberals like New York's Governor Cuomo, and it is beginning to be heard in AIDS discussions. This is not surprising, for the cost of AIDS patient care from diagnosis to death is somewhere between $35,000 and $150,000. Private funds are often quickly exhausted, and the patient ends up on the dole—harming everyone, and so allegedly warranting state coercion of the means of possible AIDS transmission.

J. S. Mill's rule-of-thumb for appraising such appeals to indirect harms is exactly on target: an indirect harm counts toward justifying state coercion only when the harm grows large enough to be considered a violation of another person's right. This understanding of harm to others is necessary so that independence is not rendered nugatory and, *as a right*, is only outweighed by something comparable to it. Now, while it is nice if products (like insurance) are cheap and taxes low, the considered opinion of our society is not that one's rights have been violated when taxes or the price of milk goes up. Indeed, in the case of taxes, the considered opinion is cast as a Constitutional provision. So arguments that smuggle coercion in through the backdoor of indirect harms are not successful. . . .

STATE PATERNALISM CONSIDERED

The important question remains whether AIDS warrants paternalistic state coercion to prevent those not-exposed from harming themselves, through banning or highly regulating the means of possible viral transmission. Usually paternalistic arguments cannot be made sensible and consistent. For example: federal AIDS funding for FY 1986 in the House came with a paternalistic rider giving the surgeon general a power he already has—to close bathhouses, gay social institutions, if they are determined to facilitate the transmission or spread of the disease, which indeed they do. (So do parks and bedrooms.) The sponsor of the rider argued that it was "a small step to help those who are unable or unwilling to help themselves" (*The Washington Blade*, 4 October 1985, p. 1). Cast so baldly, the argument simply denies independence as a value. For it is consistent with the presumption that the majority gets to determine both what the good life is and to enforce it coercively. The argument could as well be used to justify compulsory religious conversion—those who are unable or unwilling to see the light are helped to see it. . . .

PUBLIC HEALTH AND TOTALITARIANISM

Arguments offered so far by the medical community against quarantines and bathhouse closings have largely adopted the terms of mere practicality, appealing to such facts as the large number of people involved, the permanence of the virus in those exposed, and the possibility that the sexual arena may simply shift away from bathhouses where some educational efforts may be possible. I have suggested to the contrary that quarantines and closings should be opposed, not because they are impractical (though they may be), but because they are immoral.

Doctors tend to hold their unrefined view that health policy is merely a matter of strategy because they, not surprisingly, tend to see health itself as a trumping good, second to none in importance. This is a dangerous view, especially when coupled with their idea that health is an undifferentiated good. They fail to distinguish between my harming my health and my harming your health. Behind this oversight lies the further (sometimes unarticulated) presumption that you and I both are absorbed into and subordinated under something called the public health—a concept that tends to be analyzed in inverse proportion to the frequency with which it is used when trying to justify coercive acts.

No literal sense exists in which there could be such [a] thing as a public health. To say the public has a health is like saying the number seven has a color: such a thing cannot have such a property. You have health or you lack it and I have health or lack it, because we each have a body with organs that function or do not function. But the public, an aggregate of persons similarly disposed as persons, has no such body of organs with functions which work or fail. There are, however, two frequently used metaphoric senses of public health that do have a reference: one, is a legitimate use but largely inapplicable to the AIDS crisis; the other, when used normatively, is the pathway to totalitarianism.

The legitimate sense places public health in the same conceptual scheme as national defense and water purification. These are types of public goods in a technical sense—not what most people want and thus what democratic governments give them nor what tend to maximize by state means some type of good (pleasure, happiness, beauty), but what everyone wants but cannot get or get efficiently through voluntary arrangements and which thus require coercive coordinations from the state, so that each person gets what he wants. Thus, the private or voluntary arrangements of the market system do not seem likely to provide adequate national security, because a defense system that protects those who pay for it will also protect those who do not; everyone (reasonably enough) will tend to wait for someone else to pay for it, so that national security ends up not being purchased at all, or at least far less of it is purchased than everyone would agree to pay for if there were some means to manifest that agreement. The coercive actions of the state through taxation are then required to achieve the public good of national defense.

For exactly the same reason, the state is warranted in using coercive measures to drain swamps and provide vaccines against air-borne viruses, but the state is not warranted by appeal to the public good in coercing people to take the vaccine once it is freely available, for then *each* person is capable on his own—without further state coercion—of getting the protection from the disease he wants. The mode of AIDS contagion makes it relevantly like this latter case. Each person on his own—without state coercion—can get the protection from the disease that he wants through his own actions, and indeed can get it by doing himself what he might be tempted to try to get the state to force upon others, say, avoiding bathhouses. As far as the good of protection is concerned, it can be achieved with no state coercion.

Is there a public good involved simply in reducing the size of the pool of AIDS-exposed people? I see just one, the one I argued for—the ability to have a robust sex life, without fear of death. But this good does not permit every form of state coercion. Not every public good motivates every form of coercion. The public goods mentioned so far could all be achieved by *equitable* coercion (e.g., universal conscription, taxation, compensated taking of property). When equitable coercion is the means, the public good can be quite slight and still be justified (as in government support for the arts). But when the coercion is inequitably dispersed, the public good served must be considerably more compelling than the means are intrusive. Thus, dispersed coercion against select individuals that involves restricted motion and physical suffering is warranted only by unqualifiedly necessary ends: when the individuals co-erced have harmed others (as in punishment) or when it is necessary to the very existence of the country (as a partial military draft may be for a nation at defensive war). And thus too, the substantial good of civil rights protections is advanced only through the considerably weak intrusion of barring the desire of employers to indulge in whimsical and arbitrary hiring practices. The public good of an unencumbered sex life however fails this weighted ends-to-means test if the means are a dispersedly coerced sex life. For the intrusion and the good are on a par—on the one hand encumbered sex, on the other unencumbered sex. And so it appears that only equitably coercive means are available to achieve the end of reducing the pool of AIDS-exposures—taxation for preventive measures like vaccine development, but not coercive measures that affect some but not others, like closing bathhouses or banning or regulating sex practices selectively.

Those who do not find the possibility of carefree sex a public good—probably the bulk of those actually calling for state coercion—will find no legitimate help in the notion of public health for state coercion here. Those who do will find it justifies only equitable measures.

The other metaphoric sense of public health takes the medical model of the healthy body and unwittingly transfers it to society—the body politic. But this transfer (when it has any content at all) bears hidden and extremely dangerous assumptions. Plato in the *Republic* was the first thinker systematically to press the analogy of the good society to the healthy body. The state stands to the citizenry and its good, as a doctor stands to the body and its health. Society, so it is claimed, is an organism in which people are mere functional parts, ones that are morally good and emotionally well-off only insofar as they act for the sake of the organism. The analogy is alive and well today and calling out for extreme measures now. . . . On this view, the individual however harmed cannot fulfill his role. A damaged organ, the spleen for example, can be, to continue the analogy, simply cut out. By comparison, quarantines and coerced sex lives might appear as mild remedies on this analogy, but something has been lost here—persons.

The medical model of society is the conceptual engine of totalitarianism. It presumes not that the goods of individuals are final goods but that individuals are good only as they serve some good beyond themselves, that of the state or body politic. The state exists not for the sake of individuals—to protect and enhance their prospects as rational agents—but rather individuals exist for the state and are subordinated to society as a whole, the worth of which is to be determined only from the perspective of the whole. The individual, thus, is not an end in himself but exists for some social good—whether that good be some hoped-for overall happiness or some social ideal—like purity, wholesomeness, decency, or "traditional values." Unconscious obedient servicing is dressed up as virtue.

The worst political consequence of the AIDS crisis would not be simply the further degradation of gays. Gay internments would not be anything new to this century. In the European internment camps of World War II, gypsies wore brown triangle identifying badges, Jehovah's Witnesses purple, political prisoners red, race defilers black, and gays pink triangles. Worse than the further degradation of gays in America would be a general, and not easily reversed, shift in the nation's center of gravity toward the medical model and away from the position, acknowledged in America's Constitutional tradition, that individuals have broad yet determinate claims against both general welfare and social ideals. The consequence of such a shift would be that people would come to be treated essentially as resources, sometimes expendable—a determination no less frightening when made by a combined father, colonel, and doctor than by a fearful mob.

NOTE

1. See particularly the CDC's guidelines for preventing transmission in the workplace, "Recommendations for Preventing Transmission of Infection with Human T-Lymphotrophic Virus Type III/Lymphadenopathy-Associated Virus in the Workplace," *Morbidity and Mortality Weekly Report* (*MMWR*), 15 November 1985, 34: 45, 682–95.

QUESTIONS FOR COMPREHENSION AND REFLECTION

1. Mohr claims that our cherished value of independence also includes the freedom to place ourselves at risk through voluntary associations. He goes on to argue that state and government policies that interfere with this independence are coercive. Do you agree or disagree? Support your answer.
2. Do you agree with the Mohr's description of two metaphoric senses of the concept of "public health"? Support your answer. Why does the closing of gay bathhouses, in the Mohr's opinion, have little to do with public health?
3. If you were to describe the methodological analysis of Mohr's reasoning, would you find it closer to utilitarianism or deontology? Explain.
4. Compare Mohr's position to that of Rabinowitz. Which presents the more cogent argument? Which do you agree with? Give your reasons.

BONNIE STEINBOCK

Harming, Wronging, and AIDS

Bonnie Steinbock is a professor of philosophy at State University of New York in Albany. She provides a foil to Mohr's argument. After discussing the significance of Mill's
harm principle, she argues that it applies in the matter of AIDS. In contrast to Mohr,
she adds that increasing monetary costs to society are relevant considerations and that
the state can justifiably intervene in the crisis. She goes on to discuss what kinds of state
paternalism are justified. Admitting the dangers of discrimination, she holds that the
government should work to prevent discrimination while still intervening by requiring
contact tracing.

The AIDS crisis poses a number of tough questions for society. Some are medical: for example, how can we stop the spread of the disease? Others are political: what measures will people be willing to accept? But there are also moral philosophical issues raised about the legitimacy of measures that might be taken to prevent the spread of this fatal disease. Measures designed to protect some people may adversely affect the interests of others. I will examine the implications of one theory regarding legitimate state intervention—Mill's harm principle—for the AIDS crisis.

In *On Liberty,* John Stuart Mill argued that "the only purpose for which power can be rightfully exercised over any member of a civilized community, against his will, is to prevent harm to others."[1] Forcibly restricting one's behavior for one's *own* good (legal paternalism) is never justified, nor is the prohibition of behavior simply on the grounds that it is widely regarded as sinful or wicked (legal moralism). The harm principle, as it has come to be known, absolutely rejects any grounds for social or legal coercion except harm to others.

Not everyone agrees that harm to others is the sole justification for restricting freedom. It has been argued that some paternalistic intervention is not only justified, but consistent with Mill's emphasis on liberty.[2] . . . I do not intend to discuss the merits of legal paternalism or legal moralism in this paper. I propose to assume that Mill was right:

harm to others is the sole justification for limiting individual freedom. However, as we will see, acceptance of the harm principle raises as many questions as it answers.

In the first section, I shall discuss briefly the kind of harm that might plausibly be prohibited by the harm principle. Whereas disease cannot be outlawed, behavior that infects others may be. AIDS is a fatal disease. Should we regard infecting a person with AIDS as a criminal act, possibly even murder? I shall argue that, although practical difficulties regarding proximate cause would make criminal charges nearly impossible to sustain, nevertheless, infecting another person with AIDS might be considered in some cases to evidence a "depraved indifference to human life" and so be the moral equivalent of second-degree murder.

The second section discusses legitimate governmental intervention to halt the spread of AIDS. The criminal law is only one way that the state can intervene to influence behavior. Another way to restrict behavior is to limit opportunities to engage in it: e.g., closing gay bathhouses. Would such measures necessarily be a reflection of legal moralism or legal paternalism? I shall argue that this need not be the case. However, to be consistent with the harm principle, it would have to be shown both that closing the baths is likely to be effective in halting the spread of disease, and that this is the least restrictive effective method of doing so.

Another possible justification for governmental coercion is the financial cost to society as a whole. AIDS is a terribly expensive disease. I will reject the claim that the harm principle rules out consideration of the cost of AIDS and instead suggest that it calls for the least restrictive measures necessary to contain costs.

Lastly, I shall turn to the question of whether the potential harm to AIDS victims resulting from "contact-notification" is a decisive argument against it. Although the danger to AIDS victims cannot be ignored, it does not outweigh the right of their contacts to the knowledge necessary for fully informed consent to sexual activity. Instead, the state should take vigorous measures to protect AIDS victims from discrimination.

THE HARM PRINCIPLE AND THE OBLIGATIONS OF INDIVIDUALS

In its broadest sense, harm is any adverse affecting of an individual's interests. One can be harmed by natural events, such as storms, or even nonevents, such as drought, as well as by human actions. The harm principle, which justifies the restriction of human freedom, must concern harm brought about by human action. Joel Feinberg suggests that we think of harming as having two components: (1) It must lead to some kind of adverse effect, or create the danger of such an effect, on its victim's *interests;* and (2) It must be inflicted wrongfully in violation of the victim's rights.[3]

The first component makes the harm principle sufficiently broad, enabling us to recognize that people can be harmed in nonphysical ways. People have all kinds of interests, in their lives and health, in property, in their reputations, in their emotional well-being. Although certain kinds of injuries might count more heavily than others, an adequate conception of harm should do justice to the variety of kinds of harm.

The second condition is necessary to restrict the harm principle. The interests of one person may be adversely affected by the actions of another in many cases where this provides little or no reason for restricting the behavior. My taking a job that would otherwise have been offered to you does adversely affect your interests, but that is no reason for me to turn it down, much less for the state to prevent me from taking it. Another example would be a person who freely consents to plastic surgery that turns out badly, but not because of any negligence on the part of the surgeon. (That can happen, though Americans may find it difficult to believe.) The disfigured person has been harmed, but not wronged, because the physician was not at fault. There would be, on this understanding of harming, no grounds for civil, much less criminal liability.

To give someone a painful and inevitably fatal disease is clearly adversely to affect that person's interests, but is the second condition met? Do I wrong you, and do I violate your rights, if I give you AIDS? Certainly I do if I deliberately try to infect you. Although this is an unlikely scenario, it is not impossible. . . .

Few people deliberately try to infect others with fatal diseases, but carriers of disease may unknowingly infect others: Typhoid Mary is a classic example. Society must protect people from unintentional infection—a topic to which I shall return in the next section—but the unknowing carrier is not to blame (unless she is to blame for not knowing). What about the person who does know that she poses a risk to others, but does not mean to infect them? Could Typhoid Mary escape condemnation by employing double effect reasoning, and saying, "I don't mean to infect these people, just prepare their meals for them"? Certainly not. Although knowingly exposing people to harm is not usually regarded as bad as deliberately exposing them, it is still wrong and a violation of their right not to be exposed to serious health hazards. Indeed, where such exposure is not merely negligent, but reckless, and evidence of a "depraved indifference" to human life, it may even be considered to be murder in the second-degree. . . .

A dramatic example of a murder conviction for knowingly exposing people to the risk of death occurred in June, 1985, when three executives of Film Recovery Systems, Inc. were convicted of murder, and sentenced to 25 years in prison, for the death of an employee from cyanide poisoning. The murder conviction, alleged to be the first in an industrially related death, was based on the fact that the company executives were "totally knowledgeable" of the plant's hazardous conditions, and did nothing to protect, or even warn, the workers. The judge who sentenced the defendants likened their actions to leaving a time bomb on an airplane. "Every day people worked there," he said, "it kept ticking, it kept ticking."[4]

Individuals have a legal as well as moral duty not to engage in activity likely to cause the death of others. The mere fact that one did not mean to cause the death or serious bodily harm does not necessarily absolve one from criminal liability. What are the implications for the person who knows he is seropositive, but nevertheless engages in activity capable of infecting others, such as anal sex and sharing contaminated needles? If he infects someone with AIDS, which is always fatal, is that murder?

Admittedly, in most cases of AIDS, the "victim" has had numerous contacts, and so establishing the proximate causation necessary for criminal, or even civil, liability would be nearly impossible. Still, there could be cases in which the casual connection was clear. Is that murder?

Many people will be offended by the very suggestion. Seropositive individuals, if not already ill, are themselves at risk of developing AIDS. It seems very harsh to accuse the victims of a terrible disease of murder. Moreover, how can we persuade those who may be infected to submit to a test, if the result is that they are exposed to criminal liability? Is not the whole discussion of AIDS and murder entirely wrongheaded?

I am not suggesting criminal or civil liability as a practical way to deal with the AIDS crisis. However, if we think that the individual who knowingly risks infecting others seriously wrongs them, that has implications for behavior on the part of others, such as physicians and public health officials. It may be justified to infringe the rights of one person to prevent a more serious violation of the rights of another. If, on the other hand, the AIDS carrier who has sex with others does not wrong them, then violating the carrier's confidentiality will be unjustified. For this reason, we need to take seriously the charge that having sex or sharing needles with others, knowing you are seropositive, is immoral, comparable to shooting a gun into an occupied building, or driving while intoxicated.

Although AIDS carriers may be deserving of our sympathy, that fact by itself does not make their behavior in infecting others less culpable. A sick person can be as guilty of murder as a well one. Illness is relevant only if it diminishes the capacity for responsible behavior. . . .

Another possibility for diminishing responsibility for causing harm is when harm results from less than fully voluntary behavior. Sexual behavior is often less than fully voluntary, because it stems from strong feelings and drives. Still, although we may blame less the person driven by passion to do something that harms another than we would the person who does it "in cold blood," this factor does not completely exonerate. People who have the ability to conform their behavior to the requirements of morality or law have an obligation not to get into situations in which their passions are likely to rule. If they do anyway, they cannot excuse their harmful behavior by saying, "I couldn't help it." The alcoholic who cannot control his or her drinking may not be to blame for drinking, but is to blame for driving to a bar, knowing that he or she will become intoxicated and then drive home. What are the implications for seropositive individuals? In my view, they are morally required to do two things: reduce the risk of infection by practicing "safer sex" techniques, and inform their sexual contacts of their seropositive status. Are both necessary to escape moral liability? Cannot seropositive individuals fulfill their duty not to harm others simply by taking steps likely to protect them? I do not think so. Consider the case of Rock Hudson and Linda Evans, a star of the television series, *Dynasty*. Hudson, who was dying of AIDS, was scheduled to shoot a romantic scene with Evans, which required him to kiss her. At that time, neither his disease nor his homosexuality was widely known. Fearing the effect on his career if the news got out, Hudson decided to go ahead with the kiss and not tell Linda Evans.

There was little, if any, objective risk of infection to Linda Evans from that kiss. AIDS is transmitted through the direct introduction of bodily fluids, such as blood and semen, into the bloodstream of another. Does the fact make Rock

Hudson's decision morally permissible? No. This is partly because Rock Hudson was not in a position to know that he was not exposing Linda Evans to the risk of death; at that time hemophiliacs were being advised to avoid "deep kissing," because it was feared that AIDS might be transmitted through saliva. It is wrong to be willing to expose another to the risk of harm, even where there is no objective risk. Suppose Hudson had known that his kissing was extremely unlikely to infect her. Would that make kissing and not telling morally all right?

Not in my view. Intimate contact is permissible only when voluntary. When Linda Evans agreed to kiss Rock Hudson, she did not agree to kiss someone with a potentially communicable fatal disease. She could agree to that only if she knew about it. Even if the risk of catching AIDS from kissing is low, the decision whether to take that risk is hers, and hers alone. No one else, including Rock Hudson, has the right to make that decision for her. He could explain to her that there was very little danger. He could reassure her that there would be no exchange of saliva. He could press on her the damage to his career if the story got out. But to conceal from her the fact of his AIDS is to lie to her. That is a serious wrong even if his kissing her did not, as it turns out, harm her, or even run a significant risk of harming her. I do not believe that it is morally permissible to lie to someone about a matter of vital concern to avoid adverse effects on one's career.

If this is right, and Rock Hudson had a moral duty to inform Linda Evans of his condition before engaging in an activity unlikely to do her harm, how much stronger is the obligation of the seropositive individual to inform others of his or her condition before engaging in activities that may well cause them harm. The use of safer sex techniques may protect them from harm but does not meet the condition that they not be wronged. Although it is less bad to wrong but not harm than to wrong and harm, wronging is still—wrong.

Is it morally permissible merely to inform and not use safer sex techniques? It might be thought that respect for the other person's autonomy requires a mutual decision on the use of safer sex

techniques, and that it would be paternalistic for the AIDS carrier to decide unilaterally to use safer sex techniques. This has more plausibility regarding sex than it does, say, regarding the sharing of needles, because it is hard to imagine anyone who would knowingly choose to take the risk of getting AIDS from sharing an unsterilized needle. By contrast, someone might value certain unsafe sexual practices (in which semen enters the body) so highly that he or she is willing to take the risk of contracting AIDS. Nevertheless, I do not regard depriving such a person of the opportunity to take the risk as objectionably paternalistic. Respect for the autonomy of others does not require us to provide them with opportunities to hurt themselves, much less require us to inflict the harm ourselves. Your right to risk your life imposes no corresponding obligation on me to inflict harm. So although I have no right to force you to use safer sex techniques, or to prevent you from having sex with others who choose not to use them, neither do you have the right to a say in my use of such techniques. Moreover, concern for the lives of others should make the seropositive person engage only in safer sex.

To sum up, merely taking precautions probably avoids harming others, but is still morally objectionable, because the failure to disclose one's status as seropositive deprives one's sexual partners of information they have a right to know. Having unprotected sex with informed and willing partners respects their autonomy, but, given the seriousness of the risk, shows insufficient concern for their welfare. Someone who neither informs nor takes precautions, but has sex with others, knowing that he or she is seropositive, wrongs and harms, or runs the risk of harming. This displays reckless indifference to the value of human life, and, when it results in the death of a person, might reasonably be seen as the moral equivalent of murder.

GOVERNMENTAL COERCION TO PREVENT THE SPREAD OF DISEASE

What are the implications of the above section for legitimate coercive activity on the part of the state?

What measures may the state take to protect people from being infected with AIDS? In discussing coercive measures to stop the spread of AIDS, we must remember first that most of the people at risk can protect themselves by taking certain precautions. . . . Unfortunately, this is unlikely to happen with heroin addicts who are now most threatened with the massive spread of the disease. Second, although changes in voluntary behavior can protect most of those at risk, even those who are not "voluntary risk-takers" may be at risk, namely, women who have sex with men whom they do not know are homosexual or intravenous drug users, and their fetuses. What should be done to protect them? Finally, AIDS is an extremely expensive disease. Are coercive measures, which go beyond mere education, justifiable if likely to contain costs?

Obviously, the first thing the government ought to do is educate. That violates no one's rights, and is likely to be very effective in halting the spread of AIDS. The refusal to disseminate information about safer sex in places where AIDS is rampant, such as prisons, because of a moralistic and unrealistic attitude about sex, is unconscionable. Is there anything else the state would be justified in doing, along with education? Are measures that restrict the freedom of AIDS carriers ever justified? A clear requirement of justifiable coercive measures is that they are likely to be effective, since it would obviously be illegitimate, on the harm principle, to restrict freedom without good reason to believe that such restrictions protected others. Further, the protection we gain has to be significant enough to outweigh the costs of the restriction, including loss of liberty and expense.

Some of the recent proposals to combat AIDS would be unjustified, on grounds of inefficacy, even if they were not also outrageous violations of civil rights; for example, the ludicrous suggestion that those who test seropositive to AIDS be quarantined. Since AIDS carriers do not pose a danger to others through casual contact, segregation from the general population is unnecessary to prevent the spread of AIDS. Quarantine might be intended to prevent those who have been exposed to the AIDS virus from having sex or sharing needles with those who have not been exposed. However, HIV-positive individuals have the ability to infect others *forever*, whether or not they ever develop the disease themselves. To prevent those who have been exposed to AIDS from having sexual contact with others, those who test seropositive—a predicted 70% of the homosexual population of New York and San Francisco—would have to be quarantined forever—or until a vaccine or treatment is found. The idea is absurd. . . .

Less restrictive than quarantining those who test seropositive is closing places where sexual practices that spread AIDS occur, such as gay bathhouses. This was done in New York in 1985. Some people opposed this on purely pragmatic grounds: it won't stop homosexual activity, and so won't stop the spread of AIDS. In fact, it has been argued, it is counterproductive, as the baths offer an opportunity for education about techniques for avoiding the disease.

A different sort of argument against closing of the baths is offered by philosopher Richard Mohr in "AIDS, Gays, and State Coercion."[5] Mohr maintains that it is morally unjustified to close them down, even if this would retard the spread of disease, because it would be paternalistic. The reason for this is that the disease's mode of contagion assures that those at risk are those whose actions contribute to their risk of infection, chiefly through intimate sexual contact and shared hypodermic needles. If gay men choose to take risks with their health by frequenting the baths, that is their prerogative. Preventing competent adults from voluntarily taking risks with their health is paternalistic. It would no more be justified to close the baths, according to Mohr, than it would be to ban race car driving or mountain climbing.

There are two flaws in Mohr's argument. The first is that not only voluntary risk-takers are threatened by AIDS. . . . Are women who sleep with, or are even married to, gay men, unaware that they are gay, voluntary risk-takers? This is plausible only if one adopts the view that sex *per se* is a risky activity these days, so that anyone who has sex, even in an ostensibly heterosexual, monogamous marriage, must be considered to be voluntarily undergoing the risk of catching AIDS. I submit that this is implausible. A person who has sex with multiple partners, refusing to use safer sex techniques, might be regarded as a "volunteer," but not the woman unknowingly married to a bisexual. The notion of voluntary risk-taking is even more implausible when applied to the fetus who contracts the disease *in utero,* who does not act at all, much less act voluntarily. If these nonvoluntary risk-takers could be protected from getting AIDS by closing the baths, the motivation would not be paternalistic, for it is paternalism only to forcibly prevent people from doing what they wish to do and to protect them from risks they willingly undergo. To justify closing the baths on harm principle grounds, then, it remains to be shown that this is both likely to be effective and the least restrictive measure to prevent the spread of fatal disease.

The second flaw in Mohr's argument is his denial that cost may be considered on the harm principle. . . . Astonishingly, Mohr believes that these costs may not be even considered in justifying coercive measures. Referring to such costs as "indirect harm," he invokes Mill as maintaining that an indirect harm counts toward justifying state coercion only when the harm grows large enough to be considered the violation of a right. Also, although it is nice if taxes are low, no one's rights are violated when taxes go up. So we may not close the baths, forcibly preventing people from using them, even if it could be shown that this would reduce AIDS and save money.

A more antiutilitarian approach can scarcely be imagined. But one need not be a utilitarian to reject this cavalier approach toward the spending of public funds. Instead, we can recognize that an individual's right to pursue his or her life-style in the manner he or she prefers, including the taking of certain risks, is not an absolute right. If personal choices of some members of society place an enormous financial burden on others, and they cannot be persuaded by noncoercive means to change their ways, coercive measures may be justifiable. However, the least restrictive measures should be adopted. For example, we do not entirely ban mountain climbing, even though we can foresee the inevitable expensive rescues that will result from allowing it, because we acknowledge the legitimacy of an activity many people find extremely

pleasurable and meaningful. Our respect for their freedom to engage in mountain climbing does not require us to let people go wherever they choose. It is legitimate to close the riskiest routes, in order to contain costs. An alternative would be to warn people in advance that, should they get in trouble, they could expect not to get rescued. Whereas this policy has the merit of respecting autonomy, it would require callousness to carry out, and should on that ground be rejected. Instead, it is legitimate to restrict somewhat, but not entirely ban, risky behavior. Unsafe sex, with multiple partners, is risky, but attempting to legislate against it is both impractical and too great an invasion of privacy and self-determination. However, public health officials might justifiably close the riskiest places (like the notorious Mineshaft), if this were likely to halt the spread of a deadly and expensive disease, both to protect nonvolunteers at risk, and to contain costs. The freedom to have sex with anonymous, multiple partners does not seem important enough to justify great public expense.

Other possible government action includes warning the sexual partners of those who test seropositive, or "contact-notification," a program that is being carried out in San Francisco. Such programs may be objected to on the ground that the individual's right to privacy and confidentiality is violated by revealing medical information without consent. The question of how doctors should weigh their obligation of confidentiality to the patient against their obligation of protection to members of the public, especially in light of *Tarasoff,* is a large and difficult one; I do not propose to undertake it here. Instead, I will address the question of whether the adverse effects on AIDS carriers should be considered in deciding whether to reveal their seropositivity to sexual partners.

The harm done to an individual by disclosure may be private and personal, or public and institutional. An example of the first kind would be the breakup of a marriage resulting from a wife learning that her husband is gay. Examples of the second include denying infected individuals insurance, jobs, and housing.

One way to safeguard individuals from harm from disclosure is to promise confidentiality. Contacts are told that they have been exposed, but not by whom. Some are worried that confidentiality simply cannot be assured, and that if official lists are created, this will lead to discrimination. In some settings (for example, prisons), this may be the case, but it seems unduly pessimistic in general. All steps should be taken to ensure confidentiality where possible.

However, confidentiality cannot be assured where there is only one sexual contact. A monogamous woman who is told that she has been exposed to AIDS will not only figure out who has infected her, but is also likely to conclude that her husband may be gay. Unfortunately, this is also the situation in which contact-notification is most clearly justified, because the woman is not a voluntary risk-taker. Some have argued against her being informed of her exposure, on the grounds that this will likely result in great harm to him, while offering her little or no protection. She has probably already been infected, nor is there presently a cure or treatment for AIDS. Isn't this a bit like closing the barn door after the horse is gone? It has even been suggested that the real motivation for informing her that she has been exposed to AIDS is to provide her with information about her husband's possible sexual orientation, something the state has no business doing.

However, there is evidence that repeated exposure to the AIDS virus increases the chance of infection. If she is informed, she can undergo testing to see if she has been infected. She can then decide whether to become pregnant. These health considerations, combined with her right to make informed decisions regarding her own welfare, make entirely reasonable "contact-notification" programs.

There is little anyone can do about the private and personal fall-out resulting from such notification. Nor does it seem to me to have much weight in this sort of scenario. The harm that befalls the husband he has brought on himself, through his own deception. He is not entitled to compound that deception now by keeping his wife uninformed of risks to her own life and health.

Considerably more can and should be done to protect AIDS carriers from discrimination. This is another example of justifiable coercion, only here the coercion is directed at those who would discriminate against AIDS victims. AIDS victims are especially vulnerable to discrimination, "irrationally ostracized by their communities because of medically baseless fears of contagion." Therefore, they come under Section 504 of the Rehabilitation Act of 1973, according to a draft opinion prepared in April 1986 by a member of the Justice Department's Civil Rights Division. However, in June 1986 the Justice Department's Office of Legal Counsel issued a ruling, permitting the dismissal of AIDS victims based on "fear of contagion." Assistant Attorney General Charles J. Cooper held that, although the "disabling effects" of AIDS were indeed a handicap, and could not be used as a basis for discrimination by employers, the ability to transmit the disease to others is not a handicap. Mr. Cooper concluded that the law did not prohibit the dismissal of AIDS victims based on fear of contagion, however irrational. Mr. Cooper said that the Rehabilitation Act is "certainly not a general prohibition against irrational decision making by employers." Employers who discriminate against people who are left-handed or red-haired may be acting irrationally, but Congress has not yet made such discrimination illegal.

According to Mr. Cooper's interpretation of the law, a sincere belief in contagion, however irrational, is sufficient to protect the employer. On this analysis, presumably an employer who sincerely believed cancer to be catching could fire a worker with leukemia with impunity. The analysis is bogus, and so is the protection it affords handicapped people. Fortunately, a number of states have rejected the interpretation and protect AIDS victims from discrimination under state law. In June 1988, a Presidential Commission urged a Federal ban against AIDS discrimination. So far, neither the President nor Congress has acted.[6]

CONCLUSION

Individuals have a moral and legal duty not to inflict serious harms on others. Reckless infliction of harm on those who do not willingly consent is seriously wrong: indeed, it may be the moral equivalent of murder. To protect nonvolunteers from fatal disease, the government is entitled to use coercive measures, so long as these are reasonably expected to be effective and as unrestrictive as possible. However, most coercive measures so far proposed are unlikely to be effective in controlling AIDS. Many seem motivated either by panic or hatred of gays or both. A government serious about stopping the AIDS epidemic would use resources in educational campaigns and treatment programs for heroin addicts. In addition, compassion and fairness require the use of legal coercion to protect AIDS victims from discrimination.

NOTES AND REFERENCES

1. Mill, *On Liberty,* Chap. 1, para. 9.
2. Gerald Dworkin, "Paternalism," in *Morality and the Law* (Richard A. Wasserstrom, ed.), Wadsworth Publishing Company Inc., California, 1971.
3. Joel Feinberg, "Wrongful Life and the Counterfactual Element in Harming," *Social Philosophy & Policy,* vol. 4, no. 1, 1986, 145–178. See also Feinberg, *Harm to Others,* Oxford University Press, New York, 1984, Chap. 1.
4. *The New York Times,* Tuesday, July 2, 1985, A11.
5. *Bioethics,* vol. 1, no. 1, January 1987, 35–50.
6. "Federal Policy Against Discrimination Is Sought for AIDS Victims," *The New York Times,* Thursday, September 22, 1988, A35.

QUESTIONS FOR COMPREHENSION AND REFLECTION

1. Do you agree with Steinbock's application of Mill's harm principle as a basis for offering a plausible justification of legal paternalism concerning AIDS? Support your answer.
2. What are the two flaws in Mohr's argument, according to Steinbock? Are her counterarguments sound? Why would protecting nonvoluntary risk-takers not be considered paternalistic?
3. Does Steinbock's position rely more on a utilitarian or a deontological approach? Support your answer.
4. Compare Steinbock's position with that of Rabinowitz. Are they making similar claims? Are their positions different? If so, in what ways? Explain your answer.

WORKING GROUP ON HIV TESTING OF PREGNANT WOMEN AND NEWBORNS

HIV Infection, Pregnant Women, and Newborns: A Policy Proposal for Information and Testing

The Working Group consists of physicians and philosophers from the departments of health policy and management at Johns Hopkins University School of Public Health, Johns Hopkins Hospital, Georgetown University Law Center, and the Kennedy Institute of Ethics. It opposes mandatory HIV testing of pregnant women and insists that women who do test should follow strict informed-consent guidelines. It argues that, rather than mandatory testing, there should be full-fledged efforts to educate pregnant women and new mothers about the hazards of HIV infection. Furthermore, preventing the vertical transmission of HIV should not be the aim of this education since such an aim would encourage reproductive decisions that are strictly matters of personal choice, such as abortion. Along these lines, the group argues that it would be unfair to target high-risk groups for counseling because such a policy would lead to further discrimination and stigmatization of these groups.

Among the many tragic dimensions of the human immunodeficiency virus (HIV) epidemic as it moves into the 1990s is the growing number of infected women, infants, and children. Women now constitute approximately 10% of the acquired immunodeficiency syndrome (AIDS) cases thus far reported to the Centers for Disease Control. Most of these women are of reproductive age. The U.S. Public Health Service has projected that there will be approximately 3000 cases of pediatric AIDS by the end of 1991. In most of these cases, infants will have acquired the infection through vertical transmission from their mothers.

As the public health impact of HIV infection in women and children has increased, so has interest in screening pregnant women and newborns for evidence of HIV infection. Currently, however, knowing that a pregnant woman is seropositive does not necessarily indicate that her fetus is or will be affected. Human immunodeficiency virus testing of the newborn reveals only the presence or absence of maternal antibodies and thus establishes if mothers are infected, not if the infants themselves are infected. It is currently estimated that in the United States about 30% of HIV-positive mothers transmit HIV to their newborn infants.

Whether among pregnant women or newborns, HIV disproportionately affects disadvantaged women and children of color, adding yet another layer of complexity to the policy problem of who should be screened. Currently, the Centers for Disease Control reports that over 70% of women with AIDS in the United States are African-American or Hispanic. The mode of transmission in most of these cases is intravenous drug use or sexual intercourse with an intravenous drug user.

Screening of pregnant women and newborns raises profound moral, legal, and policy issues. To date, no national professional association or committee has called for the mandatory screening of either pregnant women or newborns, although arguments favoring mandatory policies have appeared in the literature. . . . Numerous national groups have advocated offering testing to either all pregnant women or all "high-risk" pregnant women. In addition, some organizations and commentators have called for directive counseling to discourage HIV-infected women from becoming pregnant or bearing children.

This article presents a detailed 10-point program of policy recommendations for both pregnant women and newborns, and develops its rationale through the examination of potential objections and criticisms.

POLICY RECOMMENDATIONS

We advocate a policy of informing all pregnant women and new mothers about the epidemic of HIV infection and the availability of HIV testing. Although screening of either pregnant women or newborns is not the central focus of our policy, because we defend a consent requirement for testing our position can be interpreted as a policy of voluntary screening. In our view, a policy of mandatory screening either for pregnant women or for newborns is not justified in the current situation on traditional public health criteria or other grounds. Moreover, we reject implementation of counseling and screening policies that interfere with women's reproductive freedom or that result in the unfair stigmatization of vulnerable social groups. Our specific policy recommendations are as follows:

1. All pregnant women and new mothers should be informed about HIV infection and the

availability of HIV testing for themselves and their newborns. Informing of pregnant women should take place at the time of registration for prenatal care. Topics to be addressed are presented in the Table. (Ideally, all women should be informed about the HIV epidemic and HIV testing in advance of pregnancy, as part of preconception care. In addition, it may shortly be advisable, either because an intrapartum intervention becomes available or because it becomes desirable to manage third trimester HIV-positive women differently, to discuss HIV testing again late in pregnancy.)

2. The information to be presented to pregnant women and new mothers may be provided through printed or audiovisual materials. However, in communities with a significant degree of HIV infection or drug use, a personal discussion is of particular importance and should be conducted. Whatever method is selected, the information disclosed should cover the same topics and content (see Table) and should be presented in a

manner and language that is meaningful and understandable to the women served.

3. The information conveyed under recommendations 1 and 2 does not substitute for either pretest or posttest counseling. All women who express an interest in HIV testing for themselves or their newborns should receive personal pretest counseling; those tested should receive personal posttest counseling.

4. Both prenatal and newborn testing are to be voluntary, with a requirement of informed consent or parental consent. Consent for testing should be solicited only after pretest counseling.

5. The involvement of state and local health departments is essential to the successful implementation of this policy. Health departments should assume responsibility for developing and updating the educational materials referred to above, assuring the availability of materials in several languages, providing protocols and training for pretest and posttest counseling, and developing evaluation mechanisms to assume the proper conduct of the program. . . .

6. Health departments should also establish standards for laboratory procedures, including a requirement that all positive tests be confirmed on an independently drawn, second blood specimen prior to communicating results to the pregnant woman or new mother.

7. Every effort should be made to secure specialized medical interventions for the management of HIV infection, appropriate social services and supports, intensive primary care and abortion services (where requested by pregnant women) for all women and infants identified as HIV positive as a result of prenatal or newborn testing. All women should be informed of any difficulties in obtaining these interventions or services for themselves or their newborns. Specific obstacles to treatment or services should be discussed during pretest counseling with any woman interested in HIV testing for herself or her newborn.

8. Once it is established whether or not infants born to mothers who are HIV positive are infected with HIV, any medical or other records including information about HIV test results should be cor-

rected to verify either that the infant has been diagnosed as infected or that the infant is not HIV-infected.

9. To assure recommendation 7, regional networks of referral services for HIV-positive women and their infants should be established. Each network should assist health care providers with the medical management and counseling of HIV-positive women and their infants, and should offer supportive social services directly to pregnant women and new mothers.

10. Existing laws regarding medical confidentiality and antidiscrimination protections should be strengthened and specifically extended to persons with HIV infection to combat the harmful consequences associated with unavoidable disclosures or public identification of HIV status. The variation between state confidentiality and antidiscrimination protections should be replaced by a uniform, national policy.

MAJOR OBJECTIONS TO POLICY RECOMMENDATIONS

Our position is subject to several powerful criticisms or objections, both from the perspective of those who favor an aggressive screening policy and from those who have serious reservations about the propriety of any type of maternal or neonatal screening or testing.

Why Pregnant Women?

Why do we need a public policy on HIV screening of pregnant women? The justification for our policy proposals reflects the importance of four goals: (1) to advance the national campaign to educate the public about HIV disease and how it can be prevented; (2) to enhance the current and future reproductive choices of women; (3) to identify women and newborns who can benefit from medical advances in the clinical management of HIV infection; and (4) to allow proper obstetrical treatment of women infected with HIV. . . .

With the exception of our fourth goal, the goals of our policy are not specific to pregnant women. Goals 2 and 3 apply to all sexually active women, and goal 1 to all persons. Nonetheless, we have focused on pregnant women in this project for several reasons. First, the issue of vertical transmission has put pregnant women into the policy spotlight. In the near future, interventions may be available to reduce the rate of vertical transmission. We were motivated to head off policy directives that viewed pregnant women as mere vessels for the unborn or vectors of disease by developing policies respectful of the reproductive rights and interests of pregnant women. Second, we believe that primary medical care is a desirable setting for educating individuals about HIV disease and the availability of HIV testing. For many women, pregnancy is the only time when they have access to comprehensive primary care services. Among women who do not receive prenatal care—which often is the situation for women who are at particular risk for HIV disease—the postpartum hospital stay is, unfortunately, often the only opportunity afforded health care providers to discuss HIV infection and to attempt referral to appropriate medical services.

Why the Requirement of Consent?

Currently, it is common practice in obstetrics to order numerous screening tests without informing the patient or obtaining informed consent. Why should testing for evidence of HIV infection be treated differently?

There are important ways in which HIV testing differs from testing for other conditions. Unlike most routine screening tests in pregnancy, HIV testing identifies a potentially fatal illness. Perhaps most important, HIV testing raises special issues of privacy, reproductive choice, and social risk that are not applicable to most other screening tests ordered in pregnancy, with the exception of toxicological screening. Unlike, for example, prenatal testing for Rh factor, it cannot be argued that testing is clearly in the best interests of pregnant women and thus that proceeding based on clinical judgment without informed consent is justified. Although the nature and extent of the harms experienced by HIV-positive women have not been well documented, recent evidence suggests that poor, minority women risk the devastation of their personal and family relation-

ships, the loss of social and medical services, the loss of control of their own medical decisions, and even the loss of their children.

There is also no public health justification for mandatory screening of pregnant women. Although the state clearly has a legitimate interest in reducing the rate of transmission of HIV infection, it is not clear how mandatory screening in general, let alone mandatory screening of pregnant women, relates to this interest.

With regard to horizontal transmission, prevention is largely a function of voluntary changes in the behavior of individuals; there is no evidence that mandatory screening alters behavior more effectively than voluntary programs of education, counseling, and the offer of testing.

We specifically did not include prevention of vertical HIV transmission among the goals for our policy. The goal of reducing vertical transmission is ethically problematic, either in the case of policies designed to prevent future pregnancies or in policies aimed at terminating current pregnancies.

Achieving the public health goal of reducing vertical transmission through the promotion of abortion is morally unacceptable, even if it is argued that an HIV-infected woman's personal decision to terminate a pregnancy is morally permissible. The question of whether to terminate a pregnancy is among the most private and significant of life's choices, but certainly without interference by the state and without unsolicited advice or other undue influence from health professionals. Promoting abortion to achieve public health goals also is imprudent and (we believe) inappropriate public policy for a society deeply divided about the morality of abortion.

Apart from the implications of our society's divisive abortion debate, we have serious reservations about the use of abortion as a means of achieving public health goals of prevention. Preventing the birth of someone who would have an illness or disability is morally different from preventing illness or disability in persons already living. Two morally relevant differences merit greater attention.

First, a public health perspective that sees the two as equivalent—a case averted is a case averted—focuses too narrowly on the moral importance of health outcome to the exclusion of the relevance of the means to their achievement. Ronald Bayer, for example, argues that while it may be rational for an HIV-infected woman to bear children when she knows that there is an approximately 70% chance that the infant will not be infected, it may not be rational from a social point of view to treat the woman's decision as one in which society must remain neutral. He concludes that, from the social or public health perspective, the fiscal and human costs associated with pediatric AIDS provide strong arguments for a policy that urges infected women not to become pregnant. However, an argument that proceeds solely from an appeal to overall social outcomes is in danger of proving too much. Although the conclusion Bayer draws is limited, his appeal to overall social consequences, without more, forces us to judge alternative public policies only on one dimension—aggregate public health benefits. It is therefore indifferent to differences in the means to the production of public health benefits and can be used equally well to argue for policies prohibiting infected women from becoming pregnant or for recommending or compelling abortion, policies that Bayer does not appear to endorse. Although attention to comparative health outcomes is a central tenet of any public health perspective, it should not be the exclusive focus.

A second objection to treating the prevention of the birth of someone who would have an illness or disability as morally equivalent to preventing illness or disability in persons already living involves a morally unacceptable view of the social worth of such persons. Public policies aimed at discouraging persons with inheritable disabilities or illnesses from having children embody highly objectionable social affirmations of individual inequality. First, it denies that such persons have an equal right to participate in a highly valued aspect of the human experience—the begetting and raising of children. Second, it says to disabled and ill persons generally that the lives of some are not worth living and hence not entitled to a share of the social resources necessary for human flourishing. Third, it conveys the message that the presence of persons with disability or illness within society is to be understood only as an economic and social drain on

the aggregate and never as a source of enrichment for the lives of others.

Some of these same concerns cause us to have moral reservations about a public policy of reducing vertical transmission by attempting to influence HIV-positive pregnant women to delay or forgo future childbearing. Although the issue of abortion is removed, the importance of protecting reproductive choice from state interference remains, as do concerns about the propriety of preventing disease by preventing the birth of people who would have the disease. Although we recognize the importance of social interests in preventing vertical transmission, and the tragic lives many infants who have AIDS experience, on balance we are not persuaded that these interests override the opposing interests of women, minorities, and persons with disabilities in restricting the state from involvement in matters of reproductive choice.

Turning from prenatal to neonatal screening, there again is no clinical or public health justification for a mandatory policy. Currently, and for the foreseeable future, programs of newborn screening are de facto programs testing for HIV infection in the mother, not the infant. Thus, any policy for newborn screening must take into account the mother's privacy and autonomy interests. In addition, newborns and their mothers are a family unit; when HIV-infected mothers experience social or institutional discrimination, their infants suffer as well. Human immunodeficiency virus–positive newborns—70% of whom are not themselves infected—face the further risk of being abandoned by their mothers, difficulties with adoption and foster home placements, and difficulties in access to day care.

At present, the expected benefits to newborns from HIV testing do not clearly outweigh these risks or the privacy and autonomy interests of their mothers. . . .

Is Not a "Targeted" Program More Appropriate?

As noted earlier, HIV infection in women and children is a highly focal epidemic. It occurs disproportionately in poor women and children of color living in the inner cities of a few metropolitan areas. Would it not be more appropriate to target information and screening resources where there is the highest concentration of infection?

We reject a "targeted" policy for several reasons. Basing the offering of testing to pregnant women on an assessment of individual risk factors has been shown to be inefficient for both hepatitis and HIV infection. As a result, targeting would need to be based on proxies for individual risk such as sociodemographic criteria. Targeting by sociodemographic criteria is, however, invidiously discriminatory on its face. Unlike certain genetic conditions, there is no biological basis for targeting HIV programs by ethnicity. Although our program only calls for informing women about the HIV epidemic and the availability of voluntary testing, the targeting of this program to only poor women of color would send the false and dangerous message that, among women, only persons of this racial and ethnic description are at risk for HIV infection. Moreover, it labels all such women—the overwhelming majority of whom are not and never will be infected—as sources of contagion. The fact that groups identified as "carrying the virus" for AIDS suffer discrimination, social prejudice, and hardship has been well documented with regard to gay men. Poor women and children of color already suffer these burdens disproportionately. Thus, to add the stigma of AIDS contagion to poor women of color is to further harm a group of persons who are already unfairly disadvantaged.

Targeting based on community prevalence rates, rather than sociodemographic criteria, is also morally problematic. Substantial efficiency is not likely to occur unless "high prevalence areas" are narrowly defined. The more narrow this definition is, the greater the potential that community prevalence rates become merely thinly veiled proxies for ethnicity and poverty. Targeting by prevalence rates would also place an inappropriate burden on women in "low prevalence areas" who have risk factors for HIV infection and for whom testing may be beneficial. In the absence of a policy such as we propose, these women may be unaware either of being at increased risk or of how to obtain testing. Certain women, such as migrant workers, might be particularly ill served.

There are also public health arguments against targeting. As noted previously, targeting may serve to create or reinforce in women who are outside the targeted group the dangerous view that they are invulnerable to HIV. Targeting thus could undermine the public health objective of universal adoption of safer sex and drug use practices. In addition, informing women about the HIV epidemic is of value in all areas of the country. There is some reason to suspect that the current epidemiological pattern of HIV infection among women and children may be shifting. . . . An informed public is our best defense against today's low-prevalence community becoming tomorrow's newest area of outbreak. Of particular concern are communities with significant drug use problems but as yet no significant HIV infection.

It might be argued that in rejecting targeting we have failed to understand what justice requires in the case of poor and minority women. Specifically, in this instance, justice may require not equal treatment but the provision of greater benefits to the worst-off members of society. Targeting, because it is more efficient, would presumably provide greater benefits to the women in the program. In order for this claim to be substantiated, however, it would first have to be established that the benefits of a targeted program to poor women of color outweigh the harms of stigma and labeling discussed earlier. Given our nation's unfortunate history with regard to the treatment of minorities, women, and the poor, it is not surprising that some read in a policy of targeting not a desire to do good, but an agenda of genocide. . . .

CONCLUSION

In the face of the complex issues and uncertainties that surround HIV infection and diagnosis in pregnant women and infants, any policy proposal is likely to be controversial and in some respects unsatisfactory. We have presented the 10 core elements of a policy that we believe represents the best compromise of competing interests and social goals. This policy is sensitive to the current medical and social facts; we examine the implications of anticipated future developments on our recommendations elsewhere.

We do not expect our policy recommendations to have any immediate or isolated effect on HIV transmission rates. It is unrealistic to expect any program of information about HIV infection and the availability of testing to, by itself, affect transmission rates, let alone a program directed at women, given the history of inequality of power and the legacy of sexual subordination that all too often still characterize relations between men and women in our society. We do believe, however, that educational programs can make a difference. With regard to smoking, it has been established that while individual education efforts were largely ineffective, the cumulative impact of multiple educational efforts in a sustained national antismoking campaign dramatically altered cultural values and reduced the prevalence of smoking. It is to be hoped that, over time, our nation will have a similar experience with HIV infection.

Nevertheless, a comprehensive policy response to controlling the HIV epidemic requires a broader focus than we have adopted herein. Human immunodeficiency virus disease in women and children is a disease of families and, as noted above, is intimately connected to relations between men and women. Any comprehensive policy must address the needs and interests of men as well as women and must address the root of the problem of HIV infection in women—drug dependency and the poverty and social isolation that make the use of drugs attractive. Without adequate drug rehabilitation services and social policies and programs that can empower both disadvantaged women and men to break the cycle of poverty that links them to drug use, policies of public information and the availability of HIV testing cannot be expected to significantly affect the pace of the HIV epidemic.

QUESTIONS FOR COMPREHENSION AND REFLECTION

1. Do you think that the group's policy recommendation to inform and advise will actually lead to preventing the spread of HIV infection? Support your answer.
2. Why is the prevention of vertical transmission of HIV not a feasible policy goal, according to the working group? Do you agree with the group's rationale? Explain.
3. Is the group's rejection of a targeting policy more in line with a utilitarian or a deontological perspective? Support your answer.
4. How would you apply the group's position to the situation of pregnant women in developing countries such as Africa?

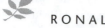

RONALD BAYER

Ethical Challenges Posed by Zidovudine Treatment to Reduce Vertical Transmission of HIV

Ronald Bayer is a professor of public health at Columbia University in New York City. Bayer argues that HIV testing of pregnant women must be voluntary and that public funds must be utilized to support treatment and counseling programs. He gives three sets of reasons—medical, ethical, and practical—why mandatory testing of pregnant women is not justified, despite the apparent success rate of zidovudine (ZDV or AZT) in reducing vertical transmission. He goes on to cite the uncertainty regarding risks associated with AZT. Moreover, he contends that any treatment for HIV must be provided in accordance with the standards of informed consent. At the same time, he supports compulsory testing of infants as long as it benefits them by either extending or saving their life.

In February 1994 the Data and Safety Monitoring Board of the National Institute of Allergy and Infectious Diseases recommended the interruption of a clinical trial designed to determine whether the administration of zidovudine to pregnant women infected with the human immunodeficiency virus (HIV) and to their newborns could reduce the rate of vertical viral transmission. Given the responsibilities of the Data and Safety Monitoring Board, there was no alternative. The difference in the rate of transmission between those receiving zidovudine and those receiving placebo was statistically significant (P = 0.00006). Women who received zidovudine had a transmission rate of 8.3 percent, as compared with 25.5 percent among those who received placebo—a reduction in the risk of transmission of 67.3 percent. The results of this trial (known as Protocol 076) appear in this issue of the *Journal*.[1]

Many questions remain unanswered. Most critically, will the administration of zidovudine to pregnant women and their newborns pose a risk to the 70 to 80 percent of children who, though born to infected women, would not themselves have been

infected? Is there some risk that the use of zidovudine during pregnancy will diminish the effectiveness of the drug when the woman's own clinical course would suggest the advisability of antiretroviral treatment.[2]

Nevertheless, in the otherwise bleak clinical picture that has surrounded AIDS, especially since the report last year that early use of zidovudine in HIV infection had no apparent effect on clinical outcome,[3] these findings represent very good news. In the clinical alert issued by the National Institutes of Health on February 20, 1994, the prospect of a "substantial potential benefit" was juxtaposed with the possibility of "unknown long-term risks."[4]

The prospect of such benefit has led many clinicians to argue that the case for testing pregnant women for HIV infection is stronger than ever. Nevertheless, many advocates for patients with AIDS and proponents of women's rights have expressed skepticism about the claims made on behalf of zidovudine treatment during pregnancy. Some have charged that an effort to modify current practice on the basis of the new finding would constitute "malpractice."[5] Driving such skepticism has been the fear that the new clinical findings would be used to override the privacy rights of pregnant women at risk for HIV, the vast majority of whom are poor black or Hispanic women.

These fears and the extent to which the new findings have produced anxiety instead of elation must be understood in the context of a history of efforts to impose treatment, even invasive procedures, on pregnant women in the interests of the offspring,[6-8] and of national surveys that indicate that the vast majority of physicians favor mandatory screening of pregnant women.[9] Mandatory screening usually refers to testing whose results can be linked to a particular woman in the absence of her consent and despite her express refusal. Most pertinently, the reaction to Protocol 076 was shaped by the fierce and widely reported debate in New York over mandatory screening of newborns for HIV. That debate and its outcome shed light on the important similarities and differences in ethics and politics between screening newborns and screening pregnant women.

In 1993 the New York state legislature considered, but ultimately rejected, a proposal by a legislator, long a defender of the reproductive rights of women, to end the mandatory blinded serologic surveillance of newborns and to replace it with a system of mandatory screening of newborns for the purposes of case finding. Opponents of blinded surveillance were appalled that it could determine how many but not which babies carried maternal antibody to HIV.[10] Yet it was the very fact that no child or mother could be identified that had, for many, rendered such surveillance without consent ethically acceptable.[11-13] On the other hand, others believed that the prospects for early clinical intervention in infected infants required that each baby who could benefit from such care receive it. To them, the right of the child to treatment was held to be more compelling than the mother's claim to privacy. Among those supporting the bill for mandatory unblinded testing of newborns were two of the three state branches of the American Academy of Pediatrics and *The New York Times,* which termed the concern about maternal privacy in this instance "theological."[14]

Undergirding the position of those who supported mandatory unblinded screening of newborns was the ethical principle that the state had a special responsibility to protect the medical interests of the child, even when such protection necessitated, in rare instances, overriding parental refusal.[15,16] This principle has long been reflected in, for example, the well-established practice of providing blood transfusions to the children of Jehovah's Witnesses despite parental objection. Even more relevant is the practice of mandatory or quasi-mandatory testing of newborns for a host of inborn metabolic conditions.[17]

Much of the opposition to mandatory unblinded testing of newborns centered on the principle that no woman should ever be compelled to undergo testing for HIV. Since the mandatory testing of newborns in fact entailed the mandatory identification of infection in their mothers, the proposed policy was deemed ethically and politically unacceptable. More important than this principle for the outcome of the debate was the fact that despite advances in the management of HIV disease, early treatment could do little to affect fundamentally the life expectancy of HIV-infected children. If it were possible to save the lives of such children or to extend them dramatically, the weight of ethical argument as well as the political picture would undoubtedly change.[18] In my view, the case for unblinded screening and treatment of newborns does not yet outweigh the privacy claims of the mother.

But if the prospect of radical improvement in the welfare of children could justify mandatory screening of newborns, why have there been so few calls for the mandatory unblinded testing of pregnant women in the light of the results of Protocol 076? Not surprisingly, intense opposition to mandatory screening during pregnancy for case-finding purposes has come from the proponents of privacy who also opposed compulsory newborn testing on principled grounds. But advocates of mandatory screening of newborns have also been loath to embrace compulsory testing of pregnant women. Why has this been so? The answer lies in the difference between the status of newborns and the status of adults. Mandatory screening of children could become justifiable if therapeutic interventions could substantially extend the lives of infected children, because treatment, regardless of parental objections, would be imperative. By contrast, the mandatory screening of pregnant women is objectionable because mandatory treatment of competent adults is virtually never acceptable. Although some states require the screening of all pregnant women for hepatitis[19] and syphilis, in general the principle of informed consent guarantees that adults have a right to refuse care, even lifesaving care. This is so even when others view the refusal of treatment as foolish or irresponsible. In view of the remaining uncertainties about the long-term consequences of zidovudine treatment during pregnancy for both the mother and her offspring, the principle of consent to both screening and treatment is even more relevant.

There are also matters of practical concern. The pragmatic aspects alone of the treatment regimen defined in Protocol 076 make the prospect of therapy without the full cooperation of infected pregnant women difficult to contemplate. Even if one sought to mandate the use of an intravenous dose of zidovudine during delivery, how could one enforce a daily regimen of five doses of zidovudine during the second and third trimesters of pregnancy? Would anything short of incarceration make such treatment possible?

Thus, both ethics and practicality dictate the rejection of compulsory treatment of pregnant women. What is needed are strong efforts to persuade women to be tested for HIV and to encourage those who are infected to undergo zidovudine treatment after being fully informed of the benefits and the uncertain, but remote, prospects of long-term negative consequences. That is precisely the conclusion reached by the Public Health Service task force convened to consider the implications of Protocol 076.[20]

If mandatory unblinded screening and treatment of pregnant women cannot be justified, ensuring access to zidovudine treatment for pregnant women does raise important issues of a different order. Obstetricians must be encouraged to offer HIV testing to pregnant women—especially those who live in communities where the seroprevalence

of the virus is high. Making that possible will require considering whether the sometimes elaborate requirements for extensive counseling before testing, mandated by law in some states, are compatible with the new clinical prospects. This issue is especially relevant in the overburdened obstetrical services of America's inner cities. Making testing routine while preserving the right of informed consent will be a great challenge.

More important, no recommendation for HIV testing would be ethical if access to the needed therapy and support was not ensured. Given the failure of the American health care system to guarantee access to health care, given that too many women at risk for HIV receive either no perinatal care or inadequate care, and given the poverty of the overwhelming majority of women who are infected, it is by no means certain that the scientific breakthrough represented by Protocol 076 will evoke the necessary social response.

No comment on the importance of the finding that zidovudine may radically reduce the rate of HIV transmission from infected women to their babies should fail to note that this major therapeutic achievement will have little or no effect on women in developing nations, where the toll of pediatric AIDS is most severe. Whether the wealthy nations of the world will be able and willing to make zidovudine available to the poorest nations will determine the course of the global epidemiology of pediatric AIDS. It will also tell us much about the extent to which our capacity for compassion can match our capacity for scientific progress.

NOTES

1. Spector S. A., Gelber R. D., McGrath N., et al. A controlled trial of intravenous immune globulin for the prevention of serious bacterial infections in children receiving zidovudine for advanced human immunodeficiency virus infection. *N Engl J Med* 331: 1181–7, 1994.
2. Zidovudine for mother, fetus, and child: Hope or poison? *Lancet* 344: 207–9, 1994.
3. Concorde Coordinating Committee. Concorde: MRC/ANRS randomised double-blind controlled trial of immediate and deferred zidovudine in symptom-free HIV infection. *Lancet* 343: 871–81, 1994.

4. Connor E. M., Sperling R. S., Gelber R., et al. Reduction of maternal–infant transmission of human immunodeficiency virus type 1 with zidovudine treatment. *N Engl J Med* 331: 1173–80, 1994.

5. HIV positive mothers know use of AZT, not approved for pregnant women, does not support unblinding newborn HIV testing. Press release of C.U.R.E. AIDS! New York, March 29, 1994.

6. Annas G. J. Forced caesareans: The most unkindest cut of all. *Hastings Cent Rep* 1982; 12(3): 16, 17, 45.

7. Kolder V. E. B., Gallagher J., Parsons M. T. Court-ordered obstetrical interventions. *N Engl J Med* 316: 1192–6, 1987.

8. Nelson L. J., Milliken N. Compelled medical treatment of pregnant women: life, liberty, and law in conflict. *JAMA* 259: 1060–6, 1988.

9. Colombotos J., Messeri P., McConnell M. B., et al. Physicians, nurses and AIDS: Findings from a national study. Research report No. 1. Rockville, Md: Agency for Health Care Policy and Research, 1994. (AHCPR publication no. 93-0043.)

10. It's a baby, not a statistic, stupid. Press release from the office of State Senator N. Meyersohn, New York, July 1993.

11. Bayer R. The ethics of blinded HIV surveillance testing. *Am J Public Health* 83: 496–7, 1993.

12. Guidelines on ethical and legal conditions in anonymous unlinked HIV seroprevalence research. Ottawa, Ont.: Government of Canada Federal AIDS Centre, May 1988.

13. Unlinked anonymous screening for the public health surveillance of HIV infections: proposed international guidelines. Geneva: World Health Organization Global Programme on AIDS, 1989.

14. AIDS babies pay the price. *New York Times*. 13 August, 1993: A26.

15. Faden R. R., Holtzman N. A., Chwalow A. J. Parental rights, child welfare, and public health: The case of PKU screening. *Am J Public Health* 72: 1396–400, 1982.

16. Screening and counseling for genetic conditions. Washington, D.C.: President's Commission for the Study of Ethical Problems in Medicine and Biomedical and Behavioral Research, 1983.

17. Institute of Medicine. Assessing genetic risks: implications for health and social policy. Washington, D.C.: National Academy Press, 1994.

18. Fleischman A. R., Post L. F., Dubler N. N. Mandatory newborn screening for human immunodeficiency virus. *Bull N Y Acad Med* 71: 4–17, 1994.

19. Maternal hepatitis B screening practices—California, Connecticut, Kansas, and United States, 1992–1993. *MMWR Morb Mortal Wkly Rep* 43: 311, 317–20, 1994.

20. Recommendations of the U.S. Public Health Service Task Force on the use of zidovudine to reduce perinatal transmission of human immunodeficiency virus. *MMWR Morb Mortal Wkly Rep* 43(RR-11): 1–20, 1994.

QUESTIONS FOR COMPREHENSION AND REFLECTION

1. Although Protocol 076 strongly suggests that a regimen of zidovudine would most likely reduce the prospects of vertical transmission of HIV, what medical concerns still exist? Are these medical unknowns sufficient and compelling reasons to prohibit mandatory screening of pregnant women? Do you agree with Bayer? Support your answers.

2. According to Bayer and others, mandatory screening would violate the privacy rights of pregnant women. Why would this be especially burdensome for poor black and Hispanic women? Do you agree with the author's position? Explain.

3. Despite his objection to the mandatory screening of pregnant women, Bayer argues that the required screening of newborns would be justified. Under what conditions does he hold this screening to be legitimate, and what is his rationale? Do you agree? Explain.

4. In light of the chapter's discussion regarding vaccine testing in Africa, do you think research efforts in the United States regarding zidovudine would have any positive outcome for women who are infected with AIDS in developing countries such as Africa? Explain.

CASES FOR ANALYSIS*

1. Gay Bathhouses

In New York City, there are a few bathhouses where gay men can meet freely for both social and sexual encounters. Here they have the opportunity to get together without fear of public approbation and stigma. Furthermore, they can meet anonymously and therefore not have to worry about their identities being revealed, with all the negative repercussions that that might entail. These bathhouses have established certain regulations that require the safe practice of sex in order to prevent the transmission of sexually transmitted diseases, particularly AIDS.

However, in the past few months, some politicians have been lobbying for a bill to close down the bathhouses. They claim that the required precautions remain virtually impossible to enforce. They argue that the clubs cannot monitor a person's sexual behavior in any meaningful way. There is strong public support to close down the bathhouses. On the other hand, gay rights advocates clearly oppose such a bill.

DISCUSSION QUESTIONS

1. Suppose you are a city council member and other politicians backing the bill request your support. What should you do? Explain.
2. How does this case relate to the exceptionalist approach to AIDS? It is well established that heavy drinking of alcohol takes place in bars and nightclubs. Should they be closed down? Explain.
3. Mohr addresses the value our society places on independence and the freedom to put ourselves at risk. He opposes the closing of gay bathhouses. How would you apply his analysis to this issue? Do you agree or disagree? Support your answer.

2. Charles Shaeffer

Charles Shaeffer is a postal worker in New York City. During the course of his routine physical exam, he had a blood test and was diagnosed as HIV positive. Charles is bisexual. Not suspecting the possibility of infection, he is shattered by the news of his condition. He is particularly angry at his male partner, Tom, with whom he shares an apartment. He suspects that he may have contracted the virus from Tom, who appears to have kept his HIV-positive condition secret.

Charles confronts Tom, who insists that he does not know his HIV status. Tom also maintains that, if he had known he was HIV positive, he would have told Charles at the beginning of their relationship. Nevertheless, Charles is so angry that he leaves Tom and moves to another apartment. Furthermore, he wants to get even and convinces himself that one way to get even is to have unprotected sex with as many strangers as possible. He decides to embark on a spree of deliberately infecting unsuspecting others.

---

*Names and cases are fictitious unless noted otherwise.

DISCUSSION QUESTIONS

1. Without any doubt, Charles's decision is irresponsible as well as unethical. Are those who engage freely in sexual relations with Charles acting irresponsibly as well? Unethically? Support your answers.
2. How would you apply the principle of informed consent to engaging in a sexual relationship? In what ways do Charles's activities make informed consent problematic?
3. Do you believe there should be laws protecting Charles's victims if he were to deliberately infect others with the AIDS virus? How would such laws reflect moral concerns in this case?

3. Gina Austin

Gina Austin is a manager at a prestigious bank in Indianapolis. She has been regularly using crack cocaine for over two years. George, Gina's sexual partner for over a year, is aware of her drug habits. In fact, he also uses crack, though not as regularly as does Gina. They live together in a small townhouse just outside the city. He has encouraged her to be tested for HIV infection. Gina has constantly refused to be tested. Finally, she agrees to be tested and tests positive.

However, Gina decides not to tell George. She does not want anything to upset their relationship, which, apart from her drug habit, has been going smoothly. She is also hoping that they can marry someday. When George inquires about the test results, Gina lies and indicates that the results were negative.

DISCUSSION QUESTIONS

1. Gina's refusal to inform her partner of her HIV status appears unethical. Does her partner have a moral responsibility to see that he is informed? Support your answer.
2. Has George contributed in any way to the risks they both run? Explain.
3. Is this case different from case 2? If so, in what way? If not, why not?

4. Dr. Tom Holbein

Thirty-six-year-old Dr. Holbein is considered by his colleagues to be one of the most promising heart surgeons in the metropolitan area. Not only is he well respected by his coworkers, but he is genuinely admired by his patients. He spends much time speaking with his patients and showing a genuine concern for their well-being. He makes every effort to respect their autonomy. As a result, he treats numerous patients.

In the course of a regular medical exam, he discovers that he is HIV positive. He believes that the only way the AIDS virus could have been transmitted to him was through infected blood while operating on a patient. Tomorrow morning, he is scheduled to perform coronary bypass surgery. He is convinced that, with proper precautions, there is no chance that he will transmit the virus to his patient. He decides to go ahead with the surgery and chooses not to disclose his status to his patient.

DISCUSSION QUESTIONS

1. Should Holbein reveal his condition to his patient before surgery? How does his resistance to disclosure affect the quality of informed consent on the part of the patient? Support your answers.

2. How would you approach this issue, utilizing a utilitarian perspective?
3. Provide a deontological examination of the issues involved. Would your deontological perspective provide a resolution different from that of the utilitarian approach? Explain.
4. How would you apply Steinbock's analysis to this case?

5. Robin Smith

Robin Smith is a twenty-seven-year-old African American. She is in her seventh week of pregnancy with her first child, and she and her husband, Aaron, are thrilled with the prospect of being parents. The state they live in has recently proposed legislation that would require HIV testing for all pregnant women. The legislation has not yet been passed, but it will soon be up for a vote. Robin is anxious about the proposal. She has never been addicted to any drug, but in the past she has occasionally tried crack cocaine. At one time, she took heroin. She fears the possibility of testing positive for HIV. Moreover, she fears the possibility of transmitting the virus, if she has it, to her baby.

In her community, advocates for women's rights are obtaining signatures to put through a referendum that would oppose the proposed bill. Advocates of the referendum are arguing that the proposed bill acts to violate the rights of pregnant women by forcing testing on them without their consent. They also claim that, even if the bill passes, there is no guarantee that treating infected women would be effective.

Robin's community representatives come to her home to obtain her signature. Aaron is very much in favor of the proposed legislation and refuses to sign the form. However, Robin believes that she should sign the petition.

DISCUSSION QUESTIONS

1. Should Robin sign the petition opposing the new bill? Support your answer.
2. Suppose you are a principal supporter of the proposed bill. What reasons would you give to defend it? How would you argue against the position stated by the Working Group on HIV Testing of Pregnant Women and Newborns?
3. Would you support a bill that required the testing of all newborns? Give your reasons. In view of this case, how would you apply and respond to Ronald Bayer's analysis?
4. Should Robin herself request that she be screened for HIV in order to lessen her chances of transmitting the virus to her child? Support your answer.

6. The Hospital and the Prison

Scripps Memorial Hospital is a community hospital that serves a community within a radius of approximately 45 miles with just over 220 beds. It is located about 20 miles from the state prison, a maximum-security prison for men that is one of the largest in the state, with over 15,000 prisoners.

There have recently been a number of cases of HIV infection among the prisoners, and they have been taken to Scripps for treatment. Eight prisoners are being treated at the community hospital. Many people in the surrounding community have protested the treatment of the prisoners in their hospital, arguing that they should be cared for elsewhere. A number of health professionals who work at the hospital agree, claiming that beds are being taken from other community members who need them. In fact, some physicians and nurses have been refused to care for the prisoners.

Many other healthcare professionals disagree. They claim that the prisoners constitute part of the community and that the aim of the hospital is to serve all needy members of the community without exception. Administrators have made it clear that all medical and nursing staff are required to care for all patients, including prisoners with AIDS.

DISCUSSION QUESTIONS

1. Suppose you are part of the medical or nursing staff. Do you think that the institutional requirement is unfair, or do you agree with it? Explain.
2. Should Scripps care for prisoners who contract the AIDS virus? Are the prisoners part of the surrounding community? Why or why not? Support your answers.
3. How would you address this issue from a deontological perspective? How would Steinbock's analysis and interpretation of Mill's harm principle apply?

7. Francis Connerton

AZT, or zidovudine, has been shown to be somewhat effective in diminishing the destructive effects of AIDS. However, the costs of AZT treatment are quite prohibitive. In addition, there seem to be highly toxic side effects. Not all patients can tolerate AZT treatment.

Francis Connerton, one of the top researchers on the effects of AZT and well respected in his field, has been consulted by a research firm to give his advice regarding the continued testing of AZT and ways to reduce its side effects. The research firm wants to conduct test trials of AZT in areas where AIDS is most prevalent, particularly sub-Saharan Africa and Southeast Asia. Because of his high standing among scientists, the firm is seeking Connerton's endorsement of these trials and is ready to pay him quite well if he himself will direct the research. Connerton, however, is well aware of some of the issues regarding conducting trials in developing countries and needs time to think about the offer.

DISCUSSION QUESTIONS

1. From a utilitarian perspective, would the benefits of conducting these trials outweigh the burdens? In your opinion, who would stand to gain the most from these trials? Explain.
2. If you were Connerton, would you accept the firm's offer? Why or why not?
3. What are some of the issues related to conducting trials in developing countries? Are such trials, to some degree, a form of exploitation? How does the issue of informed consent apply?

8. Zainabu Kasoga

Zainabu Kasoga is a twenty-six-year-old mother of three children who lives in a small village in Uganda. She was first married when she was eighteen and has had no formal education, yet Zainabu manages to take care of her family pretty much by herself. Her husband, Kessete, works for a large company 110 miles from the village. Since the family has no automobile and must rely on a bus, Kessete lives most of the time in the city.

Zainabu was diagnosed with HIV infection just over two months ago. She is convinced that she was infected by her husband, since he has been her only sexual contact. In the past few weeks, American researchers have been visiting her village in order to recruit volunteers for clinical trials they are conducting. The purpose of these trials is to test a possible AIDS vaccine. Hoping that she will eventually benefit from the new drug, Zainabu has volunteered to be a subject.

DISCUSSION QUESTIONS

1. Can Zainabu genuinely give informed consent to be a human subject for these trials? Explain.
2. What ethical issues are involved in testing Zainabu and other illiterate human subjects?
3. Contrast a utilitarian and a deontological approach to this issue. Would Zainabu and other subjects benefit from the research? If so, in what way?

C H A P T E R 1 0

Challenges in Healthcare Policy and Reform

In 1989, an estimated 400,000 Oregonians lacked health coverage. Less than 40 percent of these people were unemployed. That meant that most Oregonians who were uninsured were working and ineligible to receive **Medicaid,** the public assistance program for the poor. Each state sets its own eligibility requirements for Medicaid, and Oregon's eligibility level was set at 58 percent below the federal poverty level, which in 1989 was $12,000 per year for families. This meant that families that earned over $6,960 per year were not eligible for funding.[1] Therefore, most of the uninsured in Oregon were contributing to a system from which they could not benefit.

In order to address this inequity, the Oregon legislature passed the Oregon Basic Health Services Act in April 1989, and elaborate steps were taken to reform the state's system so it would eventually insure all its citizens. The process was complex and involved public hearings, statewide community meetings, phone surveys, and input from medical professionals in order to prioritize medical services. The goal of insuring all Oregonians required limiting the kinds of healthcare services offered. This entailed ranking medical conditions and their respective treatments in order of importance.

The controversial plan, approved in March 1993, involves a phasing-in process. Hence, it will take several years to assess its outcome. Supporters of the plan favor it for a number of reasons. To begin with, although the poor will be the ones who are initially targeted for the rationing of medical services, the plan still provides them with reasonable access to basic healthcare services. The poor will be much better off than they were before. Supporters also praise the process of seeking community consensus in a democratic fashion throughout the formulation of the plan.

Critics, however, point out that the scope of the plan, despite its aim of **universal access,** is unfair because it targets poor mothers and children by limiting their coverage under the new prioritization. Previously, poor mothers and children in the Aid to Families with Dependent Children program (AFDC) had virtually unlimited coverage. Furthermore, critics claim that targeting the poor is blatantly unfair, since it leads to a social line being drawn between the so-called poor who receive public aid and those who can afford private insurance. Critics also question whether and to what extent the public should be involved in public policy and medical decisions. They also challenge the efficacy of ranking separate conditions and treatments, since such separate ranking does not take into consideration **comorbidity,** the presence of two or more coexisting medical disorders, for example, when an individual suffers from both hypertension and diabetes. The Oregon plan ranks conditions and their treatments separately, while patients often suffer multiple, coexisting conditions. Another prominent criticism of the plan is that prioritization of healthcare services may have an adverse effect on the relationship between healthcare provider and patient in that it could reinforce a two-tiered healthcare system. This in turn could bring about a practice of sustaining two standards of healthcare: a lower standard for patients whose services are prioritized, and a higher standard for patients affluent enough to afford a wider range of services.[2]

CURRENT POLICIES IN U.S. HEALTHCARE

The crisis that Oregon faces is a microcosm of the broader crisis in the U.S. healthcare system. The healthcare system in the United States is the most expensive in the world, with healthcare costs accounting for about 14 percent of the gross national product (GNP). Are Americans reaping the benefits of this monumental investment? Nearly 40 million Americans, 20 percent of the population, have no health coverage. Yet, as Amy Gutmann points out in her article at the end of this chapter, equal and universal access to healthcare maximizes self-respect for all citizens in a democracy. Also, mortality rates, especially for infants, minorities, and the poor, are exceptionally high, and one out of every three children remains impoverished.[3] Life expectancy in the United States is lower than that of other industrialized nations.

Why is U.S. healthcare so costly and its outcome so inadequate? One reason is that the American use of medical technologies is extensive, perhaps to a large extent because of widespread public expectations regarding medicine. Many more of these new technologies seem to be touted through public advertisements. One television commercial in Pittsburgh, for example, depicted a new type of laser surgery for the eyes. Throughout the thirty-second commercial, a Gregorian chant provides the background music, a subtle way of impressing on the viewer a sort of divine sanction of the new procedure. Public exposure to medical technologies increases public expectations, and the more medical "miracles" we achieve, the more demands we place on our healthcare system.

The maximal use of medical technologies is not the same as their optimal use. For example, magnetic resonance imaging (MRI), an extremely expensive procedure, certainly constitutes a great advance in diagnosis, and healthcare professionals in the United States use these MRIs more than medical workers in any other country. Chicago alone performs more MRIs than all of Australia. Some critics charge that MRIs tend to be overused as well as inappropriately used.

Another reason why U.S. healthcare is so costly is that our medical philosophy is basically crisis-oriented, with more emphasis on rescuing than on preventing. There is certainly a growing emphasis on prevention medicine through promotion of good diet and healthy life-styles, measures that are less costly than acute care interventions. However, most research efforts and funding support still go to acute-care medicine and intervention, which in turn means more reliance on sophisticated and costly technologies. The U.S. healthcare system also has a blemished history of excessive and unnecessary use of tests and treatments, including numerous instances of unnecessary surgery such as the immoderate use of cesarean sections and radical mastectomies.

CULTURAL WINDOWS

THE CATHOLIC TRADITION OF THE COMMON GOOD

Throughout Catholic teachings, one of the most important themes is that of the **common good.** This idea of the common good is a crucial principle in Roman Catholic theology and its ongoing social teachings. What the common good means is that each individual, as well as the community as a whole, has a moral responsibility to work in ways that will develop and enhance the good of the community. The communal good necessarily entails recognizing all critical needs—physical, material, and spiritual. Since addressing our healthcare needs is a condition for individual and communal development, any attempt at healthcare reform must consider the primacy of this common good. Healthcare ethicist Mary Therese Connors puts it this way:

Health care is an instrumental good for human persons, but it must not be viewed as a separate entity apart from other community concerns which promote or impede human flourishing.[4]

In light of Catholic teachings, especially more recent statements such as the 1986 document "Economic Justice for All: Catholic Social Teaching and the U.S. Economy," from the National Conference of Catholic Bishops, this means that individual considerations of autonomy are not absolute. Despite the emphasis American culture places on individual autonomy, it does not assume priority in every given instance. Even though American healthcare ethics strongly underscores the importance of patient autonomy, Catholic teachings point out that the needs of the community must remain uppermost.

Catholic teachings endorse universal access to a decent core package of healthcare services for everyone, regardless of their socioeconomic status. This basic package must incorporate basic healthcare needs that are standard and must address the healthcare needs and priorities of the community as a whole in order to procure the common good. Yet the common good cannot be developed if the U.S. healthcare system continues to distribute healthcare on the basis of ability to pay. The document from the National Conference of Bishops specifically targets the poor as having a special moral right to services, since they have been discriminated against in the past. Working for the common good, in the Catholic tradition, means addressing the needs of the poor. This requires guaranteeing a decent core package of healthcare services for everyone.

The Catholic teaching of the common good is complemented by the equally important principle of subsidiarity. The principle of subsidiarity means that one enhances the common good by focusing most importantly on the needs of one's local community. The primary parameters, therefore, are set by the local community and its needs. Subsidiarity requires that "responsibility for an action should not progress to a higher, or less local level, than is necessary."[5] In this light, any fair attempt at healthcare reform must be primarily community-oriented.

We must keep in mind that it is often the patients who demand these tests and treatments.

Without a doubt, the U.S. healthcare system is in drastic need of reform, yet healthcare policy and reform are notoriously complex subjects. No other area in healthcare ethics more squarely confronts us with the agonizing choice between the well-being of individual patients and the welfare of the group. Issues in healthcare policy and reform force us to inspect our deep-seated values and beliefs and to rank these values in a meaningful order of priority. This chapter is about setting priorities—not simply the priorities we all have as individuals, but the collective priorities of the community in which we live. The challenge lies in finding a set of values that can provide a common ground from which we can adequately address these ethical issues in their political, economic, and social contexts.

THE CHALLENGE IN MACROALLOCATION

A city's healthcare office has limited funds for health expenditures. A local group of prominent cardiologists and cardiothoracic surgeons want to establish a heart transplant center in the city. They believe that the necessary facilities and personnel for such a center are available within the city's hospitals and that there is a genuine need for heart transplants among the region's population. They submit a formal request to use the remaining healthcare funds for their project. The same city has a consortium of nursing homes. Many of these homes require extensive repair and upgrading. The high rate of turnover among the nursing-home staff also places greater burdens on the existing staff. There have been chronic complaints about the homes and the quality of life for the residents. The consortium feels the need to upgrade conditions and increase and improve staff. It formally requests use of the city's limited funds to accomplish this upgrading. Each project requires nearly all the existing funds the city has left at its disposal, and the costs are roughly comparable. Which project should the city's health authority subsidize?[6]

This situation highlights a delicate issue. How do we weigh the value we place on the lifesaving needs of potential heart recipients against the value we place on the life-enhancing needs of the nursing-home residents? Is survival for a few more important than quality care for many?

This case and that of the Oregon experiment illustrate the problem of macroallocating healthcare resources. Macroallocation and microallocation, which we will explore below, are actually forms of rationing healthcare resources. We define **macroallocation** as the distribution of resources on a wide scale. When it comes to health services, rationing is the dreaded "r-word" among the general public. **Rationing** involves deciding who gets what and when they get it when not everyone can get what they need. Rationing implicitly occurs when healthcare services are contingent on the ability to pay or on medical insurance coverage. Rationing also takes place in Medicare programs (public assistance programs for the elderly), in which healthcare services are provided only for those who have reached a certain age. It can be based on geographical area when residents in certain areas have less access to services than those who live in other areas. People who live in poverty-stricken parts of Appalachia, for example, have less access to more technologically advanced health services than those who live in the Washington, D.C., metropolitan area.

THE UNITED KINGDOM:
QALYs and the Internal Market

In the United Kingdom, the tension between lifesaving and life-enhancing needs is addressed by **quality adjusted life years (QALYs).** The QALY is a complex formula that measures the efficacy of an intervention by considering two primary factors:

1. The length of time gained by the intervention

2. The quality of life during that time

Although this formula appears to be a neat mathematical strategy for assessment, a number of problems are associated with attempting to measure the effectiveness of a health intervention in terms of QALYs. First, it is immensely difficult to define what is meant by "quality" existence, which is a substantially subjective and arbitrary notion. Second, QALYs might make sense when applied to individuals within the same category or group, for instance, all those persons in need of a heart transplant. However, it is notoriously difficult to apply QALYs to individuals in different groups. How do we assess quality between potential heart recipients and actual nursing-home residents, for example? Furthermore, QALYs tend to favor those with a longer survival time, which means that the measurement in terms of QALYs seems somewhat prejudicial against the terminally ill and the elderly.

How does this assessment relate to the United Kingdom's introduction of what is called the internal market? Formerly, the principal healthcare philosophy behind Britain's National Health System (NHS) was that its health services would be distributed primarily according to the healthcare needs of the people. This was considered one of the great triumphs of the NHS. In this way, the NHS sought to address those areas with higher mortality and higher morbidity rates. Since 1991, however, the provision of health services in England has taken economic factors into account more seriously. Cost-containment measures and the ability to pay are turning out to be the context for determining healthcare needs. In other words, services are more often being allocated within the parameters of fixed budgets.

The internal market orientation in England is somewhat similar to the United States' practice of managed competition; however, it entails more government involvement. It is a sort of quasi-market approach to healthcare delivery combined with a far-reaching government hand. Although Britain's internal market attempts to address primarily healthcare needs, it also provides financial incentives for healthcare providers to generate profit. This incentive actually benefits healthier, more affluent populations, since treating those who are sicker and less affluent may not be as profitable. Critics point out that this factor is a subversion of the traditional thrust of the NHS and is yet another example of the global corporatization of healthcare.[7]

There are different kinds of macroallocation, or macrorationing. The most encompassing allocation measures come to communities from the government (whether state, as in the case of Oregon, or federal). The government decides how much of its budget to allocate to healthcare, defense, education, and other areas. Within the healthcare allotment, choices are then made to further partition the funding to areas such as AIDS research, organ transplantation research, antiaging research, and mental health.

Further allocation of available funds takes place among various institutions, such as deciding which organ transplant centers will receive funding or which mental health facilities will be chosen as targets of funding. The rationing becomes even more spread out as specific institutions decide which areas within their institution will receive more or less funding. Will beds from the ICU be removed in order to beef up the hospital's outpatient ward? Will maternity units be enhanced and the CCU cut back?

According to philosopher Erich Loewy, questions of macroallocation, or large-scale distribution, deal with groups of largely "unidentified lives" and should "try to bring about the greatest good for the greatest number of those lives."[8] He claims that a utilitarian rationale is an appropriate basis for dealing with these broader issues, yet his utilitarian rationale needs to be further examined. Applying a utilitarian calculus still assumes values and priorities. Are these priorities equitable? Who decides what is good for the community? Is the process of deciding these priorities a fair one?

Let us illustrate the issue of macroallocation by asking a more specific question. How should the National Institutes of Health (NIH) allocate their annual budget of $13.6 billion? For instance, which among the conditions of diabetes, AIDS, heart disease, and cancer should receive priority? Allocating resources within a utilitarian framework requires that we consider the following factors:

- How prevalent is the condition or disease?
- How is it transmitted?
- What is its mortality rate?
- How costly is the disease?

In 1996, the NIH allocated $1.4 billion to AIDS research compared to $851.6 million for research on heart disease, yet heart disease accounted for far more deaths in the United States than did AIDS. In 1996, 733,834 people died from heart disease, whereas 32,655 people died from AIDS. Furthermore, heart disease costs the United States $70 billion, while the costs of AIDS amount to $10.3 billion.[9] A similar asymmetry in allocation occurred in Canada. According to the Breast Cancer Action group in Canada, 5,000 Canadian women died of breast cancer in 1991. In that same year, 72 Canadians died of AIDS. Yet in 1991, $4 million (Canadian) was allocated for breast cancer research, while $33 million was given to AIDS research.[10] One reason for this asymmetry, at least in the United States, is the tremendous amount of media attention given to AIDS, making it more politically expedient to pursue its treatment as a top priority. However, does allocating funds in this way result in a failure to address public needs that are more real and pressing?[11]

THE CHALLENGE IN MICROALLOCATION

Sixty-three-year-old Gregory Meeson received his first heart transplant three years ago. All had gone well, and for three years he enjoyed his retirement, traveling with his wife throughout Europe. They were looking forward to a trip to Asia. His hopes were dampened, however, when he began experiencing chronic fatigue. It was discovered that his coronary arteries had significantly narrowed. His physician placed him on a waiting list for another heart. He has been on the list for over three months.

Patrick Bourke developed an acute onset of cardiomyopathy just a little over two months ago. He lives in a nearby town, and he too suffers from chronic fatigue. He eventually had to stop working. He is thirty-two years old, with a wife and two children. His physician placed him on the waiting list for a heart, and he has been on the list for close to two months. Both Meeson and Bourke weigh nearly the same and share the same blood type. When a heart becomes available, which of the two should get the heart?[12]

Whereas macroallocation deals with the broader issues of distribution, **microallocation** deals with distribution questions on a one-to-one basis with identified individuals. The case described above is a common example of the problems surrounding the allocation of scarce resources such as hearts. As the case shows, the question of microallocation goes even deeper when the issue of retransplantation is involved.

This choice is agonizing. The survival rates for patients who undergo cardiac retransplantation are poorer than the rates for patients receiving their first heart. Those who receive their first heart have an 81.7 percent survival rate for one year and a 67.8 percent survival rate for five years. The figures for retransplant patients are 57.7 percent and 41 percent, respectively.[13] If the survival rate for retransplants is lower, is it fair to retransplant Meeson's heart, especially when the likelihood of Bourke's receiving a heart in sufficient time is slim and the result may be his death?

All other things being equal, Meeson has been on the waiting list longer, which may entitle him to the next available heart. Yet this fact impacts on the wider issue. Giving hearts to patients a second or third time deprives first-time recipients. Is this fair? Consider the following recommendation of the American Medical Association's Council on Ethical and Judicial Affairs:

> A physician has the duty to do all that he or she can for the benefit of the individual patient. Policies for allocating limited resources have the potential to limit the ability of physicians to fulfill this obligation to patients. Physicians have a responsibility to participate and to contribute their professional expertise in order to safeguard the interests of patients in decisions made at the societal level regarding the allocation or rationing of health resources.
>
> Decisions regarding the allocation of limited medical resources among patients should consider only *ethically appropriate criteria relating to medical need* [italics added]. These criteria include
>
> - likelihood of benefit
> - urgency of need
> - duration of benefit
> - in some cases, the amount of resources required for successful treatment.
>
> In general, only very substantial differences among patients are ethically relevant; the greater the disparities, the more justified the use of these criteria becomes. In making quality-of-life judgements, patients should first be prioritized so that death or extremely poor outcomes are avoided; then, patients should be prioritized according to change in quality of life, but only when there are very substantial differences among patients. *Non-medical criteria, such as the following, should not be considered* [italics added]:

- ability to pay
- age
- social worth
- perceived obstacles to treatment
- patient contribution to illness
- or past use of resources.[14] (order changed)

Patient's Contribution to Illness

Traditionally, healthcare professionals have regarded treating all patients as a moral duty, regardless of their patients' personal conduct. This traditional approach is being challenged, particularly in view of scarce resources. A growing number of healthcare professionals regard personal responsibility as a morally relevant criterion in making allocation decisions.

What about patients who are habitual smokers? Drug abusers? Chronic drinkers? What about patients who are noncompliant? Some insurers charge higher premiums for people who engage in certain categories of risky behavior. On a broader societal level, there are laws concerning individuals whose risky actions result in harm to others. For example, adult drivers must see to it that young children are properly seat-belted.

One of the most contentious areas in healthcare regarding the issue of personal conduct is organ transplant. As we saw in Chapter 7, on organ transplantation, a sensitive problem concerns whether unrehabilitated alcoholics should be placed on waiting lists for liver transplants. With regard to unrehabilitated alcoholics, allocating the scarce resource of livers is a matter not simply of moral desert but of medical prognosis and likelihood of benefit.

Managed Care and Having to Choose: Patient Advocacy or Social Benefit?

Throughout the United States, several efforts to contain healthcare costs are operative, including managed care organizations and their practice of capitation (preset reimbursement for physicians based on the number of patients), group purchasing, and utilization review. To some people, containing costs seems to have become the number one goal in U.S. healthcare policy.

Yet, as emphasized throughout the text, the key moral concern of the healthcare professional in the Western Hippocratic tradition is to act in the patient's best interests. The center of concern is and always should be the patient. Thus, as they enter a new century and a new millennium, healthcare professionals face what may well be their biggest challenge. How can they act in ways that will preserve their professional and moral integrity and at the same time be effective partners in the move to contain costs? How can they balance their primary commitment to their patients with their broader moral and professional responsibility to the social good through further cost-effectiveness? How can they balance quality of care with efficient care?

Can we realistically expect a healthcare system that seems to be increasingly driven by a free-market model to put patient care and well-being as its top priority? Patients are increasingly viewed as customers or clients in this free market. Is the drive to enhance savings compatible with a patient-centered healthcare system? Can an emphasis on the bottom line be consistent with cultivating trust in a system whose providers are first and foremost advocates for their individual patients?

We appear to have gone from a system that overutilized treatment measures and tests to one that, in some cases, underutilizes them for the purpose of saving money. This is the underlying philosophy behind managed care plans. Managed care plans are essentially cooperatives between healthcare providers and insurers. They are organized clusters that work to provide quality care for patients while maintaining cost-efficiency through restricting access to tests and treatments that are both unnecessary and costly. Morreim describes the role and impact of managed care plans at length in his article at the end of this chapter.

While these efforts at cost-efficiency appear sensible in principle, they create an obvious dilemma. In cases in which added measures such as another blood test or X ray might more accurately detect a patient's problem, attempts to lower costs result in fewer procedures as well as fewer days in the hospital. This practice is often detrimental to those patients who are prematurely discharged from the hospital "sicker but quicker." Because they are discharged before they should be, their families need to provide adequate care for them at home and often are not able to do so.

Both morally and professionally, healthcare providers need to be advocates for their patients, which means doing all within their means to promote their patients' best interests. Yet these same professionals face increasing pressures—in the form of both incentives and penalties—to act in ways that will allegedly cut costs for the health system, which also means cutting costs for their patients who pay healthcare premiums. As employees of the corporatized healthcare system, physicians are pressured into being corporate agents.

This situation creates an obvious tension for the conscientious healthcare professional, who is necessarily a patient advocate. In an increasingly corporatized system that, as a corporation, focuses on acquiring profit, acting as a patient advocate may mean employing subtle strategies in order to ensure that the patient's best interests are uppermost. In other words, a system centered around cost-efficiency and profit tends to encourage forms of deception through subtle strategies on the part of providers.[15] For example, a provider may modify a diagnosis in order to keep a patient from being prematurely discharged from the hospital, or a provider may switch elderly patients from one diagnostic-related category (DRG) to another in order to justify further testing for the patients. In effect, these deceptions, while they protect patients' interests, also drive up healthcare costs and premiums.

An emphasis on cost-containment is apparent not only in the United States, but elsewhere as well. Consider the case in British Columbia in which an adult male patient died suddenly of a cerebral aneurysm. He had seen a number of physicians, but they did not immediately order a brain CT scan. The lengthy delay in getting the scan was due to the physicians' claim that, since the CT scan was expensive, they felt pressured by the health system to contain costs. The court argued that such limits worked against the patient's best interests and found the physicians involved guilty of professional negligence. The judge ruled that the primary duty of physicians must always be to their patients. Harms to the patients constitute greater loss than costs to the system.[16]

HMOs and the Elderly

Managed care actually means managed access; that is, access to more expensive types of diagnostic tests and treatments is restricted in order to control costs. Access to healthcare providers is also restricted, since patients must choose providers that are approved by the plan.

Health maintenance organizations (HMOs), the most prevalent form of managed care, are becoming the core of the market-driven healthcare system in the United States. An HMO is an organized cluster of hospitals, physicians, and insurers. The healthcare providers work within a fixed annual budget. Moreover, businesses that enroll with these plans can negotiate fees with the providers. One of the most important goals is to contain costs, including the cost of premiums paid by the public. Therein lies one of the principal merits of HMOs, since saving costs to the public is a major benefit. HMOs seek to save costs and incur profit through cutting back unnecessary tests and treatments while at the same time maintaining the provision of quality care.

The elderly are especially affected by HMO policies and practices. There are currently over 38 million Medicare recipients, of which more than 5 million are enrolled in HMOs. Because HMOs receive a fixed prior payment, some services may be limited in order to meet costs. This situation can impact negatively on Medicare patients. For example, there have been many instances of residents of nursing homes being prematurely discharged, that is, allowed to return to their homes when they still need the daily care that can be provided only at the nursing home. The extent to which services will be provided is beyond the control of the Medicare recipient.

Many elderly do have a choice—they can buy into more comprehensive plans if they are not happy with their HMO. In addition, they can pay out of pocket for extra procedures, lengthier hospital stays, and other types of coverage. Various supplemental plans cover almost all the costs associated with nursing-home care to prevent many elderly from having to use up their life savings.

On the other hand, many elderly remain on fixed incomes and are not able to afford supplemental coverage. What makes this all the more frustrating for the elderly who remain in HMOs is that the conditions for appealing treatment decisions are often restricted. In fact, patients and nursing-home residents may not even be informed that they have the option of an appeal procedure. Also, HMOs are not required to continue providing health services during an appeal process, which adversely affects patients who do appeal. The process of appeal is time-consuming. Dr. Beatrice Braun, an American Association of Retired Persons director, states:

> The biggest problem in the current appeal process is the lack of meaningful time limits. Under current regulations, an HMO can take as long as 60 days to make a formal denial of care and then an additional 60 days to reconsider its denial. This is unacceptable.[17]

WHAT CONSTITUTES A JUST HEALTHCARE SYSTEM?

What would constitute a just healthcare system? This extraordinarily complex question requires us to address a deeper question: How do we view social justice? Our answer to this question depends on how we view the nature of the relationship between individual interests and the common good. A communitarian perspective, for example, tends to assume the priority of the common good over individual freedoms. In contrast, a libertarian view tends to consider individual liberty and freedom as absolutes. A capitalist economy motivated by individual enterprise leans more toward the presupposition of individual freedom as the highest good. A socialist economy upholds communal well-being over individual freedoms. The healthcare systems of these economies reflect these respective tendencies.

To portray the tension between individual and community as irreconcilable is unfair. As philosopher Alasdair MacIntyre reminds us, all individuals belong to a historical, social, and cultural matrix. Our lives are part of an ongoing "narrative" made up of various roles contingent on various contexts. An exaggeration of individualism leads to the danger of viewing the individual as a separate, isolated entity, divorced from the communal context. Nothing could be further from the truth. While we each cultivate our individuality, we still exist within a social matrix.

Theories of Social Justice

A just healthcare system assumes a sound theory of social justice that places reasonable parameters on the rights claimed by individuals. A sound theory of social justice, then, envisions a healthy tension between individual freedom and communal well-being, a tension that exists without eliminating either interest.

Furthermore, a sound theory of justice fairly considers both relevant and irrelevant differences when it comes to distributing goods, in this case, medical resources. Deciding what is relevant and irrelevant is crucial to any fair decision. For instance, the color of one's skin or one's race is irrelevant to possessing a moral right. However, citizenship in a country is relevant to possessing legal rights in that country. Let us briefly outline some theories of social justice proposed by both classical and contemporary philosophers. The sketch is somewhat superficial, since the topic is complex.

Plato's Social Contract In Plato's dialogue *Crito*, Socrates is in prison awaiting his death. His good friend Crito visits him with an escape plan. Crito and others have seen to it that they can easily bribe the prison guards to look the other way while Socrates makes his escape. Yet Socrates can justify escaping only if he has good reason to escape, so he engages Crito in a lengthy examination of why he should escape. While Crito provides what he considers to be valid reasons for escaping, Socrates finds each reason significantly flawed. Socrates decides to remain in prison.

The fundamental reason why Socrates chooses not to escape has to do with an implicit contract he has made with the state. To escape would violate this contract, a social and legal contract by which Socrates has abided all along. Such is the **social contract:** the implicit agreement persons make to one another by virtue of living together. This contract entails mutual rights and obligations and appears to be morally binding, at least in the case of Socrates.

Aristotle's Formal Principle of Justice Aristotle carries the social contract theory a significant step further with his formal principle of justice or fairness: "Treat equals equally and unequals unequally." As a formal principle, this makes sense, yet it doesn't go far enough. We still need to ascertain what constitutes equality and on what bases "equals" can be equal and "unequals" unequal. What are the relevant differences? What makes a person equal to another? Unequal to another? How morally relevant are these differences?

John Rawls and Justice as Distribution We leap into contemporary thought with philosopher John Rawls. Rawls provides a contemporary rendition of the social contract theory through his notion of distributive justice. According to Rawls, in his classic *Theory of Justice* (1971),[18] the fairest way to view what may count as morally relevant factors for a just society would be to view things under what he calls a **veil of ignorance.** His heuristic strategy to determine "equal" and "unequal" is to arrive at a hypothetical social contract by viewing our social condition from a neutral standpoint that Rawls refers to as the original position. In this original position, we are ignorant of all advantages and disadvantages, that is, of all differences among individuals. Under this veil, we have no idea of our own particular social circumstances and are free of all biases. Thus, we would view things in the most impartial way.

Under the veil of ignorance, Rawls claims, we would end up espousing two critical principles. The first is what he calls the liberty principle, which holds that all persons should be given the same amount of liberty as all other persons regardless of each person's actual circumstances. Whether destitute or affluent, all persons ought to be accorded equal liberty.

The second principle, the difference principle, endorses the idea that it is proper to allow, and even to encourage, differences among persons. After all, persons are born into different circumstances and possess different talents and capacities. Due to such differences, inequalities will come about; but these inequalities are justified only if every effort is made to improve the lot of those in the least advantageous position. In other words, all efforts need to be made to see that those at the lowest end in society stand to gain from inequalities of circumstance.

Norman Daniels's Equality of Opportunity Rawls did not apply his theory to healthcare. His theory is a systematic, rigorous philosophical analysis on the most theoretical level. Norman Daniels, on the other hand, insightfully applies Rawls's analysis to healthcare. In his work *Just Health Care* (1985), Daniels expounds further on Rawls's liberty principle and claims that maximizing equality for all persons means seeing that all persons have an equality of opportunity. This equality of opportunity is the condition for the exercise of freedom. Illness and disease are obstacles to this equality of opportunity; therefore, they need to be eradicated. A document that reflects this idea, at least in spirit, is the United Nations Declaration of Human Rights (1948), which states, "Everyone has a right to a standard of living adequate for the health and well-being of himself and his family, including food, clothing, housing, medical care and necessary social services" (Article 25, 1).

By equality of opportunity, Daniels means using the standard of what he calls "species typical normal functioning." As far as the human species is concerned, we can establish "normal opportunity ranges" for various stages in our development. According to Daniels, we are entitled to health services that enable us to live in step with this normal opportunity range. Daniels, along with others, recently put forth a set of necessary standards for a fair healthcare system in the United States.[19] His "benchmarks of fairness for national health care reform" include, first and foremost, universal access to healthcare. He contends that all citizens, regardless of their economic status and health, must have access to a reasonable package of health services.

Daniels's analysis is rigorous and far-reaching. He applies his views of justice further in his article at the end of this chapter, "Why Saying No to Patients in the United States Is So Hard." However, critics may argue that we can utilize the normal opportunity range criterion when it comes to healthcare funding in general, but that doesn't settle more specific questions such as whether more dollars should be spent on lifesaving interventions for the few or life-enhancing interventions for the many.

Susan Sherwin's Feminist Reflective Equilibrium   Philosopher Susan Sherwin, while finding merit in Rawls's position, argues that his analysis does not go far enough in attending to more practical realities in order to construct an adequate theory of justice.[20] She proposes a methodology that she calls feminist reflective equilibrium (borrowing the idea of reflective equilibrium from Rawls). She substantiates it by alerting us to issues of power, control, and oppression within the social and institutional contexts of healthcare. This concern about oppression and power is the focus of her feminist perspective.

A Canadian, Sherwin argues that even the Canadian system, with its universalization of healthcare for its citizens, has particular problems when viewed from this feminist perspective. For instance, it does not adequately address the difficulties poor women face in gaining access to healthcare, such as finding transportation or arranging for child care.[21]

Sherwin's approach requires us to pay more attention to the relationship between economic status and health. In the United States and Canada, as in most countries throughout the world, there continue to be blatant disparities in the salaries of women and men. Furthermore, a larger proportion of women and children live in conditions of poverty. Since women on the whole are more impoverished than men, they suffer more health problems. She also states that women have more healthcare needs than do men. For instance, regarding reproductive needs, Sherwin states:

> Their [women's] reproductive needs are more frequent and more complex than are those of men and their dependence on health professionals for reproductive health care is exacerbated by the fact that all aspects of their relatively complex reproductive lives (menstruation, contraception, pregnancy, childbirth, lactation, menopause) *have been subject to medical surveillance and control.*[22] (italics added)

Despite this situation, women have a more difficult time obtaining adequate care. A 1990 study revealed that women tend to be underdiagnosed for certain conditions. For example, women are less likely than men to obtain proper medical interventions, through both diagnosis and treatment, for symptoms that normally seem to warrant standard cardiac catheterization. On the other hand, with regard to more controversial and nonstandard interventions such as psychosurgery, women are more likely to have the procedures performed on them than are men.[23] In addition, most therapeutic medical research is conducted on men, mostly for diseases men tend to suffer from. However, studies reveal that older women are just as susceptible, if not more so, to heart disease as are men; yet research regarding treatments for women is sparse. On the whole, women suffer blatant disparities in healthcare services. The situation is even worse for women who belong to minority groups. Inadequate maternal care for black women results in higher mortality rates in childbirth for both the mother and the child.[24]

Sherwin broadens the idea of healthcare to extend beyond the traditional parameters of physician services in hospitals and the like. She claims that healthcare must incorporate alternative approaches that have been proven effective. A more just healthcare system should provide access to procedures outside the conventional realm, such

ANGOLA: "Lack of Transparency" Prohibits Fair Healthcare Distribution

Luanda, the capital of Angola, is filled with costly restaurants and nightclubs and is considered one of the most expensive cities in the world. The country of Angola also possesses one of the richest reservoirs of both oil and diamonds. Experts predict that Angola will eventually outshine Nigeria as Africa's largest oil resource. Most of its oil is exported to the United States. Angola's interior is also rich in diamond mines.

Decades of civil war among rival groups in the aftermath of Angola's freedom from Portuguese control in 1975 have kept the country in constant turmoil. This turmoil has resulted in a massive inpouring of foreign aid. Billions of dollars have been given to the Angolans, much of it from the United Nations and from private organizations. However, the Angolan citizens themselves appear to have seen little of this aid. There is little accountability regarding the spending of the funds. Most of the money seems to go toward government spending, yet this spending does not benefit the ordinary Angolan. According to an International Monetary Fund (IMF) study for 1996, less than 9 percent of the aid funds spent by the government went to the social and health programs for which they were targeted. Not surprisingly, healthcare has not seen any improvement.

Angola, a country on the western side of Africa, has a population of 12 million people. Most will not live past their forty-seventh birthday. Every day, an average of sixteen children die from malaria, diarrhea, meningitis, and malnutrition. Infant mortality is exceedingly high, and hospital care lacks many essentials. In addition, the GNP per capita of $320 is below that of sub-Saharan Africa's $490. The unemployment rate is a staggering 45 percent. In many respects, the healthcare system in Angola represents the healthcare found throughout Africa: a day-to-day struggle against illness and suffering amid the ongoing encounter with poverty.

Where has the aid money gone? Without sufficient funds, Angola's healthcare system faces a losing battle against disease. Because little of the foreign aid earmarked for health and social reform reaches its intended destination, the IMF cut back its assistance program to Angola. It claimed that the government bookkeepers were guilty of what economists call lack of transparency, that is, lack of sufficient records of government spending. Members of the World Bank and the IMF have strong reason to suspect that funds are misallocated and are used essentially to line the pockets of government officials. A substantial degree of government corruption thus prohibits foreign aid from providing adequate healthcare services to Angolans.[25]

as acupuncture, herbal medicines, and massage therapy. Health services also need to address factors that contribute to health, such as environment and nutrition.

Sherwin finds merit in the theory of justice espoused by Iris Marion Young, whose book *Justice and the Politics of Difference* contends that the traditional distributive justice scheme is too narrow and certainly inadequate. The traditional paradigm ignores the social interconnectedness of persons, as well as subtle forms of oppression that exist institutionally, by viewing persons abstractly, divorced from practical realities. Sherwin and Young feel we need to incorporate these ideas into the abstract, conceptual analyses offered by Rawls and others.

Robert Nozick and Justice as Entitlement   In his classic work *Anarchy, State, and Utopia* (1974), philosopher Robert Nozick argues that a just and fair system must properly reward those who actively contribute to that system. Since those who contribute to the system are entitled to reap its rewards, a just system is one that bestows these entitlements.

Nozick recognizes that inequities exist within the U.S. socioeconomic system. However, he argues that a just system ought not to require its citizens to provide for others' needs. Acting charitably is noble; however, charity is a supererogatory act; that is, it is beyond the call of moral duty and therefore should not be imposed.

Applying Nozick's ideas of **entitlement** to healthcare means that if Americans can afford health insurance and pay for it, then they are entitled to its benefits. If some Americans are affluent enough to afford supplemental coverage, then they are entitled to what they can pay for. This point of view resonates among many Americans, especially among those who can afford health insurance. On the other hand, those unable to afford health insurance might disagree with Nozick's position, claiming that they have a right to health coverage.

How Should We Distribute Healthcare Resources?

What standards should govern how we distribute healthcare resources, particularly when these resources are scarce and the demand continues to escalate? Many commentators have proposed the following criteria as possible standards:

- Distribute according to market, that is, to those who can afford to pay.
- Distribute according to social merit.
- Distribute according to medical need.
- Distribute according to age.
- Distribute according to queuing, or first-come, first-served.
- Distribute according to random selection.

Distributing According to the Market   This distribution criterion carries significant weight within the American context of free enterprise and a market economy. It is consistent with the belief that a just system is one of entitlement, that is, reaping the benefits of what you contribute, the view of justice espoused by Robert Nozick. This approach seems popular among many Americans and is endorsed by many commentators. However, according to recent Gallup poll statistics, many more Americans appear to oppose this free-market approach. In fact, when asked which healthcare system was better, that of the United States or Canada, 62 percent of the U.S. respondents who had an opinion favored the Canadian system, a healthcare system that has universal insurance and a single payer. In other words, most Americans appeared to favor a system that is not driven by free-market concerns.[26]

A free-market approach to the distribution of healthcare services has at least three weaknesses. First, it blatantly ignores those millions of Americans who, through no fault of their own, cannot afford coverage. Those who cannot afford health coverage include not only the poor, but also many in the lower middle class as well as many who are self-employed. Health insurance becomes even more expensive for females and for older people. Lack of coverage affects not only those who cannot afford it, but their family as well. In particular, millions of women and children are penalized under this market approach to distribution.

Second, because Medicaid requirements are set by each state, many people who are not eligible for Medicaid still do not earn enough to purchase health insurance for themselves and their families. These are the working uninsured. Because they pay taxes, they contribute to the market, but they do not reap the benefits.

Third, the free-market approach ignores the needs of those who are disadvantaged due to illness. For instance, the disabled are placed at a disadvantage because they are not able to compete on a market basis with others who are healthier. In other words, a free-market approach may be fair only if there is a level playing field, yet this is not possible.

Perhaps the clearest example of this weakness is the fact that racism, still prevalent throughout American society, is strongly related to socioeconomic status. Healthcare services are unevenly distributed, with substandard services available in lower-income areas. Consider the emergency rooms at many inner-city hospitals. It is not uncommon to find the halls overflowing with indigent persons, many of them members of minority groups. Most often, they have conditions that do not necessarily warrant emergency attention but could have been attended to by a primary-care physician. However, in many cases, they do not have a primary-care physician because they do not have insurance coverage.

U.S. culture strongly emphasizes individualism and individual liberties. However, this emphasis, taken to an extreme, actually works to reinforce racism in that many poorer individuals in certain minority groups obtain far less access to health services than do those who are more affluent. Philosopher Charles J. Dougherty points out three ways in which racism in America is related to the excessive stress placed on individual freedom:

1. American healthcare providers and insurers insist on exercising their entrepreneurial liberties. That is, physicians, health institutions, insurers, pharmaceutical companies, and medical manufacturers desire to work within free-market mechanisms in order to secure their freedom to acquire profit.

2. Many American consumers insist on exercising their freedoms, especially the freedom to choose their own healthcare plans. In fact, some Americans criticize national healthcare plans elsewhere, such as in Europe and East Asia, because these plans appear to offer little or no choice.

3. Many American citizens still insist on exercising their freedom to refuse to pay the higher taxes necessary to ensure universal coverage for all citizens. Higher taxes are often viewed as tantamount to a restriction of freedom.[27]

SOUTH AFRICA:
Transformation After Apartheid?

Apartheid, with its strongly racist policies, was for many years the predominant economic ideology in South Africa. Apartheid supported the monopolization of power in the hands of the white minority of Afrikaner Nationalists. Under apartheid, in just about every corner of healthcare from infant mortality rates to life expectancy, there was a clear inequity in healthcare provision between whites and blacks. In the early 1940s in South Africa, there was one hospital bed for every 304 white people, and one for every 1,198 black people. In the major city of Cape Town, there was one doctor for every 308 whites. Meanwhile, in Zululand, there was one doctor for every 22,000 blacks. In Northern Transvaal, there was one doctor for every 30,000 blacks.[28]

Political propaganda further skewed views of the way healthcare was delivered. For instance, propaganda clearly exploited the fact that the first successful heart transplant occurred in Cape Town, pointing to this "success" as a reflection of the general health practice (the beneficiary of the transplant was white, while the donor was black). According to some commentators:

It demonstrated to the surprised world our expertise in medicine. The flag of that first transplant was waved vigorously in the faces of our critics as an example of the excellent standard of medical care practised in South Africa.[29]

This expertise was lauded despite the fact that real needs, such as the thousands of people dying daily due to malnutrition, were not being addressed. Apartheid's policies have no doubt shaped South Africa's social, cultural, and political history, and apartheid's discriminatory health policies may have some influence over current reform measures despite the overthrow of apartheid and democratic elections in 1994. The question remains, How much damage pertaining to health policy from apartheid still exists?

Two proposals for healthcare reform have emerged. In 1994, a National Health Plan (NHP) was formulated that included features such as the right of everyone to access to a broad range of health services, teamwork regarding medical care, community participation, and equitable social and economic development. The last feature was particularly emphasized, since basic economic conditions must first be met in order to ensure adequate health provision.

In the same year, the Pan Africanist Congress (PAC) proposed another draft health policy. PAC's proposals are more specific than those of the NHP and are geared to a reallocation of health services among disenfranchised black communities. The underlying principle seems similar to that of the NHP: to ensure universal and equitable access to a basic core package of health services.[30] As of 1999, there was few reliable data to measure the efficacy of the proposed programs. Time alone will reveal the long-term impact of apartheid on the equity of healthcare in South Africa.

Dougherty's last two points are arguable, since Gallup polls have indicated that many if not most Americans favor the Canadian system over the U.S. system.[31] However, taken together, these factors produce inequalities of outcomes, so that, as in any capitalist scheme hinging on the free market, there are winners and losers. Those who win win according to marketplace rules. Those who lose lose due to the same rules, and many of the losers are members of minority groups. Because many of them are at the bottom of the socioeconomic scale, they suffer the far-reaching results of inequitable health-care distribution.

Distributing According to Social Merit   This criterion holds that the litmus test for distributing scarce resources should be the degree of an individual's contribution to the social good. At first glance, this may seem to make sense. For instance, when it comes to deciding who should receive an available heart for transplantation, we may assign more weight to a judge than to a criminal. Yet we need to examine more closely the bases on which we make such judgments. For example, who should make them? Because judgments of social worth assume certain values that may not be shared by all, such a criterion can be capricious.

Consider the case of the kidney dialysis machines in Seattle. In the late 1950s, the first kidney dialysis machines were used in Seattle, Washington. Because there were not enough machines for all the patients suffering from end-stage kidney disease, an ethics committee was established to determine who would be the recipients of the treatment. The committee members considered factors such as marital status, income, education, age, gender, and occupation. The decisions of the committee were severely criticized because of the hidden biases regarding social worth. The committee was also criticized for not considering the special needs of minorities, the poor, and women. What criteria would have been the most equitable?

What about people who are partly to blame for their condition? Bringing in social merit standards inevitably brings in factors of personal merit and personal blame as well. Is the alcoholic less entitled to a liver due to his or her role in bringing about the condition? If so, where do we draw the line? Are we prepared to claim that smokers or those who engage in high-risk sports are less entitled to medical resources?

Distributing According to Medical Need   There is a strong consensus among many commentators that distributing according to medical need is perhaps the fairest approach, yet this criterion also has its share of problems. How do we determine levels of medical need? What is the relationship between urgency and need? What if the recipient's situation is so urgent that he or she desperately needs the treatment in order to survive but will survive only for a brief period of time with only marginal benefit? What if another patient stands a good chance of benefiting more and for a longer period of time, but his or her situation is not presently urgent? Because this notion of medical need is critical, it requires further clarification. We will examine it more closely in the next section.

Distributing According to Age   Consider the case of Mr. Stafford. Mr. Stafford is seventy-eight years old. He has coronary artery disease. He has also developed a progressive and apparently irreversible kidney disease. Nevertheless, he continues to be physically active. Being an avid reader, he also keeps mentally active. However, it is clear that without treatment of his kidney disease, either with dialysis or transplantation, he will most likely die within the year. Should he receive intervention?[32]

Philosopher Daniel Callahan set off a firestorm of controversy in *Setting Limits* (1987) when he suggested that age should be more seriously considered as a criterion in allocating scarce resources. Callahan did not, as some of his critics claim, advocate ageism. He pointed out, reasonably enough, that we need to make responsible choices in allocating resources. For some much older people, treatments may be marginal based on medical prognosis. Therefore, providing them with resources that could be used in more beneficial ways by younger people may not be wise. Supporters of this position also argue that it would be unfair for those who have lived out their natural life span to drain society of resources that are in diminishing supply.

In determining standards for allocating medical resources, age is certainly a realistic factor, though not the only one. Age is relevant in ascertaining medical condition, prognosis, and likelihood of recovery. For example, in the United Kingdom, patients over the age of sixty-five are less likely to receive dialysis. In New Zealand, seventy-five appears to be the cutoff point for patients receiving dialysis. It is medically likely that triple organ failure for persons in their eighties would result in progressive deterioration even if treated.

There are a number of arguments against using age as a criterion for distributing scarce healthcare resources. First, age itself is an artificial standard that stereotypes groups of people according to age categories. Generalizing about those who are chronologically old fails to consider individual instances. Some persons in their eighties are self-sufficient, mentally sharp, and physically active and healthy, just as some people in their forties and fifties are not. Second, what constitutes a "natural life span"? Implying that older persons have lived out their natural life span assumes a rather strict adherence to some natural-law standard, yet we need to be careful about such a literal natural-law position regarding healthcare. Using age as a singular basis for distribution necessarily introduces arbitrary judgment.

Distributing According to Queuing   Our society often applies the criterion of first-come, first-served. For instance, we feel wronged if someone cuts ahead of us in line at the post office. Yet should healthcare be allocated on this basis? Again, a problem arises due to inequities in socioeconomic status, among other variables. More informed patients are likely to seek healthcare earlier, and, due to various reasons including lack of transportation or child care, many people in need are not even able to seek healthcare. Those who are first in line may also have less urgent medical needs than those who show up later. This is why emergency room care and even office visits to the family physician are based on a system of triage according to degree of medical urgency.

Distributing According to Random Selection   For other medical ethicists, distributing resources according to random selection, for example, through a lottery, is the fairest method of allocation. No one individual is given preference over any other. All are viewed equally and treated equally. Factors such as socioeconomic status, income, societal contribution, personal responsibility, medical need, age, gender, race, and religion play no role. Is this the most reasonable approach? Random selection assumes that no relevant characteristics or features warrant preferential treatment regarding distribution, yet is such an assumption reasonable? Is it responsible? Or does it allow us to abdicate the responsibility of making an equitable choice? Should a serial murderer be equally entitled to receive a scarce resource? Should his or her needs be weighed equally against those of a young child?

JEWISH VIEWS ON HEALTHCARE REFORM

Guidelines for arriving at principles for healthcare reform are found in the Talmud (fifth century), the Codes of Jewish Law according to Moses Maimonides (twelfth century), and the Codes according to Shulchan Aruch (sixteenth century). According to these Jewish teachings, the professional and moral duty of the physician is to give medical care. Medical care is construed more as a duty on the part of the physician than as a right on the part of the patient. In addition, even though fees are based on time spent with the patient, a physician must provide care regardless of the patient's ability to pay.

Jewish law, or **halakhah,** supports a healthcare system that provides medical care for everyone. Furthermore, this care must meet high standards, including making treatment measures such as drugs available to everyone. Therefore, costs need to be monitored. Also, no criterion should act as a barrier to access to healthcare—there should be universal access.

Nevertheless, scarce resources are in high demand. Rationing these resources equitably necessitates distributing to those in need. At the same time, medical suitability and the likelihood of success must be considered. The only case in which age may be a factor is when age affects the medical outcome of a procedure.

Furthermore, any sound effort at healthcare reform must consider mental illness as equal in importance to physical illness. Equal attention must be given to providing care and treat-

WHAT DO WE MEAN BY HEALTHCARE NEEDS?

Molly Murphy, an independent and somewhat reclusive eighty-three-year-old widow, had been under Dr. Paul Integlia's care for some time. When Dr. Integlia eventually retired from practice, Warren Hazo became Murphy's new doctor. Murphy told Dr. Hazo that she had received regular B_{12} injections since her husband had died ten years ago. Her medical chart indicated that she did not have pernicious anemia, the only clear physiological rationale for B_{12} injections. Murphy asked Dr. Hazo to continue the injections because they had "kept me going all these years." She also requested that a home-care nurse give them to her at home because she was too old to get out much. Dr. Hazo complied with her request and filled out a home-care referral form. The next day, the physician in charge of home care called Dr. Hazo to ask him how he could justify this service.[37]

What do we mean by healthcare needs? Since we usually use the term *healthcare need* to denote what is medically necessary, such as diagnostic tests, clinical services, or preventive measures, we tend to think of healthcare needs as being defined purely in terms of medical criteria. However, healthcare needs encompass more than medical considerations. They imply all sorts of values besides purely medical ones.

ment for those suffering from mental conditions.[33]

These guidelines can be further understood in view of the Jewish understanding of justice, or **tzedakah.**[34] The notion of justice is deeply rooted in Hebrew Scripture. Rabbinic Judaism, in particular, focuses on the notion of tzedakah and underscores the importance of providing basic needs, particularly those that are life-rescuing. This notion of justice becomes the cornerstone for Jewish beliefs regarding access to healthcare. Providing for the needs of the disenfranchised, especially the poor, is an essential component of tzedakah. Moreover, all persons in the community must contribute in various ways to constructing and sustaining a just system. There is a societal and collective responsibility to ensure universal access to healthcare.

Healthcare commentator Aaron Mackler points out that the provision of healthcare services must address the basic standard of medical need. His point is comparable to Norman Daniels's standard of "species typical normal functioning" in order to enhance the "normal opportunity range," mentioned earlier.[35] At the same time, there are limits to the Jewish obligation to provide for others' needs. One is under no obligation to provide care if doing so requires endangering one's own life. The *Shulhan Arukh,* a major code of Jewish law, also alludes to situations in which providing services to save lives may be futile. Mackler states that Jewish law gives much weight to the overall well-being of the community. Excessive burdens to the community must be considered and, if possible, avoided.[36] Nevertheless, Jewish tradition seems to strongly support the need for universal access to basic healthcare services for all in the community.

On the macro level, we face the challenge of ascertaining how to rank healthcare needs in comparison with other, external, needs such as defense or education. In this case, assigning importance to healthcare is not difficult. Healthcare needs are foundational, since other needs depend on being healthy. Because healthcare needs are naturally of a higher order, they possess a greater degree of urgency. We face stickier issues when we engage in internal ranking. Among the many healthcare needs, how do we determine which needs are more important than others?

To help structure the analysis, we can think of healthcare needs as belonging to one of three categories: life-rescuing, life-sustaining, and life-improving.[38] *Life-rescuing* healthcare needs are those that prevent death. An example is surgery for a lethal head wound. These needs are the most urgent. *Life-sustaining* healthcare needs require "the extension of life over a significant period of time with at best a minimal degree of restoration to the prior state of health."[39] Palliative care for a terminally ill patient is an example. *Life-improving* needs entail a "sufficient restoration which will approximate the state of health before the onset of the condition."[40] This category includes preventive measures such as mammograms. Hip replacements are another example.

This tidy typology masks some real difficulties. Life-rescuing needs are obviously the most urgent, but are they always the most important? What if we satisfy life-rescuing needs without satisfying any of the benefits of the other two types of needs? Needs that are life-sustaining and those that are life-improving may be mutually exclusive. In this

SOLIDARITY, EQUITY, AND CLARITY CONCERNING HEALTHCARE NEEDS IN THE NETHERLANDS

All citizens of Holland, regardless of their medical condition, are covered by health insurance. Furthermore, all citizens are covered regardless of their ability to pay for care. Coverage is rather comprehensive. For example, all persons in nursing homes are covered. Therefore, nursing-home patients do not have to worry about exhausting their private funds in order to cover any medical expenses incurred for their care. This relieves family members of worries about financial burdens, in contrast to the case of nursing-home care in the United States. Another example of the comprehensive nature of Holland's coverage is that all AIDS patients without exception have access to AZT without any further charges. This is not the case in the United States, particularly given the exceptionally high costs of AZT treatment.

Holland's comprehensive and universal coverage underscores the principle of equity, a major value in Dutch culture. Furthermore, all citizens, in ways proportionate to their incomes, share in assuming the costs of providing for this care. This cost-sharing reflects the principle of solidarity, another important value among the Dutch. The values of equity and solidarity help explain the long tradition and history of tolerance in various forms, such as religious and political, in Dutch culture.

In the Dutch context of universal, comprehensive coverage, Holland has a two-tiered system. While most people are covered by mandatory insurance funded through the government based

regard, measuring benefits is problematic. How do we determine which healthcare needs are essential and which are excessive? One thing is sure—the notion of healthcare needs is not a fixed entity.

Healthcare Needs Versus Health-Related Desires

There are important differences between healthcare needs and health-related desires. Healthcare needs assume some existing or potential condition of illness or disease and seek to restore some level of normalcy, whether the need be life-rescuing, life-sustaining, or life-improving. Health-related desires, in contrast, assume a normal condition and seek to enhance this already normal condition. Thus, health-related desires do not fall under the category of genuine healthcare needs.[41]

However, there are difficulties involved in distinguishing between the two. How do we measure what is "normal," particularly if we weigh the subjective factors of pain and suffering? Suppose a person suffers from low self-esteem because he is sensitive about his nose and wants to undergo rhinoplasty. Is this a healthcare need or a health-related desire? Also, many perceived needs arise in response to expectations that are spawned by medical marketing and advertising. Advertisements—whether for new laser corneal

on taxes proportionate to people's income, other people, should they want it, are able to procure private insurance. Thus, though there is universal coverage, there is no single payer. There have been recent proposals to bring about a national health insurance plan for all citizens, which would require putting into place a **single payer system.** This would mean that the basic package of covered services would have a cutoff point not currently existing for many of those who have private, voluntary insurance.

A Committee for Choices in Health Care was established in 1990 to look into strategies regarding the allocation of scarce resources. In view of the proposals for a national health plan, a key strategy in the committee's deliberations concerned the need to be clearer about the concepts of "basic care," or "core health services." It was agreed that all citizens must have equal access to these core services, yet the committee also recognized the need to be more aware of the critical distinction between real healthcare needs and individual desires or preferences.

The committee reached the consensus that genuine healthcare needs are those that enable each citizen to more fully engage in social life. Therefore, the interests of the community, especially the interests of those who are more vulnerable, such as the elderly and the mentally disabled, supersede private interests. The elderly and the mentally disabled are considered to be valuable members of the community, whereas in the United States they are often among the more neglected groups. This communitarian approach distinguishes the Dutch healthcare system from that of the United States, which focuses more on private, individual needs. In Holland, the well-being of the community assumes priority over individualized needs.[42]

surgery, new types of growth hormone, new fertility drugs, or pills for male impotence—have a way of shaping public expectations regarding medical care. These expectations easily become needs and/or desires. Thus, clarifying what is meant by healthcare needs is a critical step in arriving at a reasonable basis for allocating resources.

Healthcare Needs and Cosmetic Surgery

The question of determining healthcare needs is especially elusive in the growing field of cosmetic surgery. For many people, the line between genuine healthcare needs and health-related desires is blurred. Cosmetic surgery has been criticized for exploiting people's narcissism rather than addressing real health needs. For example, breast augmentation for women is one of the most common procedures in the United States. (In contrast, breast reduction for women is the most popular cosmetic procedure in France.) An advertisement for breast augmentation from the Pittsburgh Institute of Plastic Surgery (PIPS) in *US Air Magazine* states, "If enlarging your breasts will help you achieve your personal goals call us at. . . ."[43] Surely, cosmetic surgery purely for the purpose of physical enhancement addresses no real healthcare need. On the other hand, cosmetic surgery provides a worthwhile service when it repairs disfigurement due to injury or to other surgeons' mistakes.

Cosmetic surgeons can find immense value in their work. In an insightful essay on the topic, philosopher Kathryn Pauly Morgan describes one surgeon who thought of his craft as "perfecting God's handiwork."[44] Some cosmetic surgeons justify their work despite limited medical resources by claiming that their services provide revenue for an institution that can be used to construct or enrich departments of service to the community, such as a mental health facility.

Although more men are having cosmetic surgery than in the past, most patients are still women. What accounts for cosmetic surgery's growing popularity? Is the fact that more women tend to seek cosmetic surgery than men a sign of women's increasing sense of autonomy? On examination, we find that biotechnologies are essentially designed and controlled by men and that most cosmetic surgeons are men. Who sets the standards for "beauty"? Is the willingness to undergo cosmetic surgery an unconscious (or conscious) submission of some women to men's "benevolence"? According to Morgan, many of these women have been seduced by the culture's ideology of beauty and fertility, an ideology formulated and fashioned by men. This takes place within a culture where "women's attractiveness is defined as attractive to men; women's eroticism is defined as non-existent, pathological, deviant, or peripheral when it is not directed to phallic goals."[45]

Healthcare Needs and Viagra

Soon after Pfizer introduced Viagra to the medical market, urologists throughout the country were writing out hundreds of thousands of prescriptions. The pills, which cost $7 to $10 each, offer temporary relief from male impotence. With an estimated 30 million American men encountering erectile problems, there has been a remarkable demand from the male population.

This demand has been great news for Pfizer. Pfizer stocks immediately soared. However, it could become an enormous financial burden for health insurers. The apparent success of the pill raises a fundamental question that has a direct bearing on the insurance industry: How necessary is sex? In other words, is a pill that treats male impotence medically necessary or merely medically desirable? Is it similar, for instance, to the antidepressant pill Prozac, which most insurance plans cover, or to Accutane, a capsule medication for acne that is covered by most plans? Or is Viagra more similar to Propecia, a pill that treats baldness, which is considered cosmetic and is therefore not covered by health plans?

Should managed care plans cover Viagra? If so, where do they draw the line? Cigna Health Care, for example, limits its coverage to six Viagra pills per month.[46] Also, how do these plans decide who is eligible? How should costs be shared? Is Viagra medically necessary? Health plans intend to cover procedures that are deemed medically necessary, while not covering those considered either experimental or cosmetic.

What compounds the issue further is that, while impotence is certainly a medical disorder, not all those who request Viagra are impotent. Those who request Viagra can claim that they are suffering from some sort of erectile dysfunction, and *dysfunction* is a slippery term. Mariann Caprino, a spokesperson for Pfizer, states that "managed-care plans cover conditions like arthritis and allergies because they *threaten people's quality of life* [italics added]. . . . That's exactly what we're talking about here."[47]

MEDICAL NECESSITY: WHERE DO HEALTH PLANS DRAW THE LINE?

Following are some examples of standard health insurance policies in the United States regarding treatment for certain conditions.

Treatments that are generally covered include

Accutane	For acne; capsule. Special permission needed.
Caverjet	For impotence; injected. Requires medical review and approval.
Muse	For impotence; penile suppository. Medical review and approval required.
Proscar	For benign prostate enlargement; pill. Actually the same drug as Propecia but covered only for this purpose.
Prozac	For depression; capsule.
Retin-A	For acne; topical cream. Can also be used for wrinkles, but only covered for treatment of acne.

Treatments that are not generally covered include

Clomid	For infertility; pill. May be covered under exceptional healthcare package.
Meridia	For diet; capsule. May be covered in cases of life-threatening obesity.
Propecia	For baldness; pill.
Protropin	For short children; recombinant growth hormone in vial. Viewed as medical procedure, and some plans may cover it.[48]

Healthcare Needs and Penile Enlargement—a Rising New Specialty

Miami physician Ricardo Samitier is credited with being the pioneer of phalloplasty, or penile enlargement. He previously performed silicone lip enlargements and eventually applied a similar process to the penis, injecting fat extracted from other body parts. Samitier's career ended after one of his patients died following a penile enlargement operation. He served time in prison on the charge of manslaughter.

Some urologists and plastic surgeons whose incomes began to diminish with managed care have found a new outlet—penile enlargement, or phalloplasty, one of the fastest-growing procedures in cosmetic surgery. Toll-free numbers can hook up potential clients with cosmetic surgeons as long as they have credit cards to pay for the procedure, which costs from $6,000 to $8,000. More than thirty Web sites pertain to penile enlargement. It is estimated that revenues from the procedure are around $24 million per year. Though this seems paltry compared to breast implants' $350 million per year, the demand for phalloplasty continues to soar.[49]

Neither the American Society for Aesthetic Plastic Surgery nor the American Urological Association has endorsed the procedure as safe and effective. In fact, there is no monitoring or regulation of the procedure. Although the Food and Drug Administration (FDA) monitors breast implants, it has no jurisdiction over phalloplasty since no drug or implant is involved.

Another household name in phalloplasty is Los Angeles urologist Melvin Rosenstein. Together with marketing specialist Ed Tilden, he founded the Men's Institute of Cosmetic Surgery, which advertised in popular magazines such as *GQ* and *Penthouse* with the slogan "Dreams do come true."[50] The institute became an overnight success as men throughout Southern California sought the procedure. However, Dr. Rosenstein fell into disrepute just as quickly as he rose to fame. Numerous complaints were filed against him by former clients as the dangers of the operation became more apparent. Some former patients charged him with negligence because they suffered severe problems such as infection, improper stitching, extreme scarring, disfigurement, shrinkage, and impotence. After the California Medical Board reviewed the complaints, Rosenstein's license was temporarily suspended.

Other complaints have been brought against other surgeons. Some lawyers even specialize in penile malpractice cases.[51] Despite all this, phalloplasty continues to be a thriving new cosmetic business.

WHERE DO WE GO FROM HERE?

We have come full circle to our earlier question: What constitutes a just healthcare system? Public policy expert Theodore Marmor insists that any reform measure must incorporate three fundamental elements: containing costs, improving access, and enhancing quality. These three concerns—costs, access, and quality—are interconnected, and all three need to be suitably considered in any genuine attempt to reform the system.[52] As it now stands, there are three possible avenues of reform that the United States can adopt: the individualist paradigm, the permissive paradigm, and the puritan paradigm.

A Free-Market System—the Individualist Paradigm

The free-market system is the current system in the United States. The free-market approach to healthcare is also called the **individualist paradigm**.[53] Only two industrialized Western countries use this paradigm: the United States and South Africa. According to this paradigm, the distribution of health services is essentially based on one's socioeconomic status. This paradigm underscores the significance of free enterprise and private ownership. The key moral principle is individual autonomy and freedom. Whether one belongs to an HMO or buys private insurance, coverage is contingent on income and employment.

Healthcare, according to this paradigm, is an entitlement. That is, it is not an innate moral right (as Norman Daniels contends) but a privilege for those who themselves contribute to the healthcare system and thereby deserve to reap its benefits. This is the view of justice espoused by Robert Nozick.

The free-market system assumes that the overall efficacy of competition within a free market will naturally reduce costs and also enhance quality care. Supporters further claim that it is the context of free enterprise that makes the United States particularly unique among nations. The critical problem with this approach is that 20 percent of the U.S. population has no healthcare coverage. A sizable proportion of the unin-

COMPARING PHYSICIANS AND TECHNOLOGIES:
The United States and Canada

If the quality of a healthcare system rests on the number of physicians and the availability of medical technologies, then the United States is superior to all other countries. The United States has often been compared to its neighbor, Canada. The following statistics indicate that, with respect to factors such as the physician population and medical technologies, the U.S. healthcare system has definite advantages, especially regarding access to certain medical technologies.[54]

Physicians per 100,000 People

Year	United States	Canada
1965	155	130
1970	159	146
1975	178	172
1980	201	184
1985	224	206
1987	234	216

(From Organisation for Economic Co-operation and Development, *Health Care Systems in Transition: The Search for Efficiency* Paris, 1990, Tables 27, 61.)

Availability of Specific Medical Technologies (units per million people)

Medical Technology	United States	Canada
Open-heart surgery	3.26	1.23
Cardiac catheterization	5.06	1.50
Organ transplantation	1.31	1.08
Radiation therapy	3.97	0.54
Extracorporeal shock wave lithoscopy	0.94	0.16
Magnetic resonance imaging	3.69	0.46

(From D. A. Rublee, "Medical Technology in Canada and the U.S.," *Health Affairs,* Fall 1989, 180.)

sured, as was the case in Oregon, work yet are not entitled to receive public funding through Medicaid.

National Health Insurance Through a Single Payer—the Permissive Paradigm[55]

Under the **permissive paradigm,** all citizens are given access to the healthcare services they genuinely need.[56] Healthcare needs are the sole determinant for obtaining services. No patients are at an advantage due to affluence; none are disadvantaged due to poverty. An example of this equal playing field is the Canadian system.

The view of distributive justice in this paradigm, espoused by John Rawls and Norman Daniels, is based on the standards of equality and need. "People should not be allowed to purchase health care which is not accessible to other people with similar needs."[57] Rawls and Daniels advocate a just society that is a moral community, recognizing the need for both equal opportunity and shared responsibility. This paradigm supports a single-tiered system contingent on the criterion of need and a single payer,

CULTURAL WINDOWS

CANADA'S HEALTHCARE SYSTEM

Canada has a national health insurance through a single payer. All Canadian citizens are covered, and there is universal access without any constraints or limits. Citizens pay no extra charges. The coverage is comprehensive, which means that all conventional treatments for conditions are insured. The coverage is also accessible in that no extra fees are charged to patients. Medical care is regulated by a centralized office. Furthermore, each of the ten provinces recognizes the coverage of all other provinces. This means that the insurance is portable and not contingent on circumstances such as change of job or location.

As a result, the Canadian system is more efficient than the complex bureaucracy in the United States. Physicians' fees are determined annually through negotiations between the provincial governments and representatives of the healthcare providers. Contrary to what critics of the Canadian system often point out, Canadians choose their own physicians, and, although there is a queuing system, the waiting lists do not tend to be long. The Canadian healthcare system has also been criticized for providing less access to more sophisticated medical technologies. However, as health policy expert Theodore Marmor points out, Canada's healthcare system does utilize high-tech medical technologies such as magnetic resonance imaging (MRI), extracorporeal shock wave lithoscopy, organ transplantation, and radiation therapy, although they are not as available or used to the same degree as in the United States. Marmor also asserts that maximal use of these technologies is not necessarily indicative of their optimal use. He claims that the Canadian system focuses on using these technologies more judiciously, since inappropriate use is not only medically risky for patients but also financially burdensome to the system.[58] Therefore, Canada's ministries of health in each province monitor the availability as well as the use of certain expensive technologies, not only to control costs but also to prevent their inappropriate use. This monitoring results in less access to and less use of certain sophisticated and expensive technologies for Canadian citizens compared to the U.S. system. For example, according to a 1989 study, the United States performed radiation therapy nearly 7.5 times more often than Canada, used extracorporeal shock wave lithoscopy nearly 6 times more than Canada, and performed magnetic resonance imaging 8 times more than Canada.[59] Despite this, the average Canadian enjoys better health than the average American and lives three to four years longer.

Rationing does occur in the Canadian system, since the supply of some scarce medical resources is less than the demand. This rationing occurs according to medical need as determined by the physician, whereas rationing in the United States is based on ability to pay. Thus, access to medical care in the United States depends in part on socioeconomic status. This is not the case in Canada.

monitored through the government. Funds come from graduated taxes so that ideally all citizens are covered.

As described earlier, recent Gallup polls show that most Americans seem to favor the Canadian system, which reflects this paradigm. Steffie Woolhandler and David U. Himmelstein, in their article at the end of this chapter, represent an American group called Physicians for a National Health Program. They claim that the Canadian health-care system is more beneficial than the U.S. system in a number of ways and that the Canadian system fairly balances equity of access with efficiency. In contrast, Ronald Bronow, who represents a group called Physicians Who Care, argues in his article that there are glaring detriments in the Canadian healthcare system. He points out that adopting the Canadian system would lead to heightened forms of rationing. Given the American ethos of individual freedom within the context of a free market, many Americans might consider this paradigm too restrictive of their personal liberties.

Multitiered System—the Puritan Paradigm

Under the **puritan paradigm,** all citizens are provided with access to a basic core package of health services.[60] However, those who are able to pay for supplemental coverage can do so and therefore have access to more services. This is the aim of the Oregon plan. It was also the aim of President Clinton's ill-fated employment-based health reform plan. Holland, France, Germany, Italy, and Japan use this approach.

Clinton's proposal was an attempt to "stretch" the current system so it eventually would cover nearly all citizens. The plan required all employers to provide coverage for their employees. Employers who refused would be levied with a tax (around 7 percent of payroll), and the funds raised from this tax would go into a public pool for funding Medicaid programs. The stretching would occur by expanding the current Medicaid programs in each state so that all who were previously uninsured would be insured. The result would be a two-tiered system of "play-or-pay."[61]

According to the puritan paradigm, everyone should have access to a basic package of health services. Thus, basic healthcare is contingent on need rather than on a free market. Managed competition plans, in principle, seek to both provide public welfare to all those in need and allow for free enterprise. For many Americans, this paradigm seems more just, especially to those who feel that they are entitled to services they can afford and have earned through their work and savings. This system also allows for freedom of choice, a key value in America.

Although this paradigm is attractive to many and seems to satisfy the need for universal access as well as the need for individual freedom, it has some flaws. Consider children who are dependent on the income of their parent(s). According to this scheme, children from families who are not affluent are deprived of services that children from affluent families have access to. Why should children and other dependents be penalized due to others' income? In this type of system, the affluent have access to superior services. Healthcare services are viewed as commodities available to the highest bidder.

Furthermore, this paradigm creates and sustains a two-tiered system that may develop into a two-tiered healthcare approach. Those on the second tier, that is, those receiving federal and state funding through the expanded Medicaid program, stand in danger of receiving second-rate healthcare services.

In conclusion, even though the United States has the embarrassing distinction of being the only industrialized nation besides South Africa that does not legally provide healthcare coverage for all its citizens, there is still hope for the United States. It can fashion for itself a fair healthcare system, but only if it is willing to undergo deep reform on many levels. The United States can learn from the experiences of other industrialized countries—both from their successes and from their mistakes. It can attempt to adapt, though not imitate, their strengths, since adaptation requires acculturation within a different context. There is hope for the U.S. healthcare system, but only if it is willing to go beyond its borders and learn from other cultures.

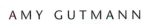

AMY GUTMANN

For and Against Equal Access to Health Care

Amy Gutmann is Laurance S. Rockefeller University Professor and founding director of the University Center for Human Values at Princeton University. Gutmann first clarifies the notion of equal access to healthcare and distinguishes it from the idea of equal consequences. In defending her principle of equal access for all citizens, she supports a single-tier healthcare system, as opposed to a market-driven system. She also discusses pertinent topics related to voluntary and involuntary diseases. She sustains her defense of a single-payer system in view of the limits it would incur on certain patient and physician freedoms. Her discussion occurs within the context of democratic and egalitarian principles.

There is a fairly widespread consensus among empirical analysts that access to health care in this country has become more equal in the last quarter century. Agreement tends to end here; debate follows as to whether this trend will or should persist. But before debating these questions, we ought to have a clear idea of what equal access to health care means. Since equality of access to health care cannot be defined in a morally neutral way, we must choose a definition that is morally loaded with a set of values.[1] The definition offered here is by no means the only possible one. It has, however, the advantage not only of clarity but also of having embedded within it strong and commonly accepted liberal egalitarian values. The debate is better focused upon arguments for and against a strong *principle* of equal access than [upon] disputes over definitions, which tend to hide fundamental value disagreements instead of making them explicit.

An equal access principle, clearly stated and understood, can serve at best as an ideal toward which a society committed to equality of opportunity and equal respect for persons can strive. It does not provide a blueprint for social change, but only a moral standard by which to judge marginal changes in our present institutions of health care.

My purpose here is not only to evaluate the strongest criticisms that are addressed to the principle, ranging from libertarian arguments for more market freedom to arguments supporting a more egalitarian principle of health care. I also propose to examine the sorts of theoretical and practical problems that arise when one tries to defend an egalitarian principle directed at a particular set of institutions within an otherwise inegalitarian society. Since it is extremely unlikely that such a society will be transformed all at once into an egalitarian one, there ought to be room within political and philosophical argument for reasoned consideration and advocacy of "partial" distributive justice, i.e., of principles that are directed only to a particular set of social institutions and whose implementation is not likely to create complete justice even within those institutions.

THE PRINCIPLE DEFINED

A principle of equal access to health care demands that every person who shares the same type and degree of health need must be given an equally effective chance of receiving appropriate treatment of equal quality so long as that treatment is available to anyone. Stated in this way, the equal access principle does not establish whether a society must provide any particular medical treatment or health care benefit to its needy members. I shall suggest later that the level and type of provision can vary within certain reasonable boundaries according to the priorities determined by legitimate democratic procedures. The principle requires that if anyone within a society has an opportunity to receive a service or good that satisfies a health need, then everyone who shares the same type and degree of health need must be given an equally effective chance of receiving that service or good.

Since this is a principle of equal *access,* it does not guarantee equal *results,* although it probably would move our society in that direction. Discriminations in health care are permitted if they are based upon type or degree of health need, willingness of informed adults to be treated, and choices of lifestyle among the population. The equal access principle constrains the distribution of opportunities to receive health care to an egalitarian standard, but it does not determine the total level of health care available or the effects of that care (provided the care is of equal quality) upon the health of the population. Of course, even if equality in health care were defined according to an "equal health" principle,[2] one would still have to admit that a just health care system could not come close to producing an equally healthy population, given the unequal distribution of illness among people and our present medical knowledge.

PRACTICAL IMPLICATIONS

Since the equal access principle requires equality of effective opportunity to receive care, not merely equality of formal legal access, it does not permit discriminations based upon those characteristics of people that we can reasonably assume they did not freely choose. Such characteristics include sex, race, genetic endowment, wealth, and, often, place of residence. Even in an ideal society, equally needy persons will not use the same amount or quality of health care. Their preferences and their knowledge will differ, as will the skills of the providers who treat them.

A One-Class System

The most striking result of applying the equal access principle in the United States would be the creation of a one-class system of health care. Services and goods that meet health care needs would be equally available to everyone who was equally needy. As a disincentive to overuse, . . . small fees for service could be charged for health care, provided that charges did not prove a barrier to entry to the poorest people who were needy. A one-class system need not, of course, be a uniform system. Diversity among medical and health care services would be permissible, indeed even desirable, so long as the diversity did not create differential access along nonconsensual lines such as wealth, race, sex, or geographical location.[3]

Equal access also places limits upon the market freedoms of some individuals, especially, but not exclusively, the richest members of society. The principle does not permit the purchase of health care to which other similarly needy people do not have effective access. The extent to which freedom of the rich must be restricted will depend upon the level of public provision for health care and the degree of income inequality. As the level of health care guaranteed to the poor decreases and the degree of income inequality increases, the equal access standard demands greater restrictions upon the market freedom of the rich. Where income and wealth are very unevenly distributed, and where the level of publicly guaranteed access is very low, the rich can use the market to buy access to health care goods unavailable to the poor, thereby undermining the effective equality of opportunity required by an equal access principle.

The restriction upon market freedoms to purchase health care under these circumstances creates a certain discomforting irony: the equal access principle permits (or is at least agnostic with respect to) the free market satisfaction of preferences for nonessential consumer goods. Thus, the rigorous implementation of equal access to health care would prevent rich people from spending their extra income for preferred medical services, if those services were not equally accessible to the poor. It would not prevent their using those same resources to purchase satisfaction in other areas—a Porsche or any other luxurious consumer good. In discussing additional problems created by an attempt to implement a principle of equal access to health care in an otherwise inegalitarian society, I return later to consider whether advocates of equal access can avoid this irony.

Hard Cases

As with all principles, hard cases exist for the equal access principle. Without dwelling upon these cases, it is worth considering how the principle might deal with two hard but fairly common cases: therapeutic experimentation in medicine, and alternative treatments of different quality.

Each year in the United States, many potentially successful therapies are tested. Since their value has not been proved, there may be good reason to limit their use to an appropriate sample of sick experimental subjects. The equal access principle would insist that experimenters choose these subjects at random from a population of relevantly sick consenting adults. A randomized clinical trial could be advertised by public notice, and individuals who are interested might be registered and enrolled on a lottery basis. The only requirement for enrollment would be the health conditions and personal characteristics necessary for proper scientific testing.

How does one apply the principle of equal access when alternative treatments are each functionally adequate but aesthetically or socially quite disparate? Take the hypothetical case of a societal commitment to adequate dentition among adults. Replacement of carious or mobile teeth with dentures may preserve dental function at relatively minor cost. On the other hand, full mouth reconstruction, involving periodontal and endodontic treatment and capping of affected teeth, may be only marginally more effective but substantially more satisfying. The added costs for the preferred treatment are not inconsiderable. The principle would seem to demand that at equal states of dental need there be equal access to the preferred treatment. It is unclear, however, whether the satisfaction of subjective desire is equivalent to fulfillment of objective need.

In cases of alternative treatments, proponents of equal access could turn to another argument for providing access to the same treatments for all. A society that publicly provides the minimal acceptable treatment freely to all, and also permits a private market in more expensive treatments, may result in a two-class system of care. The best providers will service the richest clientele, at the risk of inadequate treatment for the poorest. Approval of a private market in alternative treatments would rest upon the empirical hypothesis that, if the publicly funded level of adequate treatment were high enough, few people would choose to short-circuit the public (i.e., equal access) sector; the small additional free market sector would not threaten to lower the quality of services universally available.

Most cases, like the one of dentistry, are difficult to decide merely on principle. Proponents of equal access must take into account the consequences of alternative policies. But empirical knowledge alone will not decide these issues, and arguments for or against a particular policy can be entertained in a more systematic way once one exposes the values that underlie support for an equal access principle. One can then judge to what extent alternative policies satisfy these values.

SUPPORTING VALUES

Advocates of equal access to health care must demonstrate why health care is different from other consumer goods, unless they are willing to support the more radical principle of equal distribution of all goods. Norman Daniels provides one foundation for distinguishing between health care and other goods.[4] He establishes a category of health care needs whose satisfaction provides an important condition for future opportunity. Like police protection and education, some kinds of health care goods are necessary for pursuing most other goods in life. Any theory of justice committed to equalizing opportunity ought to treat health care as a good deserving of special distributive treatment. Equal access to health care provides a necessary, although certainly not a sufficient, condition for equal opportunity in general.

A precept of egalitarian justice that physical pains of a sufficient degree be treated similarly, regardless of who experiences them, establishes another reason for singling out certain kinds of health care as special goods.[5] Some health conditions cause great pain but are not linked to a serious curtailment of opportunity. The two values are, however, mutually compatible.

A theory of justice that gives priority to the value of equal respect among people might also be used to support a principle of equal access to health care. John Rawls, for example, argues that without self-respect "nothing may seem worth doing, or if some things have value for us, we lack the will to strive for them . . . Therefore the parties in the original position would wish to avoid at almost any cost the social conditions that undermine self-respect."[6]

Conditions of Self-Respect

It is not easy to determine what social conditions support or undermine self-respect. One might plausibly assume that equalizing opportunity and treating similar pains similarly would be the most essential supports for equal respect within a health care system. And so, in most cases, the value of equal respect provides additional support for equal access to the same health care goods that are warranted by the values of equal opportunity and relief from pain. But at least some kinds of health care treatment not essential to equalizing opportunity or bringing equal relief from pain may be necessary to equalize respect within a society. It is conceivable that much longer waiting time, in physicians' offices or for admission to hospitals, may not affect the long-term health prospects of the poor or of blacks. But such discriminations in waiting times for an essential good probably do adversely affect the self-respect of those who systematically stand at the end of the queue.

Some of the conditions necessary for equal respect are socially relative; we must arrive at a standard of equal respect appropriate to our particular society. Universal suffrage has long been a condition for equal respect; the case for it is independent of the anticipated results of equalizing political power by granting every person one vote. More recently, equal access to health care has similarly become a condition for equal respect in our society. Most of us do not base our self-respect on the way we are treated on airplanes, even though the flight attendants regularly give preferential treatment to those traveling first class. This contrast with suffrage and health care treatment (and education and police protection) no doubt is related to the fact that these goods are much more essential to our society and opportunities in life than is airplane travel. But it is still worth considering that unequal treatment in health care, as in education, may be understood as a sign of unequal respect even where there are no discernible adverse effects on the health or education of those receiving less favored treatment. Even where a dual health care system will not produce inferior medical results for the less privileged, the value of equal respect militates against the perpetuation of such a system in our society.

CHALLENGES

Equality of opportunity, equal efforts to relieve pain, and equal respect are the three central values providing the foundation of support for a principle of equal access to health care. Any theory of justice that gives primacy to these values (as do many liberal and egalitarian theories) will lend prima facie support to a health care system structured along equal access lines.

We are now in a position to consider alternative values and empirical claims that would lead someone to challenge, or reject, a principle of equal access to health care. These challenges also enable us to elaborate further the moral and political implications of the principle.

Proponents of the Market

The most radical and vocal opposition comes from those who support a pure free market principle in health care. A foundation of support for the free market principle is the idea that the relative importance of satisfying different human desires is a purely subjective matter: we can distinguish between one person's desire for good medical care and another person's desire for a good Beaujolais only by the price they are willing to pay for each. If no goods are special because there is no way of ranking desires except by individual processes of choice, then what better way than the unconstrained market to allow us to decide among the smorgasbord of goods society has to offer?[7]

Health care goods and services are likely to be more equally allocated through the market if income and wealth are more equally distributed. Several defenders of the market as a means of allocating goods and services also support a moderate degree of income redistribution on grounds of its diminishing marginal utility, or because they believe that every person has a right to a "basic minimum."[8] Neither rationale for redistribution takes us very far toward a principle of equal access to health care. If one retains the basic assumption that human preferences are totally subjective, then the market remains the best way to order human priorities. Only the market appropriately decentralizes decision-making and eliminates all nonconsensual exchange of goods and services.[9]

Although a minimum income floor under all individuals increases *access* to most goods and services, even at a higher level than that supported by Friedman and others, a guaranteed income will be inadequate to sustain the costs of a catastrophic illness. An exceptionally high guaranteed minimum might result in almost universal insurance coverage at a fairly high level. Supporters of free market allocation do not, however, press for a very high minimum for at least two reasons. They fear its effects on incentives, and they cannot justify a high guaranteed income without admitting that there are many expensive goods that are essential to all persons, and are not just mere consumer preferences.

The first reason for opposing an exceptionally high minimum is probably a good one. A principle approaching equality of income and wealth is likely to have serious disincentive effects on productive work and investment. There are also better reasons for treating health care as a special good, a good that society has an obligation to provide equally to all its members, than there are for equally distributing most consumer goods.

A significant step beyond the pure free market principle is a position that preserves the role of the market in allocating different "packages" of health care according to consumer preferences, but concedes a role for government in supplying every adult with a "voucher" of a certain monetary value redeemable exclusively for health care goods and services. Proponents of health vouchers must assume that there is something special about health care to justify government in taxing its citizens to provide universally for these goods, and not all others. But if health care is a more important good, because it preserves life and expands opportunity, then what is the rationale for effectively limiting the demand a sick but poor person can make upon the health care system? Why should access to health care be dependent upon income or wealth at all?

Opponents of equal access generally imply that more than minimal access will unjustly curtail the freedom of citizens as taxpayers, as consumers, and as providers of health care. Let us consider separately the arguments with regard to the many citizens who are taxpayers and consumers, and the few citizens who are providers of health care.

The Charge of Paternalism

Charles Fried has argued that equal access to health care is a particularly intrusive form of paternalism toward citizens. He claims further that "apart from a rather general commitment to equality and, indeed, to state control of the allocation and distribution of resources, to insist on the right to health care, where that right means a right to equal access, is an anomaly. For as long as our society considers that inequalities of wealth and income are morally acceptable . . . it is anomalous to carve out a sector like health care and say that *there* equality must reign."[10]

Would an equal access system necessarily be intrusive or paternalistic in its operation? A national health care system simply cannot be said to take away the income entitlement of citizens, since citizens are not entitled to their gross incomes. We can determine our income entitlements only after we deduct from our gross income the amount we owe the state to support the rights of others. To the extent that the rationale of an equal access principle is redistributive, those individuals who otherwise could not afford certain health care services will experience an expansion of their freedom (if we assume an adequate level of social provision). Of course, part of the justification of a national health care system is that it would also guarantee health care coverage to people who could afford adequate health care but who would not be prudent enough to save or to invest in insurance. Even if we accept the common definition of paternalistic actions as those that restrict an individual's liberty so as to further his or her interest, we still have to assess the assertion that this (partial) rationale for an equal access system entails a restriction of individual liberty. Unlike a law banning the sale of cigarettes or forcing people to wear seat belts, the institution of a national health care system forces no one to use it. If a majority of citizens decide that they want to be taxed in order to ensure health care for themselves, the resulting legislation could not be considered paternalistic: "Legislation requiring contributions to some cooperative scheme (such as medical care) . . . is not necessarily paternalistic, so long as its purpose is to give effect to the desires of a democratic majority, rather than simply to coerce a minority who do not want the benefits of the legislation."[11] It is significant in this regard that for the past twenty years the Michigan survey of registered voters has found a consistent and solid majority supporting government measures designed to ensure universal access to medical care.

The charge of paternalism levied against an equal access system is therefore dubious because it is extremely difficult, if not impossible, to isolate the self-protectionist rationale from the redistributive and the democratic rationales. Those who object to a national health care system on the grounds that it is coercing some people for their own good forget that such a system still could be justified as a means to avoid the threat to a one-class system that exempting the rich would create. To condemn such a system as paternalistic would commit us to criticizing all legislation in which a democratic majority decides to protect itself against the wishes of a minority when exemption

from the resulting policy would undermine it. Other critics wrongly assume that people have an entitlement to the cash equivalent of the medical care to which society grants them a right. People do not have such an entitlement because taxpayers have a right to demand that their tax dollars are spent to satisfy health needs, not to buy luxuries. Indeed, our duty to pay taxes is dependent upon the fact that certain needs of other people must be given priority over our own desires for more commodious living.

Other Restrictions

Nonetheless, two restrictions upon consumer freedom are entailed in an equal access system. One is the restriction imposed by the taxation necessary to provide all citizens, but especially the poorest, with access to health care goods. This restriction does not raise unique or particularly troublesome moral problems so long as one believes that the freedom to retain one's gross income is not an absolute right and that the resulting redistribution of income to the health care sector increases the life chances and thereby the effective freedom of many citizens.

But there is a second restriction of consumer market freedom sanctioned by the equal access principle: the limitation upon freedom to buy health care goods above the level publicly provided. Aside from reasserting the primary values of equality, there is at least one plausible argument for such a restriction. Without restricting the free market in extra health care goods, a society risks having its best medical practitioners drained into the private market sector, thereby decreasing the quality of medical care received by the majority of citizens confined to the publicly funded sector. The lower the level of public provision of health care and the less elastic the supply of physicians, the more problematic (from the perspective of the values underlying equal access) will be an additional market sector in health care.

Without an additional market sector, would the freedom of physicians and other providers to practice wherever and for whomever they choose be unduly restricted? The extent of such restrictions will also vary with the level of public provision and with the diversity of the health care system. Public funds already are crucial to providing many physicians with basic income (through Medicare and Medicaid fees), research opportunities through the National Institutes of Health (NIH), and many with hospitals and other institutions in which to practice (through the provisions of the Hill-Burton Act). In place of the time and resources now directed to privately purchased add-ons, an equal access system would redirect providers toward meeting previously unserved needs. These types of redirections of supply and redistribution of demand are commonly accepted in other professions that are oriented toward satisfying an important public interest. The legal and teaching professions are analogous in this regard. The equal access principle, strictly interpreted, however, adds another restriction, a limitation upon private practice that supplies health care goods not equally accessible to the entire population of relevantly needy persons. This restriction upon the freedom of providers does not have an analogue in the present practice of law or of education, although the arguments for equal access to the goods of these professions might be similar. And so, one's assessment of the strength of the case for such a restriction is likely to have implications beyond the health care system.

It is hard to see why one ought to prevent people, rich or poor, from spending money upon health care goods while permitting them to spend money on consumer goods that are clearly not essential, and perhaps even detrimental to health. One reason might be the possible systemic effect, mentioned above, that such additional expenditures would deprive the less advantaged of the best physicians. The freedom of providers as well as consumers would have to be restricted in order to curtail this effect. But beyond this empirically contingent argument for restricting any market in health care goods that are not equally accessible to all, the strict limitations upon market freedom in "extra" health care goods are hard to accept if one believes that medical services are at least as worthy items of expense as other consumer goods. One could argue that physicians ought to be free to

meet the demand for additional medical goods, especially when that demand is a substitute for demand for less important goods.

This criticism illuminates a more general problem of attempting to equalize access to any good in an otherwise inegalitarian society. The more unequal the distribution of income and wealth within our society, the more likely that the freedom of consumers and providers to buy and sell health care outside the publicly funded sector will result in inequalities that cannot properly be regarded merely as the product of differences in consumer preferences. Therefore, in an inegalitarian society, we must live with a moral tension between granting providers the freedom to leave the publicly funded sector and achieving more equality in the satisfaction of health care needs.

A principle of equal access to health care applied within an otherwise egalitarian society might give little or no reason to restrict the freedom of providers or consumers. One argument often voiced against a publicly funded system that permits a marginal free market sector is that the government is a less efficient provider of goods than are private parties. But the equal access principle does not require that the government directly provide medical services through, for example, a national health service. Government need only be a regulator of the use and distribution of essential health care goods and services. This is a role that most people concede to government for many other purposes deemed essential to the welfare of all individuals.

Government regulation may, of course, be more expensive and hence less efficient than government provision of health care services of similar extent and quality. The tradeoff here would be between the additional market choice facilitated by government regulation or private providers and the decreased public cost of government provision. Despite utilitarian claims to the contrary, no simple moral calculus exists that would enable an impartial spectator to determine where the balance of advantage lies. Philosophers ought to cede to a fairly constituted democratic majority the right to decide this issue. What constitutes a fair process of democratic decision-making is an important question of procedural justice that lies beyond the scope of this paper.

Liability for Voluntary Risks?

Another important criticism of the equal access principle cuts across advocacy of the free market and government regulation of health care. Supporters of both views might consistently ask whether it is fair to provide the same level of access for all people, including those who voluntarily adopt bad health habits, and who quite knowingly and willingly take greater-than-average risks with their lives and health. Even if it might be unjust not to provide health care for those people once the need arises, why would it not be fair to force those who choose to drink, smoke, rock climb, and sky-dive also to bear a greater burden of their ensuing medical costs than that borne by people who deliberately avoid these risky pursuits? An equal access principle seems to neglect the distinction between voluntary and nonvoluntary health risks in its eagerness to ensure that all people have an equal opportunity to receive appropriate health care.

Gerald Dworkin extensively and convincingly argues that it would not be unfair to force individuals to be financially liable for voluntarily undertaken health risks, but only under certain conditional assumptions. These include our ability (1) to determine the relative causal role of voluntary versus involuntary factors in the genesis of illness; (2) to differentiate between purely voluntary behavior and what is nonvoluntary or compulsive; and (3) to distinguish between genetic and nongenetic predispositions to illness.[12] For example, to satisfy the first condition one would have to determine the relative causal role of smoking and environmental pollution in the genesis of lung cancer; to fulfill the second, one must know when smoking (or drinking or obesity) is voluntary and when it is compulsive behavior; and to satisfy the third condition, one must distinguish among those who smoke and get cancer, and those who smoke and do not. In addition, so long as there are no good institutional mechanisms for monitoring certain risky activities or for differentiating between moderate and immoderate users of unhealthy substances, qualifying the equal access principle to

take account of voluntary health risks is likely to create more unfairness rather than less. Finally, given great inequalities in income distribution, the poor will be less able to bear the consequences of their risky behavior than will the rich, creating a situation of unfairness at least as serious as the unfairness of equally distributing the burdens of health care costs between those who voluntarily impose risks upon themselves and those who do not. With respect to the health hazards of overeating and obesity, for example, the rich have recourse to expensive programs of weight control unavailable to the poor. Since we have such scanty knowledge of situations when sickness can be attributable to voluntary health risks, criticisms of the equal access principle from this perspective have more weight in principle than they do in practice.

Equal Access to All Health Goods

All criticisms considered so far are directed at the equal access principle from a perspective suggesting that government involvement and public funding of health care would be too great and the role of the market too small in an equal access system. Now let us consider a powerful criticism of the principle for including too little, rather than too much, in the public sector. The criticism can be posed in the form of a challenge: if one crucial reason for supporting a principle of equal access is that health goods are much more essential than many other goods because they provide a basis for equalizing opportunity and relieving substantial pain, then why not require a government to provide equal access to *all* those health goods that would move a society further in the direction of equalizing opportunity and relieving pain for the physically and mentally ill? Without pretending that our society could ever arrive at a condition of absolute equality in health (or therefore strict equality of opportunity), proponents of this principle could still argue that we should move as far as possible in that direction.

In a society in which no tradeoffs had to be made between health care and other goods, equal access to *all* health goods might be the most acceptable principle of equity in health care.[13] Of course, we do not live in such a society. Given the advanced state of our medical and health care technology, and the prevalence of chronic degenerative diseases and mental disorders in our population, a requirement that society provide access to every known health care good would place an enormous drain upon social resources.[14]

Costliness per se is not the main issue. The problem with the principle of equal access to all health goods is that it demands an absolute trade-off between satisfaction of health care needs and other needs and desires. The simplest argument against this principle is that other needs, such as education, police protection, and legal aid, will be sacrificed to health care, if the principle is enforced. But this argument is too simple. A proponent of equal access to all health goods could consistently establish some priority principle among these goods, all of which satisfy needs derived in large part from a principle of equal opportunity. The weightier counterargument is that, above some less-than-maximum level in the provision of opportunity goods, it seems reasonable for people to value what, for want of a better term, one might call "quality of life" goods: cultural, recreational, noninstrumental educational goods, and even consumer amenities. A society that maximized the satisfaction of needs before it even began to provide access to "quality of life" goods would be a dismal society indeed. Most people do not want to devote their entire lives to being maximally secure and healthy. Why, then, should a society devote all of its resources to satisfying human *needs?*

Democracy and Equal Access

We need to find some principle or procedure by which to draw a line at an appropriate level of access to health care short of what is socially and technologically possible, but greater than what an unconstrained market would afford to most people, particularly to the least advantaged. I suspect that no philosophical argument can provide us with a cogent principle by which we can draw a line within the enormous group of goods that can improve health or extend the life prospects of individuals.

This problem of determining a proper level of guaranteed social satisfaction of need is not unique to health care. Something similar can be said about police protection or education in our society. Philosophers can provide reasons why police protection and education are rightly considered basic collective needs and why they should be given priority over individual consumer preferences. But no plausible philosophical principle can tell us what level of police protection or how much education a society ought to provide on an egalitarian basis.

The principle of equal access to health care establishes a criterion of distribution for whatever level of health care a society provides for any of its members. And further philosophical argument might establish some criteria by which to judge when the publicly funded level of health care was so low as to be unfair to the least advantaged, or so high as to create undue restrictions upon the ability of most people to live interesting and fulfilling lives. The remaining question of establishing a precise level of priorities among health care and other goods (at the "margin") is appropriately left to democratic decision-making. The advantage of the democratic process in determining the precise level of health care provision is that citizens have an equal and collective voice in determining a decision that, according to the equal access principle, ought to be mutually binding. Citizens not only reap the benefits; they also share the burdens of the decision to expand or limit access to health care.

There is yet another advantage to this procedural method of establishing a fair level of health care provision. If the democratic decision will be binding upon all citizens, as the equal access principle assumes it must be, then one might expect the most advantaged citizens to exercise more political pressure to increase access to health care and hence increase the opportunity of the least advantaged above the level that they could afford in a free market system, or in a system where the rich were not included within the publicly funded health care sector. One finds some evidence to support this hypothesis in comparing the relative immunity from budget cutbacks of the program under universal entitlement of Medicare compared with the income-related Medicaid program. Of course, if costliness to the taxpayer is one's only concern, this added political pressure for health care expenditures is a liability rather than a strength of a one-class system. But from the perspective of equal access, the cost of a two-class system, one privately and one publicly funded, is an inequitable distribution of quantity and quality of care according to wealth, not need. The added nonproductive costs required merely to keep the two classes apart are seldom taken into account. And from the perspective of those supporters of an equal access principle who also want to increase the total level of health care provision, the two-class system threatens to work in the opposite direction, siphoning off the pressure of citizens who have a disproportionate share of political influence. A democratic decision, the results of which are constrained by the principle of equal access, will give a relatively accurate reading of what most people believe to be an adequate level of health care protection. The major disadvantage of the equal access constraint is that the decision of the majority or its representatives binds everyone, even those people who want more than the socially mandated level of health care.

Given the great economic inequalities of our society, it is politically impossible for advocates of equal access to fulfill their task. No democratic legislator could possibly succeed in winning support for a proposal that restricted market freedom as extensively as a strict interpretation of the equal access principle requires. And it probably would be a mistake to insist upon strict philosophical standards: one thereby risks throwing the possibility of greater access to health care for the poor out with the insistence upon curtailing access for the rich.

CONCLUSION

I began by arguing that a principle of equal access to health care was at best an ideal toward which our society might strive. I shall end by qualifying that statement. A sufficiently high level of public provision of health care for all citizens and a suffi-
ciently elastic supply of health care would significantly reduce the threat to universal provision of quality health care of a private market in extra health care goods, just as a very high level of police protection and education reduces the inequalities of opportunity resulting from purchase of private bodyguards or of private school education by the rich.

In the best of all imaginable worlds of egalitarian justice, the equal access principle would be sufficiently supported by other egalitarian social and economic institutions that a market in health care would complement rather than undercut the goals of equal respect and opportunity. But philosophers ought to resist basing their political recommendations solely upon a model of the best of all imaginable worlds.

NOTES

1. N. Daniels, "Equity of Access to Health Care: Some Conceptual and Ethical Issues," paper delivered to the President's Commission for the Study of Ethical Issues in Medicine and Biomedical and Behavioral Research, Washington, DC, March 13, 1981.
2. R. Veatch, "What Is a Just Health Care Delivery," from *Ethics and Health Policy,* eds. R. Veatch and R. Bransen (Cambridge, MA: Ballinger Publishing Group, 1976).
3. P. Starr, "A National Health Program: Organizing Diversity." *Hasting Center Report* 5:11–13, 1975.
4. N. Daniels, "Health-Care Needs and Distributive Justice," *Philosophy and Public Affairs* 10 (1981), pp. 146–79.
5. A. Gutmann, *Liberal Equality* (New York: Cambridge University Press, 1980).
6. J. Rawls, *A Theory of Justice* (Cambridge, MA: Harvard University Press, 1971).
7. C. Fried, "Health Care, Cost Containment, Liberty," paper presented to the Institute of Society, Ethics, and the Life Sciences, Hastings-on-Hudson, NY, October 1979; R. Nozick, *Anarchy, State, and Utopia* (New York: Basic Books, 1974); R. N. Sade, "Medical Care as a Right: A Refutation," *New England Journal of Medicine* 285 (1971), pp. 1288–92.
8. M. Friedman, *Capitalism and Freedom* (Chicago: University of Chicago Press, 1962); C. Fried, *Right and Wrong* (Cambridge, MA: Harvard University Press, 1978).

9. Fried, *Right and Wrong*, pp. 124–26.
10. C. Fried, "Equality and Rights in Medical Care," *Hastings Center Report* 6 (1976), p. 31.
11. D. F. Thompson, "Paternalism in Medicine, Law, and Public Policy,"; D. Callahan and S. Boll (eds.), *Ethics Teaching in Higher Education* (New York: Plenum, 1980), pp. 245–75.
12. G. Dworkin, "Responsibility and Health Risks,"

paper presented to the Institute of Society, Ethics, and the Life Sciences, Hastings-on-Hudson, NY, October 1979.
13. R. Veatch, pp. 127–53.
14. A. R. Somers, *Health Care in Transition: Directions for the Future* (Chicago, IL: Hospital Research and Educational Trust, 1971).

QUESTIONS FOR COMPREHENSION AND REFLECTION

1. According to Gutmann, what are some critical differences between "equal access to medical care" and "equality of results"?
2. According to Gutmann, how does equal access bring about a maximization of self-respect for citizens in a democracy? Do you agree? Explain.
3. How does Gutmann support her proposal of equal access against the claim that cases of personal contribution to illness and disease should be treated differently from cases of involuntary illness and disease? Do you find her argument compelling? Explain.
4. Critics often point out that a single-payer system is overly paternalistic. How does Gutmann respond to this criticism? Do you agree? Explain.

NORMAN DANIELS

Why Saying No to Patients in the United States Is So Hard: Cost Containment, Justice, and Provider Autonomy

Norman Daniels is Goldthwaite Professor in the departments of philosophy and community medicine at Tufts University. Daniels tackles some critical questions concerning the relationship between cost-containment and the need to ration beneficial healthcare. He addresses this relationship on both micro and macro levels and contends that the extent of rationing will depend on fundamental principles of justice as well as on underlying views of healthcare. After comparing the U.S. experience with that of the British National Health Service, he examines the effect of economic incentives on U.S. physicians. His overriding concern is that the healthcare system in the United States as a whole does not operate according to the principle of distributive justice. For this reason, denying beneficial care is difficult to justify. All this makes the tension between cost-effectiveness and quality care more acute.

If cost-containment measures, such as the use of Medicare's diagnosis-related groups (DRGs), involved trimming only unnecessary health care services from public budgets, they would pose no moral problems. Instead, such measures lead physicians and hospitals to deny some possibly beneficial care, such as longer hospitalization or more diagnostic tests, to their own patients—that is, at the "micro" level.[1] Similarly, if the "macro" decision not to disseminate a new medical procedure, such as liver transplantation, resulted only in the avoidance of waste, then it would pose no moral problem. When is it morally justifiable to say no to beneficial care or useful procedures? And why is it especially difficult to justify saying no in the United States?

JUSTICE AND RATIONING

Because of scarcity and the inevitable limitation of resources even in a wealthy society, justice—however we elucidate it—will require some no-saying at both the macro and micro levels of allocation. No plausible principles of justice will entitle an individual patient to every potentially beneficial treatment. Providing such treatment might consume resources to which another patient has a greater claim. Similarly, no class of patients is entitled to whatever new procedure offers them some benefit. New procedures have opportunity costs, consuming resources that could be used to produce other benefits, and other classes of patients may have a superior claim that would require resources to be invested in alternative ways.

How rationing works depends on which principles of justice apply to health care. For example, some people believe that health care is a commodity or service no more important than any other and that it should be distributed according to the ability to pay for it. For them, saying no to patients who cannot afford certain services (quite apart from whether income distribution is itself just or

fair) is morally permissible. Indeed, providing such services to all might seem unfair to the patients who are required to pay.

In contrast, other theories of justice view health care as a social good of special moral importance. In one recent discussion,[2] health care was seen to derive its moral importance from its effect on the normal range of opportunities available in society. This range is reduced when disease or disability impairs normal functioning. Since we have social obligations to protect equal opportunity, we also have obligations to provide access, without financial or discriminatory barriers, to services that adequately protect and restore normal functioning. We must also weigh new technological advances against alternatives, to judge the overall effect of their introduction on equal opportunity. This gives a slightly new sense to the term "opportunity cost." As a result, people are entitled only to services that are part of a system that on the whole protects equal opportunity. Thus, even an egalitarian theory that holds health care as of special moral importance justifies sometimes saying no at both the macro and micro levels.

SAYING NO IN THE BRITISH NATIONAL HEALTH SERVICE

Aaron and Schwartz have documented how beneficial services and procedures have had to be rationed within the British National Health Service, since its austerity budget allows only half the level of expenditures of the United States.[3] The British, for example, use less x-ray film, provide little treatment for metastatic solid tumors, and generally do not offer renal dialysis to the elderly. Saying no takes place at both macro and micro levels.

Rationing in Great Britain takes place under two constraints that do not operate at all in the United States. First, although the British say no to some beneficial care, they nevertheless provide universal access to high-quality health care. In contrast, over 10 percent of the population in the United States lacks insurance, and racial differences in access and health status persist.[4, 5] Second, saying no takes place within a regionally centralized budget. Decisions about introducing new procedures involve weighing the net benefits of alternatives within a closed system. When a procedure is rationed; it is clear which resources are available for alternative uses. When a procedure is widely used, it is clear which resources are unavailable for other uses. No such closed system constrains American decisions about the dissemination of technological advances except, on a small scale and in a derivative way, within some health maintenance organizations (HMOs).

These two constraints are crucial to justifying British rationing. The British practitioner who follows standard practice within the system does not order the more elaborate x-ray diagnosis that might be typical in the United States, possibly even despite the knowledge that additional information would be useful. Denying care can be justified as follows: Though the patient might benefit from the extra service, ordering it would be unfair to other patients in the system. The system provides equitable access to a full array of services that are fairly allocated according to professional judgments about which needs are most important. The salve of this rationale may not be what the practitioner uses to ease his or her qualms about denying beneficial treatment, but it is available.

A similar rationale is available at the macro level. If British planners believe alternative uses of resources will produce a better set of health outcomes than introducing coronary bypass surgery on a large scale, they will say no to a beneficial procedure. But they have available the following rationale: Though they would help one group of patients by introducing this procedure, its opportunity cost would be too high. They would have to deny other patients services that are more necessary. Saying yes instead of no would be unjust.

These justifications for saying no at both levels have a bearing on physician autonomy and on moral obligations to patients. Within the standards of practice determined by budget ceilings in the system, British practitioners remain autonomous in their clinical decision making. They are obliged

to provide the best possible care for their patients within those limits. Their clinical judgments are not made "impure" by institutional profit incentives to deny care.

The claim made here is not that the British National Health Service is just, but that considerations of justice are explicit in its design and in decisions about the allocation of resources. Because justice has this role, British rationing can be defended on grounds of fairness. Of course, some no-saying, such as the denial of renal dialysis to elderly patients, may raise difficult questions of justice.[2] The issue here, however, is not the merits of each British decision, but the framework within which they are made.

SAYING NO IN THE UNITED STATES

Cost-containment measures in the United States reward institutions, and in some cases practitioners, for delivering treatment at a lower cost. Hospitals that deliver treatment for less than the DRG rate pocket the difference. Hospital administrators therefore scrutinize the decisions of physicians to use resources, pressuring some to deny beneficial care. Many cannot always act in their patients' best interests, and they fear worse effects if DRGs are extended to physicians' charges.[6] In some HMOs and preferred-provider organizations, there are financial incentives for the group to shave the costs of treatment—if necessary, by denying some beneficial care. In large HMOs, in which risks are widely shared, there may be no more denial of beneficial care than under fee-for-service reimbursement.[7] But in some capitation schemes, individual practitioners are financially penalized for ordering "extra" diagnostic tests, even if they think their patient needs them. More ominously, some hospital chains are offering physicians a share of the profits made in their hospitals from the early discharge of Medicare patients.

When economic incentives to physicians lead them to deny beneficial care, there is a direct threat to what may be called the ethic of agency. In general, granting physicians considerable autonomy in clinical decision making is necessary if they are to be effective as agents pursuing their patients' interests. The ethic of agency constrains this autonomy in ways that protect the patient, requiring that clinical decisions be competent, respectful of the patient's autonomy, respectful of the other rights of the patient (e.g., confidentiality), free from consideration of the physician's interests, and uninfluenced by judgments about the patient's worth. Incentives that reward physicians for denying beneficial care clearly risk violating the fourth-mentioned constraint, which, like the fifth, is intended to keep clinical decisions pure—that is, aimed at the patient's best interest.

Rationing need not violate the constraint that decisions must be free from consideration of the physician's interest. British practitioners are not rewarded financially for saying no to their patients. Because our cost-containment schemes give incentives to violate this constraint, however, they threaten the ethic of agency. Patients would be foolish to think the physician who benefits from saying no is any longer their agent. (Of course, patients in the United States traditionally have had to guard against unnecessary treatments, since reimbursement schemes provided incentives to overtreat.)

American physicians face a problem even when the only incentive for denying beneficial care is the hospital's, not theirs personally. For example, how can they justify sending a Medicare patient home earlier than advisable? Can they, like their British peers, claim that justice requires them to say no and that therefore they do no wrong to their patients?

American physicians cannot make this appeal to the justice of saying no. They have no assurance that the resources they save will be put to better use elsewhere in the health care system. Reducing a Medicare expenditure may mean only that there is less pressure on public budgets in general, and thus more opportunity to invest the savings in weapons. Even if the savings will be freed for use by other Medicare patients, American physicians have no assurance that the resources will be used to meet the greater needs of other patients. The American health care system, unlike the British one, establishes no explicit priorities for the use of resources. In fact, the savings from saying no may be used to invest in a procedure that may never

provide care of comparable importance to that the physician is denying the patient. In a for-profit hospital, the profit made by denying beneficial treatment may be returned to investors. In many cases, the physician can be quite sure that saying no to beneficial care will lead to greater harm than providing the care.

Saying no at the macro level in the United States involves similar difficulties. A hospital deciding whether or not to introduce a transplantation program competes with other medical centers. To remain competitive, its directors will want to introduce the new service. Moreover, they can point to the dramatic benefit the service offers. How can opponents of transplantation respond? They may (correctly) argue that it will divert resources from other projects—projects that are perhaps less glamorous, visible, and profitable but that nevertheless offer comparable medical benefits to an even larger class of patients. They insist that the opportunity costs of the new procedure are too great.

This argument about opportunity costs, so powerful in the British National Health Service, loses its force in the United States. The alternatives to the transplantation program may not constitute real options, at least in the climate of incentives that exists in America. Imagine someone advising the Humana Hospital Corporation, "Do not invest in artificial hearts, because you could do far more good if you established a prenatal maternal care program in the catchment area of your chain." Even if correct, this appeal to opportunity costs is unlikely to be persuasive, because Humana responds to the incentives society offers. Artificial hearts, not prenatal maternal-care programs, will keep its hospitals on the leading technological edge, and if they become popular, will bring far more lucrative reimbursements than the prevention of low-birth-weight morbidity and mortality. The for-profit Humana, like many nonprofit organizations, merely responded to existing incentives when it introduced a transplantation program during the early 1980s, at the same time prenatal care programs lost their federal funding. Similarly, cost-containment measures in some states led to the cutting of social and psychological services but left high-technology services untouched.[8] Unlike their

British colleagues, American planners cannot say, "Justice requires that we forgo this procedure because the resources it requires will be better spent elsewhere in the system. It is fair to say no to this procedure because we can thereby provide more important treatments to other patients."

The failure of this justification at both the micro and macro levels in the United States has the same root cause. In our system, saying no to beneficial treatments or procedures carries no assurance that we are saying yes to even more beneficial ones. Our system is not closed; the opportunity costs of a treatment or procedure are not kept internal to it. Just as important, the system as a whole is not governed by a principle of distributive justice, appeal to which is made in decisions about disseminating technological advances. It is not closed under constraints of justice.

SOME CONSEQUENCES

Saying no to beneficial treatments or procedures in the United States is morally hard, because providers cannot appeal to the justice of their denial. In ideally just arrangements, and even in the British system, rationing beneficial care is nevertheless fair to all patients in general. Cost-containment measures in our system carry with them no such justification.

The absence of this rationale has important effects. It supports the feeling of many physicians that current measures interfere with their duty to act in their patients' best interests. Of course, physicians should not think that duty requires them to reject any resource limitations on patient care. But it is legitimate for physicians to hope they may act as their patients' advocate within the limits allowed by the just distribution of resources. Our cost-containment measures thus frustrate a legitimate expectation about what duty requires. Eroding this sense of duty will have a long-term destabilizing effect.

The absence of a rationale based on justice also affects patients. Resource constraints mean that each patient can legitimately expect only the treatments due him or her under a just or fair distribution of health care services. But if beneficial treatment is denied even when justice does not require or condone it, then the patient has reason to feel aggrieved. Patients will not trust providers who put their own economic gain above patient needs. They will be especially distrustful of schemes that allow doctors to profit by denying care. Conflicts between the interests of patients and those of physicians or hospitals are not a necessary feature of a just system of rationing care. The fact that such conflicts are central in our system will make patients suspect that there is no one to be trusted as their agent. In the absence of a concern for just distribution, our cost-containment measures may make patients seek the quite different justice afforded by tort litigation, further destabilizing the system.

Finally, these effects point to a deeper issue. Economic incentives such as those embedded in current cost-containment measures are not a substitute for social decisions about health care priorities and the just design of health care institutions. These incentives to providers, even if they do eliminate some unnecessary medical services, will not ensure that we will meet the needs of our aging population over the next several decades in a morally acceptable fashion or that we will make effective—and just—use of new procedures. These hard choices must be faced publicly and explicitly.

REFERENCES

1. Diagnosis-related groups (DRGs) and the Medicare program: implications for medical technology. Washington D.C.: U.S. Congress, 1983. (Office of Technology Assessment OTA-TM-H-17.)
2. Daniels N. Just health care. New York: Cambridge University Press, 1985.
3. Aaron H J, Schwartz W B. The painful prescription: rationing hospital care. Washington D.C.: The Brookings Institution, 1984.
4. President's Commission for the Study of Ethical Problems in Medicine and Biomedical and Behavioral Research. Securing access to health care: ethical implications of differences in the accessibility of health services. Vol. 1. Washington D.C.: Government Printing Office, 1983.
5. Iglehart J K. Medical care of the poor—a growing problem. N Engl J Med 1985; 313:59–63.
6. Jencks S F, Dobson A. Strategies for reforming Medicare's physician payments: physician diagnosis-

related groups and other approaches. N Engl J Med 1985; 312:1492–9.

7. Yelin E H, Hencke C J, Kramer J S, Nevitt M C, Shearn M, Epstein W V. A comparison of the treatment of rheumatoid arthritis in health maintenance organizations and fee-for-service practices. N Engl J Med 1985; 312:962–7.

8. Cromwell J, Kanak J. The effects of prospective reimbursement on hospital adoption and service sharing. Health Care Finance Rev 1982; 4:67.

QUESTIONS FOR COMPREHENSION AND REFLECTION

1. According to Daniels, what factors in the United States explain why refusing treatment requests is difficult? Do you agree? Explain.
2. What ideas of justice are reflected in Daniels's analysis? Do you agree with these ideas? Explain.
3. What are some competing ideas of justice that counter Daniels's approach?
4. How does Daniels's notion of equality of opportunity underlie his analysis?

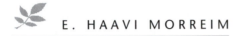

E. HAAVI MORREIM

Lifestyles of the Risky and Infamous: From Managed Care to Managed Lives

E. Haavi Morreim is a professor in the College of Medicine, University of Tennessee, Memphis. After describing three stages in the development of managed care, Morreim discusses the far-reaching implications of managed care in terms of compelling individuals to assume more responsibility for their health and thus help control healthcare expenditures. She points out the significant relationship between managing healthcare expenditures and managing personal life-styles. Furthermore, this relationship and the awareness of individual responsibility raise concerns in terms of legal, medical, and economic enforcement. Morreim also addresses pertinent issues broadening the notion of responsible use of limited healthcare resources. She concludes by supporting the application of positive economic incentives to induce more personal responsibility for one's health.

The house officer groans inwardly as the alcoholic reappears in the emergency room with his eighteenth—or is that nineteenth?—bout of acute pancreatitis. The internist sighs as she examines the obese, diabetic, hypertensive man who doesn't take his medication but still manages to take in plenty of greasy, salty foods. The surgeon is shocked as his patient, now on the mend after Medicare paid $275,000 for intensive care of his ruptured abdominal aortic aneurism, refuses to spend $75 of his own money for the new dentures that will enable him to eat solid food and regain his strength.[1] Why can't people take a little responsibility for their health, these physicians wonder.

The nation is beginning to wonder, as well. Many commentators have proposed that citizens should help tame costs by trying to stay healthy and helping to pay for their care. That move is likely to intensify and accelerate in the next few years, as managed care organizations provide an increasing proportion of citizens' health care.

According to senior analysts, managed care evolves through three stages.[2] In stage one, intensive utilization review controls expenditures via rules that limit physicians' decisions. Stage two replaces this costly, intrusive monitoring with economic incentives. Physicians regain clinical autonomy by assuming financial risk. The third stage is dubbed "true managed care": health plans "actually reduce the health risks of their enrollees. 'Plans' competitive advantages will not come from premiums, which are already nearly the same, but from proving that . . . they actually did something about health care risks.' "[3] Health plans' main vehicle for reducing health *care* risks is, of course, to reduce *health* risks. And that, inevitably, means addressing patients' lifestyles. When managed care organizations are integrated delivery systems, they provide all the health care that patients need. Reducing need is thus crucial to containing costs.

The move has already begun. Like the man who finally realized what actually causes cancer in laboratory animals—*scientists* cause the cancer!!—managed care organizations recognize that the real cause of health care costs is patients' illnesses and injuries. They are undertaking or considering a variety of lifestyle initiatives via economic, medical, and even legal means.

Economic responses to lifestyle-induced costs are becoming more common. Some employers and insurers charge higher premiums for people with unhealthy habits, or deny benefits if injuries were caused by reckless behavior like drunk driving. . . .

Medical approaches begin with preventive care, which consists of three kinds of interventions: preventing illness and injury, early detection of illness, and preventing or reducing recurrences and exac-erbations of a chronic illness. Each can involve lifestyle issues. Preventing illness and injury, for instance, almost always concerns patients' conduct outside the physician's office, since smoking, overeating, and hazardous sports all have predictable morbidities. Early detection of illness requires that patients undergo screening tests that in turn require them to spend their time, undergo some measure of discomfort if not risk, and perhaps pay for extra childcare or experience other inconveniences. Preventing recurrence or exacerbation of chronic illnesses usually requires rigorous adherence to therapy.

Such adherence can be tracked. Because the care provided by managed care organizations usually includes medications, they can (and some now do) use their computer databases to determine which patients receive immunizations and mammograms, and who fills and refills their prescriptions. Noncompliance may result in a note from the physician's office, and some organizations already use "telephone naggers" who phone often to ensure that patients are taking their medications. In other cases, managed care organizations might bypass the problem by administering treatments that do not require compliance at all—as with a one-time (but painful) injection of bicillin, instead of oral antibiotics, for a sexually transmitted disease.

In the ultimate response to noncompliance, some managed care organizations may use their data documenting patients' noncompliance to disenroll them from membership. Although fee-for-service insurers and managed care organizations more commonly disenroll patients for reasons of nonpayment or fraud (for example, by using their policies to obtain benefits for another person), documented, systematic noncompliance with medical recommendations can also be cause for removing the patient.

Legal controls can be expected as well. One managed care organization successfully lobbied a state legislature to defeat a smokers' rights bill and simultaneously secured the agreement of a local newspaper not to carry cigarette ads. Given that many managed care organizations are currently earning billions of dollars in profit,[4] well-funded lobbying on all sorts of lifestyle issues can be anticipated, ostensibly to improve public health but which also, not coincidentally, save the organizations money.

Managed care plans may look beyond the legislature in their efforts to restrict health risks. Many are already working closely with employers to institute wellness programs and health risk monitoring. While these programs in themselves may be excellent, more coercive measures could also be tried, as by charging higher premiums unless employers institute such measures as smoking bans, mandated safety measures, and the like. Here members are directly coerced, not by health care providers, but by their employers. But the impetus could come from the plan.

Managed care organizations may also raise lifestyle issues in civil litigation. In one recent case a deceased patient's family sued a health maintenance organization physician, alleging inadequate treatment of his heart condition. The physician argued that this patient had effectively committed suicide, based on his years of refusal to take his medications, eat properly, exercise, and quit smoking. The court judged these factors too remote to be the "proximate cause" of the patient's death, though it did find relevant his conduct during the hours immediately before his death—particularly his refusal to return for additional medical attention, as instructed, when his chest pain returned.[5]

This listing is not to suggest that attention to lifestyles is inevitably bad. Preventive care has been too long overlooked. And many managed care organizations are instituting voluntary programs such as exercise and nutrition classes, telephone consultation to help subscribers make intelligent use of the system, and other measures that can be a great boon to patients and plans alike. And not all attempts at lifestyle control come through managed care. Other providers and payers, including employers, can be expected to try similar approaches.

Because most of us may thus find ourselves subject to lifestyle monitoring, and because virtually all of us are concerned about the costs that others' carelessness may generate for the rest of us, it is time to take a closer look. Although there are good reasons to expect people to live prudent lifestyles and accept some consequences when they

do not, this essay argues that virtually any mechanism to enforce such responsibility—legal, medical, or economic—is seriously flawed. The more important question concerns the responsible use of resources overall, because needless expense from irresponsible living is just one of many ways to misuse health resources. A more comprehensive approach is needed.

Instead of placing financial incentives on physicians and restrictive rules on patients, patients should be brought into the financial incentives in ways that reward prudence without creating barriers to care. A variety of approaches is available, usable under traditional insurance as well as in managed care. Each lets patients experience moderate economic consequences of their health and health care decisions while, at the same time, enhancing patients' control over their care and reducing some of the economic pressures that now drive wedges between patients and physicians.

TAKING RESPONSIBILITY SERIOUSLY

There are good reasons to expect responsibility in matters of health. People can harm others directly, as careless sexual practices transmit lethal disease, or indirectly, as unhealthy living consumes limited financial and medical resources. More fundamentally, the concept of personal responsibility lies at the heart of morality. The very idea of a moral order presupposes that some actions are right, some wrong. Moral agents are not merely "encouraged" or "enabled" to be responsible.[6] They are required to and must be held to answer, perhaps to atone, if they do not.[7]

There is a catch, however. These robust responsibility requirements apply only to autonomous agents who can choose their own actions for their own reasons. We do not blame people for what is beyond their control. Disease often strikes more out of bad luck than bad behavior, and ill people may lack their usual capacity to make responsible decisions.

But there is an opposing catch. Much of our health is in our own hands. . . . In nonmedical contexts people are routinely held responsible: the bully who commits assault is not less guilty because he was drunk; the robber is no less culpable because he was high on cocaine; the lover who knowingly transmits a lethal virus can be liable. Surely we are not exempt in matters of health.

Further, although serious illness can impair decisionmaking, the majority of people visiting a physician are not seriously ill. Many medical visits are for preventive care, symptomatic relief of self-limited illnesses like colds and flu, and routine management of chronic illnesses such as diabetes and hypertension. Most of these people are just as capable of being responsible in health care as they are elsewhere in life.

Unfortunately, although enforcing lifestyle responsibility through law, medicine, or economics can perhaps have some limited legitimate role, there are also major problems.

LEGAL ENFORCEMENT

Enforcement of healthy lifestyle choices through the courts or legislation might prohibit or require specified conduct, as with motorcycle helmet laws or smoking bans. These restrictions have long been controversial. . . . Such intrusions can penetrate beyond conduct, into private beliefs and values. Optimal health is just one value, alongside others ranging from risky sports for entertainment to unhealthy ethnic diets. And not everyone agrees what health is. . . . Enforcement itself could also be highly intrusive—spying and prying to see who's smoking on the sly.

Still, law does have some legitimate voice regarding personal responsibility in health care. In contract negotiations, the law regards medical patients as vulnerable and gives them a strong benefit of the doubt in their interactions with health insurers, hospitals, and physicians.[8] Nevertheless, patients are expected to be responsible adults. They must not deliberately or intentionally harm others, and their contributory negligence, such as noncompliance with medical instructions, can reduce or preclude damage awards for malpractice injuries.[9] Sometimes a patient who knowingly consents to risks, such as an unconventional medical treatment, may simply have to live with the bad outcome, with no right of recovery for injuries.

And if a patient consistently refuses to cooperate with therapy, eventually the physician is no longer obligated to care for her.

In sum, though these limited legal measures seem appropriate, the problems caused by irresponsible living do not generally warrant the coercive power of the state. Unfortunately, once we agree that people should mostly be permitted to live as they wish, we face the burdens their freedom can impose on the rest of us. Since the idea of responsibility requires people to live with the consequences of their decisions, perhaps we should expect them to bear the natural consequences of their unhealthy lifestyles by denying medical rescue.

MEDICAL ENFORCEMENT

Lifestyle-based restrictions on medical care are not limited to managed care organizations. . . . Today, some physicians refuse to offer coronary bypass surgery to patients who refuse to stop smoking,[10] while others might deny multiple valve replacements to a patient whose continued intravenous drug use keeps reinfecting his heart.[11]

It is generally wrong to deny medical care because of patients' lifestyles for four reasons. First, denying treatment can be unreasonably harsh. Many ostensibly voluntary behaviors are mediated by genetic predispositions, while other bad habits have an addictive dimension, and chronic illnesses can render some patients psychologically less able to act rationally according to their values.[12] The harshness goes further. Requiring someone to live with the consequences of his actions can, in medicine, be deadly. Failing to use a seatbelt is foolish—especially if one is driving to a store to buy cigarettes and greasy junk food. But the person does not deserve to die for it, which is just what may happen if the offender is denied medical care after his auto accident. If we are unwilling to criminalize such activity, we should not seek to make its consequences even worse than incarceration.

Second, medical punishment for lifestyle vices raises important problems of science and evidence. Just as there is insufficient evidence to determine when bad habits have been caused by factors other than voluntary choice, those habits in turn may play an uncertain role in the actual development of illness. Triggers for lung cancer, for instance, can include genetic and environmental factors, and it may be impossible to determine which factors play what role.

The problem runs deeper. Epidemiological evidence is too frequently overthrown. . . . Moderate caffeine during pregnancy might—or then again might not—be harmful.[13] Women in their forties should get a mammogram every year or two—until new evidence suggests that it does not save lives in this age group, and one (but not another) cancer agency changes its screening recommendations.[14] Alcohol can be good for your health, while exercise can kill you.[15]

Sometimes our beliefs about patients are even flimsier. It would be easy to assume that liver transplant for an alcoholic is pointless—surely the person will ruin a second liver the same way he did the first. Yet studies suggest these patients' one-year survival after the procedure appears comparable to other patients', and return to alcohol is uncommon.[16]

Using science as the basis for behavior control is also a hazard to science itself. The more forcefully science is used to curtail people's behavior, the more it is resented when the mandate later turns out to be wrong. Reciprocally, science that shapes medical, political, and economic policy is itself in danger of being shaped more by economic mandates and political correctness than by intellectual rigor.

Problem number three arises if, at the policy level, we construct broad rules forbidding certain resources for certain kinds of patients, as by refusing liver transplant for alcoholics. Aside from possibly offending antidiscrimination laws, such policies would ignore potentially important differences between patients. One person may be only a minimal smoker whose cancer was primarily caused by hereditary factors, while another may truly have smoked his way into a heart attack. Under a policy denying surgeries to smokers, both would be denied care. . . .

The alternative, namely expecting physicians to determine case-by-case which patients truly caused their own problems, raises the fourth even more

serious concern. Denying medical care for lifestyle vices conflicts with a deep moral conviction of medicine: compassion for the patient as a human being in need. Let judges condemn the guilty, but let physicians help the suffering. The physician who denies medical care as a penalty for irresponsible conduct is no longer a healer with a fiduciary commitment to each patient, but an enforcer of social policy.

Moreover, the enforcer role can be medically counterproductive. Good care requires a complete and honest history from the patient, a requirement so important that stout principles of confidentiality assure patients that disclosures to physicians will not find their way to third parties who could do them harm. Where the physician stands as judge and jury of the patient's failure to live responsibly, as by denying bypass surgery to smokers, the enemy threatening harm is the physician himself. Here, the patient who tells his physician the truth is a fool.

This is not to say that physicians cannot expect patients to be responsible partners within their relationship. Patients are obligated to provide an accurate history, to participate in decisions about treatment, and to carry out or else renegotiate their agreements. The patient who routinely deceives, or refuses to comply with treatment and yet demands unflagging devotion, unfairly manipulates the physician and demeans his integrity.

Determining just how physicians should respond, however, poses a challenge. The physician's personal or professional integrity may require him to refuse some patient demands. And sometimes it may be acceptable to deny specified medical services if a patient is unwilling to provide cooperation that is essential to the treatment's success. A patient who refuses to take antirejection medications has exempted himself from organ transplant. On the whole, however, such denials are hazardous. They can tempt the physician to exercise his superior knowledge and power of prescription as a weapon to manipulate patients into submission, bypassing the necessary discussion, negotiation, and free consent. The patient should not fear abandonment every time he disagrees with the physician.

At the same time, the physician should not be expected indefinitely to pick up the pieces left by abusively irresponsible patients. In such cases it is probably best for the physician simply to withdraw from the relationship, with appropriate notice and perhaps an explanation that circumstances have shown he is unable to meet this particular patient's needs.

In the final analysis, patients should not generally have to pay for lifestyle indiscretions by forfeiting medical care, either by social policy or by physician discretion. Medical vigilantism is repugnant.

ECONOMIC ENFORCEMENT

Economic responsibility can be imposed prior to unhealthy conduct or concurrently with its consequences. Taxes on cigarettes and alcohol, for example, aim to deter the unwanted conduct and to collect in advance the money to treat the anticipated health problems, as do higher insurance premiums for people with high-risk habits.

These levies seem partly fair, partly not. The more one smokes, the higher the risks and taxes. Stop smoking, and pay no more taxes. On the other hand, it is difficult to tax other vices, such as overeating. And cigarette taxes are also paid by smokers who never become ill. . . .

There are other problems. A heavy tax on cigarettes can spawn a ferocious black market, consuming more money to catch crooks than it raises for health care. Higher insurance premiums either require risk takers to be honest in ways that will raise their premiums or necessitate unsavory intrusions into privacy to overcome the expected dishonesty. Furthermore, economic facts don't always support the taxes. Smokers do generate health care costs. Yet they often die of relatively inexpensive causes, right around the time of retirement—saving considerably on pension plans.[17]

The pay-as-you-go approach is already in place to some extent. When insurers require substantial cost sharing, those who are ill more, pay more. Similarly, coverage for behavior-caused illnesses and injuries might be reduced. . . . Here, however, familiar problems arise, such as determining whether the illness was caused by truly voluntary conduct. In other cases high costs levied on pa-

tients could bar them from health care altogether, an unduly punitive outcome. Incentives, such as paying regular bonuses to a pregnant cocaine user for remaining drug free until delivery, can perversely backfire. Paying only those who originally test positive for drugs would be a powerful incentive to take up drugs as soon as one knows one is pregnant; but paying everyone to "be good" would be prohibitively costly.

BROADER CONCEPTS OF RESPONSIBLE RESOURCE USE

For better or worse, then, it seems there is little we should do to enforce clean living. Annoying though it is to see common resources depleted by people who will not behave as responsible adults, the price of coercing goodness may be even worse for us all. Limiting patients' recovery in civil suits for the consequences of their own foolishness is only right. But legally prohibiting risky conduct, while justifiable in a few circumstances, invades important liberties. And if an activity is not pernicious enough to be declared illegal, punishing it by withholding medical care would be harsh, ill-founded, and contrary to medicine's most cherished values. And economic remedies, such as heavy taxes and *post hoc* fees for health vices, can often be unfair, impractical, and empirically unjustified. Thus, these various measures offer a few legitimate ways to enforce limited accountability, but hardly a satisfactory comprehensive solution.

Perhaps we must resign ourselves to rescue and resent. Common decency will not let us turn someone away, bleeding or dying, just because he was foolish. In this way we partly generate our own problem. It is difficult to take seriously an admonition to behave if one knows he will be rescued. A washed-out homeowner may be told that if he rebuilds his home on a flood plain, we will not bail him out of the next flood. But if we take pity on his suffering after that next flood and cover his losses again, we have taught him that irresponsibility pays, exacerbating the free-rider problem for future disasters. We may believe that individuals should experience the consequences of their choices, yet we must find a way that is not so punitive that it either harms suffering individuals or triggers our own urge to rescue regardless of irresponsibility.

A better answer requires us to reformulate the question. Lifestyle issues are just one part of a larger challenge: more responsible use of health care resources, generally. There are many ways to use health care resources irresponsibly—doing too much, too little, or the wrong thing—and virtually anyone in the health care system can behave irresponsibly. Patients can fail to wear bike helmets or demand antibiotics for viral infections. Physicians can order tests and treatments more justified by habit than by science or to ward off purely hypothetical malpractice liability. Hospitals may open more beds than they can fill or acquire technology they cannot fully use. Administrative inefficiency can waste time and money without enhancing care or profits.

Currently, health plans are largely in charge of resource use. Businesses and governments insist on moderate premium prices and good quality of care, but the health plans usually determine the specifics. Health plans have two basic ways to contain costs: *direct controls,* in which they directly determine which interventions will be authorized for which patients under what conditions, and *incentives* inspiring physicians and other providers toward conservative resource use.

Recently plans have begun to realize that these utilization controls can be expensive, intrusive, economically ineffective, and medically harmful. Hence we see the shift described above, from stage one to stage two in the evolution of managed care, in which clinicians are left to deliver care as they see fit, but under the pressures of economic incentives. Increasingly, those incentives are not cash rewards for specific cost-saving decisions, but broad constraints such as capitation, in which all patients' care is covered by a flat fee, and profiling of physicians' overall performance with the threat of being "deselected," or fired, by the managed care organizations. These arrangements attempt to bring physicians into the plans' overall goals for containing costs without dictating the specifics of care.

The *langue du jour* speaks of "aligning" incentives among physicians, employers, managed care organizations and other payers.[18] Significantly in these discussions, patients are not listed among the financial players. . . .

Of course, managed care organizations do not ignore patients in containing costs. Just as with physicians, such plans and other payers have two basic options regarding patients' role: they can control, or they can offer incentives. Currently, controls on patients' choices of plans, providers, and treatments are the main instrument. Most patients have little or no choice among health plans. . . .

Within plans, patients' choices of providers and treatments are likewise limited, except where they can afford to pay substantial out-of-pocket costs for out-of-plan options. Limiting patients' choices is essential to managed care.[19] Patients may even find controls exerted by their own physicians. . . .

But patients' role in containing costs will not be limited to controlling choices among plans, physicians, and treatments. Lifestyle management will inevitably enter. Such measures can, of course, be medically beneficial. However, the very idea of patient autonomy suggests that patients are entitled to have a different opinion about their best interests, medical and otherwise. The hypertensive patient may find that the medications permitted by his managed care organization's stringently limited formulary have unacceptable side-effects; or the inner-city dweller may find that walking for exercise in his neighborhood is far more dangerous than being overweight.

Equally ominous, many managed care organizations are beginning to require physicians to police these lifestyle rules. For example, many plans now have incentives rewarding physicians for quality of care. The concept is laudable, but in many cases quality is measured in part by how successfully the physician gets his patients to come in for designated services and to comply with their medications.[20] The physician must demand ever more insistently that patients follow all sorts of medical orders that may or may not suit their preferences.

Perhaps most disturbing of all, under current economic arrangements, successful regulation of patients' health habits translates directly into cash in the pockets of employers, payers, health plans, and physicians. The patient gives up his favorite vices so that others can pocket the savings.

Currently most patients have little or no incentive toward cost-consciousness, particularly in managed care, where copays are almost negligible. But it is also true elsewhere in the health care system, where cost sharing is generally modest, and many patients purchase "gap" insurance, or urge physicians to waive the copays, or simply refuse to pay them. So long as this is true, patients will inevitably be subject to others' control—because there are only the two options: controls and incentives.

If patients are to avoid being subjected to extensive, offensive, and often rather insidious forms of health care limits and lifestyle coercion, it would seem that the only alternative is to bring them into the same "alignment" of incentives that now is beginning to unify all the other players in the health care scene. At the same time, such economic involvement should not pose barriers to care. Fortunately, several approaches are available, and some are already being successfully used.

ECONOMIC ACCOUNTABILITY

The objective of these approaches is to place patients systematically in closer contact with the economic consequences of all their health care decisions, not just those associated with unhealthy habits. They do so not by installing financial barriers to care, but by rewarding prudent resource use. Thus the incentives are positive, not negative.

For example, a Medical Savings Account is a tax-free fund, perhaps $3,000, to cover the routine costs of care, while catastrophic insurance covers health care exceeding that amount. The fund might be filled by the individual, the employer, or even the government so that everyone—including the poor—could afford it. In one version, money left at the end of each year would roll over into the next year's account for future medical expenses. . . . In another version, patients keep the remainder at the end of each year. Medical savings accounts have been endorsed by the American Medical Association and a number of political leaders.

Managed care organizations could do something similar. One approach would place a specified number of points (say, 3,000) into an account for each subscriber at the beginning of the year.

The patient would "spend" those points, for example for ordinary physician visits or medications that are costlier than those on the formulary. Reciprocally, extra points might be awarded to encourage important preventive care such as immunizations and prenatal care, or needed follow-up for chronic illness or serious injury. Points remaining at the end of the year might be returned as cash or reduced premiums, banked for the next year, or perhaps spent in a catalogue of goods such as health club memberships or household items.[21]

Such approaches have important advantages. Financial barriers to care are eliminated as patients enjoy either first-dollar coverage through a dedicated account or all needed care directly from the managed care organizations. At the same time, patients have a real reward for prudent resource use, unlike the current situation. Managed care patients with minimal copayments sometimes make needless visits for minor or self-limited problems ("it's free, so I might as well go"), or insist on exotic treatments that are not medically indicated ("I paid my premium, so I'm entitled"). Patients with indemnity insurance sometimes urge their physicians to extract extra resources by "gaming the system."

In contrast, deducting such care directly from patients' medical savings accounts or managed care points could prompt more careful use of resources. Similarly, the indigent person with a government-funded account would be rewarded for seeking care from a primary care physician rather than an emergency room. Additionally, these incentives would expose patients to some of the costs of unhealthy habits. As those with a medical savings account pay directly for the first $3,000 of their care, fellow subscribers don't have to. The account would cover most if not all of the physician visits necessitated by smokers' extra respiratory infections, for example. Similarly, managed care points diminish as extra illnesses from unhealthy habits require more physician visits. And on both approaches, patients may be less likely to demand unnecessary care, such as antibiotics for viral ailments. In the process, people with serious or chronic illnesses would enjoy what, for them, is the best prize of all: more and better health care. A system less clogged with demands for marginal care can be more fully dedicated to those who really need it.

Reciprocally, such a system need not foster another kind of irresponsibility: forgoing necessary care in order to save money. There are several reasons.

First, the money or points in these accounts cannot be directly traded for beer or other commodities. More importantly, the principle of autonomy permits competent patients to forgo care for whatever reason they see fit, and people are entitled to define for themselves what care is "necessary" and what is not. If they are entitled to refuse care on religious, personal, or even frivolous grounds, surely they are entitled to do so on economic grounds if they have determined that some other use of their money is more important. No rule requires that health needs must be met before all other needs, any more than all people must buy the safest possible automobile regardless of the cost. A society in which Prudent Purchase Police barred the door to fast-food stands would be oppressive indeed.

Further, greater patient cost-consciousness should diminish the need for outside micromanagement, with commensurate reductions in administrative costs of care, annoying hassle factor, and even premium costs. More important, if patients help curb overutilization, then insurers and managed care organizations may find less need for the financial incentives that place physicians in conflicts of interest by encouraging them to cut back on care. Indeed, when the money at stake is the patient's rather than the physician's, the physician who discusses costs is not an adversary guarding his and third parties' money, but an ally looking at the patient's broader interests, helping him both to ensure that the value of care is worth its cost and to avoid medically short-sighted cost-cutting.

Just as compelling, perhaps, is evidence indicating that people who are actually in such systems use them well. Several corporations use variations of medical savings accounts with significant success. Golden Rule Insurance Company, for example, instituted a savings account option for its own

employees, in addition to their usual indemnity option. The 80 percent who chose the medical savings account during the first year received a total of $468,000 in rebates at the end of the year. The following year, with even more employees enrolled, the plan returned $743,000, or over $1,000 per worker. The savings came several ways. Some individuals needing outpatient diagnostic testing, for instance, did price-shopping that revealed wide variations in the costs of the same test from one provider to the next, with no identifiable difference in quality. Higher-priced providers began cutting their rates to compete. Claim costs on catastrophic insurance decreased, with subsequent lowering of premiums. And equally important, some health care utilization actually increased. For many low-wage families, the typical indemnity deductible of several hundred dollars effectively prohibited many forms of preventive care. . . .

DOING THE BEST WE CAN

There would be little reason to care about bad habits that harm only the individual if it weren't for the fact that the rest of us pay for the repairs. Admittedly, the mild incentives in this approach do not solve the problem of irresponsible lifestyles. Deducting a few dollars or points from an account is unlikely to transform smokers and drinkers into paragons of health virtue. But there is no fully satisfactory solution. Any serious legal, medical, or economic enforcements against unpalatable lifestyles will usually be worse than the vices they attack. Fortunately, this recognition does not constitute a defeat, for it helps us to redirect our focus.

The real question is much broader: how do we ensure that all those with an important stake in the health care system—payers, providers, and patients alike—use its resources more wisely? The value of greater economic accountability for patients is found not in its power to change their lifestyles, but in its capacity to foster more responsible use of health care resources generally, to return to patients a greater measure of control over their health care, and to avert the potentially major and illegitimate intrusions into personal lives that are surely around the corner if patients are not brought into resource management in more constructive ways. It is no panacea, but it is probably the best we can do.

REFERENCES

1. J. P. Weaver, "The Best Care Other People's Money Can Buy," *Wall Street Journal*, 19 November 1992.
2. Anita J. Slomski, "Maybe Bigger Isn't Better After All," *Medical Economics* 72, no. 4 (1995): 55–58.
3. Slomski, "Maybe Bigger Isn't Better," p. 58.
4. George Anders, "HMOs Pile Up Billions in Cash, Try to Decide What to Do with It," *Wall Street Journal*, 21 December 1994.
5. Van Vacter v. Hierholzer, 865 S.W.2d 355 (Mo. App. W.D. 1993).
6. Reinhold Priester, "A Values Framework for Health System Reform," *Health Affairs* 11 (1992): 84–107, at 99.
7. E. Haavi Morreim, "Impairments and Impediments in Patients' Decision Making: Reframing the Competence Question," *Journal of Clinical Ethics* 4 (1993): 294–307.
8. E. Haavi Morreim, "Redefining Quality by Reassigning Responsibility," *American Journal of Law and Medicine* 20 (1994): 79–104.
9. Barry R. Furrow, Sandra H. Johnson, Timothy S. Jost, and Robert L. Schwartz, *Liability and Quality Issues in Health Care* (St. Paul: West Publishing Co., 1991) at 188–98.
10. M. J. Underwood and J. S. Bailey, "Coronary Bypass Surgery Should Not Be Offered to Smokers," *British Medical Journal* 306 (1993): 1047–48.
11. Lance K. Stell, "The Noncompliant Substance Abuser," *Hastings Center Report* 21, no. 2 (1991): 31–32.
12. Roger Higgs, "Human Frailty Should Not Be Penalised," *British Medical Journal* 306 (1993): 1049–50; David Orentlicher, "Denying Treatment to the Noncompliant Patient," *JAMA* 265 (1991): 1579–82.
13. Brenda Eskenazi, "Caffeine During Pregnancy: Grounds for Concern?" *JAMA* 270 (1993): 2973–74.
14. Marilyn Chase, "Mammogram Starting Age Rises to 50 Under New Federal Recommendations," *Wall Street Journal*, 6 December 1993.
15. Gary D. Friedman and Arthur L. Klatsky, "Is Alcohol Good for Your Health?" *NEJM* 329 (1993): 1882–83; Gregory D. Curfman, "Is Exercise Beneficial—or Hazardous—to Your Health?" *NEJM* 329 (1993): 1730–31.
16. Kenneth R. McCurry, Prabhaker Baliga, Robert M. Merion et al., "Resource Utilization and Outcome for Liver Transplantation for Alcoholic Cirrhosis," *Archives of Surgery* 127 (1992): 772–77; Carl Cohen et al., "Alcoholics and Liver Transplantation," *JAMA* 256 (1991): 1299–1301.
17. W. G. Manning, B. K. Emmett, J. P. Newhouse et al., "The Taxes of Sin: Do Smokers and Drinkers Pay Their Way?" *JAMA* 261 (1989): 1604–9.
18. E. Haavi Morreim, "The Ethics of Incentives in Managed Care," *Trends in Health Care, Law & Ethics* 10 (1995): 56–62.
19. B. Weise, "Managed Care: There's No Stopping It Now," *Medical Economics* 72, no. 5 (1995): 26–43.
20. C. Appleby, "HEDIS: Managed Care's Emerging Gold Standard," *Managed Care* 4 (1995): 19–24; Slomski, "Maybe Bigger Isn't Better."
21. E. Haavi Morreim, "Diverse and Perverse Incentives in Managed Care"; forthcoming in *Widener Law Symposium Journal*, 1995.

QUESTIONS FOR COMPREHENSION AND REFLECTION

1. What are the three phases of managed care? In the opinion of Morreim, how does managed care challenge the traditional view of precluding personal contribution to illness as a relevant factor in treatment decisions?
2. How do economic, medical, and legal controls reinforce the need for personal responsibility for one's health? Are these controls justifiable? Support your answer.
3. Morreim broadens her analysis of personal responsibility to incorporate institutional responsibility. How does managed care reflect this broader issue? How can managed care redress some of the problems?
4. What moral principles underlie Morreim's proposal regarding economic accountability in managed care? Do you agree with her analysis? Explain.

STEFFIE WOOLHANDLER AND
DAVID U. HIMMELSTEIN

A National Health Program: Northern Light at the End of the Tunnel

Steffie Woolhandler is an assistant professor of medicine and adjunct associate professor of public health at Harvard Medical School. David U. Himmelstein is an associate professor of medicine at Harvard Medical School. Both are cofounders of Physicians for a National Health Program in Cambridge, Massachusetts. They argue that the fairest way to ensure equity of access to healthcare in the United States is to adopt a single-payer system along the lines of the Canadian model. This would save costs and, in the long term, would be more efficient than the current, multitiered system. They contrast the fragmentary quality of U.S. healthcare coverage with the administrative effectiveness demonstrated in Canada. Citing what they believe are practical and substantive benefits in the Canadian system, they propose a sweeping reform of U.S. healthcare financing and administration.

Few would dispute that our health care system is deeply troubled. Thirty-seven million Americans are uninsured, health care costs continue their exuberant growth, and bureaucracy increasingly intrudes in the examining room. Opinion on solutions is more divided.

We and many colleagues have proposed a sweeping reform of health care financing[1] because we are convinced that lesser measures will fail, as they have for the past quarter century. Expanding Medicaid,[2] mandating that employers provide health benefits,[3] setting up state risk pools, and similar piecemeal attempts to expand access either fuel inflation or install intrusive cost-management bureaucracies—usually both.[4] Providing more care to those currently uninsured must raise costs if resources are not diverted from elsewhere in the system. Unless bureaucracy is trimmed, these resources will be siphoned from existing clinical care, a process invariably overseen by yet another layer of bureaucrats.

Medicare epitomizes the problem. It improved access for the elderly, but costs soared and diagnosis related groups resulted.[5] Moreover, cost-management bureaucracies are not only intrusive but expensive, leading to a steady fall in the care-bureaucracy ratio, which is now little better than 3 : 1.[6] For each dollar spent for the clinical components of care, 30 cents is spent for administrators and their tools.[6] Resources seep silently but inexorably from the clinic to the administrative suite. The shortage of bedside nurses coexists with a proliferation of Registered Nurse utilization reviewers and preadmission screeners. Few physicians now escape the pleasure of their scrutiny.

Such an enormous bureaucratic burden is a peculiarly American phenomenon. Our insurance companies take 12% of their premiums for overhead[7]; Canada's program runs for less than 3% overhead.[6] We devote more than 18% of hospital spending to administration and billing; Canada devotes 8%.[6,8] United States physicians spend 45% of gross income for professional expenses, much of it for billing; our Canadian colleagues spend 36%.[9,10] Overall, we spend 2.6% of our gross national product for health care bureaucracy, while Canada spends 1.1%.[6] Reducing our health administrative apparatus to the Canadian level would have saved about $2 billion this year.

Unfortunately, piecemeal tinkering cannot reverse bureaucratic hypertrophy. The key to administrative simplicity in Canada is the single-source system of payment[11]: in each province, virtually all bills are paid by the provincial insurance plan. Hospitals do little or no billing and need not keep track of the charges for individual patients.[12] They are paid a global annual budget to cover all costs, much as a fire department is funded in the United States. Physicians bill by checking a box on a simple insurance form and submitting it to the provincial plan. Fee schedules are negotiated annually between the provincial medical associations and governments.[12,13] All patients have the same (complete) coverage.

The fragmentation of insurance coverage in the United States (with > 1500 different plans) requires the current herculean administrative efforts. Hospitals must determine eligibility, keep track of charges, and bill for each patient individually; coverage and regulations vary widely. Each insurer employs legions (6000 people work for Blue Cross of Massachusetts alone) to market their plans and minimize their costs, often by simply shifting those costs onto patients, other insurers, the government, or hospital red ink. Physicians must deal with an increasingly complex tangle of insurance forms and requirements. Our group practice pays about 10% of gross revenues to a billing service, a typical figure.[6]

The national health program (NHP) we propose would create a single tax-funded comprehensive insurer in each state, federally mandated but locally controlled.[1] Everyone would be fully insured for all medically necessary services and private insurance duplicating the NHP coverage would be proscribed, as would patient copayments and deductibles. The current byzantine insurance bureaucracy with its tangle of regulations and wasteful duplication would be dismantled. Instead, the NHP in each state would disburse all funds, and central administrative costs would be limited by law to 3% of total health spending. Cost-shifting efforts would be pointless—there would be nowhere to shift costs to. Marketing of insurance plans, health maintenance organizations, and hospitals would also be eliminated, saving billions of dollars annually.

We expect that initially the NHP would cause little change in the total cost of care, with savings on administration and billing approximately offsetting the costs of expanded care.[14] The Canadian experience suggests the increase in use of care would be modest after an initial surge,[15] with most of the rise occurring among the poor and those with serious symptoms.[16,17]

Demonstration projects in one or more states might precede nationwide implementation. In these demonstrations, and during the phasing in of a nationwide system, funding would mimic existing patterns to minimize economic disruption—but all payment would be funneled through the NHP. Thus, Medicare and Medicaid monies would go to the NHP; employers would pay an NHP tax equivalent to the average now spent for health benefits; and individuals would pay a tax equivalent to the current average out-of-pocket expenditure.

The NHP would pay each hospital and nursing home a global budget to cover all operating expenses. This operating budget would be negotiated annually based on past expenditures, previous financial and clinical performance, projected changes in costs and use, and proposed new and innovative programs. Capital projects would be funded through separate appropriations from the NHP, and the use of operating funds for capital purchases or profits would be prohibited to minimize incentives for hospitals to skimp on care. Under this payment scheme, many administrative tasks would disappear. There would be no hospital bills to keep track of, no eligibility determination, and no need to attribute costs and charges to individual patients.

Physicians would enjoy a free choice of practice settings and styles. They could elect to be paid on a fee-for-service basis or receive salaries from health maintenance organizations, hospitals, or other institutional providers. The representative of the fee-for-service practitioners (perhaps the state medical society) and the state's NHP board would negotiate a simplified binding-fee schedule. Practitioners who accepted payment from the NHP could bill patients directly only for uncovered services (as is done for cosmetic surgery in Canada). The effort and expense of billing would be trivial: stamp the patient's NHP card on a billing form, check a box, send in all the bills once a week, and receive full payment for virtually all services—with an extra payment for any bill not paid within 30 days. Health maintenance organizations and group practices could elect to be paid a capitation fee to cover all services except inpatient hospitalization, which would be funded through hospitals' global budgets. Regulations on capital funding and profits would be similar to those for hospitals. Financial incentives for physicians based on the health maintenance organization's financial performance would be prohibited.

A similar system has worked well in Canada for nearly 20 years.[4,12,18] There are virtually no financial barriers to care and fewer nonfinancial barriers than in our country.[19] Health spending per capita, though 30% below the US figure, is the second highest in the world.[20] It has remained stable as a proportion of gross national product largely because bureaucracy has not hypertrophied and because the NHP, as the sole source of funds for health care, is able to set and enforce overall budgetary limits.[11] Despite disputes about the adequacy of funding for high-technology care,[21] most observers agree that quality of care has remained on a par with the United States and health status is at least as good as in our country.

Regulation of practice in Canada consists mainly of setting ceilings on aggregate physician reimbursement, hospital budgets, and capital spending and monitoring for outlandish abuses (e.g., a single family physician who billed for $250,000 for urinalyses in 1 year).[11,13] Detailed oversight of the clinical encounter has proved unnecessary and clinical freedom is better preserved than in our country.[22,23] Although Canadian physicians have battled government over adequate funding, physician incomes are high and have more than kept pace with inflation.[13] Overall, 69% of Canadian physicians rate their NHP good or excellent, 61% believe it has improved health status, and the same proportion express satisfaction with their own practices.[24] Medicine remains a much sought after career, attracting nearly three times as many applicants per medical school place (and per capita) as in the United States.[25-27]

The Canadian system enjoys overwhelming support among patients.[19] Indeed, only 3% of Canadi-

ans would go back to the US-style system that predated their NHP.[19] In contrast, 61% of Americans favor a Canadian-style reform,[19] more than twice as many as support patchwork approaches like extending Medicaid.[28] United States corporations are also increasingly interested in fundamental health policy reform. Thus, Chrysler's health insurance costs ($700 per car in the United States vs $223 in Canada) have spurred Lee Iacocca to consider supporting an NHP (*Baltimore Sun*. April 16, 1989:2D).

Despite such popular and powerful support, the NHP we propose faces important political obstacles. The virtual elimination of private health insurance will meet stiff opposition from the insurance industry and necessitate a large-scale retraining program for employees of insurance companies (many might be employed as support personnel to free nurses for clinical tasks). Although business as a whole would see no rise in its health care costs, firms not now providing health benefits would face increased taxes without the offset provided by the elimination of health insurance premiums.

The long-term financial viability of the system we propose is critically dependent on achieving and maintaining administrative simplicity. The Canadian macromanagement approach to cost control—setting overall budgetary limits—is inherently less intensive administratively than the current US micromanagement approach that depends on case-by-case scrutiny of billions of individual expenditures and encounters. However, even in a Canadian-style system, vigilance and statutory limits on administrative spending will likely be needed to curb the tendency of bureaucracy to reproduce and amplify itself.

An NHP would solve the cost-vs-access conflict by slashing bureaucratic waste and improving health planning. It would reorient the way we pay for care and eliminate financial barriers to access, but preserve the physician-patient relationship. An NHP would offer patients a free choice of physicians and hospitals, and physicians a free choice of practice style and hospital affiliation. How many failed patchwork reforms, how many patients turned away from care they can't afford, how many dollars spent on bureaucracy, before we arrive at the only viable solution—a universal, comprehensive, publicly administered national health program?

REFERENCES

1. Himmelstein D U, Woolhandler S, the Writing Committee of the Working Group on Program Design. A national health program for the United States: a physicians' proposal. *N Engl J Med.* 1989; 320: 102–108.
2. Thorpe K E, Siegel J E, Dailey T. Including the poor: the fiscal impacts of Medicaid expansion. *JAMA.* 1989; 261:1003–1007.
3. The National Leadership Commission on Health. *For the Health of a Nation: A Shared Responsibility.* Ann Arbor, Mich: Health Administration Press; 1989.
4. Evans R G. Finding the levers, finding the courage: lessons from cost containment in North America. *J Health Polit Policy Law.* 1986; 11:585–615.
5. Aiken L H, Bays K D. The Medicare debate: round 1. *N Engl J Med.* 1984; 311:1196–1200.
6. Himmelstein D U, Woolhandler S. Cost without benefit: administrative waste in U.S. health care. *N Engl J Med.* 1986; 314:441–445.
7. Levit K R, Freeland M S. National medical care spending. *Health Aff.* 1988; 7(5):124–136.
8. *Administrative and Supportive Services.* Ottawa, Canada: Health Information Division, Dept of Health and Welfare; 1981.
9. Reynolds R A, Ohsfeldt R L, eds. *Socioeconomic Characteristics of Medical Practice.* Chicago, Ill: American Medical Association; 1984.
10. *Estimates of Physicians' Earnings, 1973–1982.* Ottawa, Canada: Health Information Division, Dept of National Health and Welfare; 1983.
11. Evans RG, Lomas J., Barer ML, et al. Controlling health expenditures: the Canadian reality, *N Engl J Med.* 1989; 320:571–577.
12. Iglehart JK. Canada's health care system. *N Engl J Med.* 1986; 315:202–208, 778–784.
13. Barer M L, Evans R G, Labelle R J. Fee controls as cost control: tales from the frozen north. *Milbank Q.* 1988; 66:1–64.
14. Himmelstein D U, Woolhandler S. Free care: a quantitative analysis of the health and cost effects of a national health program. *Int J Health Serv.* 1988; 18:393–399.
15. LeClair M. The Canadian health care system. In: Andreopoulos S, ed. *National Health Insurance: Can We Learn From Canada?* New York, NY: John Wiley & Sons Inc; 1975:11–92.
16. Enterline P E, Salter V, McDonald A D, McDonald J C. The distribution of medical services before and after 'free' medical care: the Quebec experience. *N Engl J Med.* 1973; 289:1174–1178.
17. Siemiatycki J, Richardson L, Pless I B. Equality in medical care under national health insurance in Montreal. *N Engl J Med.* 1980; 303:10–15.
18. Taylor M G. *Health Insurance and Canadian Public Policy: The Seven Decisions That Created the Canadian Health Insurance System and Their Outcomes.* Montreal, Canada: McGill-Queens University Press; 1987.
19. Blendon R J. Three systems: a comparative survey. *Health Manage Q.* 1989; 11:1–10.
20. Scheiber G J, Poullier J-P. Recent trends in international health care spending. *Health Aff.* 1987; 6(3): 105–112.
21. Task Force on the Allocation of Health Care Resources. *Health: A Need for Redirection.* Ottawa: Canadian Medical Association; 1984.
22. Hoffenberg R. *Clinical Freedom.* London, England: Nuffield Provincial Hospitals Trust; 1987.
23. Relman A S. American medicine at the crossroads: signs from Canada. *N Engl J Med.* 1989; 320:590–591.
24. Stevenson H M, Williams A P, Vayda E. Medical politics and Canadian Medicare: professional response to the Canada Health Act. *Milbank Q.* 1988; 66:65.
25. Jonas H S, Etzel S I. Undergraduate medical education. *JAMA.* 1988; 260:1063–1071.
26. Ryten E. Medical schools in Canada. *JAMA.* 1988; 260:1157–1161.
27. US Bureau of the Census. *Statistical Abstract of the United States: 1989.* Washington, DC: Government Printing Office; 1989.
28. Seaver D J, Huske M S. *Health Care Attitude Survey Shows Surprising Results.* Cambridge, Mass: Arthur D Little; 1988.

QUESTIONS FOR COMPREHENSION AND REFLECTION

1. According to the authors, how does Medicare epitomize the bureaucratic burdens with respect to health reform?
2. In the opinion of the authors, how does the Canadian system rectify these bureaucratic obstacles?

3. Woolhandler and Himmelstein propose a national health plan (NHP) that would adopt some of the approaches utilized within the Canadian plan. How would their proposed plan redress the inequities that exist within the current U.S. system? Do you agree with their design? Explain.
4. Does Woolhandler and Himmelstein's analysis incorporate more utilitarian theory or deontology? Do you see any flaws in their analysis? Explain.

RONALD BRONOW

A National Health Program: Abyss at the End of the Tunnel—the Position of Physicians Who Care

Ronald Bronow is president of Physicians Who Care in San Antonio, Texas. Bronow sharply disagrees with Woolhandler and Himmelstein. He argues that if the United States were to adopt the Canadian system, it would bring about more harm than benefit. In his opinion, there would be real problems involving the underfinancing of healthcare, as well as difficulties associated with rationing healthcare delivery. He points out that these problems are currently being faced in parts of Canada, and he highlights these shortcomings in the province of Saskatchewan. Bronow concludes by laying out two different scenarios for the future of American medicine, indicating that the deciding factor will be the role played by American physicians.

Doctors Woolhandler and Himmelstein,[1] in their Commentary in the October 29, 1989, issue of *The Journal,* argue that a national health program based on the Canadian system is the best solution to the crisis in American health care financing. The authors, however, fail to recognize the negative repercussions of such a system, the consequences of which are now being fully realized in Canada.

The province of Saskatchewan started compulsory universal health insurance in 1961. The same province was among the first to announce it had run out of money for medical care services for 1987 and would be unable to pay for them for the rest of the year. Following a funding freeze imposed by Premier Grant Devine's Conservative government, Saskatchewan's hospitals faced a critical shortage of beds, with 1870 patients waiting for

surgery at Saskatoon's University Hospital alone (*Macleans.* February 13, 1989:32). At the present time, health care in most provinces consumes more than one third of the total provincial budget, and the costs continue to rise. The province of Ontario shows projected expenditures for 1989 and 1990 of close to $14 billion, on total government revenues of $40 billion (W. Goodman, MD, oral communication, January 1990). Canadian provincial health and finance ministers recently issued a report arguing that the future quality of the system is threatened because the rate of growth in federal transfer payments to the provinces has averaged 9%, while health care expenditures are rising at an average rate of 11.3%—a familiar scenario. But, despite this, Prime Minister Mulroney has proposed a 2-year freeze on federal payments to the

10 provinces, moneys needed to help finance health care programs (*New York Times*, January 28, 1990:F13). A heated debate is raging over whether Canada can continue to afford the 20-year-old publicly funded universal system. The Canadian Medical Association and Canadian Hospital Association have warned that underfinancing and rationing have created a two-tiered health care system in which those with money go to private clinics or the United States, while those without political connections and/or financial resources wait in "long queues." Moore[2] has warned that "unless a financing system creates incentives to dampen consumer demand, expenditure caps will only result in more rationing, reductions in the use of new technologies, and the further subjection of health care budgets to special interest group politics." Canada is faced with a system in which the funding is finite and limited, while the demands of the patients are not. The mounting strains on the system of medical care have raised the prospect that so-called user fees may eventually be needed to discourage Canadians from making needless medical visits (*Globe and Mail.* November 17, 1989:A12).

The politicians, to cope with the crisis, are restricting access to medical care. Hospitals across the country are taking beds out of service, limiting the number of operations they perform, and cutting back on other services, as provincial governments battle to keep down health care costs. There is a shortage of critical care and neonatal beds in Ontario. The Ontario Medical Association confirms that there has been a net decrease of about 2000 beds in the province during the past 1 to 2 years.[3] In Toronto an estimated 1000 people are facing waits of as long as a year for bypass operations at three hospitals. In Ontario the normal wait for cataract surgery is 5 to 6 months (*Financial Post.* January 20, 1989:11). During the past 2 years, most of the provinces have sought to curb costs by telling hospitals they will no longer pay for operating deficits (*Macleans.* February 13, 1989:32). Emergency departments in large hospitals in major Canadian cities have been shut down because of lack of beds. Important teaching hospitals have been unable to purchase new equipment without cutting back on traditional services.[4] More

and more Canadian hospital beds are being occupied by elderly patients who stay there longer than 60 days, and whose costs are well below average. This prevents physicians from using the beds to treat short-term, acutely ill patients, exactly the opposite of the US system.[5]

Canadian politicians have blamed physicians for the mounting crisis. The Canadian government is arguing that physicians are refusing to advise their patients to use medical procedures that are the best value, but insist on advising patients on the best possible treatment. Certainly, physicians in Ontario have freely admitted this. Dr Henry Gassman, speaking on behalf of Ontario doctors, was quoted in the *Toronto Sun* on February 4, 1989: "Your doctor will not enter into any agreement which will sacrifice the accessibility or quality of care in favor of the government's agenda of cost reduction." The conflict arises because the government wants the physicians to serve as the "gatekeeper" who controls the rationing of medical services, and the physicians do not want the job.[6] Also in Ontario, the Health Ministry has told two hospital administrations that for them to receive desperately needed funding, the physicians on the staff must accept "alternative payment methods." The alternatives being considered include fixed salary for physicians and capitation. Ontario Health Minister Elinor Caplan stated, "We have said for quite some time that, as we look at alternative approaches to delivery of services, that there should be options available for both providers and consumers." She said, "We've been encouraging communities to look at innovative and creative proposals for the delivery of those kinds of services" (*Globe and Mail.* January 18, 1989:A8).[7] In Quebec, the government has put a ceiling on certain categories of income. Any fees earned by a general practitioner in excess of $164,108 (Canadian) a year are reimbursed at a rate of 25%.[8] In 1987, the Manitoba government disposed of the system of binding arbitration for fee negotiations with the Manitoba Medical Association after physicians had been awarded a 5.7% fee increase. British Columbia has capped growth of physicians' payments at 3% per year.[5]

It has been argued that the above stories are merely anecdotal. If so, their sheer number demands attention. Our primary concern is that health care decisions are being made by the state, not the individual.

Considering the many Canadian problems and the rescinding here of the Medicare Catastrophic Coverage Act, it is unlikely that Congress will pass any major health care financing legislation in the immediate future. Our government, in struggling with its own budget deficits, will not be willing to transfer a very large segment of private financing to the tax rolls.[9] It would then have to finance health care for large poverty populations, a nonexistent situation in Canada. And, the price tag for a Canadian-style health care system? At least $339 billion in additional taxes, according to a study prepared for the National Center for Policy Analysis (*Business Insurance.* March 5, 1990:B8). Despite this, I see two quite different scenarios as to where American medicine will be by the turn of the century.

SCENARIO 1

There will be increased funding for health care for the poor. This will come from either state, county, or federal funds and will be funded by a direct tax increase, either federal or state. Other possibilities include a value-added tax, sales tax, or taxes on alcohol and tobacco consumption. There will be basic levels of health care coverage for the indigent. This coverage will be determined by guidelines worked out from treatment outcomes analysis, funds available, and value to society.

(During the early 1990s, the costs of American technology continued to overwhelm the short-term saving from managing of health care.[10] The following system of financing evolved, following extensive public debate.)

Every working American will be covered by a basic employer-funded program. Policies will be based on a $250 (or higher) yearly deductible payment. This will create less third-party interference and make insurance costs more predictable. If the employee decides to buy his or her own policy, the employer will contribute the same amount as for the employer-funded plan. Premiums, deductibles, and copayments will be tax deductible by the person paying the bill. But, the employer-funded premiums will be treated as taxable income to the employee (*New York Times,* February 21, 1990:A5). State pools and tax credits will help to ease the burden on small businesses. Health care decisions, again, will be made by the physician and the patient rather than the third party. The increased deductible will discourage overutilization, both by the patient and by the physician.[11] The costs of managing care will be dramatically decreased as insurance companies pay health benefits according to scientific guidelines used in medicine. The results of scientific outcomes analysis will be disseminated to the practicing physician. The insurance companies will use these guidelines to determine payment rather than questioning the physician's decision step-by-step, creating paperwork and increased bureaucratic costs. This shift in policy will have been initiated by the 1989 study from the National Academy of Science, which showed that utilization review, by managing site and duration of treatment rather than the need for services, did not alter the pattern of continued high rates of increase in health care costs. All savings had been largely offset by administrative costs and increased use of outpatient services.[12, 13]

Health maintenance organizations will be limited to Kaiser-style staff-model plans. Independent practice associations based in physicians' offices will disappear as the health maintenance organizations find it impossible to make a profit in such groups without excessively rationing care.

The malpractice system will be reorganized into a workers' compensation-style commission. Claims will be heard, fault determined, and money awarded based on injuries and loss of further earning potential. Billions of dollars in unnecessary tests and procedures will be saved by taking malpractice out of the tort system.

Medicine will devise effective systems to punish bad physicians, while Congress will pass legislation to protect those who sit on peer review panels from charges of anticompetitiveness.

Outcomes and practice-pattern analysis of individual physicians will identify cost-effective, quality providers who will be rewarded by the payers. Physicians who overcharge and overutilize will also be identified. They will be advised to change their practice patterns or not continue on insurance company panels.

SCENARIO 2

Frustrations from the failure of managed care to slow medical inflation, along with the push of Congress to blame physicians for the health care crisis, will create a government one-payer system. Patients will believe they will be entitled to complete, free medical care. This will create a credit-card mentality among the American public. As in Canada, there will be unlimited demand for services with finite resources.[12] This will create delays in diagnostic testing and therapy, particularly surgical. As the money runs out of the "global budget," physicians will be blamed for overutilizing resources to increase their personal income. Punitive measures will then be instituted, such as salary caps and decreased future payments based on the budget deficit.

The overall quality of care in the United States will decrease as costs skyrocket and physicians lose their autonomy and their decision-making power. Patients who can afford it will seek private care, although most people will accept the system because it's free, and, as in Canada and England, public expectations will be significantly diminished.[14]

As was noted in the late 1980s, the quality of incoming medical students will continue to decrease. As doctors lose their decision-making power, they will also lose the joy of practicing medicine. Congress and the news media will answer by stating that physicians are basically greedy and will [go] on to other fields when they realize they cannot make as much money in medicine.

Who could tip the balance between the two scenarios? American physicians. Will they lead, or watch from the sidelines? We will see what happens.

REFERENCES

1. Woolhandler S, Himmelstein D U. A national health program: northern light at the end of the tunnel. *JAMA.* 1989; 262:2136–2137.
2. Moore S. America's current love affair with the Canadian health system. *Health Care Trends Rep.* February 1989:1, 15, 16.
3. Nesdoly D. Guest editorial. *Fam Pract.* November 25, 1989:4.
4. Reece R. The Canadian health care system model. *Reece Rep.* April 1989:6.
5. Six tough questions. *Calif Phys.* October 1989:32–49.
6. Slemon C. *Health Care in Ontario: Ontario Libertarian Party Position Paper,* Toronto, Canada: Ontario Libertarian Party: 1989.
7. Berube B, McAllister J. Blackmailed: Ontario doctors held to ransom over hospital. *Med Post.* January 14, 1989:1.
8. Lemieux P. Socialized medicine: the Canadian experience. *Freeman.* March 1989:97.
9. Kirshner E. Insider interview with Bernard S. Tresnwki. *Healthweek.* December 4, 1989:12–15.
10. Iglehart J. A conversation with William B. Schwartz. *Health Aff.* Fall 1989:71–73.
11. Manning W, Newhouse J, Duan N, et al. Health insurance and the demand for medical care: evidence from a randomized experiment. *RAND Health Insurance Experiments Series.* Santa Monica, Calif: RAND Corp: February 1988:24.
12. Moore S. The future of utilization management. *Health Care Trends Rep.* November 1989:1, 15, 16.
13. *Controlling Costs and Changing Patient Care? The Role of Utilization Management.* Washington, DC: National Academy Press: October 1989.
14. Iglehart J. A conversation with William B. Schwartz. *Health Aff.* Fall 1989:64–67.

QUESTIONS FOR COMPREHENSION AND REFLECTION

1. According to Bronow, what are the negative repercussions for Canadians of the Canadian healthcare system?
2. According to Bronow, why have Canadian politicians blamed Canadian physicians for the problems that have come about in implementing the Canadian system?
3. Compare and contrast the two scenarios that Bronow foresees as most likely to occur in the American system. Do you agree with his forecasts? Explain.
4. Does Bronow's analysis reflect a more utilitarian approach to the issues, or is it more deontological? Support your answer.

❧ CASES FOR ANALYSIS*

1. Cutbacks at Phipps

Phipps Memorial Hospital is a community hospital with 500 beds. It offers services to the community in family medicine, internal medicine, gynecology and obstetrics, surgery, pediatrics, and psychiatry. These areas also have small resident-training programs. Transplants—usually kidney and heart—are also performed in this hospital. The outpatient department is rather extensive, and there is a new service devoted to drug addiction.

Administrators are putting together five- and ten-year plans. Although Phipps receives a certain amount of federal funding, most of its revenue comes from private sources. Administrators are aware that federal funding will be cut back in the years ahead, and additional funds from private sources will need to fill in the gaps. This means that reimbursement over the next several years will be diminished and that plans for physical growth and for hiring new personnel need to be frozen. Administrators realize these measures are not enough. Hospital personnel will have to be cut back, as will some programs and services.

DISCUSSION QUESTIONS

1. If you were involved in making the budget decisions, what cutbacks would you advise? How would you justify them? What moral principles would you appeal to?
2. Should cutbacks be across the board throughout the hospital, or should certain areas be targeted? If the latter, which ones, and why?
3. How much weight would you give to each of the proposed criteria for distributing resources? What would be your most important criterion for making specific cutbacks?

2. Danielle Marsh[62]

Danielle Marsh is a thirty-five-year-old single mother with three young children, ages seven, nine and fourteen. She has been on welfare for the past two years. Marsh last worked as a checkout clerk at the local grocery store. She was fired from this job because she consistently showed up for work at least thirty minutes late, and customers often complained that she was rude to them. A year ago, she was diagnosed with breast cancer, and she underwent a radical mastectomy. Things seemed to be going well until two months ago, when the tumor reappeared despite various aggressive treatments. After exhausting all other options, her physician recommended a bone marrow transplant. Her fourteen-year-old daughter, Pamela, appears to be a suitable match.

Since Marsh is covered by Medicaid, a state review board meets to decide whether it will pay for the operation. The review board determines that the procedure is an unproven technique, even though private insurers in the state fund the procedure.

---

*Names and cases are fictitious unless noted otherwise.

DISCUSSION QUESTIONS

1. Is the judgment of Medicaid's state review board fair? What might be the rationale behind its decision?
2. Should Marsh's personal behavior and difficulty holding a job be relevant factors in reaching a moral resolution regarding her treatment? Explain.
3. Does this case reflect broader ethical issues pertaining to a two-tiered health system? If so, in what ways? Explain.

3. Anthony Almado

Seventy-three-year-old Anthony Almado has emphysema. Over the past seven years, ever since retiring from his job at the post office, he has experienced chronic respiratory difficulty. He has been admitted to the hospital four times, each time for a brief stay. A few days ago, he contracted a severe cold. It was so serious that he was again admitted to the hospital.

At 3 A.M., Almado's attending nurse, Connie Johnson, who was new to the hospital, noticed that he was becoming extremely lethargic, and she was convinced that he would most likely experience respiratory failure unless he was placed on a respirator. Johnson initiated efforts to place him on a ventilator after speaking with Almado's physician. When she discussed this treatment with her supervisor, the supervisor alerted Johnson to the hospital's current policy of using respirators only in the ICU. There is only one bed available in the ICU, and the general practice in the hospital is to keep one bed open in the ICU in case of emergency.

DISCUSSION QUESTIONS

1. What should the nurse do? Support your response.
2. Whose rights take priority: Almado's right to medical treatment or society's claim on a scarce health resource?
3. Is the hospital policy regarding the use of respirators justifiable? Is the hospital practice regarding leaving one bed open in the ICU justifiable? Support your answers.

4. Medical Necessity and Home Care[63]

Jenny Riggi, a seventy-nine-year-old retired widow, belongs to the Optima HMO. She lives alone. Riggi lives on a fixed income and cannot afford to buy into any supplemental healthcare plans. She has recently had episodes of congestive heart failure and atrial fibrillation. These episodes have required her to take regular medication and to be on a salt-free diet. She has also shown signs of progressive loss of short-term memory and orientation. Her condition has made it necessary for a visiting nurse to come to her home.

The visiting nurse came to Riggi's home for a brief period and then stopped coming when Riggi appeared stable. Riggi again experienced congestive heart failure. Her physician ordered a series of home visits to make sure that she was cooperating with her regimen. After six weeks, her congestive heart failure cleared.

Her HMO covers "medically necessary" treatments. Home care is covered if certain criteria are met:

- The service is an essential part of active treatment.
- There is a defined medical goal that the patient expects to gain.
- The patient is homebound for medical reasons.
- Home care is not for "custodial" reasons.

Given Riggi's mental and physical state, she may experience more episodes of congestive heart failure due to inability to comply with the regimen unless home visits are regularly provided. But, now that Riggi is stable, her physician wonders whether her HMO would consider such visits "medically necessary."

DISCUSSION QUESTIONS

1. Is there sufficient evidence that Riggi's home care is "medically necessary"? Support your answer.
2. From the point of view of Optima HMO, it could claim that checking up on Riggi to ensure that she follows her regimen could be done by neighbors and is not necessarily "medically" necessary. How would you respond?
3. Do you think the phrase "medically necessary" assumes criteria that are more than simply medical? Explain.

5. James Coleman[64]

When forty-three-year-old James Coleman, a construction worker, had his regular physical exam, he was discovered to have a ventricular heart arrhythmia that appeared serious enough to be possibly life-threatening. After taking the prescribed disopyramide, an antiarrhythmic drug, he began to experience severely blurred vision and a dry mouth. His physician prescribed propranolol to be used with the disopyramide, and the side effects disappeared. He continued to take the combined drugs.

Two years later, Coleman moved to another town and joined the local HMO. His primary physician referred him to a cardiologist when Coleman requested that his prescription be refilled. The cardiologist, Dr. Schmidhofer, at first considered the possibility of prescribing propranolol alone but reconsidered based on the slight risk of a heart attack. However, he also noticed, on reviewing Coleman's financial chart, that the cost of prescribing disopyramide was exceedingly higher than the cost of propranolol—over $400 annually compared to less than $30 per year. Prescribing only the cheaper medication would save the HMO money, and the risk of heart failure taking only propranolol was very slight.

DISCUSSION QUESTIONS

1. In this case, should Dr. Schmidhofer strive to save the HMO money? How does this obligation weigh against his obligation to act in the best interests of his patient? Support your answer.
2. How morally relevant are cost factors when it comes to physicians' fulfilling their traditional duty to their patients? Is the traditional duty being challenged or in any way compromised in this case? Explain.

3. What reasons can you give in support of prescribing only propranolol? What reasons can you give in support of prescribing both drugs together? Explain your reasons.

6. Turning Away Patients[65]

Dr. Laurence Andrews has a thriving private practice in an affluent area just north of Palm Springs, California. He has just hired a new office assistant, after firing the former assistant, Barbara Brown, for refusing to turn away potential patients who do not have health insurance. Brown refused to comply with this directive on the grounds that it was unethical to turn away patients for lack of insurance. Andrews, on the other hand, claims that his policy is entirely justified because his private practice and office, with overhead including salaries, office space, medical equipment, and the like, require that his patients have adequate coverage. In addition, he has his bills from medical school to pay, as well as costly premiums for malpractice insurance. He has a family to care for, and their care rests on his income.

Andrews has made it clear to his new assistant, Janice Molinaro, that she must determine potential patients' health coverage status. If they do not have coverage, he will refer them to other physicians. Molinaro at first has no problem with this arrangement and agrees to comply with it. However, after turning away some people who have come to the office in genuine need of medical care, she rethinks Andrews's policy. She speaks with Andrews about her concerns, yet he remains adamant. He will not take on any patient who does not have insurance. Molinaro does not want to lose her job. She is recently divorced and is now a single parent with two young children to provide for. Her former husband has left the country and has stopped paying alimony, leaving her with a huge amount of debt.

DISCUSSION QUESTIONS

1. Is Dr. Andrews's policy unethical? Why or why not?
2. What utilitarian and deontological arguments can you give that, on the one hand, justify his policy, and, on the other hand, oppose his policy? Explain in detail.
3. How should Molinaro deal with her predicament? Support your answer.

7. Limiting Emergency Room Hours[66]

Grand Valley Community Hospital serves a rural community of about 12,000 in Montana. It has recently had to deal with diminishing budgets requiring that certain services be cut back or eliminated. A group of external financial assessors was invited to conduct a feasibility study of various departments in terms of their financial stability. The assessors concluded that one of the most expensive departments in the hospital was the emergency room. Hospital administrators then decided to limit the services offered by the emergency room. They announced that the emergency room would be closed regularly from 10:00 P.M. until 6:00 A.M. They felt that this would save a sizable amount of money for the hospital. Otherwise, the hospital would stand in danger of going bankrupt.

The announcement by Grand Valley's administration evoked an uproar among the local residents that has led to all sorts of public forums. Administrators for the hospital defend their position and claim that, since patients in need of emergency medical attention during the late evening and early morning hours can seek medical care at a state-run hospital approximately 35 miles from Grand Valley, access to emergency treatment is not being denied to the community. However, the rural community comprises a population of around 2,500 indigent residents. Opponents of limiting Grand Valley's emergency room hours claim that most of these indigent residents are not able to obtain the transportation necessary to travel to the state hospital. They argue that closing the emergency room during these hours seriously restricts these poor residents' access.

DISCUSSION QUESTIONS

1. The decision to close the emergency room during certain hours was a decision reached by Grand Valley's administrators after consultation with the financial advisors. Could the administrators have empowered the general community to take a more active part in resolving the financial solvency problem? Explain.
2. Is the decision of the administrators ethically justifiable? Support your answer.
3. How would you address this issue using a utilitarian calculus? How would you apply a deontological approach in reaching a justifiable resolution? Explain.

8. Leslie Franck[67]

In many people's eyes, Leslie Franck is an attractive woman. In her mid-thirties, she continues to work as a fashion model for a number of modeling agencies. Although she appears attractive to many, she herself is particularly conscious of her nose, which she is convinced is too large. In fact, she has been self-conscious about her nose since she was a teenager.

Deciding to remedy her appearance and boost her self-esteem, she visits a local cosmetic surgeon to ask his advice. The surgeon points out to Franck the inconveniences and possible risks associated with rhinoplasty, the technical term for a nose lift. He also points out that the procedure is relatively expensive. He concludes that the financial burdens, as well as the slight risks involved, may argue against having the procedure. Moreover, he assures Leslie that her nose is normal and there is no real need for surgery. He refuses to perform the procedure on Franck.

Franck visits another cosmetic surgeon to get a second opinion—one that supports her own beliefs. The second surgeon agrees with the first that Franck's nose is normal. However, he believes that her self-esteem is a critical issue and therefore justifies the procedure on the grounds of its hoped-for positive psychological benefits for Franck. He agrees to perform the operation.

DISCUSSION QUESTIONS

1. Was the first surgeon justified in refusing to operate on Franck? Support your answer.
2. Do you think that Franck's rhinoplasty is "medically necessary"? Why or why not? Explain.
3. Do you think the opinions of others count in determining what is medically the norm? Should they count more than the opinion of Franck herself? Explain.

Appendix: Living Will Samples

My Living Will
To My Family, My Physician, My Lawyer and All Others Whom It May Concern

Death is as much a reality as birth, growth, maturity and old age—it is the one certainty of life. If the time comes when I can no longer take part in decisions for my own future, let this statement stand as an expression of my wishes and directions, while I am still of sound mind.

If at such a time the situation should arise in which there is no reasonable expectation of my recovery from extreme physical or mental disability, I direct that I be allowed to die and not be kept alive by medications, artificial means or "heroic measures". I do, however, ask that medication be mercifully administered to me to alleviate suffering even though this may shorten my remaining life.

This statement is made after careful consideration and is in accordance with my strong convictions and beliefs. I want the wishes and directions here expressed carried out to the extent permitted by law. Insofar as they are not legally enforceable, I hope that those to whom this Will is addressed will regard themselves as morally bound by these provisions.

(Optional specific provisions to be made in this space — see other side)

DURABLE POWER OF ATTORNEY (optional)

I hereby designate _____ to serve as my attorney-in-fact for the purpose of making medical treatment decisions. This power of attorney shall remain effective in the event that I become incompetent or otherwise unable to make such decisions for myself.

Optional Notarization:

"Sworn and subscribed to

before me this _____ day

of _____, 19_____."

_____
Notary Public
(seal)

Signed_____

Date _____

Witness _____

_____
Address

Witness _____

_____
Address

Copies of this request have been given to _____

_____

(Optional) My Living Will is registered with Concern for Dying (No. _____)

Distributed by Concern for Dying, 250 West 57th Street, New York, NY 10107 (212) 246-6962

Living Will Declaration

Society for the Right to Die

250 West 57th Street/New York, NY 10107

To My Family, Doctors, and All Those Concerned with My Care

This declaration sets forth your directions regarding medical treatment.

I, _____, being of sound mind, make this statement as a directive to be followed if I become unable to participate in decisions regarding my medical care.

If I should be in an incurable or irreversible mental or physical condition with no reasonable expectation of recovery, I direct my attending physician to withhold or withdraw treatment that merely prolongs my dying. I further direct that treatment be limited to measures to keep me comfortable and to relieve pain.

You have the right to refuse treatment you do not want, and you may request the care you do want.

These directions express my legal right to refuse treatment. Therefore I expect my family, doctors, and everyone concerned with my care to regard themselves as legally and morally bound to act in accord with my wishes, and in so doing to be free of any legal liability for having followed my directions.

You may list specific treatment you do not want. For example:

Cardiac resuscitation
Mechanical respiration
Artificial feeding/fluids by tubes

Otherwise, your general statement, top right, will stand for your wishes.

I especially do not want: _____
_____
_____
_____
_____
_____

You may want to add instructions for care you do want—for example, pain medication; or that you prefer to die at home if possible.

Other instructions/comments: _____
_____
_____
_____

If you want, you can name someone to see that your wishes are carried out, but you do not have to do this.

Proxy Designation Clause: Should I become unable to communicate my instructions as stated above, I designate the following person to act in my behalf:

Name_____

Address_____

If the person I have named above is unable to act in my behalf, I authorize the following person to do so:

Name_____

Address_____

Sign and date here in the presence of two adult witnesses, who should also sign.

Signed:_____Date:_____

Witness:_____Witness:_____

Keep the signed original with your personal papers at home. Give signed copies to doctors, family, and proxy. Review your Declaration from time to time; initial and date it to show it still expresses your intent.

Notes

CHAPTER 1

1. See Daniel Goldhagen, *Hitler's Willing Executioners* (New York: Knopf, 1996).
2. Hannah Arendt, *Eichmann in Jerusalem: A Report on the Banality of Evil* (New York: Viking, 1963), 95.
3. Andrew C. Ivy, "Nazi War Crimes of a Medical Nature," *Federation Bulletin* 33 (1947): 133–146.
4. Eva Mozes Kor, "Nazi Experiments as Viewed by a Survivor of Mengele's Experiments," in Arthur L. Caplan, ed., *When Medicine Went Mad: Bioethics and the Holocaust* (Totowa, NJ: Humana Press, 1992), 3–5.
5. Stanley Milgram, *Obedience to Authority* (New York: Harper & Row, 1974), 6.
6. Veatch, *Cross Cultural Perspective*, 111.
7. From *Hippocrates*, vol. 1, trans. W. H. S. Jones, Loeb Classical Library (Cambridge: Harvard University Press, 1923), 164–165.
8. Daniel Bonevac, William Boon, and Stephen Phillips, *Beyond the Western Tradition: Readings in Moral and Political Philosophy* (Mountain View, CA: Mayfield Publishing Co., 1992), 147.
9. Quoted from Robert M. Veatch, ed., *Cross Cultural Perspective in Medical Ethics: Readings* (Boston: Jones and Bartlett Publishers, 1989), 128–129.
10. Some philosophers refer to theoretical ethics as "metaethics"; however, others consider metaethics to be a subdivision of theoretical ethics.
11. Some philosophers refer to applied ethics as "normative ethics"; however, others distinguish between the two, considering applied ethics to be the application of ethical norms.
12. Nahid Toubia, *Female Genital Mutilation: A Call for Global Action* (New York: New York Women, 1993).
13. Olayinka A. Koso-Thomas, "Female Circumcision," in Warren Thomas Reich, ed., *Encyclopedia of Bioethics*, vol. 1 (New York: Simon & Schuster Macmillan, 1995), 386.
14. See Chapter 6 for further discussion of the Tuskegee Study.
15. Ruth Benedict, "Anthropology and the Abnormal," *Journal of General Psychology* 10 (1933), 73.
16. Gontran de Poncins, *Kabloona* (New York: Reynal & Hitchcock, 1941).
17. Karen McCarthy Brown, "Afro-Caribbean Spirituality: A Haitian Case Study," in Lawrence E. Sullivan, *Healing and Restoring: Health and Medicine in the World's Religious Traditions* (New York: Macmillan, 1989), 255–285.
18. Kofi Appiah-Kubi, "Religion and Healing in an African Community," in Sullivan, *Healing and Restoring*, 203–224.
19. See the work of Lawrence Kohlberg, *Essays in Moral Development*, vol. II, *The Psychology of Moral Development* (San Francisco: Harper & Row, 1984).
20. Hannah Arendt, *Eichmann in Jerusalem: A Report on the Banality of Evil* (New York: Viking, 1963), 104–112.
21. Kohlberg, *Essays in Moral Development*, vol. II.
22. Donnie J. Self and DeWitt C. Baldwin, Jr., "Moral Reasoning in Medicine," in James Rest and Darcia Narvaez, *Moral Development in the Professions: Psychology and Applied Ethics* (Hillsdale, NJ: Lawrence Erlbaum Associates, 1994), 147–162.
23. D. J. Self, J. D. Skeel, and N. S. Jecker, "A Comparison of the Moral Reasoning of Physicians and Clinical Medical Ethicists," *Academic Medicine* 68, no. 11 (1993): 855–859.
24. Self and Baldwin, "Moral Reasoning in Medicine," 156.
25. D. J. Self, N. S. Jecker, and D. C. Baldwin, Jr., "A Preliminary Study of the Moral Orientation of Justice and Care Among Graduating Medical Students" (unpublished manuscript, 1993).
26. D. J. Self and M. Olivarez, "The Influence of Gender on Conflicts of Interest in the Allocation of Limited Critical Care Resources: Justice vs. Care," *Journal of Critical Illness* 8, no. 1 (1993): 64–74.
27. James Rest, "Research on Moral Development: Implications for Training Counseling Psychologists," *The Counseling Psychologist* 12, no. 2 (1984): 19–29.
28. Sarah A. Tooley, *The Life of Florence Nightingale* (New York: Macmillan, 1905), 39–40.
29. Muriel J. Bebeau, "Influencing the Moral Dimensions of Dental Practice," in James Rest and Darcia Narvaez, *Moral Development in the Professions: Psychology and Applied Ethics* (Hillsdale, NJ: Lawrence Erlbaum Associates, 1994), 121–146.
30. Carol Gilligan and Jane Attanucci, "Two Moral Orientations: Gender Differences and Similarities," *Merrill-Palmer Quarterly* 34, no. 3 (1988): 223–237.

31. Self, Jecker, and Baldwin, "A Preliminary Study."

32. C. D. Cook, "Influence of Moral Reasoning on Attitudes Toward Treatment of the Critically Ill," *Proceedings of the 17th Annual Conference on Research in Medical Education* 17 (1978): 442–443.

33. D. J. Self, D. E. Schrader, D. C. Baldwin, Jr., and F. D. Wolinsky, "The Moral Development of Medical Students: A Pilot Study of the Possible Influence of Medical Education," *Medical Education* 27 (1993): 26–34.

34. Self and Baldwin, "Moral Reasoning in Medicine."

35. See chart in Rest and Narvaez, *Moral Development in the Professions*, 14.

36. D. A. Baab, and M. J. Bedeau, "The Effect of Instruction on Ethical Sensitivity," *Journal of Dental Education* 54, no. 1 (1990): 44.

37. Laura J. Duckett and Muriel B. Ryden, "Education for Ethical Nursing Practice," in Rest and Narvaez, *Moral Development in the Professions*, 51–69.

38. "Counseling and Social Role Taking," in Rest and Narvaez, *Moral Development in the Professions*, 85–99.

39. D. C. Baldwin, Jr., E. Adamson, D. J. Self, and T. J. Sheehan, "Moral Reasoning and Malpractice: A Study of Orthopedic Surgeons" (unpublished manuscript, 1994).

40. T. J. Sheehan, S. Husted, D. Candee, C. D. Cook, and M. Bargen, "Moral Judgment as a Predictor of Clinical Performance," *Evaluation and the Health Professions* 3 (1980): 393–404.

41. Self and Baldwin, "Moral Reasoning in Medicine," 152.

42. D. E. Benor, N. Notzer, T. J. Sheehan, and G. R. Norman, "Moral Reasoning as a Criterion for Admission to Medical School," *Medical Education* 18 (1984): 423–428.

43. For exact citation, check out Walters, *Encyclopedia of Bioethics*, vol. 4 (1985), 2125.

44. From Karo's Shulchan Aruch, *Yore Deah* 336:1, as quoted in "A Jewish Perspective on the Four Principles," in Raanan Gillon, ed., *Principles of Health Care Ethics* (New York: John Wiley & Sons, 1994), 67.

45. "Definition of Medical Profession," in *Islamic Code of Medical Ethics Kuwait Document* (Islamic Organization of Medical Sciences, 1981).

46. Case study from Judith A. Boss, *Perspectives on Ethics* (Mountain View, CA: Mayfield Publishing Co., 1998), 168.

47. Stacy Teicher, "When Minors Refuse Medical Treatment," *Christian Science Monitor* 91 (9 February 1999): 3.

48. Kwame Gyekye, *An Essay on African Philosophical Thought: The Akan Conceptual Scheme* (New York: Cambridge University Press, 1987).

49. "Kevorkian: Convicted of Second-Degree Murder," *American Health Line*, 29 March 1999.

50. Thomas Johnsen, "Healing and Conscience in Christian Science," *The Christian Century* 111 (29 June 1994): 640.

51. David Sanders and Jessee Dukeminier, Jr., "Medical Advance and Legal Lag: Hemodialysis and Kidney Transplantation," *UCLA Law Review* 15 (February 1968): 366–380.

52. John Stuart Mill, "Utilitarianism," in Mary Warnock, ed., *Utilitarianism* (New York: Meridian, 1962), 257.

53. George Will, "Life and Death at Princeton," *Newsweek*, 13 September 1999.

54. Robert S. Pozos, "Scientific Inquiry and Ethics: The Dachau Data," in Arthur L. Caplan, ed., *When Medicine Went Mad: Bioethics and the Holocaust* (Totowa, NJ: Humana Press, 1992), 99.

55. Kor, "Nazi Experiments," 8.

56. Ann Harrison, Ahmed M. H. Al-Saadi, Ali S. O. Al-Kaabi, Mohammed R. S. Al-Kaabi, Saif S. M. Al-Bedwawi, Saiof O. M. Al-Kaabi, and Salem B. S. Al-Neaimi, "Should Doctors Inform Terminally Ill Patients? The Opinions of Nationals and Doctors in the United Arab Emirates," *Journal of Medical Ethics* 23 (1997): 101–107.

57. "Curing Health Care," *Newsweek*, 18 October 1999, 24–25; "Minorities Are Most Uninsured," *USA Today*, 20 October 1999, 1.

58. See *The World Almanac Book of Facts 1999* (Mahwah, NJ: Funk and Wagnalls Corp., 1998).

59. See *The World Almanac Book of Facts 1998* (Mahwah, NJ: Funk and Wagnalls Corp., 1997).

60. See *The World Almanac Book of Facts 1999*.

61. Aristotle, *Nicomachean Ethics*, trans. H. Rachman (Cambridge: Harvard University Press, 1975), 1095a, 8–10.

62. Guo Zhaojiang, "Chinese Confucian Culture and the Medical Ethical Tradition," *Journal of Medical Ethics* 21 (September 1995): 239–246.

63. "History of Medicine," *Encyclopedia of Chinese Medicine* (Shanghai: Shanghai Science and Technology Publishing House, 1987), 88.

64. Guo Zhaojiang, "Chinese Confucian Culture," 239.

65. Ministry of Health, People's Republic of China, "Regulations for Medical Ethics and Their Implementation" (1988).

66. Aristotle, *Nicomachean Ethics*, 13.

67. Eduardo Osuna, Maria D. Perez-Caceles, Miguel A. Esteban, and Aurelio Luna, "The Right to Information for the Terminally Ill Patient," *Journal of Medical Ethics* 24 (1998): 106–109.

68. Renee Fox and Judith Swazey, "Medical Morality Is Not Bioethics: Medical Ethics in China and in the United States," in *Perspectives in Biology and Medicine* 27 (Chicago: University of Chicago Press, 1984), 336–360.

69. P. Benner and J. Wrubel, *The Primacy of Caring* (Menlo Park, CA: Addison-Wesley, 1989).

70. See R. M. Hare, "Methods of Bioethics: Some Defective Proposals," *Monash Bioethics Review* 13 (1994), for an excellent discussion on balancing the different theories.

71. National Commission for the Protection of Human Subjects of Biomedical and Behavioral Research, *The Belmont Report: Ethics Principles and Guidelines for the Protection of Human Subjects of Research* (Washington, D.C.: National Institutes of Health, 1979).

72. Emiko Ohnuki-Tierney, "Health Care in Contemporary Japanese Religions," in Lawrence E. Sullivan, *Healing and Restoring: Health and Medicine in the World's Religious Traditions* (New York: Macmillan, 1989), 59–87.

73. Nancy S. Jecker et al., *Introduction to the Methods of Bioethics* (Sudbury, MA: Jones & Bartlett, 1997), 115.

74. Quoted in Norman Daniels, "Wide Reflective Equilibrium in Practice," in L. W. Sumner and Joseph Boyle, eds., *Philosophical Perspectives on Bioethics* (Toronto: University of Toronto Press, 1996), 105.

CHAPTER 2

1. Donald Oken, "What to Tell Cancer Patients: A Study of Medical Attitudes," *Journal of the American Medical Association* 175 (1961): 1120–1128.

2. C. Eugene Emery, Jr., "Deception OK, Some Doctors Say," *Providence Journal*, 26 May 1986, A1.

3. Robert Pool and Marc Tauss, "Saviors," *Discover* 19 (May 1998): 52–56.

4. Judith Jarvis Thomson, "A Defense of Abortion," *Philosophy and Public Affairs* 1, no. 1 (1971):

5. Judy Monroe, "Binge Drinking," *Current Health 2* 22 (May 1996): 26.

6. Stanley Joel Reiser, "Technology," in Warren Thomas Reich, ed., *Encyclopedia of Bioethics* (New York: Simon and Schuster Macmillan, 1995), 2477.

7. Sogyal Rinpoche, *The Tibetan Book of Living and Dying* (San Francisco: HarperCollins, 1992), 8–9.

8. M. Janet Lux-Barger and Robert P. Heaney, "For Better or Worse: The Technological Imperative in Health Care," *Social Science and Medicine* 22 (1986): 1313–1320.

9. Rinpoche, *Tibetan Book of Living and Dying*, 242.

10. Rinpoche, *Tibetan Book of Living and Dying*, 243.

11. See Kenneth Ring, *Heading Towards Omega: In Search of the Meaning of Near-Death Experience* (New York: Quill, 1985).

12. Chris van Weel and Joop Michels, "Dying, Not Old Age, to Blame for Cost of Health Care; Ageing Today and Tomorrow," *Lancet* 350 (18 October 1997): 1159.

13. Rosner, 1967. Warren Thomas Reich, ed. (New York: Simon and Schuster Macmillan, 1995).

14. R. P. Sloan and E. Bagiella, "Religion, Spirituality, and Medicine," *Lancet* 353 (20 February 1999): 664–667.

15. Sloan and Bagiella, "Religion, Spirituality, and Medicine," 664.

16. Peter Jaret, "Can Prayer Heal? Researchers with Their Feet on the Ground Say It Can—but Not in the Way You Might Think," *Health* 12 (March 1998): 48.

17. Sloan and Bagiella, "Religion, Spirituality, and Medicine," 666.

18. Hassan Hathout, "Contemporary Arab World," in *The Encyclopedia of Bioethics*, vol. 3 (1995).

19. See Judith A. Boss, *The Birth Lottery: Prenatal Diagnosis and Selective Abortion* (Chicago: Loyola University Press, 1993).

20. Robert Weir, *Selective Non-Treatment of Handicapped Newborns* (New York: Oxford University Press, 1984), 129.

21. Gina B. Kolata, "Mass Screening for Neural Tube Defects," *Hastings Center Report* 10 (December 1980): 9.

22. Ed McGaa (Eagle Man), *Mother Earth Spirituality: Native American Paths to Healing Ourselves and Our World* (San Francisco: Harper & Row, 1990), 203–204.

23. Sam Blowsnake, *The Autobiography of a Winnebago Indian*, trans. Paul Radin (New York: Dover, 1963 [1923]), 75.

24. Arthur Kleinman, "Medicine, Anthropology of," in Warren Thomas Reich, ed., *Encyclopedia of Bioethics*, vol. 3 (New York: Simon & Schuster, 1995), 1669.

25. "Medical Ethics, History of: South and East Asia," in Reich, ed., *Encyclopedia of Bioethics*, vol. 3, 1496.

26. Leigh Turner, "An Anthropological Exploration of Contemporary Bioethics: The Varieties of Common Sense," *Journal of Medical Ethics* 24 (1998): 127–133.

27. "Medical Ethics, History of: South and East Asia," 1496.

28. Atwood D. Gaines, "Race and Racism," in Reich, ed., *Encyclopedia of Bioethics*, 2197.

29. Peter Singer, *Animal Liberation*, 2d ed. (New York: Random House, 1990).

30. Jaret, "Can Prayer Heal?" 48.

31. Ibid.

32. Ibid.

33. Jacques Soustelle, *Daily Lives of the Aztecs on the Eve of the Spanish Conquest*, trans. Patrick O'Brian (New York: Macmillan, 1955), 196–197.

34. The Defining Issues Test (DIT) is based on Lawrence Kohlberg's stage theory of moral development. See Lawrence Kohlberg, *Essays in Moral Development*, vol. II, *The Psychology of Moral Development* (San Francisco: Harper & Row, 1984), and James Rest, "Research on Moral Development: Implications for Training Counseling Psychologists," *The Counseling Psychologist* 12, no. 2 (1984).

35. D. C. Baldwin, Jr., E. Adamson, D. J. Self, and T. J. Sheehan, "Moral Reasoning and Malpractice: A Study of Orthopedic Surgeons" (unpublished manuscript, 1994).

36. Elliot Turiel, Carolyn Hildebrandt, and Cecilia Wainryb, "Judging Social Issues: Difficulties, Inconsistencies, and Consistencies," *Monographs of the Society for Research in Child Development* 56, no. 2 (1991).

37. The term *rhetoric* is being used in the narrower sense of Sophist-type rhetoric rather than in the broad sense of any type of persuasive argument.

38. We need not concern ourselves at this point with learning how to determine whether the form of a deductive argument is correct, since this would require a course in logic.

39. A method of scientific investigation in which neither the subjects nor the investigator working with the subjects or analyzing the data knows what treatment, if any, the subjects are receiving. In a typical double-blind study, half of the subjects get the treatment, and the other half get a placebo.

40. John Rawls, *A Theory of Justice* (Cambridge, MA: Harvard University Press, 1971), 49.

41. Courtland Milloy, "St. Peter Won't Stop for Body Count at Heaven's Gates," *The Washington Post*, 4 April 1989, B3.

42. James Rest, "Research on Moral Development," 19–29.

43. Stanley Milgram, *Obedience to Authority* (New York: Harper & Row, 1974).

44. Arthur Jensen, "How Much Can We Boost IQ and Scholastic Achievement?" *Harvard Educational Review* 39 (Winter 1969): 1–23.

45. George E. Ehusani, *An Afro-Christian Vision* (Lanham, MD: University Press of America, 1991), 216.

46. "Infants: History of Infanticide," in Reich, ed., *Encyclopedia of Bioethics*, 1202–1203.

47. James Sorenson, "Some Social and Psychological Issues in Genetic Screening," in Daniel Bergsma, ed., *Ethical, Social and Legal Dimensions of Screening for Human Genetic Disease* (Miami: Symposium Specialists, 1974), 176.

48. Rosalyn Darling, *Families Against Society: A Study of Reactions to Children with Birth Defects* (London: Sage Publications, Ltd., 1979), 150–152.

49. Mary Benedict, Roger White, and Donald Cornely, "Maternal Perinatal Risk Factors and Child Abuse," *Child Abuse and Neglect* 9 (1985): 222.

50. Marc Miringoff, *The Index of Social Health, 1989, Measuring the Well Being of Children* (New York: Fordham Institute for Innovation in Social Policy, Fordham University, 1989), 6–7.

51. "U.S. Weighs Suing Tobacco Firms over Medicare Costs," *The Providence Sunday Journal*, 16 August 1998, A15.

52. Lawrence Kohlberg, *The Philosophy of Moral Development* (New York: Harper & Row, 1981.)

53. Robert Pool and Marc Tauss, "Saviors," *Discover* 19 (May 1998): 53–54.

54. Martin Luther King, Jr., *Strength to Love* (Philadelphia: Fortress Press, 1963), 19.

CHAPTER 3

1. Adapted from Samuel Gorovitz, *Doctors' Dilemmas* (New York: Macmillan, 1982).

2. Lewis Mehl-Madrona, *Coyote Medicine* (New York: Scribner, 1997), 28.

3. Robert M. Veatch, "Models for Ethical Medicine in a Revolutionary Age," *Hastings Center Report* 2, no. 3 (1972): 5–7.

4. See Vardit Rispler-Chaim, "Doctor-Patient Relations," in *Islamic Medical Ethics in the Twentieth Century* (Leiden: E. J. Brill, 1993), 62–71.

5. The example and passage are taken from Geri-Ann Galanti, *Caring for Patients from Different Cultures: Case Studies from American Hospitals*, 2d ed. (Philadelphia: University of Pennsylvania Press, 1997), 25–26.

6. Galanti, *Caring for Patients*, 65.

7. William F. May, "Code, Covenant, Contract, or Philanthropy?" *Hastings Center Report* 5, no. 6 (1975): 29–38. See also his *The Physician's Covenant: Images of the Healer in Medical Ethics* (Philadelphia: Westminster Press, 1983).

8. "Prayer of Moses Maimonides," trans. H. Friedenwald, *Bulletin of the Johns Hopkins Hospital* 28 (1927): 260–261.

9. From Janet Kraegel and Mary Kachoyeanos, "Just a Nurse," cited in Daniel F. Chambliss, *Beyond Caring: Hospitals, Nurses, and the Social Organization of Ethics* (Chicago: University of Chicago Press, 1996), 108.

10. Chambliss, *Beyond Caring*, 7.

11. Chambliss, *Beyond Caring*, 90.

12. Chambliss, *Beyond Caring* (from an interview), 107. See the discussion here from pp. 104–110.

13. Gina Kolata, "Where Marketing and Medicine Meet," *New York Times* (10 February 1998): A14.

14. Ibid.

15. "Oath of Initiation (*Caraka Samhita*)," in Warren T. Reich, ed., *Encyclopedia of Bioethics*, vol. 4 (New York: Free Press, 1978), 1732.

16. See Prakash N. Desai, "Medical Ethics in India," *Journal of Medicine and Philosophy* 13 (August 1988): 244–246.

17. This is not to discount the existence of pressures placed on physicians who operate more independently and are not under the aegis of a managed care plan. There are quite a few cases of physicians who have a vested financial interest in medical companies whose products these physicians utilize. Therefore, they have a direct financial incentive to order tests or use equipment, since they stand to make a profit from such use. The question is whether the tests and usage are genuinely medically necessary for the patient.

18. See A. Enthoven and R. Kronick, "A Consumer-Choice Health Plan for the 1990s: Universal Health Insurance in a System Designed to Promote Quality and Economy," *New England Journal of Medicine* 320 (1989): 29–37, 94–101.

19. Ezekiel J. Emanuel and Allan S. Brett, "Managed Competition and the Patient-Physician Relationship," *New England Journal of Medicine* 329, no. 12 (1993): 880.

20. Ibid.

21. This example is based on a similar case offered by Richard S. Liner, "Physician Deselection: The Dynamics of a New Threat to the Physician-Patient Relationship," *American Journal of Law & Medicine* 23, no. 4 (1997): 511–512.

22. See "Study Finds Dip in Income of Doctors," *New York Times* (3 September 1996): D9.

23. For an interesting and comprehensive discussion, see "Ethical Issues in Managed Care," *Journal of the American Medical Association* 273, no. 4 (1995): 330–335.

24. See Liner, "Physician Deselection," 517.

25. In Amihay Levy and Abraham Ohry, "The Physician's Oath Today: Necessity or Anachronism?" *Medicine and Law* 6 (1987): 221–222.

26. Levy and Ohry, "Physician's Oath," 219–225.

27. In Philip C. Hebert, *Doing Right: A Practical Guide to Ethics for Physicians and Medical Trainees* (Oxford: Oxford University Press, 1966), 66.

28. Ibid.

29. K. P. Dalla-Vorgia, K. Katsouyanni, T. N. Garanis, G. Touloumi, P. Drogari, and A. Koutselinis, "Attitudes of a Mediterranean Population to the Truth-Telling Issue," *Journal of Medical Ethics* 18 (1992): 67–74.

30. This case is taken from Hebert, *Doing Right*, 48.

31. Hebert, *Doing Right*, 52.

32. See John W. Douard and William J. Winslade, "*Tarasoff* and the Moral Duty to Protect the Vulnerable," in R. I. Simon, ed., *Review of Clinical Psychiatry and the Law*, vol. 1 (American Psychiatric Press, Inc., 1990), 163–176.

33. Cited in Douard and Winslade, "*Tarasoff*," 61.

34. In A. Haddard and L. Dougherty, "Whistleblowing in the OR," *Today's OR Nurse* (March 1991): 30–31.

35. See the discussion in Charles M. Culver and Bernard Gert, *Philosophy in Medicine* (New York: Oxford University Press, 1982), 52ff.

36. Case cited in Hebert, *Doing Right*, 94.

37. Taken from Dan C. English, *Bioethics: A Clinical Guide for Medical Students* (New York: W. W. Norton and Company, 1994), 62.

38. This case and the questions following are taken from Judith Boss, *Analyzing Moral Issues* (Mountain View, CA: Mayfield Publishing, 1998).

39. Taken from Galanti, *Caring for Patients*, 70.

CHAPTER 4

1. The term *fetus* will be used throughout this text to refer to the unborn human throughout the nine months of gestation.

2. Marji Gold, Denise Luks, and Matthew R. Anderson, "Medical Options for Early Pregnancy Termination," *American Family Physician* 56 (August 1997): 533–538.

3. "Abortion: After Long Downswing, Numbers Climb Again," *American Health Line*, 2 August 1999.

4. Gold, Luks, and Anderson, "Medical Options," 533–539.

5. "Advocate Lied on Late-Term Method," *Facts on File World News Digest* (20 March 1997): 195F3.

6. *The World Almanac 1999* (Mahwah, NJ: Funk and Wagnalls).

7. Major Garrett, "China's Forced Population Limits," *U.S. News & World Report* 124 (22 June 1998): 47.

8. Ren-Zong Qiu, "Medical Ethics and Chinese Culture," in Edmund Pellegrino, Patricia Mazzarell, and Pietro Corsi, eds., *Transcultural Dimensions in Medical Ethics* (Frederick, MD: UPG, 1997), 159–173.

9. Gail Weiss, "Sex-Selection Abortion: A Relational Approach," *Hypatia* 10, no. 1 (Winter 1995): 202–217.

10. Elisabeth Rosenthal, "For One-Child Policy, China Rethinks Iron Hand," *New Republic* 219 (23 November 1998): 6.

11. Satrughna Behera, "Ethical Problems in Medical Practice—an Indian Perspective," *Darshana International* 33 (October 1993): 47.

12. Paul U. Unschuld, "Confucianism," *Encyclopedia of Bioethics*, vol. 1 (1995): 465–468.

13. Allan Rosenfield and Sara Iden, "Abortion: Medical Perspectives," in Warren T. Reich, ed., *Encyclopedia of Bioethics*, vol. 1 (Simon & Schuster Macmillan, 1995), 1–5.

14. "African Religion," *Encyclopedia of Bioethics*, vol. 1 (1995), 83.

15. Richard Nyberg, "Pro-life Activists Deplore Liberal Abortion Law: South Africa," *Christianity Today* 41 (6 January 1997): 60.

16. Helen Carter, "Pro-Choice vs. Pro-Life," *The Guardian* (London), 24 September 1998, 5.

17. "Bitter Pill: Japan," *The Economist* 344 (8 November 1997): 42–43.

18. Miura Domyo, *The Forgotten Child: An Ancient Eastern Answer to a Modern Problem* (Henley-on-Thames, GB: Aidan Ellis, 1983).

19. Elaine Martin, "Rethinking the Practice of Mizuko Kuyo in Contemporary Japan: Interviews with Practitioners at a Buddhist Temple in Tokyo," paper presented at the Association for Asian Studies, Honolulu, 11–14 April 1996.

20. Brief of 281 American Historians as *Amici Curiae* Supporting the Appellees in *Webster v. Reproductive Services*, 1988.

21. James C. Mohr, *Doctors and the Law: Medical Jurisprudence in Nineteenth-Century America* (New York: Oxford University Press, 1993), 42–43.

22. Reva Siefel, "Reasoning from the Body: A Historical Perspective on Abortion Regulation and Questions of Sexual Protection," *Stanford Law Review* 44 (January 1992), 286.

23. Elizabeth Cady Stanton, "Child Murder," *The Revolution* 1(10) (12 March 1868): 146–147.

24. Elizabeth Cady Stanton, "Infanticide," *The Revolution* 1(4) (29 January 1868): 57–58.

25. Susan B. Anthony, "Marriage and Maternity," *The Revolution* 4(1) (8 July 1869): 4.

26. Judith Blake, "Abortion and Public Opinion: The 1960–1970 Decade," *Science* 171 (1971): 540–548.

27. Today about 25 percent of pregnancies are ended by abortion, from a high of one-third in 1988. Gold, Luks, and Anderson, "Medical Options," 533.

28. "Abortion Surveillance: Preliminary Data—United States, 1993 (from the Centers for Disease Control and Prevention)," *Journal of the American Medical Association*, 275 (10 April 1996): 1073; and Vrazo Fawn, "Abortions Drop Significantly, Study Reports," *Knight-Ridder/Tribune News Service*, 19 June 1994; "Experts Try to Explain Declining Abortion Rate," *CQ Researcher* 44 (28 November 1997): 1038.

29. Hassan Hathout, "Contemporary Arab World," *Encyclopedia of Bioethics*, vol. 3 (1995), 1452–1457.

30. Ibid.

31. Carroll Bogert, "Abortion and the Fight of God: Many Doctors Willing to Perform Abortions Are Strongly Religious," *Newsweek* 124 (17 October 1994): 40.

32. For more on the Islamic perspective on abortion, see "Abortion: Religious Traditions," in Warren T. Reich, ed., *Encyclopedia of Bioethics*, vol. 1 (New York: Simon & Schuster Macmillan, 1995), 38–42.

33. Alison M. Jaggar, "Regendering the U.S. Abortion Debate," *Journal of Social Philosophy* 28 (Spring 1997): 131. For a more in-depth analysis of this argument, see "Abortion and Feminism," *Social Theory and Practice* 16 (Spring 1990): 1–17.

34. For a more in-depth analysis of this argument, see "Abortion and Feminism," *Social Theory and Practice* 16 (Spring 1990): 1–17.

35. Geoge J. Gallup, *The Gallup Poll: Public Opinion 1996* (Wilmington, DE: Scholarly Resource, Inc., 1997), 112–113.

36. Gallup, *The Gallup Poll 1996*, 110–111. See also *The Gallup Poll: Public Opinion 1990*, 45.

37. Barbara Weiss, "*Roe vs. Wade* at 25: The Tough Questions Linger," *Medical Economics* 75 (10 August 1998): 138.

38. *ABC Nightly News*, 16 January 1997.

39. "Fewer Doctors Performing Abortions," *Facts on File World News Digest* (12 October 1995): 766B2.

40. For a more detailed discussion of the concept of personhood, see pages 00–00 in Chapter 1, "Moral Theory."

41. S. Cromwell Crawford, *Dilemmas of Life and Death; Hindu Ethics in North American Context* (Albany: State University of New York, 1995), 21.

42. Crawford, *Dilemmas of Life and Death*, 19.

43. Robert J. White, "Partial-Birth Abortion: A Neurosurgeon Speaks," testimony by U.S. House Committee on the Judiciary, 19 June 1996.

44. For a defense of this definition of personhood, see Baruch Brody, "The Morality of Abortion," in *Abortion and the Sanctity of Human Life: A Philosophical View* (Cambridge, MA: MIT Press, 1975).

45. Clifford Grobstein, *Science and the Unborn* (New York: Basic Books, 1988), 109.
46. Weiss, "*Roe vs. Wade* at 25," 138.
47. See, for example, Gallup, *The Gallup Poll 1996*.
48. Jaggar, "U.S. Abortion Debate," 136.
49. See Judith A. Boss, "Pro-Child, Pro-Choice: An Exercise in Doublethink?" *Public Affairs Quarterly* 7 (April 1993): 85–91.
50. *A Dictionary of Philosophy*, 2d ed. (New York: St. Martin's Press, 1979), 97.
51. Winny Koster-Oyekan, "Why Resort to Illegal Abortion in Zambia? Findings of a Community-Based Study in Western Province," *Social Science and Medicine* 46, no. 10 (1998): k1303–1312.
52. Ibid.
53. The term *selective abortion* is also used for cases involving more than two or three fetuses, usually because of the use of fertility drugs. In these cases, a mother may request that one or more of the fetuses be killed so that the others will have a better chance of surviving. However, these are not strictly abortions since the pregnancy is not terminated nor is the body of the dead fetus expelled before birth.
54. Nicholas D. Kristof, "The Chosen Sex: Peasants of China Discover New Way to Weed Out Girls," *New York Times*, 21 July 1993, A1.
55. Lynn Odell, "Researchers Study Safer Protocols to Detect Fetal Anomalies," *Medical Industry Today*, Medical Data International, Inc., 17 November 1998.
56. See Judith A. Boss, "First Trimester Prenatal Diagnosis: Earlier Is Not Necessarily Better," *Journal of Medical Ethics* 20 (1994): 146–151.
57. Paul Sachdev, ed., *International Book on Abortion* (Chicago: Greenwood, 1988), 102.
58. Lydia Saad, "Americans Divided over Abortion Debate," *Gallup Poll Week in Review*, 18 May 1999.
59. See *Statistical Abstract of the United States, 1997* (Washington, D.C.: U.S. Bureau of the Census, 1997), 75.
60. Dorothy Wertz and John Fletcher, "Ethics and Medical Genetics in the United States," *American Journal of Medical Genetics* 29 (April 1988): 823–825.
61. Helen Carter, "Pro-Choice vs. Pro-Life," *The Guardian* (London), 24 September 1998, 5.
62. *The Economist* 336 (5 August 1995): 43.
63. See Susan Nicholson, "Abortion: On Fetal Indications," in Thomas A. Shannon, ed., *Bioethics* (Ramsey, NJ: Paulist Press, 1981), 73–93.
64. H. Tristam, "Ethical Issues in Aiding the Death of Young Children," in Marvin Kohl, ed., *Beneficent Euthanasia* (Buffalo, NY: Prometheus Books, 1982), 186.
65. Since then, there have been a mounting number of wrongful-birth lawsuits, in which OB/GYNs are sued by parents claiming that they would have had an abortion had prenatal diagnosis detected the fetal abnormality. See "Wrongful Birth: Will OB/GYNs Face More and More Lawsuits?" *American Health Line*, 9 August 1999.
66. Wertz and Fletcher, "Ethics and Medical Genetics," 823–825.
67. Jerome Lejeune, "On the Nature of Man," *American Journal of Human Genetics* 22 (March 1970): 121–128.
68. For more discussion on Huntington's disease see Chapter 5, "Genetic Engineering, Reproductive Technologies, and Cloning."
69. See Chapter 5 for more on genetic research on a "gay gene."
70. John Fletcher, "The Brink: The Parent-Child Bond in the Genetic Revolution," *Theological Studies* 33 (September 1972): 482.
71. Paul A. Logli, "Drugs in the Womb: The Newest Battlefield in the War on Drugs," *Criminal Justice Ethics* (Winter/Spring 1990), 25.
72. Karen Rafinski, "Fetal Alcohol Syndrome: The Risk Is Real," *Providence Journal*, 15 July 1998, E3.
73. Logli, "Drugs in the Womb," 23–24.
74. Ernest L. Abel, *Fetal Alcohol Syndrome* (Oradell, NJ: Medical Economic Books, 1990), 104.
75. Katherine Beckett, "Fetal Rights and 'Crack Moms': Pregnant Women in the War on Drugs," *Contemporary Drug Problems* 22 (Winter 1995): 587–612.
76. Ibid.
77. The term *partial-birth abortion* was first used in 1995 in the Federal Partial-Birth Abortion Ban Act. Dr. James McMahon, whose use of the procedure fueled the debate, invented the term *intact dilation and evacuation* for the procedure. However, most physicians, ethicists, and legislators use the term *partial-birth abortion*.
78. Diane M. Gianelli, "Medicine Adds to Debate on Late-Term Abortion: Abortion Rights Leader Urges End to 'Half Truths,' " *American Medical News*, 3 March 1997, 3, 28.
79. Cases from Gloria Peldt and Ralph Reed, "The Abortion Debate: Opposing Views on Partial-Birth Abortion," *Cosmopolitan* 223 (July 1997): 155–156.
80. *Keeler v. Superior Court*, 2 Cal. 3d 619, 637 (1970).
81. *Casey*, 505 U.S. at 870.
82. Diane Gianelli, "Shock Tactic Ads Target Late-Term Abortion Procedure," *American Medical News*, 5 July 1993, 3.
83. Leslie Cannold, "Women, Ectogenesis and Ethical Theory," *Journal of Applied Philosophy* 12, no. 1 (1995): 58–61.
84. Weiss, "*Roe vs. Wade* at 25," 138.
85. Ibid.
86. Ibid.
87. Thomas M. Garrett, Harold W. Baillie, and Rosellen M. Garrett, *Health Care Ethics: Principles and Problems* (Englewood Cliffs, NJ: Prentice Hall, 1993), 171–172.
88. David Grimes, "RU-486: Politics and Science Collide," *Los Angeles Times*, 17 June 1991, B5.
89. "Abortion-Related Crime Increased in 1997," *Providence Journal*, 18 January 1998, F5.
90. Lois Margaret Nora and Mary B. Mahowald, "Neural Fetal Tissue Transplants: Old and New Issues," *Zygon* 31 (December 1996): 615–633.
91. "Ultrasound Effects," *Economist* 336 (5 August 1995): 34.
92. P. A. Jacobs, J. A. Strong, and M. Melville, "Aggressive Behavior, Mental Subnormality and the XYY Male," *Nature* 208 (25 December 1965): 1351.
93. Celeste McGovern, "A Taboo Broken but Not Forgotten," *Alberta Report/Western Report* 15 (10 October 1998): 43.

94. Karen Rafinski, "Fetal Alcohol Syndrome: The Risk Is Real," *Providence Journal*, 15 July 1998, E3.
95. This case analysis is based on an actual case.
96. Federal Legislative Office of the National Right to Life Committee, "Why Are Partial-Birth Abortions Performed?" http://www.nric.org/abortion/ pba/hypba-performed.html.
97. "Blasts Probed at Atlanta Family Clinics," *U.S. News*, 16 January 1997.
98. "AMA Praises Decision on Abortion-Related Web Site," *Medical Data International Inc.*, 4 February 1999.

CHAPTER 5

1. Plato, *Republic*, bk III (410), bk IV (456–461).
2. "Ethical and Religious Directives for Catholic Health Care Services," Directive #20 (1994).
3. D. J. Kevles, *In the Name of Eugenics: Genetics and the Uses of Human Heredity* (New York: Knopf, 1985), 100.
4. Kenneth Garver and Rick Santorum, "Eugenics and Catholic Medicine," *Ethics and Medics* 23, no. 7 (July 1998): 1–3.
5. Frank C. Dukepoo, "Commentary on 'Scientific Limitations and Ethical Ramifications of a Non-representative Human Genome Project: African American Response': An American Indian Perspective," *Science and Engineering Ethics* 4, no. 4 (1998): 172.
6. John Carey, "Playing God in the Lab," *Business Week*, 26 April 1999, 83.
7. "Life Sciences' Harvest of Hopes," *Business Week*, 12 April 1999, 138.
8. Quoted in Jeremy Rifkin, "The Biotech Century: Human Life as Intellectual Property," *Nation* 266 (13 April 1998): 13–23.
9. Dick Thompson, "The Gene Machine," *Time* 15 (24 January 2000): 58.
10. See Mary Rosner and T. R. Johnson, "Telling Stories: Metaphors of the Human Genome Project," *Hypatia* 10 (Fall 1995): 104–129.
11. For a complete copy of the Mataatua Declaration, see *Cultural Survival Quarterly*, Summer 1996, 52–53.
12. See Henry T. Greely, "Genes, Patents, and Indigenous Peoples," *Cultural Survival Quarterly*, Summer 1996, 54–57.
13. For an excellent discussion of this issue, see Barbara Looney, "Should Genes Be Patented? The Gene Patenting Controversy: Legal, Ethical, and Policy Foundations of an International Agreement," *Law and Policy in International Business* 26 (22 September 1994): 231 ff.
14. Dukepoo, "An American Indian Perspective," 172.
15. Ibid.
16. Dukepoo, "An American Indian Perspective," 173.
17. LeRoy Walters, "Genetics and Reproductive Technologies," in Veatch, ed. (1989), 212.
18. Alex Brooks, "Mentally Ill Patients Need Protection from Inappropriate Genetic Testing," *British Medical Journal* 317 (3 October 1998): 903.
19. The Council on Ethical and Judicial Affairs, American Medical Association, "Multiplex Genetic Testing," *Hastings Center Report* 28 (July/August 1998): 15–21.
20. Council on Ethical and Judicial Affairs, "Multiplex Genetic Testing," 17–18.
21. Ingrid Krueger, "Weeding Out the Disabled," *Alberta Report/Western Report* 24 (13 October 1997): 44.
22. "Ethical and Religious Directives for Catholic Health Care Services," Directive #54 (1994).
23. See Ruth Chadwick, Henk ten Have, Jorgen Husted, Mairi Levitt, Tony McGleenan, Darren Shickle, and Urban Wiesing, "Genetic Screening and Ethics: European Perspectives," *Journal of Medicine and Philosophy* 23, no. 3: 259.
24. Dorothy Wertz, "Medical Genetics: Ethical and Social Issues," in *Encyclopedia of Bioethics*, vol. 3 (1995), 1652–1655.
25. John Fletcher, "Moral Problems and Ethical Guidances in Prenatal Diagnosis: Past, Present and Future," in Aubrey Milunsky, ed., *Genetic Disorders and the Fetus*, 2d ed. (New York: Plenum Press, 1986), 848.
26. E. Virginia Lapham, Chahira Kozma, and Joan O. Weiss, "Genetic Discrimination: Perspectives of Consumers," *Science* 274 (October 1996): 621.
27. Theresa M. Marteau and Robert T. Croyle, "Psychological Responses to Genetic Testing," *British Medical Journal* 316 (February 1998): 694.
28. Anneke Lucassen, "Ethical Issues in Genetics of Mental Disorders; Commentary," *Lancet* 352 (26 September 1998): 1004.
29. Theresa M. Marteau and Robert T. Croyle, "Psychological Responses to Genetic Testing," *British Medical Journal* 316 (28 February 1998): 693–696.
30. Council of Europe, Parliamentary Assembly, Recommendation 934, "On Genetic Engineering" (Strasbourg, France, 1982).
31. Robin M. Henig and Terry Miura, "Tempting Fates," *Discovery* 19 (May 1998): 58.
32. Richard Jerome and Lyndon Stamber, "Life from Death," *People Weekly*, 19 April 1999, 60–63.
33. Robert Snowden and Elizabeth Snowden, "Ethical Problems in Infertility Treatment," in Raanan Gillon, ed., *Principles of Health Care Ethics* (London: John Wiley & Sons, Ltd., 1994), 601.
34. Karen Wright, "Human in the Age of Mechanical Reproduction," *Discover* 19 (May 1998): 74–81.
35. Geoffrey Crowley and Andrew Muir, "Ethics and Embryos," *Newsweek* 125 (12 June 1995): 66.
36. Henig and Miura, "Tempting Fates," 58.
37. Royal Commission on New Reproductive Technologies, *Final Report: Proceed with Care* (Ottawa, Canada, 1993).
38. Leigh Hopper, "Eleven-Month-Old Chukwus Honored," *Houston Chronicle*, 7 November 1999.
39. Ezekiel Emanuel, "Eight Is Too Many," *New Republic* 220 (1 January 1999): 8.
40. Hasan Hathout, "Islamic Concepts and Bioethics," in *Bioethic Yearbook: Center for Ethics, Medicine and Public Issues*, vol. 1 (London: Dordrech and Kluwer, 1991).
41. Surzh, *Shurz* (Consultation) XL11: 99-50.
42. Sherifa Zuhur, "Of Milk-Mothers and Sacred Bonds: Islam, Patriarchy, and New Reproductive Technologies," *Creighton Law Review* 25 (1992): 1725–1738.
43. Ibid.

44. Shelley Lau, "Report from Hong Kong," *Cambridge Quarterly of Healthcare Ethics* 4 (1995): 364–366.

45. Marilyn Gardner, "Should Children Know Donor Parents?" *Christian Science Monitor* 90 (28 October 1998): B5.

46. See Segun Gbadebesin, "Bioethics and Culture: An African Perspective," *Bioethics* 7, no. 2/3 (1993): 257–262.

47. Barbara Rothman, *Recreating Motherhood: Ideology and Technology in a Patriarchal Society* (1989).

48. Karen Wright, "Human in the Age of Mechanical Reproduction," 74–81.

49. James Bernasko et al., "Twin Pregnancies by Assisted Reproductive Techniques: Maternal and Neonatal Outcomes," *Obstetrics and Gynecology* 89, no. 3 (1997): 368–372.

50. James Webb, "Cloning Plans Breed Skepticism, Outrage," *Providence Journal Bulletin*, 8 January 1998, A1, A11.

51. Mark Johnson, "From Hubris and Hysteria, a Global Furor over Cloning," *New York Times*, 24 January 1998, A1.

52. "The Bad Seed," editorial, *New York Times*, 9 January 1998.

53. Nick Nuttall, "Scientists Take a Giant Step Towards Cloning Humans," *The Times*, 23 July 1998.

54. "Human Hybrid," *Discover* 20 (January 1999): 62.

55. "Cloning Success Spurs Debate; Other Developments," *Facts on File World News Digest*, 3 April 1997, 235E2.

56. *The Opinion of the Advisers to the President of the European Commission on the Ethical Implications of Biotechnology*, 28 May 1997.

57. E. V. Kontorovich, "Asexual Revolution," *National Review* (9 March 1998): 30.

58. Stephan Herrera, "Monster Mice," *Forbes* 63 (8 March 1999): 136.

59. Quoted in Bob Harris, "Second Thoughts About Cloning Humans," *The Humanist* (May–June 1997): 43.

60. Quoted in Charles Marwick, "Put Human Cloning on Hold, Say Bioethicists," *Journal of the American Medical Association* 278, no. 1: 14.

61. Jennifer Couzin, "What's Killing Clones?" *U.S. News & World Report* 126 (24 May 1999): 65.

62. "Many U.S. Animals Pregnant with Clones," *Providence Journal*, 28 June 1997, A4.

63. Wayne Kondro, "Canadian Government Will Revisit Human-Cloning Legislation," *Lancet* 353 (8 May 1999): 1599.

64. John Carey, "Playing God in the Lab," *Business Week*, 26 May 1999, 84.

65. John Grogan and Cheryl Long, "The Problem with Genetic Engineering," *Organic Gardening* 47 (January/February 2000): 42–44.

66. "The Moo Two: Any Way You Splice It," *Newsweek*, 2 February 1998, 65.

67. Rosamond Rhodes, "Genetic Links, Family Ties, and Social Bonds: Rights and Responsibilities in the Face of Genetic Knowledge," *Journal of Medicine and Philosophy* 23, no. 1 (1998): 10–30.

68. Anne Taylor Fleming, "Why I Can't Use Someone Else's Eggs," *Newsweek*, 12 April 1999, 12.

69. Glenn Zorpette, "Off with Its Head!" *Scientific American* (January 1998), 41.

70. Richard Stone, "Cloning the Woolly Mammoth," *Discover* 20 (April 1999): 56–62.

71. Stone, "Cloning the Wooly Mammoth," 56.

CHAPTER 6

1. Stephen B. Thomas and Sandra C. Quinn, "The Tuskegee Syphilis Study, 1932–1972: Implications for HIV Education and AIDS Risk Education Programs in the Black Community," *American Journal of Public Health*, 81, no. 11 (1991): 1501.

2. Clayton L. Thomas, ed., *Taber's Cyclopedic Medical Dictionary* (Philadelphia: R. A. Davis, 1989), 637.

3. For an excellent summary of the history of human experimentation, see David Rothman, "Human Research: Historical Aspects," in Riech, *Encyclopedia of Bioethics*, 2248–2258.

4. Margaret Moreland Stathos, "The History of the New England Anti-Vivisection Society," *NEAVS Members Magazine, 1995 Centennial Issue*, 80, no. 1 (1995): 2–3.

5. Ibid.

6. See also Robert J. Lifton, *Nazi Doctors*.

7. Allen M. Hornblum, "They Were Cheap and Available: Prisoners as Research Subjects in Twentieth Century America," *British Medical Journal*, 315, no. 7120 (1997): 1437.

8. Conference on Clinical Trials in Correctional Settings, October 1999, Providence, RI.

9. Rihito Kimura, "Medical Ethics, History of: Contemporary Japan," in Warren Thomas Reich, ed., *Encyclopedia of Bioethics*, New York: (Simon & Schuster Macmillan, 1995), 1496.

10. Paul M. McNeill, *The Ethics and Politics of Human Experimentation* (Cambridge, UK: Press Syndicate of the University of Cambridge, 1993), 23–26.

11. Japan was not the only country conducting secret weapons experiments. The United States and Australia also carried out secret, potentially fatal experiments on their own citizens. In Australia, mustard gas experiments were carried out on 1,000 "volunteers," many of whom suffered long-term health problems as a result. In the United States, thousands of citizens were used as unwitting subjects in radiation experiments.

12. "More Efforts Needed to Enroll Prisoners in AIDS Trials," *AIDS Weekly*, 21 November 1994, 15.

13. Ibid.

14. Medical Data International, Inc., "South African Authorities OK Trials of AIDS Drug," *Medical Industry Today*, 8 September 1999.

15. Sandra D. Lane, "Research Bioethics in Egypt," in Raanan Gillon, ed., *Principles of Health Care Ethics* (West Sussex, England: John Wiley & Sons, 1994), 885–894.

16. Arthur L. Caplan, ed., *When Medicine Went Mad: Bioethics and the Holocaust* (Totowa, NJ: Humana Press, 1992).

17. Ibid.

18. Sarah Ramsay "WMA Postpones Decision to Revise Declaration of Helsinki," *Lancet*, 354 (11 September 1999): 928.

19. "Protection of Human Subjects in Research Questioned," *Issues in Science and Technology* 15, no. 1 (Fall 1998): 27.

20. Sheila Kaplan and Shannon Brownlee, "Duke's Hazards," *U.S. News & World Report* 126 (24 May 1999): 66.

21. G. I. Serour, "Islam and the Four Principles," in Gillon, *Principles of Health Care Ethics*, 87–89

22. First International Conference on Islamic Medicine, "Islamic Code of Medical Ethics," *World Medical Journal* 29, no. 5 (1982): 80.

23. National Commission for the Protection of Human Subjects of Biomedical and Behavioral Research, *The Belmont Report: Ethics Principles and Guidlines for the Protection of Human Subjects of Research* (Washington, D.C.: National Institutes of Health, 1979).

24. Stathos, "New England Anti-Vivisection Society," 10.

25. Arjun Makhijani and Bette-Jane Crigger, "Enger Enters Guilty Plea," *Bulletin of the Atomic Scientists* 50, no. 2 (March 1994): 18.

26. See John Arras, "Noncompliance in AIDS Research," *Hastings Center Report* 20, no. 5 (September–October 1990): 24–32.

27. For a discussion and analysis of this study, see Robert M. Veatch, "'Experimental' Pregnancy," *Hastings Center Report*, no. 1 (June 1971): 2–3.

28. Veatch, "'Experimental' Pregnancy," 3.

29. The National Journal Group, Inc., "New York: Advocates for Mentally Ill Oppose Guidelines," *American Health Line*, 19 January 1999.

30. Stephen Haimowitz, Susan J. Delano, and John M. Oldham, "Uninformed Decisionmaking; The Case of Surrogate Research Consent," *Hastings Center Report* 27, no. 6 (November 1997): 9.

31. "Schizophrenia: Consenting Adults," *Science News*, 154 (5 December 1998): 367.

32. Kurt Eichenwald and Gina Kolata, "Drug Trials Hide Conflicts for Doctors," *New York Times*, 148 (16 May 1999): 1, 34.

33. Eichenwald and Kolata, "Conflicts for Doctors," 35.

34. Medical Data International, Inc., "U.N. Calls on Donor Countries to Boost AIDS Funding," *Medical Industry Today*, 23 April 1999, and "Conspiracy Theories Pose Challenge to African AIDS Workers," *Medical Industry Today*, 16 August 1999.

35. See Geoffrey Sea, "The Radiation Story No One Would Touch: Media's Unwillingness to Cover the Story of Government Experimentation on Human Beings Without Their Informed Consent," *Columbia Journalism Review* 32, no. 6 (March 1994): 37.

36. Vanessa Merton, "The Exclusion of Pregnant, Pregnable, and Once-Pregnable People (a.k.a. Women) from Biomedical Research," *American Journal of Law & Medicine* 12, (January 1993): 369–451.

37. Devra Davis et al., "Male-mediated Teratogenesis and Other Reproductive Effects," *Reproductive Toxicology* 6, no. 289 (1992): 289–292.

38. Stephanie Stapleton, "Trying to Get More Women in Clinical Trials", *American Medical News* 40, no. 4 (3 November 1997): 1–3.

39. Lucy Johnson and Ruaridh Nicoll, "AIDS Drugs Cut to 'Guinea Pigs'," *Review of African Political Economy* 24 (September 1997): 388–389.

40. See Pinit Ratanakul, "Medical Ethics, History of: South and East Asia," in Reich, *Encyclopedia of Bioethics*, 1507–1509.

41. See Sharon Begley and Daniel Glick, "Eying the Fetal Future: In the Shadows, a Controversial Search for Cures," *Newsweek*, 14 December 1998, 54–55.

42. For a more in-depth discussion of this case and the use of primates in experiments, see Deborah Blum, *The Monkey Wars* (New York: Oxford University Press, 1994).

43. Peter Singer, *Animal Liberation* (New York: Random House, 1990), 37.

44. The Vegetarian Society, "Gene Genius?" *The Vegetarian*, Spring 1993.

45. Dan Vergano, "Of Transgenic Mice and Men," *USA Today*, 25 May 1999: 11D.

46. Mukerjee Madhusree, "Trends in Animal Research, *Scientific American* 276, no. 2 (February 1997): 86.

47. Adapted from *PETA Factsheet on Animal Experiments*, #1.

48. Madhusree Mukerjee, "Trends in Animal Research," *Scientific American*, 276 (February 1997): 86.

49. Thomas Aquinas, *Summa Contra Gentiles*, book 3, part 2, chap. 112, trans. the English Dominican Fathers (Chicago: Benziger Brothers, 1928).

50. Basant K. Lai, "Hindu Perspective on the Use of Animals in Science," in Tom Regan, ed., *Animal Sacrifice: Religious Perspective on the Use of Animals in Science* (Philadelphia: Temple University Press, 1986), 208.

51. Jeremy Bentham, *Principles of Morals and Legislation* (London: Clarendon Press, 1907), 1.

52. Singer, *Animal Liberation*, 6.

53. Susanne Althoff, "Cruelty-free Research," *Vegetarian Times*, August 1993, 74.

54. Jack H. Botting and Adrian R. Morrison, "Animal Research Is Vital to Medicine," *Scientific American*, 276 (February 1997): 83.

55. Medical Data International, Inc., "Days of the Lab Rat May Soon Be Numbered," *Medical Industry Today*, 26 July 1999.

56. ABC Evening News, 6 May 1999.

57. "Drug Firm Sued by Auschwitz 'Guinea Pig.'" *The Guardian* (London), 19 February 1999, 12.

58. Robert S. Pozos, "Scientific Inquiry and Ethics: The Dachau Data," in Caplan, *When Medicine Went Mad*, 99.

59. Eva Mozes Kor, "Nazi Experiments as Viewed by a Survivor of Mengele's Experiments," in Caplan, *When Medicine Went Mad*, 8.

60. Dick Thompson, "Real Knife, Fake Surgery," *Time*, 22 February 1999, 66.

61. Thompson, "Real Knife, Fake Surgery," 66.

62. For more on this case, see Eichenwald and Kolata, "Conflicts for Doctors," 1, 34–35.

63. Nancy Neveloff Dubler and Victor W. Sidel, "On Research on HIV Infection and AIDS in Correctional Institutions." *Milbank Quarterly*, 67, no. 2 (22 June 1989): 171.

64. "High AIDS Rates, Other Infectious Diseases Reported in U.S. Prisons," *AIDS Weekly Plus*, 13 September 1999.

65. For more on this argument, see A. J. Bronstein, "Oral Remarks Given at the Conference on Research on HIV Infection and AIDS in Correctional Institutions," New York City, 28 June 1988.

66. Dan Vergano, "Of Transgenic Mice and Men: Human Touch Turns Rodents into Pioneers of Medical Research," *USA Today*, 25 May 1999, 11D.

67. Ibid.

68. This is a fictional case study.

CHAPTER 7

1. Christiaan Barnard and C. Pepper, *Christiaan Barnard: One Life* (New York: Macmillan, 1969); cited in Jay Katz, *The Silent World of Doctor and Patient* (New York: Free Press, 1984), 136. Katz provides a fascinating account of the conversations between Barnard and each of his first two heart transplant patients.

2. Ibid., cited in Katz, 138.

3. Philip Blaiberg, *Looking at My Heart* (New York: Stein and Day, 1968), 66; cited in Katz, 172.

4. Robert Sells, "Clinical Transplantation," in David C. Thomasma and Thomasine Kushner, eds., *Birth to Death: Science and Bioethics* (Cambridge: Cambridge University Press, 1996), 103.

5. Gregory Pence, *Classic Cases in Medical Ethics*, 2d ed. (New York: McGraw-Hill, 1990), 262–264.

6. See the discussion in Pence, *Classical Cases*, 263.

7. Quran 17, 36; cited in Vardit Rispler-Chaim, "Organ Transplant," *Islamic Medical Ethics in the Twentieth Century* (Leiden: E. J. Brill, 1993), 32. See his discussion in pp. 28–43.

8. Rispler-Chaim, "Organ Transplant," 35–37.

9. Department of Health and Human Services, in Stephanie Stapleton, "HHS Wants to Change How Organs Are Allocated for Transplant," *American Medical News* 41, no. 11 (16 March 1998): 11.

10. See Helen Hardacre, "Response of Buddhism and Shinto to the Issue of Brain Death and Organ Transplant," *Cambridge Quarterly of Health Care Ethics*, 3 (1994): 594–597. For another fine discussion, see Rihito Kimura, "Japan's Dilemma with the Definition of Death," *Kennedy Institute of Ethics Journal*, 1, no. 12 (June 1991): 123–131.

11. See also Michael Brannigan, "A Chronicle of Organ Transplant Progress in Japan," *Transplant International* 5 (1992): 180–186.

12. Sheryl WuDunn, "Death Taboo Weakening, Japan Sees 1st Transplant," *New York Times* (1 March 1999).

13. Rispler-Chaim, "Organ Transplant," 35–40.

14. Stapleton, "HHS Wants to Change How Organs Are Allocated for Transplant," 11.

15. Ibid.

16. Ibid.

17. Stapleton, "HHS," 12.

18. From "A Gift for a Stranger," *Omaha World-Herald*, 6 September 1991, cited in Mary Ann Lamanna, "Giving and Getting: Altruism and Exchange in Transplantation," *Journal of Medical Humanities* 18, no. 3 (1997): 170.

19. Renee C. Fox and Judith P. Swazey give an absorbing and fascinating account in *Spare Parts: Organ Replacement in American Society* (New York: Oxford University Press, 1992).

20. This case is taken from Jameson Forster, William G. Bartholome, and Romano Delcore, "Should a Patient Who Attempted Suicide Receive a Liver Transplant?" *Journal of Clinical Ethics* 7, no. 3: 257–258.

21. Forster et al., "Liver Transplant," 260.

22. Colin E. Atterbury, "Anubis and the Feather of Truth: Judging Transplant Candidates Who Engage in Self-Damaging Behavior," *Journal of Clinical Ethics* 7, no. 3 (Fall 1996): 273.

23. Ibid.

24. Jaspar Becker, "Lethal Injection May Assist Organ Trade," *South China Morning Post*, 23 April 1996, 9.

25. David Rothman, "Body Shop," *The Sciences*, November/December 1997, 19.

26. "Thais Going to China for Secret Organ-Transplant Operations," *The Straits Times* (Singapore), 7 January 1997, 16.

27. David Tracy, "Foreign Organs Dilemma," *South China Morning Post*, 17 August 1997, 8.

28. Cesar Chelala, "Organ Trade Violates Human Rights," *Newsday*, 6 March 1998, A43.

29. Cited in Rothman, "Body Shop," 18.

30. James F. Blumstein, "Legalizing Payment for Transplantable Cadaveric Organs," in Thomasma and Kushner, ed., *Birth to Death*, 122. Blumstein discusses his position in pp. 119–132.

31. Blumstein, "Cadaveric Organs," 129.

32. Blumstein, "Cadaveric Organs," 126.

33. J. B. Dossetor and V. Manickavel, "Ethics in Organ Donation: Contrasts in Two Cultures," *Transplantation Proceedings*, 23, no. 5 (October 1991): 2508.

34. Dossetor and Manickavel, "Ethics in Organ Donation," 2510–2511.

35. *New York Times*, 30 June 1992, B6.

36. *Pittsburgh Tribune-Review*, 1 July 1992, A5.

37. Tom Regan, "The Other Victim," *Hastings Center Report* 15, no. 1 (February 1985): 9–10.

38. Taken from Dan English, *Bioethics: A Clinical Guide for Medical Students* (New York: W. W. Norton & Co., 1994), 134.

39. This real case and the questions following are taken from Judith Boss, *Analyzing Moral Issues*, (Mountain View, CA: Mayfield, 1999), 481.

40. Case and questions taken from Boss, *Analyzing Moral Issues*, 838. The case and the names are real.

CHAPTER 8

1. See Ren-Zong Qiu, "Chinese Medical Ethics and Euthanasia," *Cambridge Quarterly of Healthcare Ethics* 2 (1993): 73.

2. Kazumasa Hoshino, "Euthanasia: Current Problems in Japan," *Cambridge Quarterly of Healthcare Ethics* 2 (1993): 45–46.

3. Ad Hoc Committee of the Harvard Medical School to Examine the Definition of Brain Death, "A Definition of Irreversible Coma," *Journal of the American Medical Association* 205, (1968): 337–340.

4. Multi-Society Task Force on Persistent Vegetative State, "Medical Aspects of the Persistent Vegetative State," *New England Journal of Medicine* 330 (1994): 1499–1508, 1572–1579.

5. Actually, there are three terms that are distinguished from one another: voluntary, nonvoluntary, and involuntary. Involuntary euthanasia occurs when the patient is able to make a voluntary choice but does not do so, and a decision is made to end the patient's life. Involuntary euthanasia is never morally justifiable.

6. Alan Meisel, "The Legal Consensus About Forgoing Life-Sustaining Treatment: Its Status and Its Prospects," *Kennedy Institute of Ethics Journal* 2, no. 4 (December 1995): 309–345.

7. The terms *difference position* and *nondifference position* are modeled after applicable commentaries and positions argued by James Rachels and Dan Brock, among others.

8. This is why Aristotle postulated at least four distinct types of causes: material, efficient, formal and final.

9. Cited in Qiu, "Chinese Medical Ethics," 71.

10. Qiu, "Chinese Medical Ethics," 71–71.

11. Dan English, *Bioethics: A Clinical Guide for Medical Students* (New York: W. W. Norton & Co., 1994), 175.

12. In Afaf Ibrahim Meleis and Albert Jonsen, "Ethical Crises and Cultural Differences," *Western Journal of Medicine* 138, no. 6 (June 1983): 889–892.

13. This was a key notion in the work of Louis Janssens and was later refined and clarified by Joseph Selling.

14. K. N. Siva Subramanian, "In India, Nepal, and Sri Lanka, Quality of Life Weighs Heavily," *Hastings Center Report* (August 1986), 20–21.

15. Subramanian, " Quality of Life," 21.

16. Cited in Judith Boss, *Analyzing Moral Issues* (Mountain View, CA: Mayfield, 1999), 243.

17. Paula Span, *Washington Post*, 14 November 1996, B1.

18. *In re Conroy*, 486 A.2d 1209 (New Jersey App. Div., 1985).

19. This is the point stressed by Damien Keown and John Keown in "Killing, Karma and Caring: Euthanasia in Buddhism and Christianity," *Journal of Medical Ethics*, 21 (1995): 265–269.

20. See Pinit Ratanakul, "Bioethics in Thailand: The Struggle for Buddhist Solutions," *Journal of Medicine and Philosophy* 13, no. 3 (August 1988): 309–310.

21. Roy W. Perrett, "Buddhism, Euthanasia and the Sanctity of Life," *Journal of Medical Ethics* 22 (1996): 309–313.

22. A fine treatment of hospice is in Sandol Stoddard, *The Hospice Movement—A Better Way of Caring for the Dying* (New York: Random House, 1978).

23. Cited in Boss, *Analyzing Moral Issues*, 247.

24. Richard Leiby, *Washington Post*, 11 August 1996, F1.

25. Ibid.

26. Ibid.

27. Timothy Quill, "Death and Dignity: A Case of Individualized Decision Making," *New England Journal of Medicine* (7 March 1991): 691–694.

28. See the August 12, 1998, edition of the *Journal of the American Medical Association*.

29. See the discussion of this issue in Kary L. Moss, ed., *Man-Made Medicine: Women's Health, Public Policy, and Reform* (Durham, NC: Duke University Press, 1996).

30. Eliza W. Farnham, from *Woman and Her Era*, cited in Thomas R. Cole and Mary G. Winkler, eds., *The Oxford Book of Aging: Reflections on the Journey of Life* (New York: Oxford University Press, 1994), 37–38.

31. Ellen Newton, from *This Bed My Centre*, cited in Cole and Winkler, *Oxford Book of Aging*, 156.

32. Lawrence J. Schneiderman and Nancy S. Jecker, *Wrong Medicine: Doctors, Patients, and Futile Treatment* (Baltimore: Johns Hopkins University Press, 1995): 51–54.

33. Howard Brody give s this example in Schneiderman and Jecker, *Wrong Medicine*, 10.

34. Schneiderman and Jecker, *Wrong Medicine*, 11

35. Schneiderman and Jecker, *Wrong Medicine*, 155, 156.

36. This is a real case.

37. This is a real case; the name has been changed to protect privacy.

38. Case and questions taken from Boss, *Analyzing Moral Issues*, 307–308. The case and the name are real.

39. From Geri-Ann Galanti, *Caring for Patients from Different Cultures: Case Studies from American Hospitals* (Philadelphia: University of Pennsylvania Press, 1997), 109–110.

40. Ibid.

41. This is a real case from Schneiderman and Jecker, *Wrong Medicine*, 83–84.

42. From Bette-Jane Crigger, ed., *Cases in Bioethics*, 3d ed. (New York: St. Martin's Press, 1998), 101.

CHAPTER 9

1. "College HIV Rate Holds Steady, but Risk of Exposure Remains High," *AIDS Alert* 9, no. 11 (November 1994): 153–156.

2. "The Growing Specter of AIDS in the Young," *Medical Update* 17, no. 9 (March 1994): 3.

3. "AIDS Is Leading Killer of Americans from Age 25 to 44," *Jet* 87 (20 February 1995): 22.

4. See the Web site http://www.avert.org/usastats.htm.

5. See the Web site http://www.avert.org/worldstats.htm.

6. William J. Castello/Associated Press, *Pittsburgh Post-Gazette*, 27 November 1997, A10.

7. Gregory E. Pence, *Classic Cases in Medical Ethics*, 2d ed. (New York: McGraw-Hill, 1995), 420.

8. G. D. Comstock, *Violence Against Lesbians and Gay Men* (New York: Columbia University Press, 1991), 171–172.

9. Comstock, *Violence Against Lesbians and Gay Men*, 31–55.

10. David L. Kirp and Ronald Bayer, eds., *AIDS in the Industrialized Democracies: Passions, Politics, and Policies* (New Brunswick, NJ: Rutgers University Press, 1992), 149, 159, 165, 294, 260.

11. Cited in J. Gordon Melton, *The Churches Speak on: AIDS* (Detroit: Gale Research, 1989), xviii.

12. Chandler Burr, "The AIDS Exception: Privacy vs. Public Health," *Atlantic Monthly* (June 1997): 64–65.

13. This is arguable and remains controversial among scientists. Many American researchers hold this position, while quite a number of their European counterparts disagree.

14. Bernard Rabinowitz, "The Great Hijack," *British Medical Journal*, 313, no. 7060 (28 September 1996): 826.

15. See R. Denenberg, *Gynecological Care Manual for HIV Positive Women* (Durant, OK: Essential Medical Information

Systems, 1993), and D. J. Cotton, "AIDS in Women," in S. Broder, T. C. Merigan, and D. Bolognesi, eds., *Textbook of AIDS Medicine* (Baltimore, MD: Williams & Wilkins, 1994); 161–68.

16. Centers for Disease Control and Prevention (CDC), *HIV/AIDS Surveillance Report* 6, no. 2 (1995): 12.

17. Philip S. Rosenberg, Robert J. Biggar, and James J. Goedert, "Declining Age at HIV Infection in the United States," *New England Journal of Medicine* 330 (1994): 789.

18. S. Sanchez, "AIDS Extradition OK'd," *USA Today*, 11 September 1991, 1A.

19. This is according to the Centers for Disease Control and Prevention HIV/STD/TB Prevention New Update, reported in *Cleveland Live News Flash/Plain Dealer Online*, 10 February 1999.

20. "College HIV Rate Holds Steady, but Risk of Exposure Remains High," *AIDS Alert* 9, no. 11 (November 1994): 153–156.

21. Burr, *AIDS Exception*, 61.

22. Michael Ornstein, *AIDS in Canada: Knowledge, Behaviour, and Attitudes of Adults* (Toronto: Institute for Social Research, York University, 1989), 65.

23. Cited in Kirp and Bayer, *AIDS in Industrialized Democracies*, 264–265.

24. "AIDS Study: Many at Risk Not Tested," *Chicago Tribune*, 20 August 1991, sec. 1, p. 10.

25. Christopher Burns, "AIDS Rages with Africa Hit Worst," *Pittsburgh Post-Gazette*, 27 November 1997, A10. The figures in the selection are taken from pp. A1, A10.

26. Information from the Centers for Disease Control and Prevention, National AIDS Clearinghouse, reported in *PANA Wire Service*, 13 January 1999.

27. See Nicholas A. Christakis, "The Ethical Design of an AIDS Vaccine Trial in Africa," *Hastings Center Report* (June/July 1988): 31–37.

28. Pence, *Classic Cases*, 430.

29. Sheryl Gay Stolberg, "Epidemic of Silence: A Special Report; Eyes Shut, Black America Is Being Ravaged By AIDS," *New York Times*, 29 June 1998, A1.

30. Cited in ibid.

31. Carlos del Rio et al., "Premarital HIV Testing: The Case of Mexico," *AIDS & Public Policy Journal* 10, no. 2 (Summer 1995): 104–106.

32. Cited in del Rio et al., "Premarital HIV Testing," 106.

33. Ronald Bayer, "Ethical Challenges Posed by Zidovudine Treatment to Reduce Vertical Transmission of HIV," *New England Journal of Medicine*, 331, no. 18 (3 November 1994): 1223–1225.

34. Ronald Nakasone, "Illness and Compassion: AIDS in an American Zen Community," *Cambridge Quarterly of Healthcare Ethics*, 4 (1995): 488–493.

35. Ibid.

36. Katherine Butler, "Modern Plague Ravages Urban Eskimos," *The Independent*, London, 6 June 1998, 18.

37. Cited in ibid.

38. Julie Hamblin, 1994, cited in Alastair Campbell, Max Charlesworth, Grant Gillett, and Gareth Jones, *Medical Ethics* (Auckland: Oxford University Press, 1997), 113.

39. This is an estimate from the Uganda Women's Lawyers Association. Cited in Jane Perlez, "Uganda's Women:

Children, Drudgery, and Pain," on Christina Sommers and Fred Sommers, *Vice and Virtue in Everyday Life*, 4th ed. (Fort Worth: Harcourt Brace College Publishers, 1985), 229.

40. This is according to the United Nations Children's Fund study, cited in Perlez, "Uganda's Women," 227. The account of Safuyati Kawuda is from this article.

41. Burr, *AIDS Exception*, 65.

42. Tim Golden, "Dental Patient Torn," by AIDS Calls for Laws," *New York Times*, Associated Press, 21 June 1991.

43. American Medical Association, Council on Ethical and Judicial Affairs, *Code of Medical Ethics: Current Opinion and Annotations* (Chicago, IL: American Medical Association, 1997), sec. 9.131, 157.

44. J. Thorton and C. Mount, "AIDS Error Confirmed by Hospital" *Chicago Tribune*, 26 April 1991, sec. 2, p. 2.

45. P. Gorner and M. L. Millenson, "Organ Transplant Doctors Try to Calm Fears on AIDS," *Chicago Tribune*, 18 May 1991, sec. 1, pp. 1, 4.

46. J. F. Sullivan, "Judge Rules Surgeon Infected with AIDS Must Tell Patients," *New York Times*, 26 April 1991, 13.

47. Mary Chamberland et al., "Health Care Workers with AIDS," *Journal of the American Medical Association* 266, no. 24 (25 December 1991).

48. Tom Ehrenfeld, "AIDS Heroes and Villains," *Newsweek*, 14 October 1991, 66.

49. A. R. Jonsen, "Is Individual Responsibility a Sufficient Basis for Public Confidence?" *Archives of Internal Medicine* 151 (1991): 660–662.

50. Jonsen, "Individual Responsibility," 662.

51. David C. Thomasma and Patricia Marshall, "Ethical Pitfalls and Benefits of Disclosure of HIV-Positive Status," in John F. Monagle and David C. Thomasma, *Health Care Ethics: Critical Issues for the 21st Century* (Aspen Publishing, 1997), 196.

CHAPTER 10

1. Michael Brannigan, "Oregon's Experiment," *Health Care Analysis*, 1, no. 1 (June 1993): 15. See the discussion on pp. 15–32.

2. These arguments for and against the plan are discussed in Brannigan, "Oregon's Experiment," 25–30.

3. Physician's Task Force on Hunger in America, *Hunger in America: The Growing Epidemic* (Middletown, CT: Wesleyan University Press, 1985).

4. Mary Therese Connors, "Health Care Reform: A Catholic Perspective," in *Critical Interval*, (Pittsburgh: St. Francis Health System, 1994). See her insightful discussion on pp. 5–6.

5. Connors, "Health Care Reform," 6.

6. Adopted from Campbell et al., *Medical Ethics* (Auckland: Oxford University Press, 1997), 187.

7. See Allyson Pollock, "The Politics of Destruction: Rationing in the UK Health Care Market," *Health Care Analysis*, 3, no. 4 (November 1995): 299–308.

8. Erich H. Loewy, *Textbook of Healthcare Ethics* (New York: Plenum Press, 1996), 240.

9. Robert Pear, "Health Agency Is Urged to Re-evaluate Spending Priorities," *New York Times*, 9 July 1998.

10. Montreal *Gazette*, 27 April 1992, B2. Cited in Susan Sherwin, "Theory Versus Practice in Ethics: A Feminist Perspective on Justice in Health Care," in L. W. Sumner and Joseph Boyle, eds., *Philosophical Perspectives on Bioethics* (Toronto: University of Toronto Press, 1996), 208.

11. The National Health Council consists of more than 100 advocacy groups, such as the American Heart Association. The council's president, Myrl Weinberg, recently pointed out that representatives from these groups need to sit on NIH committees to help ensure that the allocation of funds is fair.

12. This is a rendition of a case used in Eileen G. Collins and Gerald J. Mozdzierz, "Cardiac Retransplantation: Ethical Issues," *Heart and Lung* 22, no. 3 (May/June 1993): 209.

13. Collins and Mozdzierz, "Cardiac Retransplantation," 208.

14. American Medical Association, Council on Ethical and Judicial Affairs, *Code of Medical Ethics: Current Opinions and Annotations* (Chicago, IL: American Medical Association, 1997), "Ethical Considerations in the Allocation of Organs and Other Scarce Medical Resources Among Patients," *Archives of Internal Medicine*, 155 (1995): 29–40.

15. See Arthur Caplan, *Am I My Brother's Keeper? The Ethical Frontiers of Biomedicine* (Bloomington: Indiana University Press, 1997), 148.

16. From Philip C. Hébert, *Doing Right: A Practical Guide to Ethics for Physicians and Medical Trainees* (Toronto: Oxford University Press, 1996), 150.

17. Ibid.

18. John Rawls, *A Theory of Justice* (Cambridge, MA: Harvard University Press, 1971).

19. Norman Daniels, Donald W. Light, and Ronald L. Caplan, *Benchmarks of Fairness for Health Care Reform* (New York: Oxford University Press, 1996); see especially pp. 35–69.

20. Susan Sherwin, "Theory Versus Practice in Ethics: A Feminist Perspective on Justice in Health Care, in L. W. Sumner and Joseph Boyle, eds., Philosophical Perspectives in Bioethics (Toronto: University of Toronto Press, 1996), 187–209.

21. Sherwin, "Theory Versus Practice," 198.

22. Ibid.

23. Richard J. McMurray, "Gender Disparities in Clinical Decision-Making," report to the American Medical Association Council on Ethical and Judicial Affairs, 1990; cited in Sherwin, "Theory Versus Practice," 199.

24. See Ruth H. Gordon-Bradshaw, "A Social Essay on Special Issues Facing Poor Women of Color," in Cesar A. Perales and Lauren S. Young, eds., *Too Little Too Late: Dealing with the Health Needs of Women in Poverty* (New York: Harrington Park Press, 1986); cited in Sherwin, "Theory Versus Practice," 199.

25. Taken from Dean E. Murphy, "Angola's Victims of Peace," *Los Angeles Times* 18 June 1998, 1.

26. See George Gallup, Jr., *The Gallup Poll: Public Opinion 1997* (Wilmington, DE: Scholarly Resources, 1998), 152–153.

27. Charles J. Dougherty, "Equality and Inequality in American Health Care," in Monagle and Thomasma, *Health Care Ethics*, 306.

28. Michael A. Simpson, "Reforming Health Care in South Africa," in David Seedhouse, ed., *Reforming Health Care: The Philosophy and Practice of International Health Reform* (West Chichester: Wiley 1995), 104. See his article on pp. 101–119.

29. See J. A. Odell and J. G. Brink, "Heart Transplantation in South Africa—A Critical Appraisal," *South African Medical Journal* 82 (1992): 394–396. Cited in Simpson, "Reforming Health Care," 110.

30. See Soloman R. Benatar and H. C. J. van Rensburg, "Health Care Services in a New South Africa," *Hastings Center Report* 25, no. 4 (July/Aug. 1995): 16–21.

31. See Gallup, *Public Opinion 1997*, 152–153.

32. Adapted from Hibert, *Doing Right*, 138.

33. Rabbi Moshe Kletenik, "Health Care Reform: A Jewish Perspective," *Critical Interval* 4, no. 2 (1994): 10.

34. Aaron L. Mackler, "Judaism, Justice, and Access to Health Care," *Kennedy Institute of Ethics Journal* 1, no. 2 (June 1991): 143–161.

35. Mackler, "Judaism," 151.

36. Mackler, "Judaism," 153.

37. From Hibert, *Doing Right*, 140.

38. See the discussion in Michael Brannigan, "Health Care Needs: The Riddle Behind the Mask," *Health Care Analysis* 3, no. 4 (November 1995): 309–312.

39. Brannigan, "Health Care Needs," 311.

40. Ibid.

41. See Charles Dougherty, *American Health Care: Realities, Rights, and Reforms* (New York: Oxford University Press, 1988).

42. See H. A. M. J. ten Have and H. J. Keasberry, "Equity and Solidarity: The Context of Health Care in the Netherlands," *Journal of Medicine and Philosophy* 17 (1992): 463–477.

43. *US Air Magazine* November 1993, 118.

44. Kathryn Pauly Morgan, "Gender Rights and Rites: The Biopolitics of Beauty and Fertility," in Sumner and Boyle, *Philosophical Perspectives in Bioethics*, 217.

45. Morgan, "Gender Rights and Rites," 225.

46. Geoffrey Cowley, "Is Sex a Necessity?" *Newsweek*, 11 May 1998, 63.

47. Cited in Cowley, "Is Sex a Necessity," 62.

48. Newsweek Research, First Databank, Inc., *Newsweek*, 11 May 1998, 63.

49. Lisa Bannon, "Growth Industry: How a Risky Surgery Became a Profit Center for Some L.A. Doctors," *Wall Street Journal*, 6 June 1996, 1, 48–49.

50. Bannon, "Growth Industry," 48.

51. Ibid.

52. Theodore R. Marmor provides an invaluable discussion in *Understanding Health Care Reform* (New Haven, CT: Yale University Press, 1994).

53. This term is based on Judith A. Boss, "Paradigms of Justice in Access to Health Care," a paper presented at a 1995 Mt. Sinai Medical Center conference on "Access to Health Care," New York City.

54. Both tables are cited in Seedhouse, *Reforming Health Care*, 64, 65.

55. See D. Himmelstein and S. Woolhandler, "A National Health Program for the United States: A Physicians' Pro-

posal," *New England Journal of Medicine* 320 (1989): 102–108. See also Catholic Health Association, *Setting Relationships Right: A Working Proposal for Systemic Healthcare Reform* (St. Louis, MO: Catholic Health Association, 1992).

56. See Boss, "Paradigms of Justice."

57. Boss, "Paradigms of Justice," 5.

58. Theodore R. Marmor, "Patterns of Fact and Fiction in the Use of Canadian Experience," in a chapter by Lawrence D. Brown, and Theodore R. Marmor, "Health Care Reform in the United States: Clinton or Canada?" in Seedhouse, *Reforming Health Care*, 63–65.

59. The source for this study in D. A. Rublee, "Medical Technology in Canada and the U.S.," *Health Affairs*, Fall 1989, 180. See the discussion in Brown and Marmor, "Health Care Reform in the United States," 63–65.

60. See Boss, "Paradigms of Justice."

61. See John D. Rockefeller, IV, "The Pepper Commission Report on Comprehensive Health Care," *New England Journal of Medicine* 323 (1990): 1005–1007.

62. Adapted from John Hoyt, "Allocation of Health Care: Micro vs. Macro Decision Making," in *Critical Interval*, 11.

63. Adapted from Bette-Jane Crigger, ed., *Cases in Bioethics: Selections from the Hastings Center Report*, 3d ed. (New York: St. Martin's Press, 1998), 282.

64. This case is adapted from Crigger, *Cases in Bioethics*, 244.

65. The main idea behind this case is adapted from Thomas M. Garrett, Harold W. Baillie, and Rosellen M. Garrett, *Health Care Ethics: Principles and Problems*, 3d ed. (Upper Saddle River, NJ: Prentice Hall, 1998), 108.

66. Adapted from Garrett et al., *Health Care Ethics*, 108.

67. Adapted from Garrett et al., *Health Care Ethics*, 77.

Credits

with Human Subjects," Spring 1969, Vol. 98, No. 2. P. 373 Arthur Caplan, "How Did Medicine Go So Wrong?" from *When Medicine Went Mad: Bioethics and the Holocaust*, Arthur Caplan, ed., Humana Press, 1992, pp. 53, 58–59, 64–77. Reprinted with permission from the publisher. P. 379 George Annas and Michael Grodin, "Human and Maternal-Fetal HIV Transmission Prevention Trials in Africa," *American Journal of Public Health*, April 1998, Vol. 88, No. 4, pp. 560–563. With permission from The American Public Health Association. P. 384 Carl Cohen, "Do Animals Have Rights?" in *Ethics and Behavior*, Vol. 7, No. 2, 1997, 103–111. Copyright © 1997 Carl Cohen. Reprinted with permission from the author. P. 392 Judith A. Boss and Alyssa V. Boss, "Paradigm Shifts, Scientific Revolutions and the Moral Justification of Experimentation on Nonhuman Animals," *Between the Species*, Summer & Fall 1994, 119–130. Reprinted with permission from the publisher.

Chapter 7 p. 437 Kevin O'Rourke, O. P., "Research with Fetal Tissue," *Ethical Issues in Health Care*, Vol. 9, No. 1, September 1987. Reprinted with permission from the author. P. 439 Tracy E. Miller, "Multiple Listing for Organ Transplantation: Autonomy Unbounded," *Kennedy Institute of Ethics Journal*, Vol. 2, No. 1, March 1992, 43–59. Copyright © 1992 The Johns Hopkins University Press. Reprinted with permission from the publisher. P. 449 Alvin H. Moss and Mark Siegler, "Should Alcoholics Compete Equally for Liver Transplantation?" *Journal of the American Medical Association*, Vol. 265, No. 10, March 13, 1991, 1295–1298. Reprinted with permission from American Medical Association. P. 456 Carl Cohen and Martin Benjamin, "Alcoholics and Liver Transplantation," *Journal of the American Medical Association*, Vol. 265, No. 10, March 13, 1991, 1299–1301. Reprinted with permission from American Medical Association. P. 462 The Working Group on Genetic Engineering in Non-Human Life Forms, Church of Scotland, "The Ethics of Xenografting—Transplanting Animal Organs into Human," 1995. Reprinted with permission.

Chapter 8 p. 508 James Rachels, "Active and Passive Euthanasia," *New England Journal of Medicine*, Vol. 292, January 9, 1975. Reprinted with permission from Massachusetts Medical Society. P. 512 Tom L. Beauchamp and James F. Childress, "Rachels on Active and Passive Euthanasia," in Tom L. Beauchamp and Robert M. Veatch, *Ethical Issues in Death and Dying, Second Edition*, Prentice-Hall, 1996. Reprinted with permission from the author. P. 516 Michael C. Brannigan, "Re-Assessing the Ordinary/Extraordinary Distinction in Witholding/Withdrawing Nutrition and Hydration," *Contemporary Philosophy*, Vol. 13,

No. 6, November/December, 1990. Reprinted with permission from the author. P. 523 Margaret Pabst Battin, "Physician-Assisted Suicides," in *Ethical Issues in Suicide*, Prentice-Hall, 1995. Reprinted with permission from the author. P. 532 Susan M. Wolf, " A Feminist Critique of Physician-Assisted Suicide," in Susan Wolf, ed., *Feminism and Bioethics*, Oxford University Press, 1996.

Chapter 9 p. 574 Bernard Rabinowitz, "The Great Hijack," *British Medical Journal*, Vol. 313, No. 7060, September 28, 1996, p. 826. Reprinted with permission from BMJ Publishing Group. P. 576 Richard D. Mohr, "AIDS, Gays, and State Coersion," *Bioethics*, Vol. 1, No. 1, 1987, 35–50. Copyright © 1987 Richard D. Mohr. Reprinted with permission from the author. P. 581 Bonnie Steinbock, "Harming, Wrongdoing, and AIDS," in James M. Humber and Robert F. Almeder, *Biomedical Ethics: 1988*, Humana Press, 1989. Reprinted with permission from Bonnie Steinbock and Humana Press. P. 588 Working Group on HIV Testing of Pregnant Women and Newborns, "HIV Infection, Pregnant Women, and Newborns: A Policy Proposal for Information and Testing," *Journal of the American Medical Association*, Vol. 264, No. 18, November 14, 1990. Reprinted with permission of American Medical Association. P. 596 Ronald Bayer, "Ethical Challenges Posed by Zidovudine Treatment to Reduce Vertical Transmission of HIV," *The New England Journal of Medicine*, Vol. 331, No. 18, November 3, 1994. Reprinted with permission from Massachusetts Medical Society.

Chapter 10 Amy Gutmann, "For and Against Equal Access to Health Care," *Milbank Quarterly*, Vol. 59, No. 4, 1981, 542–560. Reprinted with permission from Blackwell Publishers. P. 645 Norman Daniels, "Why Saying No to Patients in the U.S. Is So Hard," *New England Journal of Medicine*, May 22, 1986. Reprinted with permission from Massachusetts Medical Society. P. 650 E. Havi Morreim, "Lifestyles of the Risky and Famous: From Managed Care to Managed Lives," *Hastings Center Report*, Vol. 25, No. 6, November/December 1995. Reprinted with permission from The Hastings Center. P. 660 Steffi Woolhandler and David U. Himmelstein, "A National Health Program: Northern Light at the End of the Tunnel," *Journal of the American Medical Association*, Vol. 262, No. 15, October 20, 1989, 2136–2137. Reprinted with permission from the American Medical Association. P. 664 Ronald Bronow, "A National Health Program: Abyss at the End of the Tunnel—The Position of Physicians Who Care," *Journal of the American Medical Association*, Vol. 263, No. 18, May 9, 1990, 2488–2489. Reprinted with permission from the American Medical Association.

Glossary/Index

Africa (*continued*)
AIDS and HIV in, *560–561,*
567–568
AIDS research in, 351, 379–384
contraception in, *195*
infertility in, *274*
informed consent in, *561*
surrogate mothers in, *274*
women in, *567–568*
African Americans
AIDS and, 555, 561, 563
healthcare access for, 617
life span of, 34
in medical experimentation, 350
sickle cell screening of, 263
Afterlife, 60
Age
organ transplantation and, 422
resource allocation and,
622–624
Aging
in America, *504*
in China, *489*
Hinduism on, *489*
Ahimsa: Buddhist and Hindu principle of nonhurting, 189, *190, 354,
358, 497*
AIDS: Viral disease that causes the
breakdown of white blood cells, especially T cells, so that the immune system is considerably
weakened, exposing the individual
to fatal viral and bacterial infections. *See also* human immunodeficiency virus (HIV), 549–604. *See
also* HIV positivity
in Africa, 351, 379–384, *560–561,
567–568*
African Americans with, 555,
561, 563
in Australia, *553, 557*
in Canada, *557*
codes of ethics for, *570*
confidentiality and, 553, 555,
556, 569–573
in Denmark, *553*
discrimination against, 41
drug development for, 333, 344,
349
education for, 565
exceptionalism: Phenomenon
whereby measures typically
taken to prevent the spread of
infectious disease are not applied, as a general rule, to the
prevention of AIDS, 552–556,
553, 558

in Greenland, *566*
guidelines for, 572–573
health insurance and, 559
healthcare professionals with,
569–573
in Holland, *553, 558*
homosexuality and, 552–555
incidence of, 550, *551,* 555, 561,
566, 571
in Islamic cultures, *554*
public welfare and, 555, 571
readings on, 574–604
religions and, *554,* 561, 564–565
as a reportable disease, 556
research, 351, *354,* 379–384, 610
risk of, 555, 556, 569–571
testing, 556–563
transmission of, 550–551, 561,
568, 571, 596–599
treatment of, 558, 559, *560–561,*
563–564
universal precautions for, 570,
572
vaccines, *560*
women and, 555–556, 561, 563
AIDS, Gays and State Coercion,
576–580
Akan tribe, 23
Alcoholics and Liver Transplantation,
456–461
Alcoholics, organ transplants for,
426–427, 449–456, 456–461
Alexion Pharmaceuticals, Inc., 282
An Almost Absolute Value in History,
208–211
Alternative medicine, 617, 619
Altruism, in organ donation, 431
Alzheimer's disease, 346, 501–502
AMA. *See* American Medical Association
American Civil Liberties Union, on
HIV screening, 568
American College of Obstetricians
and Gynecologists, on abortion,
203
American Dental Association, on
AIDS, 569, 573
American Hospital Association, on
patient's rights, 116
American Medical Association
on abortion, 181, 182, 203
on AIDS, 569, *570,* 573
on black physicians, 12
codes of ethics, 3
on end-of-life decisions, *475*
on euthanasia, 479
on HIV screening, 559

on informed consent surrogates,
347, 353
on life support, 474
on organ transplantation,
422–423
on research, 342
on resource allocation, 611–612
on therapeutic privilege, 345
American Nurses Association, codes
of ethics, 35
Analogies: Comparison between two
similar things or events, 78, 91–93
Analysis, in critical thinking: Process
of critically examining our worldview, using reason and logic,
67–68, 91–94
Ancient medicine, *69*
Anencephaly: Congenital condition
in which the cerebral hemispheres
are significantly lacking, 199, 413,
416, 507
Anger, 71, *72*
Angola, healthcare access in, *618*
Animal experimentation (nonhuman), 327, 356–362, *357,* 392–400.
See also Animals (nonhuman)
as anthropocentrism, 67
Buddhism on, 38, *358*
distributive justice and, 31
Hinduism on, *357, 358*
history of, 330
Jainists on, *358*
replacements for, 362
as speciesism, 27
Animal Liberation Front, 356
Animals (Nonhuman). *See also* Animal experimentation (nonhuman)
Buddhism on, 34, 38, 67, *358*
cloning, 249, *277, 279,* 281,
282–283
duty to, 361
euthanasia of, 501
genetic engineering of,
282–283, 356, *357,* 434, 436
Hinduism on, 67, *357, 358*
Jainists on, 67, *358*
naturalistic fallacy and, 89
as organ donors (*see* Xenografts)
vs. persons, 14
pleasures and, 27
rights of, 34, 356–361, 384–392,
434–435
suffering of, 330
value of, 436
Annas, George J., 329, 349, 351,
379–384
Anthony, Susan B., 181

Anthropocentrism: Belief that human beings are the central or most significant entity of the universe, 14, 67, 358–359

Anti-semitism, 11

Antipsychotic drugs, 346

Antivivisection movement, 333

Apartheid, *621*

Appeal to inappropriate authority: Fallacy that occurs when someone appeals to an expert or authority in a field other than the one under discussion, 84

Appeal to tradition: Fallacy that occurs when someone argues that a practice or attitude is morally acceptable because it is a tradition or a cultural norm, 89

Applied ethics: Subdivision of ethics, also known as normative ethics, concerned with giving practical guidelines or behavioral norms, 6

Aquinas, Thomas
    on ensoulment, 186
    on natural law, 24
    on nonhuman animals, 357–358
    on suicide, *494*

Arab culture
    informed consent in, *487*
    treatment refusal in, *486–487*

Arguments: Type of reasoning composed of two or more propositions, one of which is claimed to follow logically from or be supported by the others, 73–80, 81

Aristotle
    on casuistry, 42
    on character, 114
    on natural law, 24
    on nonhuman animals, 357
    on social justice, 615
    on virtues, 37, 43–47, 114

Armstrong, Paul, 474

Arnold, Robert, 427

Artificial feeding, 484

Artificial insemination: Mechanical placement of a man's sperm into a woman's reproductive tract; the sperm used can be that of the husband or partner (AIH) or that of a donor (AID), *269, 271, 272*
    with surrogate, *270*

Asch, Ricardo, 275

Ashrama: Literally, "rest-stop," the Hindu stages along life's journey, *488–489*

Assisted reproduction. *See* Reproductive technology

Assisted suicide, 13, 28, 30, 473–474. *See also* Euthanasia; Physician-assisted suicide

Assumptions, 56, 68, 86–88

Atman: Hindu term for true self or soul, 489

Atomic Energy Commission experiments, 343–344

Attempted suicide, 495

Aulisio, Mark, 427

Auschwitz-Birkenau concentration camp, 1, *2*

Australia
    active euthanasia in, *500*
    AIDS and HIV in, *553, 557*

Authority figures
    inappropriate, 84–85, *90*
    in Japan, *134–135*
    in medical experimentation, *334–335*
    obedience and, 1, 3, 6, 18–19, 85
    physicians as, 84–85, 109
    torture and, 3

Autonomy: Capacity to make rational and free choices; principle of self-rule or self-determination, 4, 40–41
    in abortion, 187, 193–194, 205–206
    Buddhism on, 40
    in China, *477–478*
    common good vs., 40
    vs. community, 32, 40, 63–64
    dignity and, 29, 32
    genetic engineering and, 256, 261–262, 283
    genetic testing and, 262, 264–265
    of healthcare professionals, 40, 41, 122–123
    in human research, 39
    in Japan, *477–478*
    vs. materialism, 73
    vs. medical futility, 505–507
    of organ donors, 417–418, 430
    vs. paternalism, 40, 576–580
    reproductive technology and, 273–274
    self-determination and, 126, *478*
    suicide and, 496

Autopsies, *413, 414*

Autosomal recessive inheritance, *259*

Avoidance, 70–71, *72*

Ayurvedic medicine: System of Hindu medicine, derived from the classic text *Carakasamhita,* that stresses the relationship between health, spiritual progress, and moral behavior, *120–121*

Azidothymidine (AZT): Treatment for HIV infection that is somewhat effective in slowing down the effects of AIDS if the infected person is treated early enough; also known as zidovudine, 559, 563–564, 596–599

AZT. *See* Azidothymidine (AZT)

Baboons, as organ donors, 415, 432–434, 435

Baby AIDS Compromise, 568

Baby Doe Rules, 31, 490–491

Baby Fae, 352, 433–434, 435

Bacon, Francis, 358

Badger, Rebecca, 502

Bailey, Leonard, 434

Bandwagon approach, 84

Barnard, Christiaan, 409–410, 413

Bastable, Austin, 502–503

Battin, Margaret Pabst, 496, *500,* 523–532

Bayer Company research, 362

Bayer, Ronald, 564, 596–599

Beauchamp, Tom L., 39, 481, 512–515

Beauty, 628

Beecher, Henry, 340

Begging the question: Fallacy, also known as circular reasoning, that occurs when the premise and conclusion are actually different wordings of the same proposition, 88, *90*

Behavior
    high-risk, 555, 556
    moral, 18–19
    self-destructive, 425–427

The Belmont Report, 39–42, 341

Benedict, Ruth, 11

Beneficence: Duty to do good and benefit others
    authority figures and, 109
    in deontology, 32
    as a duty, 39–40, 93–94
    in Greece, *127*
    in human research, 39–40
    in paternalism, 202
    in utilitarianism, 26

Benefits
    vs. burdens, 491
    vs. harm, 361
    of life support, 507
    of medical experimentation, 328, 351, 359
    resource allocation and, 612

Benjamin, Martin, 456–461

Bentham, Jeremy, 26–27, 359

Egg donors, 273

Egypt, medical experimentation in, *337*

Eichmann, Adolf, 15

Eightfold path, 37

Elderly patients
HMOs and, 613–614
in Holland, *626–627*

ELISA test, for AIDS: Conventional test used to detect the presence of HIV, 559

Emanuel, Ezekiel, 122

Embryo research, 355

Embryo splitting, 276

End-of-life decisions, 473–548
AMA on, *475*
in China, *477–478*
incompetent adults and, 483–491
in Japan, *477–478*
self-determination in, 481

Endangered species, cloning, *277*

Engineering model, of physician-patient relations, 111

England. *See* Great Britain

Ensoulment, 185, 186, 189

Entitlement: Theory of justice that states that a just society is one that sufficiently compensates those who actively contribute to that society, 619

Epidemics, 551–552

Equilibrium, reflective, 80, 617, 619

Equivocation: Fallacy that occurs when the meaning of an ambiguous term shifts during the course of the argument, 80–81, *90*

Erectile dysfunction, 628

Eskimos, euthanasia and, *13*, 13

Ethical and Social Issues in Prenatal Sex Selection, 226–236

Ethical Challenges Posed by Zidovudine Treatment to Reduce Vertical Transmission of HIV, 596–599

Ethical relativism: Moral theories that claim that morality is created by people rather than being universal and that moral systems can be different for different people, 7–15

Ethicists, 6

Ethics. *See also* Codes of ethics
applied, 6
healthcare (*see* Healthcare ethics)
theoretical, 6

Ethics committees, 505

Eugenics: Science of improving the genetic quality of offspring; act of intentionally ending the life of a patient with an incurable disease. *See* Genetic engineering

Euthanasia, 75, 473–548, *483*. *See also* Assisted suicide
active (*see* Active euthanasia)
Buddhism on, *493, 497–498*
in China, *483*
dangers of, 76
duty and, 30
Eskimos and, *13*, 13
fetal, 199
justice and, 32
litigation on, 474–476, 492–493, 502
of the mentally ill, 1
of nonhuman animals, 501
nonvoluntary, 78, 479–480
passive, 479, 480–483, *483*, 508–515
physician-assisted (*see* Physician-assisted suicide)
pleasures and, 27
readings on, 508–548
slippery slope argument in, 499, 501
types of, 479–480, *480*
voluntary: Euthanasia as a result of a patient's expressed wishes, 479, 496

Experience, in critical thinking, 57–67

Experimentation: Scientific procedure used to test a hypothesis or increase scientific knowledge. The primary purpose of *therapeutic experimentation* is to benefit the subject; the primary purpose of *nontherapeutic experimentation* is to contribute to knowledge. *See* Medical experimentation

Experts, inappropriate, 84–85

Faith healing, 25

Faith vs. science, 68

Fallacies: Argument that is psychologically or emotionally persuasive but logically incorrect.
abusive, 81
of accident, 83–84
ad hominem, 81–82, *90*
of appeal to tradition, 89–91, 184
of begging the question, 88, *90*
circumstantial, 81–82

in critical thinking, 80–93
of false cause, 86–88, 363
of ignorance: Fallacy committed when someone argues that a conclusion is true simply because it has not been proved false, or that it is false simply because it has not been proved true, 85–86, *90*
informal, 80
naturalistic, 89, *90*, 282

False cause: Fallacy that occurs when someone mistakes something for the cause of an event that, in fact, is not the cause, 86

Family. *See also* Community
in China, *477*
cloning and, 280–281
in decision-making, 63–64, *66*
genetic information and, 264, 265, 283
in Japan, *135, 477*
organ transplantation and, 417–418, 427

Family planning, abortion for, *178, 185*

Farnham, Eliza, *504*

Fathers, abortion and, 193

FDA. *See* Food and Drug Administration

Feelings, 7–8, 26

Feminists
on abortion, 181, 219–225
on caring, 38–39
on physician-assisted suicide, 499, 532–543
on physician-patient relations, 154–163
on reproductive technologies, 274
on social justice, 617, 619

Fertility treatment. *See* Reproductive technology

Fetal alcohol syndrome, 200–201

Fetal tissue transplants
abortion and, 206, 420
procuring, 420
research on, 355, 437–439

Fetuses
development of, 191–193, *192*
euthanasia of, 199
gene therapy for, 267
harm to, 200–203
maternal rights and, 200–202
medical experimentation on, 349–350, 355
as patients, 202–203

Fetuses (*continued*)
personhood of, 91, 188, 189–193, 191–193
potentiality of, 189–190
research on, 349–350, 355, 437–439
rights of, 185–186, 191
viability of, 192

Fidelity, duty of: Duty to honor past commitment and promises, 30

Fieger, Geoffrey, 503

Filial piety: Key teaching in Confucianism regarding family members' right and duties to one another, 477

Finkbine, Sherrie, 174

Fitzsimmons, Ron, 203

Fletcher, John, *197,* 200, 226–236

Food and Drug Administration
on HIV screening, 552
on penile enlargement, 629–630
on women research subjects, 351

Food, genetic engineering of, 253, *277*

For and Against Equal Access to Health Care, 635–645

Foreign aid, to Angola, *618*

Four Moral Principles Approach, 39–42

Four Noble Truths: Heart of Buddha's teachings regarding suffering and liberation from suffering, 497

Fox, Joseph, 486–487

Fox, Renee, 424

Free-market approach, to resource allocation, 619–623, 630–631, 633

Freed, Curt, 355

Fundamental Principles of the Metaphysic of Ethics, 49–53

Futility, medical, 505–507

Gaines, Atwood, 67

Galen, *69*

Galton, Francis, 249

Gamete intrafallopian transfer, *269, 270, 272, 273*

Gandhi, Mahatma, *252,* 359

Gender role, paternalism and, 89

Gene pool
commercialization of, 253
deterioration of, 251–252
gene therapy for, 266–267

Gene therapy, 265–267

Genealogy, Sacredness and the Commodities Market, 285–290

Generalization, 79, 82–83, *90*

Genes: Basic unit of heredity; each gene occupies a specific location on a chromosome.
commercialization of, 254, 256–258
definition of, 253
patents on, 254, 256–258
Genetic counseling, 261–262
Genetic disorders
abortion for, 198
congenital, *64,* 86–87
definition of, 261
diagnosis of, 259–265
in the gene pool, 251–252
from reproductive technology, 275

Genetic diversity, cloning and, 283

Genetic engineering: Alteration of genetic material by artificial means, 265–268, 283–284
for animal-to-human transplants, 434, 436
autonomy and, 256, 261–262, 283
with cloning, 279–280
dangers of, 76
of food, 253, *277*
history of, 249–253
indigenous people and, 254–255, *255, 257,* 285–290
informed consent in, *257,* 257–258, 266
of nonhuman animals, 282–283, 356, *357,* 434, 436
for perfect humans, 267–268, 274, 279, 313–326
prenatal, 268
readings on, 285–326
reductionism in, 59
religions on, *252, 256*

Genetic enhancement: Manipulation of genes in to order improve a being's genetic code, 267–268, 274, 279, 313–326

Genetic Links, Family Ties, and Social Bonds, 291–298

Genetic screening and testing, 258–265
autonomy and, 262, 264–265
discrimination and, 263–264
health insurance and, 261, 263–264
for homosexuality, 261
multiplex, 260
prenatal, 196, 198, 260–261, 262
privacy and, 264–265

Gennarelli, Thomas, 356

Genocide, selective abortion as, 194

Genome: Genetic blueprint contained in a complete set of chromosomes. *See also* Human Genome Project
cloning of, *277*
commercialization of, 256–258

Genotype: Basic combinations of genes of a particular organism, 249
definition of, 253

Germ line therapy: Introduction of normal genes into the germ cells—ova and sperm—to replace deleterious genes, 266, 283

German measles, 181

Germany. *See also* Nazi Germany
abortion in, 179
human experimentation in, *332*

GIFT. *See* Gamete intrafallopian transfer

Gift exchanges, 423–424, 428

Gilligan, Carol, 16–18, 38

God, 20, 281–282

The Golden Rule, 29

Goldhagen, Daniel, 11

Good Samaritans, 94

Goodbye Dolly, 298–303

Graham, Walter, 423

Gratitude, duty of: Duty to express appreciation for past or unearned services received, 30

Great Britain
abortion in, 177
healthcare access in, *609*
HIV screening in, *557*
medical experimentation in, 346, 356
radiation experiments by, 344

The Great Hijack, 574–575

Greece
beneficence in, *127*
disclosure in, *127*
nonmaleficence in, *127*
terminally ill patients in, *127*
truth in, *127*

Green Screen: Term referring to the practice of investigating whether a patient who is a candidate for an organ transplant is in fact eligible through insurance coverage, 421

Greenland, AIDS in, *566*

Griswold v. Connecticut, 182

Grodin, Michael, 329, 349, 351, 379–384

Grossman, Howard, 492

Groups
control, 329
high-risk, 555, 556, *562*

Needs (Healthcare), 622, 625–630, *626–627*
  basic, 633
  vs. desires, 627–628
  health insurance plans on, *629*
  in Holland, *626–627*
Negligence, 131
Nelson, Hilde Lindemann, 154–163
Neonates
  heart transplantations for, 353, 413, 433–434
  HIV screening of, 564, 568
  seriously ill, 355, 490–491, *492–493*
Nepal, burdens in, *492–493*
Netherlands. *See* Holland
New England Anti-Vivisection Society, 330
Nicomachean Ethics, 43–47
Nightingale, Florence, *35*
NIH. *See* National Institutes of Health
Ningen: Japanese term for "human," which conveys the idea of being "in between" others, thereby assuming a relationship, 477
Noguchi, Hideyo, 331
Nondisclosure, 124–125, 126, 128
Nonmaleficence: Duty to avoid harm, 26, 32
  fetal, 202
  in Greece, *127*
  in physician-assisted suicide, 496, 498
  prenatal testing and, 262
  reproductive technology and, 275
  in research, 39–40, 362
  right not to know and, 265
Nonpersons, 15
Nonviolence, *190*
Noonan, John, Jr., 189, 191, 208–211
Norbet, Sheila, 129
Normality, 261
Nozick, Robert, 619, 630
Nuclei transfer, 276–277, *279*
Nuremberg Charter, 24–25
Nuremberg Code, 333, 335–337, *336*, 338
Nurse-patient relations, 114–116
Nurse-physician relations, 115–116, 139–143
Nurses
  abortion and, 205
  caring and, 38, 114
  codes of ethics for, 3–4, *35*, 35
  education of, 115–116

hierarchies of, 117
in Islamic culture, *112–113*
societal view of, 114
virtue and, 35
Nursing homes, 614

Obedience, authority figures and, 1, 3, 6, 18–19, 85
Office for Scientific Research and Development, 333
Ohry, Abraham, *125*
O'Leary, Hazel, 343
On Liberty, 47–49
On Telling Patients the Truth, 152–154
Opinions: Statement based on feeling rather than on fact or reason, 7, 67, 67–68
Opportunity, equality of, 616–617
Oregon Basic Health Services Act, 605
Organ donors, 416–420
  AIDS from, 570–571
  autonomy of, 417–418, 430
  cadaver, 411, 418, 431
  in Canada, 418, 428
  in China, *483*
  Christianity on, 81
  commercialization of, 428–432
  family and, 417–418
  in India, *432–433*
  in Islamic cultures, *414*, *419*
  living, 418, *419*
  nonhuman animal (*see* Xenografts)
  religions on, 411
  socioeconomic status of, 428, 430, 431, *432–433*
  vulnerable populations as, 411, 418, *429–430*
Organ transplantation, 409–472, 611, 622
  for alcoholics, 426–427, 449–456, 456–461
  commercialization of, 428–432
  corneal, 410
  criteria for, 421–422, 423, 425–427
  cross-species (*see* Xenografts)
  immunosuppressant agents for, 413, 434
  incidence of, 416
  informed consent in, 411–412, 435
  in Japan, *412–413*
  Judaism on, *413*
  kidney, *432*, 434
  liver, 422–423, 425–427, 432–433, 434, 456–461

mentally disabled persons and, 418, 421
neonatal, 352, 413
readings on, 437–472
resource allocation and, 412, 415
survival rates for, 410
waiting lists for, 421–422, 424–425, 439–449
Organizational policy, 116–117, 118
O'Rourke, Kevin, 437–439
Orphans, experiments on, 333
Owens, Walter, 490

Pain, 330, 498
Palliative care, 625
Paradigm Shifts, Scientific Revolutions and the Moral Justification of Experimentation on Nonhuman Animals, 392–400
Paradigms: Overall way of regarding and explaining phenomena within a particular discipline, 57, 68
  individualistic, 630
  permissive, 631
  puritan, 633
Parenting in an Era of Genetics, 313–326
Parents. *See also* Mothers
  cloning and, 280–282
  genetic enhancement and, 313–326
  rights of, 40, *185*, 187, 200–202, 490–491
  surrogate consent by, 341, 346–347, *347*, 353
Partial-birth abortion: Late-term form of abortion that involves partial delivery of a live fetus; also known as intact dilation and evacuation (IDE), 176, 203–205
Passive euthanasia: Withholding or withdrawing treatment, resulting in a patient's death, 479, 480–483
  in China, *483*
  nonvoluntary vs. voluntary, *480*
  Rachels on, 508–512, 512–515
Pasteur, Louis, 330
Patents
  on cell lines, 254, 256, 281
  on genes, 254, 256–258
  information and, 258
Paternalism: Relationship in which the physician, because of his or her greater medical knowledge and authority, overrides the patient's own decision making and

Prescriptive statements: Statement that tells us what *ought to be*, 55, 56–57

Presumed consent: Practice whereby it is presumed that an individual consents to donate his or her organs unless otherwise indicated, 418

Preventive medicine, 360, 606

Price, Craig, 8

Priestly model: One of Veatch's four models of the physician/patient relationship; in this model, the physician assumes all decision making for the patient, 111

Prima facie duty: A duty that is morally binding unless it conflicts with a more pressing moral duty, 30

Principle of Descending Order, 348–349

Principle of double effect, 194, 196

Principle of proportionality: Standard by which the benefits of treatment or nontreatment outweigh the burdens, 491

Principle of subsidiarity, *607*

Principlism: Claim that the general moral principles provide a common language for ethicists and that we can best formulate useful rules for healthcare ethics by beginning with general principles and applying them to specific situations, 39, 42

Prisoners
    experiments on, 331, 333, *335*, 338
    informed consent and, 338
    as organ donors, *429–430*

Privacy. *See also* Confidentiality
    abortion and, 182, 183
    collective, 256
    dying and, 474–475
    genetic engineering and, 256
    genetic testing and, 264–265
    HIV status and, 552, 559, 568, 574–575
    right to, 182, 183, 291–298

Probability, 78

Prognosis, resource allocation and, 612, 623

Projected judgment, 488–489

Proposition: In logic, a statement that expresses a complete thought and that can be true or false, 161, 474

Propositions, in critical thinking, 73

Prostaglandins, 176–177

Protease inhibitors: Treatment for HIV that may block or slow down transmission of HIV to infants, 560

Protection, right to, 129

Protestants, on abortion, 186

Proxy consent: Situation in which someone else, such as a parent or guardian, gives consent on behalf of a patient, 137

Psychological research, *357*

Psychotherapists, confidentiality and, 130–131

Public good. *See* Common good

Public opinion, 84
    on abortion, 188–189
    on nonhuman animal research, 356–358
    on physician-assisted suicide, 502

Public policy, 605–634, 635–672

Public safety, vs. patients rights, 128–129

Puritan paradigm: Healthcare model in which all citizens have access to a basic package of healthcare services, with additional services contingent on ability to pay, 633

Quality adjusted life years: Strategy, used in the United Kingdom, to measure the effectiveness of healthcare treatment by calculating the length of improvement time and the quality of life, *609*

Quality of life
    abortion and, 198–200
    AMA on, 611
    evaluating, 491, *492*, 501
    in Great Britain, *609*
    pleasures and, 27
    Viagra and, 628

Quarantines, for HIV positive individuals, *562*

Queuing, 624

Quill, Timothy, 503

Quinlan, Karen, 56, 474–476

Rabies experiments, 330

Rabinowitz, Bernard, 555, 558, 574–575

Rachels, James, 481, 482, 508–512, 512–515

Racism, 64–67, 85, 620
    abortion and, 194
    genetic engineering for, 250–251

vs. individual freedom, 620, 622
in medical experimentation, 350, 351

Radiation experiments, 343–344

Ramsey, Paul, 20, 251

Ranagimachi, Ryuzo, 278

Randomized clinical trials: Matching of a randomly selected experimental group, who receive the treatment, and a control group, who receive either a placebo or no treatment, as a means of controlling variables, 329

Rationing (Healthcare): Distribution of limited resources, such as transplant organs or healthcare technology, on the basis of specific criteria, 608, 610, *632*, 645–650

Rawls, John, 31–32, 80, 616, 631

Re-Assessing the Ordinary/Extraordinary distinction in Withholding/ Withdrawing Nutrition and Hydration, 516–522

Reasoning
    circular, 88
    deductive, 76–80, 91
    inductive, 76–80, 91–92
    moral, *17*, 17–18, 20, 54–55, 67–68, 125

Reductionism, 59

Reed, Walter, 331

Reflective equilibrium, 80, 617, 619

Refusal of treatment. *See* Treatment refusal

Regan, Tom, 34, 361, 435

Reincarnation, 67, *190, 493*

Relativism
    cultural, 9–15
    ethical, 7–15
    sociological, 9

Religions, 20–23, 25, 85. *See also* specific religions
    on abortion, 179, *180,* 185–187, 189, *190*
    on AIDS, *554,* 561, 564–565
    on cloning, 278, 281–282
    fundamentalist, 186
    on genetic engineering, *252,* 256
    healing power of, *62,* 63
    on medical experimentation, 38, *341, 354, 358*
    on organ donation, 411
    on treatment refusal, *22*

Reparation, duty of: Duty to make amends for past harms done to others, 30–31

Reportable diseases, 128, 552–553, 556

Reproductive compensation, 262

Reproductive rights, 34, 275–276, 281, 298–303

Reproductive technology, 268–276, 277
- Confucianism on, *272*
- genetic damage from, 275
- in Hong Kong, *272*
- informed consent in, 273
- in Islamic cultures, *271*
- types of, *269*, 269–273

Required request: Practice whereby healthcare professionals are required to request the family's consent in order to use organs from a deceased patient, 418

Research: Orderly investigation, experimentation, or scientific study of a phenomenon in order to gain new knowledge and analyze the significance of the findings. *See also* Medical experimentation
- on AIDS, 351, *354*, 379–384, 610
- American Medical Association on, 342
- on breast cancer, 610
- cause/effect relationships in, 363
- classified, 344
- cloned animals for, *277*
- definition of, 327
- design, 329
- on embryos and fetuses, 355
- financial incentives in, 348, 349
- funds for, 342
- informed consent and, 134
- intent of, 328–329
- multinational, 351, *354*
- by physicians, 341–342, 348, 349
- politics in, 342
- psychological, *357*
- species differences in, 360
- subjects, 39–42, 348–353, *352–353*
- unethical, *341*, 362–364
- on women, 350, 351, 617

Research with Fetal Tissue, 437–439

Resistance: Use of immature defense mechanisms—such as ignorance, avoidance, anger, clichés, jargon, and conformity—as a means of preventing our worldview from being analyzed, 69–73, 80

Resource allocation, 619–625
- by age, 622–624
- AMA on, 611–612
- benefits and, 612
- free-market approach to, 619–623, 630–631, 633
- Judaism on, *623–624*
- macroallocation, 608, 610
- by managed care programs, 612–613
- by medical need, 622
- microallocation, 610–614
- by multitiered systems, 633–634
- organ transplantation and, 412, 415
- prognosis and, 612, 623
- by queuing, 624
- by random selection, 624–625
- by social worth, 622

Rest, James, 18

Resurrection, *414*

Rewarded gifting, *433*

Rhetoric: A means of defending a particular worldview rather than analyzing it. Unlike a logical argument, rhetoric uses only statements that support a particular opinion and disregards any statements that do not support this opinion, 67, 74

Rhodes, Rosamond, 265, 291–298

Rifkin, Jeremy, 253

Right to Die Society of Canada, 503

Right(s), 32–34, 81
- to be cloned, 298–303
- to be well born, 200
- of children, 34
- to commit suicide, 33, 473
- to die, 474–475
- vs. duties, 32, 33–34
- fetal, 185–186, 191
- to health, 33
- of healthcare professionals, 205–206
- HIV screening and, *562*
- of incompetent patients, 361
- of individuals, 47–49
- to information, *272*
- legal vs. moral, 32–33, 81, 90–91
- liberty, 33–34, 40–41
- to life, 34, 91, 92, 188
- in medical experimentation, 337
- of nonhuman animals, 34, 356–361, 384–392, 434–435
- not to know, 264–265
- parental, 40, *185*, 187, 200–202, 490–491
- of patients (*see* Patient rights)
- to privacy (*see* Privacy)
- to protection, 129
- to refuse treatment, 480–481, 485
- reproductive, 34, 275–276, 281, 298–303
- severance, 194, 196, 204
- of terminally ill patients, 37
- United Nations on, 616
- welfare, 33–34, 193–194
- of women, 76, 188, 193–194, 202–203

Rights ethics: Ethical theory that moral entitlements are the basis of ethics, 33

Risk
- of AIDS, 555, 556, 569–571
- in medical experimentation, 328

Roe v. Wade, 174, 177, 183–184
- challenges to, 187
- excerpts from, *182–183*
- on fetal viability, 192
- on liberty rights, 193–194

Roman Catholic Church
- on abortion, 179, 186, 189, 194
- on AIDS, *554*
- on cloning, 278
- on the common good, *607*
- on contraception, 24
- on life support, 474, 481–482
- on prenatal diagnosis, 261
- on reproductive technologies, 275
- on sexual sterilization, 250

Rose, Gerhard, 333

Rosenstein, Melvin, 630

Roslin Institute, 278

Ross, W.D., 30–31

Rothman, Barbara, 274

Rothman, Cappy, 268

RU-486. *See* Mifepristone

Rules, exception to, 83–84

Russell, William, 361–362

Rzepkowski, Neal, 571, 572

Sachedina, Abdulaziz, 278

Saikewicz, Joseph, 489–490

Salgo v. Leland Stanford Board of Trustees, 109, 111

Samitier, Ricardo, 629

Samples, representative, 79

Sandoz Pharmaceutical Corporation, 256

Sanger, Margaret, 182

Saunders, Cicely, 499

Schizophrenia, 346

Schneiderman, Lawrence, 506

Science vs. faith, 68

ISBN 1-55934-976-X

90000

9 781559 349765